Systemic Sclerosis: An Autoimmune Disease

Systemic Sclerosis: An Autoimmune Disease

Edited by Billy Patterson

AMERICAN
MEDICAL PUBLISHERS
www.americanmedicalpublishers.com

American Medical Publishers,
41 Flatbush Avenue,
1st Floor, New York,
NY 11217, USA

Visit us on the World Wide Web at:
www.americanmedicalpublishers.com

ISBN: 978-1-63927-215-0

Cataloging-in-Publication Data

Systemic sclerosis : an autoimmune disease / edited by Billy Patterson.
p. cm.
Includes bibliographical references and index.
ISBN 978-1-63927-215-0
1. Systemic scleroderma. 2. Autoimmune diseases. 3. Multiple sclerosis.
4. Collagen diseases. I. Patterson, Billy.
RC924.5.S34 S97 2022
616.544--dc23

Table of Contents

Preface

Systemic sclerosis or systemic scleroderma is an autoimmune disease of the connective tissue. The condition is characterized by the thickening of the skin due to a deposition of collagen and injuries to small arteries. Systemic sclerosis is of two types- localized and systemic. The localized condition affects the skin of the hands, feet and the face, while the systemic condition involves the heart, lungs, kidneys and gastrointestinal tract. Death due to sclerosis often occurs due to heart, lung and kidney involvement. Sclerosis is also considered to be a risk factor for cancer. The diagnosis of sclerosis is based on clinical examination, biopsy and presence of autoantibodies. There is no known cure for sclerosis. Treatment consists of NSAIDs, calcium channel blockers and topical therapies for improving pain and ulceration, and relieving other symptoms. This book elucidates the concepts and innovative models around the management of systemic sclerosis. It presents researches and studies performed by experts across the globe. Students, researchers, experts and all associated with immunology will benefit alike from this book.

The information contained in this book is the result of intensive hard work done by researchers in this field. All due efforts have been made to make this book serve as a complete guiding source for students and researchers. The topics in this book have been comprehensively explained to help readers understand the growing trends in the field.

I would like to thank the entire group of writers who made sincere efforts in this book and my family who supported me in my efforts of working on this book. I take this opportunity to thank all those who have been a guiding force throughout my life.

Editor

1

Stress granules and RNA processing bodies are novel autoantibody targets in systemic sclerosis

Michael E. Johnson[1], Andrew V. Grassetti[1], Jaclyn N. Taroni[1], Shawn M. Lyons[2], Devin Schweppe[1], Jessica K. Gordon[3], Robert F. Spiera[3], Robert Lafyatis[4], Paul J. Anderson[2], Scott A. Gerber[1] and Michael L. Whitfield[1,5*]

Abstract

Background: Autoantibody profiles represent important patient stratification markers in systemic sclerosis (SSc). Here, we performed serum-immunoprecipitations with patient antibodies followed by mass spectrometry (LC-MS/MS) to obtain an unbiased view of all possible autoantibody targets and their associated molecular complexes recognized by SSc.

Methods: HeLa whole cell lysates were immunoprecipitated (IP) using sera of patients with SSc clinically positive for autoantibodies against RNA polymerase III (RNAP3), topoisomerase 1 (TOP1), and centromere proteins (CENP). IP eluates were then analyzed by LC-MS/MS to identify novel proteins and complexes targeted in SSc. Target proteins were examined using a functional interaction network to identify major macromolecular complexes, with direct targets validated by IP-Western blots and immunofluorescence.

Results: A wide range of peptides were detected across patients in each clinical autoantibody group. Each group contained peptides representing a broad spectrum of proteins in large macromolecular complexes, with significant overlap between groups. Network analyses revealed significant enrichment for proteins in RNA processing bodies (PB) and cytosolic stress granules (SG) across all SSc subtypes, which were confirmed by both Western blot and immunofluorescence.

Conclusions: While strong reactivity was observed against major SSc autoantigens, such as RNAP3 and TOP1, there was overlap between groups with widespread reactivity seen against multiple proteins. Identification of PB and SG as major targets of the humoral immune response represents a novel SSc autoantigen and suggests a model in which a combination of chronic and acute cellular stresses result in aberrant cell death, leading to autoantibody generation directed against macromolecular nucleic acid-protein complexes.

Keywords: Systemic sclerosis, Scleroderma, Autoantibody, RNA processing bodies, Stress granules

Background

Systemic sclerosis (SSc) is a rare systemic autoimmune disease of unknown etiology characterized by skin fibrosis, internal organ involvement, vascular abnormalities, and autoantibody production. Patients are broadly classified as having either limited (lSSc) or diffuse (dSSc) disease based primarily upon the extent of skin involvement and autoantibody profiles. While a wide array of autoantibodies have been described for SSc, only a small number of these targets are used for clinical diagnosis and stratification. Autoantibodies targeting RNA polymerase III (RNAP3), topoisomerase 1 (TOP1; commonly referred to as Scl70), and centromere proteins (CENP) represent the three the most common, clinically measured autoantibodies observed in SSc [1, 2]. Other autoantibodies, including fibrillarin (U3RNP), Pm/Scl, Ku, U1RNP, U11/U12, and Th/To have also been described [1, 3] but are not routinely measured for clinical subtyping.

* Correspondence: michael.l.whitfield@dartmouth.edu
[1]Department of Genetics, Geisel School of Medicine at Dartmouth, Hanover, NH, USA
[5]Dartmouth Medical School, Hinman Box 7400, Hanover, NH 03755, USA
Full list of author information is available at the end of the article

While the processes underlying autoantibody production in SSc remain poorly understood, the presence of certain autoantibodies is strongly predictive of clinical outcomes [1–3]. TOP1 and RNAP3 autoantibodies are almost exclusively seen in dSSc, while CENP, Th/To, and U1RNP antibodies are more commonly associated with lSSc [1, 3]. U3RNP autoantibodies are not associated with either clinical subset, and are often found in conjunction with other autoantibodies, including both TOP1 and CENP [3]. Certain antibodies, such as TOP1 and U11/12, have been shown to be predictive of poorer overall prognosis, including increased likelihood of pulmonary fibrosis [4] and cardiac involvement, while RNAP3 autoantibodies have recently been linked to co-occurrence of SSc with cancer [5].

Despite the importance of autoantibodies in SSc, the vast majority of target identification and phenotypic screening has been performed using methods targeting only a single autoantibody, with little ability to detect novel or low abundance autoantibodies. Furthermore, these methods fail to address the possibility of co-occurrence of multiple autoantibodies within a patient, which may have important clinical implications. Autoantigen microarrays have proven successful for screening large numbers of autoantibodies in parallel, however target identification is limited to those antigens produced and printed on the antigen microarrays [6]. To address these limitations, we performed immunoprecipitations (IP) of HeLa whole cell lysates using sera from RNAP3-, CENP-, and TOP1-positive patients, as well as healthy controls, followed by mass spectrometry (LC-MS/MS) to provide an unbiased assessment of all autoantibodies present in these SSc patients. This method provides a better view of the full range of autoantibodies present in SSc, including both novel and established targets, and provides insights into the general processes underlying autoantibody production.

Methods

Clinical samples

Patient serum was obtained from Boston University Medical School, Boston (BUMC), MA, USA and the Hospital for Special Surgery (HSS), New York, NY, USA. All relevant study protocols were approved by the Dartmouth College committee for the protection of human subjects, and the internal review boards of both BUMC and HSS. Informed consent was obtained from all patients prior to sample collection. Patients were diagnosed with either dSSc or limited SSc, as determined using the 1980 American College of Rheumatology classification criteria. Detection of major autoantibody reactivities was performed using standard clinical assays.

Human cell lysates

HeLa cells were cultured in DMEM supplemented with 10 % fetal bovine serum (FBS) (v/v) and 100 IU/mL penicillin-streptomycin. Cells were grown to approximately 80 % confluence, harvested in IP lysis buffer (150 mM NaCl, 50 mM Tris pH 7.5, 1 mM $MgCl_2$, 1 mM EDTA, 0.5 % Triton X-100, 2.5 mM β-mercaptoethanol, 1 mM sodium molybdate, 1 mM sodium fluoride, 1 mM sodium tartrate, 1 mM dithiothreitol (DTT), and protease inhibitors (Roche, Indianapolis, IN, USA)), lysed by passage through a pre-chilled high-gauge syringe, and centrifuged for 15 minutes to pellet debris. Lysates were then clarified by incubating for 4 h at 4 °C on a rotating platform. Protein concentrations were quantified using a standard bicinchoninic acid (BCA) protein assay kit (Thermo Scientific, Waltham, MA, USA).

Serum immunoprecipitation

Patient serum was cross-linked to Protein G Dynabeads (Invitrogen, St. Louis, MO, USA) prior to IP. First, 100 μL serum (approximately 1 mg IgG) was added to 50 μL Protein G beads and incubated for 5 h at 4 °C. Samples were then washed in PBS, equilibrated in cross-linking buffer (50 mM HEPES, pH 8.2), and cross-linked to Protein G beads by the addition of 20 mM dimethyl pimelimidate and 300 mM HEPES (DMP) solution for 10 minutes at room temperature (repeated three times). The crosslinking reaction was then terminated by the addition of 50 mM ammonium bicarbonate, and the resulting antibody bead mixture added to 500 μL cell lysate (diluted to 4 mg/mL in IP lysis buffer). Samples were incubated overnight at 4 °C on a rotating platform, washed in cold IP lysis buffer, and eluted in a buffer containing 2 % SDS, 75 mM NaCl, 50 mM Tris pH 8.1, and 20 % glycerol at 65 °C for 5 minutes. Eluates were reduced by the addition of 0.1 M dithiothreitol (DTT) (to a final concentration 5 mM), and incubated at 80 °C for 5 minutes. Samples were then resolved by SDS-PAGE, split into high (>60 kDa) and low (<60 kDa) molecular weight fractions and analyzed by mass spectrometry.

Mass spectrometry

Proteins contained in Coomassie-stained gel regions were digested overnight with trypsin (1:200 w/v) at 37 ° C. Following digestion, peptides were extracted from the gels, dried, and analyzed by nanoscale LC-MS/MS. LC-MS/MS analyses were performed on either LTQ Orbitrap Classic or Orbitrap Fusion LC-MS/MS platforms. LTQ Orbitrap Classic analyses were conducted as described previously [7].

For Orbitrap Fusion analyses, samples were loaded onto an EASY-nLC 1000 Liquid Chromatograph (Thermo Scientific, Waltham, MA, USA) and separated by reverse-phase high pressure liquid chromatography (RP-HPLC) using an approximately 36-cm column with a 100-μM inner diameter packed with 3 μm 120 Å C_{18} particles (Dr. Maisch GmbH, Ammerbuch-Entringen, Germany). The resultant peptide eluate was directed into an Orbitrap Fusion Tribrid Mass Spectrometer operating in a data-dependent sequencing acquisition mode across a 30-minute reverse-phase gradient (6 % acetonitrile, 0.1 % formic acid to 30 % acetonitrile, 0.1 % formic acid) at 350 nL/min flow rate. The Orbitrap Fusion was operated with an Orbitrap MS1 scan at 120 K resolution, followed by Orbitrap MS2 scans of higher energy collision-induced dissociation (HCD) fragment ions (30 % HCD energy) at 15 K resolution using a maximum cycle type of 2 s, precursor ion dynamic exclusion window of 15 s, +2, +3, and +4 precursor ions selected for LC-MS/MS, and maximum ion injection times of 100 ms (MS1) and 50 ms (MS2). The resulting tandem mass spectra were data-searched using the COMET search engine [8] against a *Homo sapiens* proteome database (source: Uniprot; download date: 2 July 2013) with a precursor ion tolerance of +/- 1 Da [9] and a fragment ion tolerance of 0.02 Th. Peptide spectra matches (PSMs) were filtered to <1 % false discovery rate using the target decoy strategy [10], and reported.

IP-western blots

Anti-UPF1 antibody was kindly provided by Dr. Lynne Maquat (University of Rochester Medical Center, Rochester, NY, USA). Antibodies to MOV10 and CAPRIN1 were purchased from Proteintech (Chicago, IL, USA); antibodies to G3BP1 and USP10 were purchased from Santa Cruz Biotechnology (Santa Cruz, CA, USA). Serum immunoprecipitation of HeLa lysates was performed as described above; 50 % of each eluate (15 μL) was then run on a 10 % bis-tris precast gel (Life Technologies, Carlsbad, CA, USA). HeLa whole cell lysate (100 μg) was used as a positive control; no loading control was performed due to the absence of viable targets present in all IP eluates. Western blots were then run following standard protocols, and visualized using Western Lightning ECL Pro or Ultra substrate (Perkin Elmer Inc., Waltham, MA, USA), as necessary.

Data analysis

Non-redundant peptide hits, defined as mass spectra mapping exclusively to a given peptide fragment, were used for all downstream analyses. Pairwise comparisons between samples were performed by Fisher's exact test using the Bonferroni correction for multiple hypothesis testing. Venn diagrams were generated using VENNY [11]. Network analysis was performed using the Genome-scale Integrated Analysis of gene Networks in Tissues (GIANT; http://giant.princeton.edu/) global network [12] and visualized using Cytoscape [13]. Communities in the network were detected using fast-greedy modularity as implemented in igraph. Functional annotation of individual communities was performed using g:Profiler [14]. Semiquantitative enrichment of SSc-associated autoantibodies was determined using a binary assessment of autoantibody presence or absence in a sample. Preferential enrichment in SSc was defined as all proteins detected in >50 % of all patient samples at a frequency >1.5-fold relative to controls. Enrichment of biological processes and cellular components was determined using g:Profiler using the g:SCS threshold correction for multiple hypothesis testing and a functional category size ≤500 genes. Hierarchical clustering was performed using Cluster 3.0 [15], and visualized using Java TreeView [16].

Immunofluorescence

The day prior to the experiment, 10^5 U2OS cells were seeded onto 11 mm glass coverslips and allowed to attach overnight at 37 °C/5 % CO_2 in DMEM containing 10 % FBS (Gibco). Cells were treated with 100 μM sodium (meta)arsenite (Sigma Aldrich) for 1 h to induce the formation of stress granules and then with 4 % paraformaldehyde solution at room temperature for 15 - minutes followed by blocking and permeabilization with 5 % normal horse serum, 0.1 % digitonin in Tris-buffered saline. Staining was performed with anti-eIF3b (Santa Cruz), anti-SK1-Hedls (Santa Cruz), and patient sera for 1 h at room temperature. Secondary antibodies (anti-goat-Cy3, anti-mouse-Cy2, and anti-human-Cy5) were purchased from Jackson Laboratories and incubated at room temperature for 1 h. Conventional fluorescence microscopy was performed using a microscope (model Elipse E800, Nikon, Tokyo, Japan) with epifluorescence optics with a digital camera (model CCD-SPOT RT; Diagnostic Instruments, Sterling Heights, MI). Images were compiled using Adobe Photoshop software (CS6; Adobe Systems, San Jose, CA).

Results

Identification of proteins cross-reacting to serum antibodies

Immunoprecipitations (IP) of HeLa whole cell lysates were performed using sera obtained from 13 SSc patients and 4 healthy controls. HeLa cells were chosen based upon their consistent, high level of expression of a broad range of proteins from the human genome [17].

SSc patients were divided into three groups, TOP1, RNAP3, and CENP, as measured in a reference laboratory; clinical data for each patient are shown in Table 1. These groups were chosen based upon their relative frequency, and their importance in clinical diagnosis. Immunoprecipitated proteins were analyzed by LC-MS/MS, and the resulting spectra aligned to the reference human proteome (UCSC version hg19). Data are presented in two ways; first to identify the total number of

Table 1 Clinical information for patients involved in this study

Sample	Group	Age (years)	Sex	Race	Disease type	ILD/PAH	Disease duration (years)	ANA pattern	ANA titer	MRSS
SSc 1	TOP1	36	F	White	Diffuse	mild ILD	2.5		1:320	43
SSc 132	TOP1	49	F	White	Diffuse	No		Homogeneous	1:640	27
SSc 218	TOP1	55	F	White	Diffuse	ILD		Homogeneous/nucleolar	1:2560	18
SSc 208	TOP1	64	M	White	Diffuse	No		Nucleolar	1:1280	37
SSc 5	RNAP3	53	M	White	Diffuse	No	0.75	Speckled	1:80	36
SSc 7	RNAP3	45	F	Black	Diffuse	No	0.5	Speckled	1:80	27
SSc 10	RNAP3	52	M	White	Diffuse	No	0.5		0	22
SSc 18	RNAP3	69	F	White	Diffuse	ILD	0.5	Nucleolar	1:160	44
SSc 159	CENP	54	F	Mixed	Limited	No	7	Centromere	1:1280	2
SSc 177	CENP	64	F	White	Limited	No	15	Discrete speckled	4+	
SSc 194	CENP	66	F	White	Limited	No	18	Discrete speckled	4+	6
SSc 238	CENP	53	F	White	Limited	No	6	Centromere	1:640	5
SSc 226	CENP	55	F	Asian	Diffuse	No		Centromere	1:1280	6
HC 162	Control	24	M	White						
HC 400	Control	21	M	White						
HC 117	Control		M							
HC 118	Control		M							

Blank cells indicate information not available at the time of sample collection. *ILD* interstitial lung disease, *PAH* pulmonary arterial hypertension, *ANA* anti-nuclear antibody, *MRSS* modified Rodnan skin score, *SSc* systemic sclerosis, *M* male, *F* female

peptides that could be aligned to each protein (total hits), and second to identify all non-redundant peptides that mapped exclusively to a given protein (non-redundant hits). A complete list of all data can be found in Additional file 1: Table S1.

Exclusivity and co-occurrence of SSc autoantibodies

We observed a high degree of reproducibility between patients within their respective autoantibody groups (TOP1, RNAP3, and CENP; Fig. 1). The greatest degree of overlap between peptides was observed among RNAP3 patients (Fig. 1a and c), with 420 proteins (54.1 %) detected in all four patients (Fig. 1c). The remaining groups exhibited significant overlap in three of four (TOP1) and four of five (CENP) patients, respectively (Fig. 1a), along with a single outlier that showed either higher (SSc 208; TOP1) or lower (SSc 226; CENP) total peptide hits relative to other samples in these groups. Within TOP1, 111 proteins (14.2 %) were detected in all four patients (Fig. 1d), while CENP exhibited 48 proteins (10.5 %) common to all patients (Fig. 1c). The least overlap was seen in healthy controls, with only 40 proteins (7.6 %; Fig. 1b) common across individuals.

Across all samples, 283 proteins (25.0 %) were detected in at least one patient in each of the four autoantibody groups (Fig. 1e, Additional file 2: Table S2). Some of these proteins likely represent background signals (serum albumin (ALB), β-tubulin (TUBB), and ribosomal proteins), while others are considered specific to SSc despite trace level detection in controls. For example, multiple SSc autoantibody targets, including Ku (XRCC5 and XRCC6), Ro52/TRIM21, and nucleophosmin/B23 (NPM1) were present in this set of proteins. In contrast, 87 proteins (7.7 %) were detected in all three SSc groups, but were absent in controls (Fig. 1e; Additional file 2: Table S2). Functional analyses of these proteins revealed strong enrichment of proteins involved in oxidative stress responses and nucleic acid processing (Additional file 3: Table S3B).

Of the 1,130 non-redundant proteins identified, 473 (41.8 %) were unique to a given autoantibody group (Fig. 1f); however, the vast majority of these proteins were exclusive to a single patient, with only 111 (23.5 %) detected in two or more patients. These results suggest a wide range of autoantibody responses within each of the clinical autoantibody groups beyond what has already been described.

Among the major autoantibody groups, immunoprecipitation of RNAP3 was exclusive to the RNAP3 group, with no RNAP3 peptides detected in any of the other samples (Table 2). In contrast, TOP1 peptides were consistently highest among TOP1 patients, but were also detected at low levels in all four RNAP3$^+$ patients, and in two controls (Table 2). As these patients were negative for TOP1 autoantibodies by clinical testing, these results indicate a higher degree of sensitivity for our IP/MS protocol compared to standard ELISA-based methods used clinically. In contrast, CENP was only

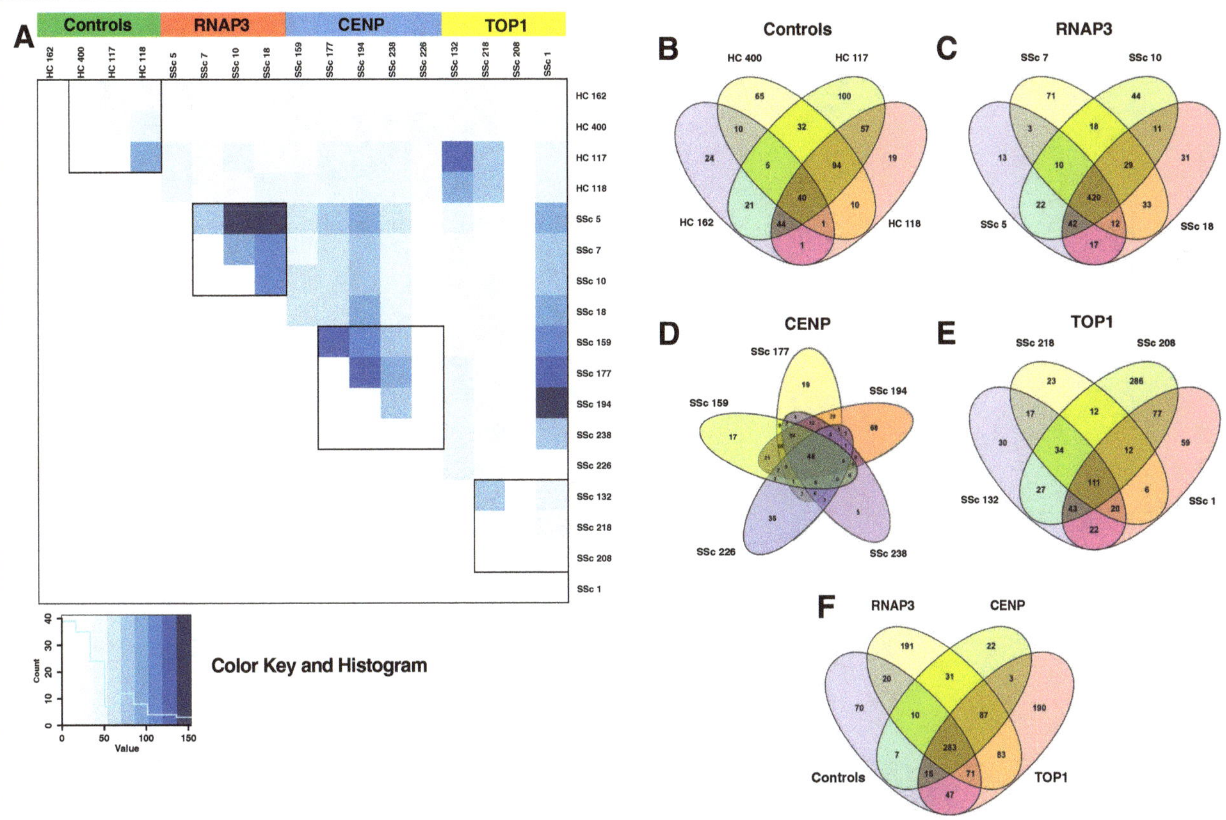

Fig. 1 Overview of mass spectrometry results. **a** Correlation matrix of non-redundant protein hits for all patients and controls. Comparisons were performed using Fisher's exact test with the Bonferroni correction. *Black boxes* indicate intra-group comparisons for each of the four clinically defined groups. *Green* controls; *red* RNA polymerase III (*RNAP3*); *blue* centromere protein (*CENP*); *yellow* topoisomerase I (*TOP1*). **b-f** *Venn diagrams* depict overlap in non-redundant peptide hits within and between groups. **b** healthy controls, **c** RNAP3, **d** CENP, **e** TOP1, and **f** overlap between groups

detected at low levels in the CENP group, likely because it remained bound to the tightly packed centromere complex of chromatin.

Other known SSc autoantigens were also detected. RuvBL [18] was strongly detected in all SSc samples, while virtually absent in controls. Ku and Su, along with a wide array of anti-tRNA synthetases [19] were routinely detected in both the RNAP3 and TOP1 subsets, but were only weakly present in the CENP and control groups (Table 2).

Several autoantigens previously implicated in SSc were found at low, background levels in both SSc and control samples. Ro52/TRIM21 [20] and nucleophosmin/B23 [21] were widely detected across all four groups, suggesting widespread reactivity to these proteins in SSc and controls. We did not find evidence in SSc of enrichment of Pm/Scl autoantibodies, which target exosome components EXOSC1-10 [22]. Peptides for these proteins were absent in the CENP group, but were detected at low levels in other subsets, including controls. Autoantigens not detected here include many of the URNPs, PDGFR, matrix metalloproteinases, tissue plasminogen activator, and vascular receptor antibodies (Table 2).

Functional clustering of identified proteins

To identify functional interactions among autoantigens, all 763 non-redundant protein hits were submitted as a query to the GIANT global average network. This approach included both SSc-specific targets and those detected at background levels in controls, to better understand the full range of autoreactive proteins and complexes. Nine distinct communities were identified within the resulting network, in which each gene is represented by a node, and two genes share an edge if they are predicted to functionally interact (Additional file 4: Figure S1). Analysis of each of these communities by g:Profiler revealed functional enrichment for a wide range of biological processes associated with important disease processes and components (Additional file 4: Figure S1). Community 1 is dominated by ribosomal proteins, eukaryotic initiation factor 3 (eIF3) subunits, and includes the SSc autoantibody target nucleophosmin/B23. Communities 2 and 8 show strong enrichment for Gene Ontology (GO) terms mRNA processing, ribonucleoprotein complex, and cytosolic stress granule. Community 2 is dominated primarily by DEAD box

Table 2 SSc-associated autoantibodies observed in this study

Alias	Associated proteins	Disease subset	Clinical associations	Prevalence in this dataset (avg/freq)				Reference
				Control (n = 4)	RNAP3 (n = 4)	TOP1 (n = 4)	CENP (n = 5)	
Major autoantibodies								
RNA Pol III	POLR3A	dSSc	Renal crisis, cancer	-	+++ (28/4)	-	-	Graf, et al. 2012 [1]; Mehra, et al. 2013 [3]
Scl70	TOP1	dSSc	Poor prognosis, internal organ involvement, and proteinuria	+ (3/2)	+ (4/4)	+++ (19/4)	-	Mehra, et al. 2013 [3]
Centromere	**CENPB**, CENPH	lSSc/CREST	PAH, ILD	-	-	-	+ (1/2)	Mehra, et al. 2013 [3]
Other SSc autoantibodies present in our dataset								
Endothelial Cell	TUBB, **VCL**, LMNA, RPLP0	SSc	PAH	+ (1/1)	++ (6/4)	+ (4/2)	+ (0/1)	Dib, et al. 2012 [34], Naniwa, et al. 2007 [35]
Fibroblast	ENO1, G6PD, **HSPA1A**, HSPA1B, VIM	SSc	PAH	+ (3/4)	+++ (12/4)	++ (5/3)	++ (8/5)	Terrier, et al. 2008 [36], Terrier, et al. 2009 [37]
Histone	H1FX, HIST1H1B, **HIST1H4A**	SSc	PF, internal organ involvement, decreased survival	+ (1/1)	+ (3/3)	+ (1/1)	-	Mehra, et al. 2013 [3]
B23	NPM1	dSSc, CENP- lSSc	PAH	+ (4/4)	++ (7/4)	++ (5/4)	++ (6/5)	Mehra, et al. 2013 [3]
Ku	**XRCC5**, XRCC6	lSSc	Myositis	+ (3/3)	+++ (12/4)	++ (8/4)	+ (2/3)	Graf, et al. 2012 [1]; Mehra, et al. 2013 [3]
Su	AGO2	SSc, PM/Scl	Unknown	-	+ (1/2)	+ (3/1)	-	Satoh, et al. 2013 [38]
Mitochondrial (M2)	**DLD**, PDHB	lSSc	Strong association with primary biliary cirrhosis	+ (1/1)	+ (2/3)	+ (1/1)	-	Mehra, et al. 2013 [13]
Pm/Scl	EXOSC1-**10**	SSc	PF, digital ulcers; decreased risk of PAH and GI symptoms	+ (2/2)	++ (5/3)	+ (2/2)	-	Mehra, et al. 2013 [13]
hnRNPs	**HNRNPA1**-3, HNRNPL	SSc	Common in SARDs	+ (0/1)	++ (7/4)	+ (3/4)	+ (2/4)	Siapka, et al. 2007 [39]
U1	**SNRNPA**, SPRNP70	SSc	Co-occurrence with SS-A/SS-B, PAH, overlap syndrome	-	+ (2/4)	+ (1/2)	+ (0/1)	Graf, et al. 2012 [1]; Mehra, et al. 2013 [3]
U5	SNRNP200	SSc, PM/Scl	Unknown	++ (6/3)	++ (9/4)	++ (8/3)	+ (1/2)	Kubo, et al. 2002 [40]
RO52/TRIM21	TRIM21	SSc	ILD, other autoimmune diseases	++ (6/3)	+++ (12/4)	++ (6/4)	++ (8/4)	Mehra, et al. 2013 [3]
RuvB	**RUVBL1**, RUVBL2	dSSc	Common in SARDs, older age at onset, male sex	+ (1/1)	++ (7/4)	+ (3/4)	+ (2/4)	Kaji, et al. 2014 [18]
Annexin V	ANXA5	dSSc, CENP- lSSc	Digital ischemia	+ (2/2)	++ (7/4)	+ (4/3)	+ (3/4)	Mehra, et al. 2013 [3]
SS-B/LA	SS-A, **SS-B**	SSc	ILD, other autoimmune diseases	-	+ (3/4)	+ (2/2)	+ (0/1)	Mehra, et al. 2013 [3]
Peroxiredoxin	PRDX1	SSc	Disease duration, PF, cardiac involvement, TOP1+ patients	+ (2/4)	++ (8/4)	+ (3/3)	+ (4/4)	Mehra, et al. 2013 [3]
hUBF/NOP90	UBTF	lSSc	Mild organ involvement, favorable prognosis	-	+ (1/2)	-	-	Mehra, et al. 2013 [3]
Th/To	POP1	lSSc	PF, renal crisis, poor prognosis, myositis, PAH	+ (1/2)	+ (1/1)	+ (3/3)	-	Graf, et al. 2012 [1]; Mehra, et al. 2013 [3]

Table 2 SSc-associated autoantibodies observed in this study *(Continued)*

PL-12	AARS	SSc, PM/DM	ILD without myositis	-	-	+ (1/1)	+ (1/1)	Hamaguchi, et al. 2013 [19]
OJ	IARS	SSc, PM/DM	ILD without myositis	+ (1/1)	-	+ (3/3)	-	Hamaguchi, et al. 2013 [19]
EJ	GARS	SSc, PM/DM	ILD, myositis	-	+ (3/4)	+ (2/2)	+ (0/1)	Hamaguchi, et al. 2013 [19]
Jo-1	HARS	SSc, PM/DM	ILD, myositis	-	+ (1/4)	-	-	Hamaguchi, et al. 2013 [19]
PL-7	TARS	SSc, PM/DM	ILD, myositis	+ (2/2)	++ (8/4)	++ (6/4)	+ (2/4)	Hamaguchi, et al. 2013 [19]
Ha	YARS	SSc, PM/DM	Interstitial pneumonia	-	+ (0/1)	-	-	Hashish, et al 2005 [41]
Zo	**FARSA**, FARSB	SSc, PM/Scl	Anti-synthetase syndrome	-	+ (2/4)	-	-	Betteridge, et al. 2007 [42]
SSc autoantibodies not detected in our dataset								
Fibrillarin	U3RNP	dSSc	More frequent in blacks; severe disease, poor prognosis	-	-	-	-	Mehra, et al. 2013 [3]
U11/U12 RNP	SNRNP35	SSc	Lung fibrosis, gastrointestinal involvement	-	-	-	-	Mimori, 1999 [43]
PDGFR	PDGFR	SSc	Unknown	-	-	-	-	Svegliati Baroni, et al. 2006 [44]
MMP	MMP family	dSSc	Skin, lung, and vascular fibrosis	-	-	-	-	Mehra, et al. 2013 [3]
tPA	PLAT	lSSc	PAH	-	-	-	-	Mehra, et al. 2013 [3]
IFI16	IFI16	lSSc	Common in SARDs	-	-	-	-	Mehra, et al. 2013 [3]
Fibrillin 1	FBN1	dSSc	Choctaw and Japanese patients; absent in Caucasians	-	-	-	-	Mehra, et al. 2013 [3]
Vascular Receptors	AGTR2, EDN1	SSc	TOP1+ patients, renal crisis	-	-	-	-	Mehra, et al. 2013 [3]
ATF2	ATF2	SSc	Longer disease duration, decreased lung function	-	-	-	-	Mehra, et al. 2013 [3]

Data are presented as the average of all peptide hits across each autoantibody group, followed by the frequency of peptide detection within the group. For autoantibodies known to target more than one protein or subunit, data for a single representative protein are shown, with the specific protein highlighted in bold. Associated proteins indicate specific protein targets identified in this study; among autoantibodies not identified here, the most common targets are listed. Symbols: -, +, ++, and +++ indicate an average of 0, 1–4, 5–9, and ≥10 peptide hits per group, respectively

SSc systemic sclerosis, *lSSc* limited cutaneous SSc, *dSSc* diffuse cutaneous SSc, *PAH* pulmonary arterial hypertension; *ILD* interstitial lung disease; *CREST* CREST syndrome (calcinosis, Raynaud phenomenon, esophageal dysmotility, sclerodactyly, and telangiectasia); *PM/Scl* polymyositis/scleroderma, *PM/DM* polymyositis/dermatomyositis

helicases proteins, while community 8 contains a diverse array of proteins including multiple SSc autoantibodies, including TOP1, SSB, Pm/Scl proteins, URNPs, and HNRNPs, and numerous serine/arginine-rich splicing factors. Community 3 consists primarily of aminoacyl tRNA synthetases, a cluster often targeted in autoimmune diseases [19, 23]. Communities 4, 5, and 9 are strongly associated with a variety of GO processes known to play a major role in SSc, including wound healing, IFN signaling, and response to oxidative stress. Major proteins include CD44, HLAs, myosins, and filamin proteins in community 4 and tricarboxylic acid cycle proteins in community 5. Community 9 contains multiple protein disulfide isomerases and peroxiredoxins, protein folding enzymes such as calnexin (CANX) and calreticulin (CALR), and the major collagen processing enzyme prolyl 4-hydroxylase beta (P4HB). Community 6 contains multiple annexin and 14-3-3 proteins; enriched GO processes include ribonucleoprotein complex assembly, mitochondrial transport, RNA processing, and anchoring junction. Community 7 associated with GO terms include cell cycle, RNA polymerase III complex, DNA-PK-Ku complex, and antigen processing and presentation. Community 7 includes several SSc autoantibody targets including Ku proteins XRCC5 and 6, RUVBL1 and 2, RNA polymerase I and II subunits, multiple proteasomal subunits, and T-complex proteins.

Preferential detection of autoantibodies in SSc

Subsequent comparisons between groups were performed in a semiquantitative manner based on the presence or absence of a given protein in an immunoprecipitant, with quantitative analyses limited to comparisons within an individual sample. To identify biological processes and cellular components differentially targeted in SSc, with minimal to no background detection in controls, we examined all proteins detected in >50 % of SSc samples at a frequency >1.5-fold relative to controls, resulting in a list of 137 differentially detected proteins (Fig. 2; Additional file 2: Table S2). Enriched biological processes included *ncRNA metabolic process*, response to oxygen radical, and triglyceride-rich lipoprotein particle remodeling. Preferentially targeted cellular components include cytosolic stress granule, lipid-protein complex, pigment granule, and anchoring junction; molecular functions include antioxidant activity and mRNA binding (Additional file 3: Table S3C).

RNA processing centers are major targets of SSc autoantibodies

The strong enrichment for GO terms associated with mRNA processing and stress response, as well as the identification of cytosolic stress granule as an enriched cellular component, led us to further investigate the role of stress granules (SG) and RNA processing bodies (PB) in the autoantibody response of SSc. SG and PB represent distinct, non-membranous cytoplasmic entities, which arise in response to different cellular stresses including oxidative stress, hypoxia, viral infection, unfolded proteins, and amino acid deprivation [24]. These structures exist in constant flux, driven by the availability of constituent mRNPs, regulating the fate of untranslated mRNAs in response to translational arrest [25]. While SG are generally absent under normal conditions, PB are constitutively present at low levels due to their role as microRNA processing centers. Both structures have been shown to arise in response to cellular stresses, including oxidative stress, ischemia, and cancer [26], all of which are known to be important in SSc pathogenesis [5, 27].

In addition to the 137 differentially detected proteins described above, a wide range of PB/SG constituents were readily detected across most SSc samples (Additional file 5: Table S4). Substantial reactivity was seen against PB components such as UPF1 and MOV10, and SG proteins FXR1 and FXR2, G3BP1 and G3BP2, and USP10. Only background levels of reactivity were seen in healthy controls.

Validation of PB/SG antibodies in SSc

In order to validate the differential abundance of PB/SG proteins identified by LC-MS/MS, HeLa whole cell lysates were immunoprecipitated using antibodies from each patient as described in the LC-MS/MS analyses. Western blots were performed by resolving equal volumes of IP eluates by SDS-PAGE and transferring to nitrocellulose. Blots were then probed with antibodies targeting PB/SG proteins UPF1, MOV10, CAPRIN1, G3BP1, and USP10. These targets were chosen based upon their high level of detection across SSc groups, as determined based on our LC-MS/MS data. Strong reactivity was seen against all five proteins in SSc with only trace levels detected in controls (Fig. 3a), indicating widespread immune responses against these protein complexes.

Further validation was performed using immunofluorescence (IF) staining of U2OS cells maintained under conditions of oxidative stress to induce PB/SG formation. Cells were probed with patient sera in combination with PB and SG markers SK1-Hedls and eIF3b, respectively. Co-localization between patient sera and PB/SG markers was observed in six of nine SSc patients, with at least one positive sample in each of the three autoantibody groups; no staining was seen for any of the three healthy controls (Fig. 3b). These results are consistent with that seen on LC-MS/MS, particularly among RNAP3 patients, who exhibited the strongest and most consistent autoantibody responses across both methods. Taken together, these data strongly implicate PB/SG as novel targets of SSc autoantibody responses.

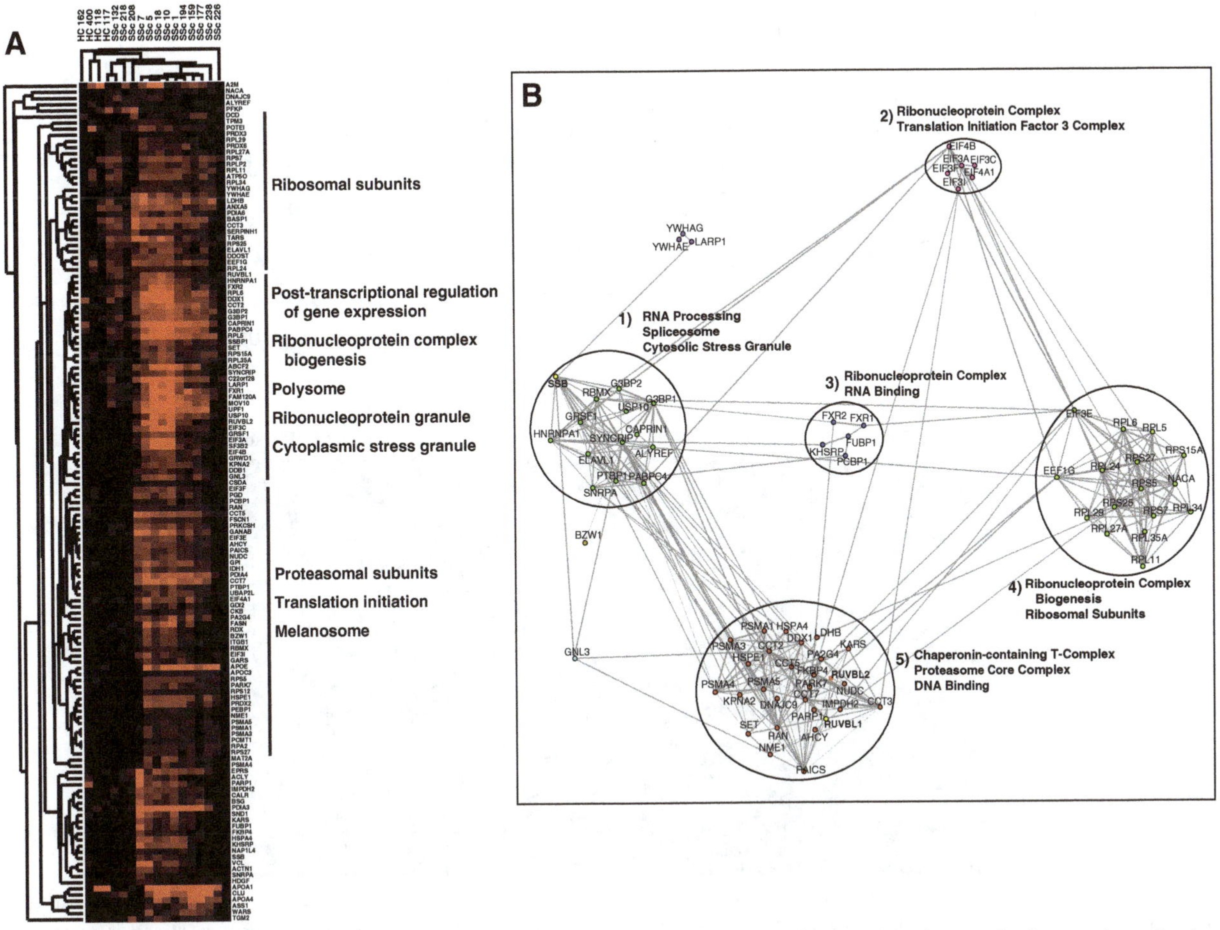

Fig. 2 Proteins differentially detected in systemic sclerosis (*SSc*). Semiquantitative enrichment of SSc-associated autoantibodies was determined using a binary assessment of autoantibody presence or absence in a sample. Preferential enrichment in SSc was defined as all proteins detected in >50 % of all patient samples at a frequency >1.5-fold relative to controls. **a** Heat map of proteins differentially detected in SSc. **b** Network analysis of differentially detected proteins. Community detection was performed using the GIANT global network; functional annotation was performed using gProfiler

Discussion

Autoantibodies have long been used in the diagnosis of SSc, with different autoantibodies predictive of clinical outcomes, including interstitial lung disease, pulmonary arterial hypertension, and skin involvement. While a wide array of SSc-associated autoantibodies have been described, diagnoses are often performed based upon the presence or absence of reactivity against three proteins: RNAP3, TOP1, and CENP. The data presented here suggest a much broader autoantibody response, which is reflective of underlying disease pathologies. Strong subset-specific reactivity was evident against both RNAP3 and TOP1, with no RNAP3 peptides detected in any of the other groups; however, all four RNAP3 patients exhibited modest reactivity against TOP1, indicating a degree of overlap between these two autoantibody groups. When peptides recovered are extended beyond the three major targets, we found substantial overlap across the three major SSc groups. We found peptides from the autoantigens of RuvBL1/2, which appear to act as general markers of SSc, with consistent detection across all SSc groups, with almost no reactivity seen in controls. In contrast, some common SSc autoantigens such as B23 and Ro52/TRIM21 were recovered in virtually all samples, and in controls, indicating an important degree of baseline reactivity against some of the more common autoantibody targets.

In this proof-of-concept study, we do not attempt to address the clinical implications of the autoantibody responses described here due to the limited number of patients analyzed, nor are we able to speculate on the presence or absence of these autoantibodies in other SSc autoantibody groups. Our depth in this study comes from the number of potential antigens analyzed, which cover the full proteome. Future studies examining a much larger cohort of SSc patients, along with representatives of other

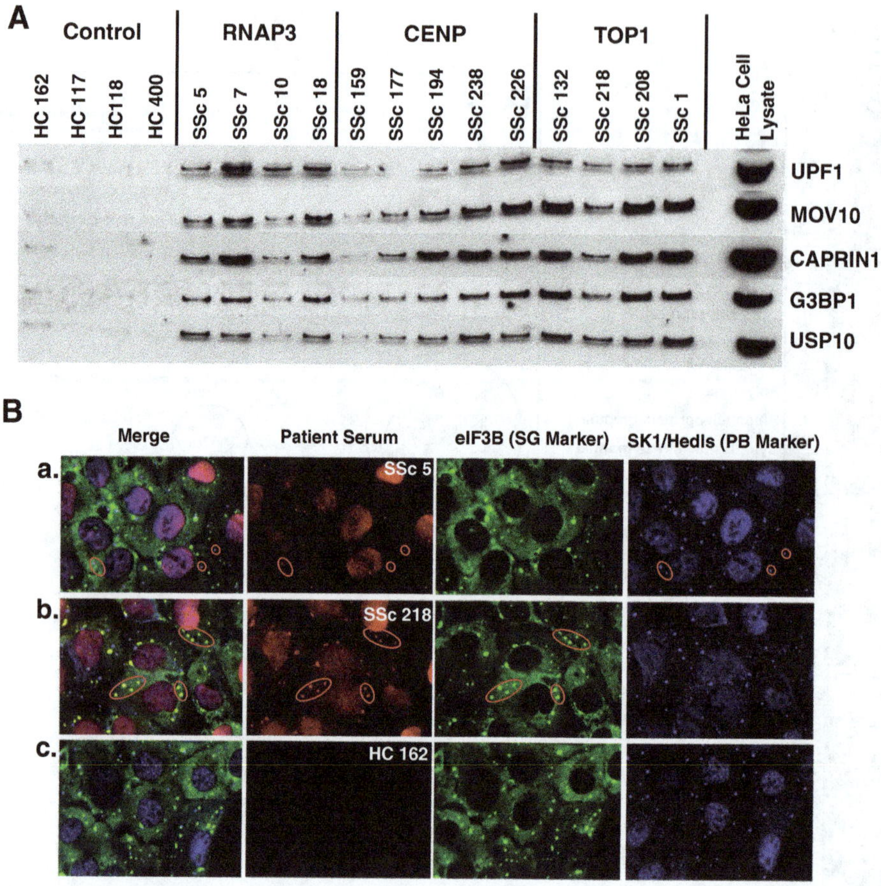

Fig. 3 Validation of RNA processing bodies (*PB*)/stress granules (*SG*) as a target of the SSc autoimmune response. **a** HeLa cell lysates were immunoprecipitated using patient sera, resolved by SDS-PAGE, and probed with antibodies targeting known PB and SG proteins; HeLa whole cell lysate was used as a control. **b** Immunofluorescence was performed in U2OS cells treated with sodium (meta)arsenite to induce the formation of SG. Cells were then fixed with 4 % paraformaldehyde and permeabilized with 5 % normal horse serum and 0.1 % digitonin in Tris-buffered saline. Staining was performed with anti-eIF3b (SG marker), anti-SK1-Hedls (PB marker), and patient sera. Representative images depicting co-localization between patient sera and SG/PB markers are shown, with sites of co-localization circled in *red*. *RNAP* RNA polymerase, *CENP* centromere protein *TOPI* topoisomerase I

autoimmune diseases, will be necessary to determine the clinical value of these potential autoantibodies.

This is not the first study to suggest the presence of multiple autoantibodies in SSc. Immunoassays performed by Op De Beeck, et al. revealed the presence of multiple autoantibodies in a small subset of SSc patients [28]. A similar analysis by Graf et al. using the EUROLINE immunoassay revealed the presence of multiple autoantibodies in 11 % of patients [1].

Autoantibodies against extracellular immune signaling receptors and extracellular matrix proteins were conspicuously absent in these data; this includes the absence of numerous autoantibodies previously implicated in SSc pathogenesis, such as anti-fibrillin 1, anti-MMP, and anti-PDGFR [29]. Additional analyses in other cell types, such as fibroblasts or endothelial cells, and cells maintained under physiologically relevant growth conditions, such as immune activation or oxidative stress, may be useful for identifying other proteins and complexes which may play a role in disease pathogenesis.

In addition to identifying novel autoantibody targets, the unbiased nature of mass spectrometry provides additional insights into the processes potentially underlying autoimmunity. The preferential detection of proteins associated with RNA processing and oxidative stress as a general feature of SSc autoantibodies may be indicative of their origins. Combined with the consistent targeting of PB/SG described here spanning all SSc patients, these data suggest a basic model in which disease-specific pathologies give rise to specific autoantibodies. Strong induction of SGs is observed in response to cellular stresses, including oxidative stress and ischemia, two well-established phenomena in SSc [27]. SG/PB are also readily induced in response to the tumor microenvironment, consistent with recent evidence linking RNAP3-positive SSc and cancer [5, 30]. Combined with evidence linking transforming growth factor (TGF)-β signaling with an increase in PB formation [31], many of the major processes underlying SSc pathogenesis appear broadly consistent with an immune response against cells undergoing a stress response. PBs are also known to associate with other cytoplasmic structures, such as U bodies [32], which house an number of well-established SSc autoantibody targets, including U1, U5, and U11/U12. Taken together, these data suggest a model in which autoantibodies arise as a secondary phenotype in response to SSc-related processes already underway.

Some evidence suggesting a link between PBs and autoimmunity has been described previously. Bhanji, et al. observed reactivity against a number of PB-associated proteins, including GE1/*Hedls*, GW182, and Ago2 in a range of autoimmune diseases, including SSc [33]. Among these autoantigens, only Ago2 was also identified in this analysis, suggesting a persistent, yet diverse response against this complex. A similar analysis of SG-associated proteins has not been performed; however given the reactivity to PB proteins seen in other autoimmune diseases, reactivity in other autoimmune diseases is possible. A detailed analysis using both mass spectrometry and other methods will be necessary to understand the degree to which autoantibodies to SG/PBs are seen in other autoimmune diseases, and the clinical implications of these findings.

This work has several limitations. First, we cannot eliminate the possibility that some proteins found in our mass spectrometry data result from co-IP of multiprotein complexes by a single autoantibody; however, we were able to confirm the presence of multiple PB/SG autoantibodies by other means (Fig. 3). We also cannot rule out the possibility that some targets were missed due to their being sequestered into tightly packed molecular complexes associated with chromatin. For example, the presence of CENP autoantibodies within these samples had been established using clinical methods, indicating its absence in our mass spectrometry data is likely a result of its sequestration into large macromolecular complexes with limited solubility. A lack of age- and gender-matched controls likely underestimates the degree of baseline reactivity seen in unaffected controls. Finally, the small number of patient samples used in this study prevents any clinical interpretation, and the variability in the number of peptides recovered between experiments limits direct quantitative comparisons between autoantibody groups.

Conclusions

The data presented here provide evidence of diverse immune reactivities in SSc targeting a wide array of protein complexes. Among these complexes, autoantibodies targeting PB/SG were consistently identified across both clinical SSc subsets and major autoantibody groups, suggesting a potential novel autoantibody target. Taken together, these data suggest immune responses to proteins involved in cellular stress may be a common mechanism for autoantibody generation.

Additional files

Additional file 1: Table S1. Complete list of peptides identified in this analysis. *TP* number of total peptides mapping to a protein, *UP* number of unique peptides mapping to a protein, *UM* number of non-redundant peptides mapping exclusively to a protein, *MW* molecular weight, *Length* protein length in amino acids. (XLS 639 kb)

Additional file 2: Table S2. Gene lists used in these analyses. (XLSX 17 kb)

Additional file 3: Table S3. Systemic sclerosis (SSc)-specific enrichment of processes and components. Proteins differentially detected in SSc were analyzed using gProfiler. Statistically significant processes and components are shown. A) Peptides detected at any level across all four groups. B) Peptides identified in all SSc groups, but absent in controls. C) Analysis of 137 proteins differentially detected in SSc. *BP* biological process, *CC* cellular component, *MF* molecular function, *ke* KEGG pathway, *re* REACTOME pathway. (ODS 70 kb)

Additional file 4: Figure S1. Network analysis of systemic sclerosis (SSc) autoantigens. All 763 non-redundant peptide hits identified in two or more patients were analyzed using the Genome-scale Integrated Analysis of gene Networks in Tissues (GIANT) global network to identify functionally associated protein networks. Analysis of community function was performed using gProfiler. SSc-associated autoantibodies are highlighted in *yellow*. (EPS 1902 kb)

Additional file 5: Table S4. Processing body and stress granule proteins identified in this analysis. *Proteins with multiple subunits. Data indicate non-redundant peptide hits. (ODS 20 kb)

Abbreviations

CENP: centromere protein; DMEM: Dulbecco's modified Eagle's medium; dSSc: diffuse systemic sclerosis; ELISA: enzyme-linked immunosorbent assay; FBS: fetal bovine serum; GIANT: Genome-scale Integrated Analysis of gene Networks in Tissues; IFN: interferon; kDa: kiloDalton; LC-MS/MS: liquid chromatography tandem-mass spectrometry; IP: immunoprecipitation; lSSc: limited systemic sclerosis; PB: RNA processing bodies; PBS: phosphate-buffered saline; RNAP3: RNA polymerase III; SG: stress granules; SSc: systemic sclerosis; TOP1: topoisomerase I.

Competing interests

Dr. Whitfield has received royalties for patents regarding gene expression biomarkers in Scleroderma and is a scientific founder of Celdara Medical LLC. Dr. Lafyatis has received both grants and consulting fees from Genzyme/Sanofi, Shire, Regeneron, Biogen, BMS, Inception, Precision Dermatology, PRISM, UCB, Pfizer and Roche/Genentech; he received consulting fees from Lycera, Novartis, Celgene, Amira, Celdara, Celltex, Dart Therapeutics, Idera, Intermune, Medimmune, Promedior, Zwitter, Actelion, EMD Serono, Akros, Extera, Reneo, Scholar Rock, and HGS. No authors have any non-financial conflicts of interest to report.

Authors' contributions

MEJ conceived of the study, performed experiments, analyzed data, and wrote the manuscript. AVG performed mass spectrometry and helped to revise the manuscript. JNT performed data analysis and helped to revise the manuscript. SML performed immunofluorescence experiments, and helped to revise the manuscript. DS performed mass spectrometry, and revised the manuscript. JKG, RFS, and RL provided clinical samples, and revised the manuscript. PJA designed experiments, provided technical assistance, and revised the manuscript. SAG and MLW conceived of the study, participated in its design, and helped to revise the manuscript. All authors read and approved the final manuscript.

Acknowledgements

This work was supported by grants from the NIH National Institute of Arthritis and Musculoskeletal and Skin Diseases (NIAMS) Center of Research Translation (P50 AR060780 to MLW and RL), the Department of Defense (PR130908 to MLW), and a SYNERGY grant from the Geisel School of Medicine at Dartmouth (to MLW). JNT is supported in part by a grant from the National Institute of General Medical Sciences (NIGMS; T32GM008704). SAG is supported by grants R01-CA155260 and S10-OD016212 from the NIH. JKG is supported by a Kellen Foundation Clinician Scientist Development Award from the Hospital for Special Surgery. Written informed consent was obtained from all participants for publication of their individual details in this manuscript. All consent forms are held by the respective authors' institutions and are available for review by the Editor-in-Chief.

Author details

[1]Department of Genetics, Geisel School of Medicine at Dartmouth, Hanover, NH, USA. [2]Division of Rheumatology, Immunology, and Allergy, Brigham and Women's Hospital, Boston, MA, USA. [3]Department of Rheumatology, Hospital for Special Surgery, New York, NY, USA. [4]Boston University School of Medicine, Boston, MA, USA. [5]Dartmouth Medical School, Hinman Box 7400, Hanover, NH 03755, USA.

References

1. Graf SW, Hakendorf P, Lester S, Patterson K, Walker JG, Smith MD, et al. South Australian Scleroderma Register: autoantibodies as predictive biomarkers of phenotype and outcome. Int J Rheum Dis. 2012;15:102–9.
2. Steen VD. Autoantibodies in systemic sclerosis. Semin Arthritis Rheum. 2005; 35:35–42.
3. Mehra S, Walker J, Patterson K, Fritzler MJ. Autoantibodies in systemic sclerosis. Autoimmun Rev. 2013;12:340–54.
4. Fertig N, Domsic RT, Rodriguez-Reyna T, Kuwana M, Lucas M, Medsger TA, et al. Anti-U11/U12 RNP antibodies in systemic sclerosis: A new serologic marker associated with pulmonary fibrosis. Arthritis Care Res. 2009;61:958–65.
5. Joseph CG, Darrah E, Shah AA, Skora AD, Casciola-Rosen LA, Wigley FM, et al. Association of the autoimmune disease scleroderma with an immunologic response to cancer. Science. 2014;343:152–7.
6. Robinson WH, DiGennaro C, Hueber W, Haab BB, Kamachi M, Dean EJ, et al. Autoantigen microarrays for multiplex characterization of autoantibody responses. Nat Med. 2002;8:295–301.
7. Yore MM, Kettenbach AN, Sporn MB, Gerber SA, Liby KT. Proteomic analysis shows synthetic oleanane triterpenoid binds to mTOR. PLoS ONE. 2011;6:e22862.
8. Eng JK, Jahan TA, Hoopmann MR. Comet: An open-source MS/MS sequence database search tool. Proteomics. 2013;13:22–4.
9. Hsieh EJ, Hoopmann MR, MacLean B, MacCoss MJ. Comparison of database search strategies for high precursor mass accuracy MS/MS data. J Proteome Res. 2009;9:1138–43.
10. Elias JE, Gygi SP. Target-decoy search strategy for increased confidence in large-scale protein identifications by mass spectrometry. Nat Methods. 2007;4:207–14.
11. Oliveros JC. VENNY. An interactive tool for comparing lists with Venn Diagrams. 2007.
12. Greene CS, Krishnan A, Wong AK, Ricciotti E, Zelaya RA, Himmelstein DS, et al. Zaslavsky E. Understanding multicellular function and disease with human tissue-specific networks. Nat Genet. 2015;47:569–76.
13. Shannon P, Markiel A, Ozier O, Baliga NS, Wang JT, Ramage D, et al. Cytoscape: a software environment for integrated models of biomolecular interaction networks. Genome Res. 2003;13:2498–504.
14. Reimand J, Arak T, Vilo J. g: Profiler—a web server for functional interpretation of gene lists (2011 update). Nucleic Acids Res. 2011;39:W307–15.
15. Eisen MB, Spellman PT, Brown PO, Botstein D. Cluster analysis and display of genome-wide expression patterns. PNAS. 1998;95:14863–8.
16. Saldanha AJ. Java Treeview—extensible visualization of microarray data. Bioinformatics. 2004;20:3246–8.
17. Novoradovskaya N, Perou C, Whitfield M, Basehore S, Pesich R, Aprelikova O, et al.: Universal human, mouse and rat reference RNA as standards for microarray experiments. In: Mol Bio Cell: 2002: Amer Soc Cell Biology 8120 Woodmont Ave, STE 750, Bethesda, MD 20814-2755 USA; 2002: 241A-241A.
18. Kaji K, Fertig N, Medsger TA, Satoh T, Hoshino K, Hamaguchi Y, et al. Autoantibodies to RuvBL1 and RuvBL2: A novel systemic sclerosis-related antibody associated with diffuse cutaneous and skeletal muscle involvement. Arthr Care Res. 2014;66:575–84.
19. Hamaguchi Y, Fujimoto M, Matsushita T, Kaji K, Komura K, Hasegawa M, et al. Common and Distinct Clinical Features in Adult Patients with Anti-Aminoacyl-tRNA Synthetase Antibodies: Heterogeneity within the Syndrome. PLoS ONE. 2013;8:e60442.
20. Fujimoto M, Shimozuma M, Yazawa N, Kubo M, Ihn H, Sato S, et al. Prevalence and clinical relevance of 52-kDa and 60-kDa Ro/SS-A autoantibodies in Japanese patients with systemic sclerosis. Ann Rheum Dis. 1997;56:667–70.
21. Ulanet DB, Wigley FM, Gelber AC, Rosen A. Autoantibodies against B23, a nucleolar phosphoprotein, occur in scleroderma and are associated with pulmonary hypertension. Arth Care Res. 2003;49:85–92.
22. Brouwer R, Vree Egberts WTM, Hengstman GJD, Raijmakers R, van Engelen BGM, Peter Seelig H, et al. Autoantibodies directed to novel components of the PM/Scl complex, the human exosome. Arth Res. 2002;4:134–8.
23. Lega J-C, Fabien N, Reynaud Q, Durieu I, Durupt S, Dutertre M, et al. The clinical phenotype associated with myositis-specific and associated autoantibodies: A meta-analysis revisiting the so-called antisynthetase syndrome. Autoimmun Rev. 2014;13:883–91.
24. Kedersha N, Ivanov P, Anderson P. Stress granules and cell signaling: more than just a passing phase? Trends Biochem Sci. 2013;38:494–506.
25. Kedersha N, Anderson P. Regulation of translation by stress granules and processing bodies. Prog Mol Biol Transl Sci. 2009;90:155–185.
26. Anderson P, Kedersha N. Stress granules: the Tao of RNA triage. Trends Biochem Sci. 2008;33:141–50.
27. Katsumoto TR, Whitfield ML, Connolly MK. The pathogenesis of systemic sclerosis. Annu Rev Pathol-Mech. 2011;6:509–37.
28. Op De Beéck K, Vermeersch P, Verschueren P, Westhovens R, Mariën G, Blockmans D, et al. Antinuclear antibody detection by automated multiplex immunoassay in untreated patients at the time of diagnosis. Autoimmun Rev. 2012;12:137–43.
29. Chung L, Utz P. Antibodies in scleroderma: Direct pathogenicity and phenotypic associations. Curr Rheumatol Rep. 2004;6:156–63.
30. Anderson P, Kedersha N, Ivanov P. Stress granules, P-bodies and cancer. Biochim Biophys Acta. 2015, 1849, 861–870.
31. Blanco FF, Sanduja S, Deane NG, Blackshear PJ, Dixon DA. Transforming growth factor β regulates P-body formation through induction of the mRNA decay factor tristetraprolin. Mol Cell Bio. 2014;34:180–95.
32. Liu J-L, Gall JG. U bodies are cytoplasmic structures that contain uridine-rich small nuclear ribonucleoproteins and associate with P bodies. PNAS. 2007; 104:11655–9.
33. Bhanji RA, Eystathioy T, Chan EKL, Bloch DB, Fritzler MJ. Clinical and serological features of patients with autoantibodies to GW/P bodies. Clin Immunol. 2007;125:247–56.
34. Dib H, Tamby MC, Bussone G, Regent A, Berezné A, Lafine C, Broussard C, Simonneau G, Guillevin L, Witko-Sarsat V, et al. Targets of anti-endothelial cell antibodies in pulmonary hypertension and scleroderma. Eur Respir J. 2012;39(6):1405–1414.
35. Naniwa T, Sugiura Y, Banno S, Yoshinouchi T, Matsumoto Y, Ueda R. Ribosomal P protein P0 as a candidate for the target antigen of anti-endothelial cell antibodies in mixed connective tissue. Clin Exp Rheumatol. 2007;25:593–598.
36. Terrier B, Tamby MC, Camoin L, Guilpain P, Broussard C, Bussone G, et al. Identification of target antigens of antifibroblast antibodies in pulmonary arterial hypertension. Am J Resp Crit Care Med. 2008;177(10):1128–1134.
37. Terrier B, Tamby MC, Camoin L, Guilpain P, Bérézné A, Tamas N, et al. Anti-fibroblast antibodies from systemic sclerosis patients bind to α-enolase and are associated with interstitial lung disease. Ann Rheum Dis. 2009.
38. Satoh M, Chan JY, Ceribelli A, del-Mercado MV, Chan EK. Autoantibodies to Argonaute 2 (Su antigen). In: Ten Years of Progress in GW/P Body Research. Springer. 2013:45-59.
39. Siapka S, Patrinou-Georgoula M, Vlachoyiannopoulos PG, Guialis A. Multiple specificities of autoantibodies against hnRNP A/B proteins in systemic rheumatic diseases and hnRNP L as an associated novel autoantigen. Autoimmunity. 2007;40(3):223–233.
40. Kubo M, Ihn H, Kuwana M, Asano Y, Tamaki T, Yamane K, Tamaki K. Anti-U5 snRNP antibody as a possible serological marker for scleroderma–polymyositis overlap. Rheumatol. 2002;41(5):531–534.

2

Increased serum levels of fractalkine and mobilisation of CD34$^+$CD45$^-$ endothelial progenitor cells in systemic sclerosis

Audrey Benyamine[1,2,3*†], Jérémy Magalon[3,4†], Sylvie Cointe[2,3], Romaric Lacroix[2,3], Laurent Arnaud[2], Nathalie Bardin[3,5], Pascal Rossi[1,3], Yves Francès[1], Fanny Bernard-Guervilly[1], Gilles Kaplanski[3,6], Jean-Robert Harlé[7], Pierre-Jean Weiller[7], Philippe Berbis[8], David Braunstein[9], Elisabeth Jouve[9], Nathalie Lesavre[9], Françoise Couranjou[9], Françoise Dignat-George[2,3], Florence Sabatier[3,4], Pascale Paul[2,3] and Brigitte Granel[1,3]

Abstract

Background: The disruption of endothelial homeostasis is a major determinant in the pathogenesis of systemic sclerosis (SSc) and is reflected by soluble and cellular markers of activation, injury and repair. We aimed to provide a combined assessment of endothelial markers to delineate specific profiles associated with SSc disease and its severity.

Methods: We conducted an observational, single-centre study comprising 45 patients with SSc and 41 healthy control subjects. Flow cytometry was used to quantify circulating endothelial microparticles (EMPs) and CD34$^+$ progenitor cell subsets. Colony-forming unit-endothelial cells (CFU-ECs) were counted by culture assay. Circulating endothelial cells were enumerated using anti-CD146-based immunomagnetic separation. Blood levels of endothelin-1, vascular endothelial growth factor (VEGF) and soluble fractalkine (s-Fractalkine) were evaluated by enzyme-linked immunosorbent assay. Disease-associated markers were identified using univariate, correlation and multivariate analyses.

Results: Enhanced numbers of EMPs, CFU-ECs and non-haematopoietic CD34$^+$CD45$^-$ endothelial progenitor cells (EPCs) were observed in patients with SSc. Patients with SSc also displayed higher serum levels of VEGF, endothelin-1 and s-Fractalkine. s-Fractalkine levels positively correlated with CD34$^+$CD45$^-$ EPC numbers. EMPs, s-Fractalkine and endothelin-1 were independent factors associated with SSc. Patients with high CD34$^+$CD45$^-$ EPC numbers had lower forced vital capacity values. Elevated s-Fractalkine levels were associated with disease severity, a higher frequency of pulmonary fibrosis and altered carbon monoxide diffusion.

Conclusions: This study identifies the mobilisation of CD34$^+$CD45$^-$ EPCs and high levels of s-Fractalkine as specific features of SSc-associated vascular activation and disease severity. This signature may provide novel insights linking endothelial inflammation and defective repair processes in the pathogenesis of SSc.

Keywords: Systemic sclerosis, Fractalkine, Endothelial progenitor cells, Endothelial microparticles, Circulating endothelial cells, Vascular endothelial growth factor, Endothelin-1, Endothelial homeostasis

* Correspondence: audrey.benyamine@ap-hm.fr
†Equal contributors
[1]Internal Medicine Department, Assistance Publique-Hôpitaux de Marseille (APHM), CHU Nord, 13015 Marseilles, France
[2]Haematology and Vascular Biology Laboratory, APHM, CHU Conception, 13005 Marseilles, France
Full list of author information is available at the end of the article

Background

Systemic sclerosis (SSc) is a systemic autoimmune disease characterised by vascular damage and fibrosis [1]. The blood vessel is the primary target for both initiating and propagating the local immune activation and fibrosis. This vascular hypothesis has been underscored by the impairment of the flow-mediated dilation (FMD) of the brachial artery, a validated, non-invasive physiological measure of endothelial function [2].

The disruption of endothelial integrity involves an altered balance between lesion and repair processes that can be assessed by non-invasive endothelium-derived biomarkers which our group has contributed to identify and standardise [3, 4]. These markers include circulating endothelial cells (CECs) that enter the bloodstream following detachment of stressed endothelial cells from the vessel wall and endothelial microparticles (EMPs) that are shed during the membrane remodelling of activated or apoptotic endothelial cells. These markers have been shown to have diagnostic and prognostic value in cardiovascular diseases [4–6], but their significance in inflammatory and autoimmune diseases is less well established [7–9].

In response to vascular injury, endothelial repair mechanisms have been shown to involve the recruitment of progenitor cells (PCs) [10]. In their pioneering work, Asahara et al. [10] identified a bone marrow-derived circulating population of PCs expressing CD34 and kinase insert domain receptor (KDR, vascular endothelial growth factor receptor 2 [VEGFR-2]) antigens that displays the capacity to differentiate into an endothelial phenotype and contribute to physiological or pathological neovascularisation. These cells were referred to as *endothelial progenitor cells* (EPCs).

From that time, extensive research has led to the recognition that EPCs represent a highly heterogeneous cell compartment. Indeed, various circulating subpopulations with different stages of maturation, lineage origin and functional properties contribute to the "EPC pool" [11, 12]. Following the first report of decreased levels of circulating EPCs in SSc [13], several controversial studies have addressed their quantitative and functional alterations [14–23]. These discrepancies may arise from the clinical characteristics of the enrolled patients with SSc and the disparate methodologies used to analyse EPCs. Indeed, despite the effort to find a consensus [22], these methods based on flow cytometric analyses or on ex vivo culture protocols have sometimes led to the assessment of distinct cell populations.

Importantly, most of the literature in the SSc field has focused on cells that belong to the haematopoietic lineage [23]. Indeed, recent clarifications in EPC identity indicate that a combination of CD34, CD133 and KDR markers enumerate mostly bone marrow-derived haematopoietic cells or progenitors that correlate with vascular endothelial status [11]. These cells are now designated as circulating angiogenic cells (CACs) to reflect their potential to sustain angiogenesis but lack de novo vessel-forming activity [24]. Additionally, the colony-forming unit-endothelial cell (CFU-EC) assay introduced by Hill et al. allowed for the description of the CFU-ECs as relevant biomarkers of cardiovascular risk [25]. Increased CFU-EC formation was also associated with the inflammatory response to endothelial injury [26]. These CFU-ECs exhibit characteristics of monocytes/macrophages and contribute to a paracrine support of endothelial lining repair [26].

By contrast, "true EPCs" have been identified within the $CD45^-$ non-haematopoietic fraction of the $CD34^+$ circulating PCs and are capable of forming highly proliferative late-outgrowth endothelial colonies. These cells, also named *endothelial colony-forming cells* (ECFCs), behave as angioblasts with a specific ability to achieve endothelial differentiation and contribute to de novo vessel formation [24]. They are unlikely derived from bone marrow, but rather belong to a pool of vascular wall-resident precursors [11]. Owing to the extreme scarcity of EPCs in peripheral blood, very few clinical studies have tackled this cell population. These investigations were restricted mainly to the cardiovascular field and suggested the potential relevance of $CD34^+CD45^-$ EPC quantification as a reflection of inflammatory [27] or mechanical vascular injury [28]. To our knowledge, this $CD34^+CD45^-$ EPC subset has never been investigated in patients with SSc.

In addition, several soluble inflammatory endothelial mediators, such as endothelin-1 [29] and soluble fractalkine (s-Fractalkine) [30], have been associated with SSc pathogenesis. Elevated endothelin-1 levels were shown to induce endothelial cell activation, fibroblast differentiation and vascular remodelling [29]. This discovery allowed for the therapeutic targeting of the endothelin-1 pathway, which led to a real clinical benefit in patients with pulmonary arterial hypertension [31] and digital ulcers [32]. Fractalkine (chemokine [C-X3-C motif] ligand 1 [CX3CL1]) is an endothelial membrane-bound adhesion molecule and a soluble chemokine after metalloprotease cleavage [33]. Increased endothelial cell surface expression and circulating s-Fractalkine levels have been described in inflammatory contexts of vascular injury, such as atherosclerosis [34] and immune diseases, including SSc [30]. The upregulation of fractalkine on activated endothelial cells allows for the recruitment and activation of immune cells expressing chemokine (C-X3-C motif) receptor 1 (CX3CR1) [35]. Polymorphisms of CX3CR1 have been associated with SSc-associated pulmonary arterial hypertension [36]. Accordingly, the disruption of the interaction between fractalkine and CX3CR1 has been shown to dampen the fibrotic process in a murine model of cytokine-induced SSc [37].

For this reason, we sought to provide an integrative view of the endothelial status based on the combined assessment of circulating biomarkers of endothelial inflammation, injury and repair. Our objective was to delineate specific profiles associated with SSc disease and severity.

Methods

Patients

Forty-five consecutive, unselected patients with SSc were recruited at the Department of Internal Medicine, Assistance Publique-Hôpitaux de Marseille (APHM). All the enrolled patients had a score ≥9 for SSc according to the 2013 American College of Rheumatology/European League Against Rheumatism criteria [38]. Among the patients were 44 women and 1 man with a median age of 60.38 years (IQR 51.45–72.38 years) (Table 1). Healthy volunteers ($n = 41$) were recruited for the study by the Centre d'Investigation Clinique Marseille, APHM, and used as control subjects. The control group consisted of 38 women and 3 men with a median age of 55.97 years (IQR 53.56–59.64 years) (Table 1). Written informed consent was obtained according to the Declaration of Helsinki, and the study was approved by the local ethics committee review board of Marseilles.

Clinical and standard biological assessment

All subjects had a physical examination and underwent laboratory tests. Characteristics of the study population are summarised in Table 1. Arterial stiffness was assessed by measuring the right carotid-radial pulse wave velocity (PWV) using a validated, non-invasive, automated method. The FMD of the brachial artery was measured as previously reported [2].

Patients with SSc were classified as having limited cutaneous SSc or diffuse cutaneous SSc according to the criteria established by van den Hoogen et al. [38]. The disease duration, the presence of Raynaud's phenomenon, pitting scars, digital ulcers, digital gangrene or telangiectasia were recorded. The modified Rodnan skin score (mRSS) was graded on a scale of 0–3 with a maximum total score of 51. Disease severity was measured on a scale of 0–4 according to the Medsger severity scale [39]. Two groups of patients were segregated on the basis of severity state: Group 1 comprised grades 0, 1 and 2, and group 2 consisted of grades 3 and 4 (Table 2).

Concomitant treatments of patients with SSc are described in Additional file 1: Table S1. Biological data comprised white blood cell count, haemoglobin rate, platelets count, low-density lipoprotein cholesterol, high-density lipoprotein cholesterol, triglycerides, creatinine level and C-reactive protein (CRP) level (Additional file 1: Table S2).Pulmonary involvement was determined by pulmonary function tests, including forced vital capacity (FVC), diffusing capacity of the lung for carbon monoxide (DLCO) and DLCO divided by alveolar volume (DLCO/VA). Fibrosis was diagnosed on the basis of chest computed tomography, with qualitative criteria consisting of the presence of honeycombing, ground-glass opacities, reticular abnormalities, traction bronchiectasis and septal thickening. Systolic pulmonary arterial pressure was measured by transthoracic echocardiography, and pulmonary hypertension was confirmed by right heart catheterisation. Anti-nuclear antibodies were assessed by indirect immunofluorescence analysis of HEp-2 cells. Anti-centromere and anti-topoisomerase I antibodies were measured by enzyme-linked immunosorbent assay (ELISA).

Flow cytometric enumeration of endothelial microparticles

Control and patient samples for EMP analysis were collected and processed according to the current International

Table 1 Demographic characteristics and cardiovascular risk factors of the subjects

	Patients with SSc ($n = 45$)	Control subjects ($n = 41$)	*P* value
Sex, male/female, *n*	1/44	3/38	0.3437
Age, years, median [IQR]	61.49 (±11.95) 60.4 [51.5–72.4]	56.09 (±7.82) 56 [53.6–59.6]	0.0375
BMI, kg/m^2, median [IQR]	23.05 (±4.63) 22.5 [20.2–23.8]	25.3 (±3.75) 24.9 [22.8–28.3]	0.0022
Systolic blood pressure, mmHg	119.11 (±16.95) 120 [105–130.25]	127.7 (±14.1) 126 [119.25–135.25]	0.0141
Diastolic blood pressure, mmHg	71.86 (±8.91) 72.5 [67.75–78.25]	79.15 (±9.71) 79 [73–84.25]	0.0006
Resting heart rate, beats/minute	71.25 (±10.24) 70.5 [64–76.25]	68.95 (±9.93) 70 [62.75–74]	0.3001
LDL cholesterol, g/L	3.29 (±1.32) 3.2 [2.36–4.28]	3.69 (±0.79) 3.59 [3.17–4.13]	0.0978
HDL cholesterol, g/L	1.72 (±0.43) 1.71 [1.4–1.95]	1.59 (±0.43) 1.51 [1.34–1.85]	0.1848
Triglycerides, g/L	1.14 (±0.47) 0.93 [0.81–1.48]	1.4 (±0.74) 1.25 [0.88–1.66]	0.1303
Carotid-radial pulse wave velocity, m/second	11.05 (±3.32) 10.5 [8.16–13]	10.11 (±3.01) 9.46 [7.62–12.05]	0.1855
Flow-mediated dilation, %	9.87 (±6.97) 9.3 [5.8–14.76]	15.29 (±8.75) 12.35 [9.09–21.38]	0.0084

Abbreviations: BMI Body mass index, *HDL* High-density lipoprotein, *LDL* Low-density lipoprotein, *SSc* Systemic sclerosis
Variables are described using mean (±SD) and median [IQR]

Table 2 Clinical characteristics of patients with systemic sclerosis

	Patients with SSc ($n = 45$)
Diffuse/limited cutaneous subtype	16 (35.6%)/29 (64.4%)
Anti-centromere/anti-topoisomerase I	21 (46.7%)/19 (42.2%)
Disease duration ≤3 years/˃3 years	15 (34.1%)/29 (65.9%)
Medsger severity scale	
Grades 0, 1 and 2	1 (2.2%), 14 (31.1%) and 7 (15.6%)
Grades 3 and 4	22 (48.9%) and 1 (2.2%)
Pitting scars	24 (53.3%)
Digital ulcers	18 (40.0%)
Digital gangrene	4 (8.9%)
Telangiectasia	29 (64.4%)
Pulmonary function tests	
DLCO, %	97.3 [88.8–103.5]
DLCO/VA, %	67.4 [61.35–78.2]
FVC, %	99.3 [84.1–115.6]
Pulmonary fibrosis	7 (18.9%)
Systolic pulmonary arterial pressure[a]	33 [27.8–37.5]

DLCO Diffusing capacity of the lung for carbon monoxide, FVC Forced vital capacity, VA alveolar volume
Qualitative variables are described using counts and percentages. Quantitative variables are described using median [first quartile–third quartile]
[a]Transthoracic echocardiography assessment

Society on Thrombosis and Haemostasis guidelines [40]. Briefly, blood samples collected into 5-ml BD Vacutainer tubes containing 0.129 mol/L sodium citrate (BD Diagnostics, Franklin Lakes, NJ, USA) were subjected to two successive centrifugations ($2500 \times g$ for 15 minutes at room temperature), and platelet-free plasma (PFP) was prepared. The PFP was homogenised before being aliquoted and stored at −80 °C until use. Annexin V-fluorescein isothiocyanate (FITC) and the following fluorescent antibody reagents were procured from Beckman Coulter (Villepinte, France): CD31-phycoerythrin (PE) (clone 1 F11) and CD41-PE-cyanine 7 (CD41-PC7) (clone P2), as well as their respective isotype controls.

EMPs were enumerated by high-sensitivity flow cytometry following standardisation as previously described [41]. In brief, 30 μl of PFP was incubated with the appropriate amount of specific antibody or isotype control matched in terms of final concentration and fluorescence backgrounds, plus 10 μl of annexin V-FITC. Each stained sample was analysed on a NAVIOS-3 laser instrument (Beckman Coulter Life Sciences, Miami, FL, USA) following a protocol standardised with Megamix-Plus FSC beads (BioCytex, Marseille, France) with sizes ranging from 0.3 to 0.9 μm. EMPs were defined as annexin V^+/$CD31^+CD41^-$ events. The absolute EMP counts (events per microlitre) were determined using ad hoc counting beads (CytoCount™; Dako, Glostrup, Denmark).

Enumeration of circulating endothelial cells

CECs were isolated by immunomagnetic separation using Dynabeads coated with anti-CD146 monoclonal antibody (Life Technologies, Carlsbad, CA, USA) from 1 ml of blood samples collected into 5-ml ethylenediaminetetraacetic acid (EDTA) Vacutainer tubes. CECs were identified on the basis of previously described consensual morphologic and immunologic criteria [42]: rosette cell staining with acridine orange, size >15 μm, bearing more than five beads, and *Ulex europeaus* lectin-1 binding. Counting was performed with a fluorescence microscope.

Assessment of colony-forming unit-endothelial cells

CFU-ECs were produced according to the protocol initially described by Hill et al. [25] and adapted by Smadja et al. [43]. Mononuclear cells (MNCs) were obtained by density gradient isolation and cultured with the EndoCult® Liquid Medium Kit (STEMCELL Technologies, Vancouver, BC, Canada) according to the manufacturer's instructions. In short, MNCs were re-suspended in complete EndoCult® medium and seeded at 5×10^6 cells/well in fibronectin-coated tissue culture plates (BD Biosciences, San Jose, CA, USA). After 48 h, to obtain CFU-ECs, non-adherent cells were collected and plated in EndoCult® buffer at 10^6 cells/well in 24-well fibronectin-coated plates. CFU-EC colonies were counted after another 3 days, as recommended by the manufacturer.

Enumeration and characterisation of circulating progenitor cells by flow cytometry

Blood samples were collected into 5-ml, EDTA-coated BD Vacutainer tubes. $CD34^+CD45^+$ haematopoietic progenitor cells ($CD34^+CD45^+$ HPCs) and $CD34^+CD45^-$ EPCs were enumerated with a whole-blood flow cytometry protocol adapted from the standardised International Society of Hematotherapy and Graft Engineering single-platform sequential gating strategy [44]. Briefly, 100 μl of blood was stained with FITC-CD45 antibody, PE-CD34 antibody or PE-immunoglobulin G1 (IgG1), and 7-aminoactinomycin D (7-AAD) (Stem-Kit Reagents; Beckman Coulter Life Sciences), according to the manufacturer's instructions. After lysis of erythrocytes, flow count beads were added to each sample for absolute value determination, and samples were analysed with a NAVIOS flow cytometer equipped with CXP software (Beckman Coulter Life Sciences). At least 75,000 $CD45^+$ cells were acquired per run. $CD34^+CD45^+$ HPCs and $CD34^+CD45^-$ EPCs were identified within 7-AAD-negative viable cells displaying forward scatter (FSC)/side scatter (SSC) characteristics corresponding to the lymphocyte cluster and $CD45^{dim}$ or $CD45^-$ expression. The results were expressed as absolute numbers of $CD34^+CD45^+$ HPCs and $CD34^+CD45^-$ EPCs per millilitre of blood. The gating strategy is illustrated in Additional file 2: Figure S1.

Because $CD34^+CD45^+CD133^+$ PCs and $CD34^+CD45^+KDR^+$ PCs, identified as CACs, are present in low levels in peripheral blood, these progenitor subsets were quantified using a four-color flow cytometry strategy after direct immunolabelling of isolated peripheral blood mononuclear cells (PBMCs). PBMCs were isolated from 7 ml of heparinised peripheral blood by density gradient centrifugation with lymphocyte separation medium (PAA Laboratories, Pasching, Austria), and they were labelled with 10 µl of 7-AAD viability dye, 10 µl of FITC-CD34 antibody (Beckman Coulter), 10 µl of ECD-CD45 antibody (Beckman Coulter) and 10 µl of PE-CD133 antibody (Miltenyi Biotec, Bergisch Gladbach, Germany) or PE-KDR antibody (R&D Systems, Abingdon, UK). A 10-µl quantity of concentration-matched, PE-conjugated murine IgG1 antibody was used as a fluorescence minus one control. After incubation for 20 minutes at room temperature, cells were washed and re-suspended in 500 µl of PBS, and then analysed using a NAVIOS flow cytometer.

After selection of 7-AAD-negative cells, $CD133^+$ and KDR^+ cells were identified within $CD34^+CD45^+$ cells displaying FSC/SSC characteristics corresponding to the lymphocyte cluster. At least 5×10^5 viable cells were acquired per run. The percentage of $CD133^+$ or KDR^+ cells among $CD34^+CD45^+$ cells was determined. Results were expressed as absolute values per millilitre of blood of $CD34^+CD45^+CD133^+$ PCs, and $CD34^+CD45^+KDR^+$ PC values were obtained by multiplying the percentage of each cellular subpopulation by the absolute values of $CD34^+CD45^+$ HPCs determined as described above. The literature-based identification criteria and characteristics of the endothelial cell populations of the endothelial cell population investigated in the present study are summarised in the Additional file 1: Table S3.

Analysis of circulating vascular endothelial growth factor, endothelin-1 and soluble fractalkine levels

Circulating levels of vascular endothelial growth factor (VEGF), endothelin-1 and s-Fractalkine (CX3CL1) were measured in serum using commercially available ELISA kits obtained from R&D Systems Inc. (Minneapolis, MN, USA). Assays were performed according to the manufacturer's instructions.

Statistical analysis

Quantitative variables were described using mean (±SD) or median and IQR [first quartile–third quartile] according to their distribution. The normality of the distribution was assessed graphically. Qualitative variables were described using counts and percentages. The correlations between quantitative variables were performed using Spearman's correlation. Student's t test and the Mann-Whitney U test were performed to compare using quantitative variables of the two groups. The chi-square test or Fisher's exact test was used to compare qualitative variables. P values <0.05 were considered significant.

A multivariate model based on logistic regression with a robust estimator (generalised estimating equation with M-estimator) was used to assess independent factors associated with SSc. A stepwise backward elimination procedure was performed to conserve variables with an adjusted P value <0.05. Variables first introduced into the univariate model were those with a P value <0.20.

To analyse the association of the variables with clinical characteristics (cutaneous subtype, disease duration groups of severity of patients with SSc defined by Medsger severity scale), we first used quantitative values of these biomarkers. We next aimed to deepen the analysis in an exploratory prospect evaluation by segregating groups. We used decision trees with the chi-square automatic interaction detection (CHAID) method to assess whether cut-off values of these biomarker levels could enable us to discriminate these two groups of severity states in a dichotomous manner. Analyses were performed using Prism 5.0 (GraphPad Software, La Jolla, CA, USA) and IBM SPSS Statistics version 20.0 (IBM, Armonk, NY, USA) software.

Results

Characteristics of the study population

The characteristics of the study population, including cardiovascular risk factors and vascular phenotypes, are summarised in Table 1. SSc-related features are shown in Table 2, and the ongoing treatments are reported in Additional file 1: Table S1. The patient sample comprised 44 women and 1 man with a median age of 60.38 years [IQR 51.45–72.38 years] and median disease duration of 15 years. The control group of healthy volunteers consisted of 38 women and 3 men with a median age of 55.97 years [IQR 53.56–59.64 years]. Sixteen patients (35.6%) had diffuse cutaneous SSc, and 29 patients (64.4%) had limited cutaneous SSc. The demographic characteristics of patients with SSc were comparable to those of the healthy control subjects, except for higher mean age, lower body mass index (BMI) and lower arterial blood pressure observed in the patients with SSc (Table 1). The prevalence of cardiovascular risk factors, including diabetes, tobacco consumption, familial history of coronary disease, hypercholesterolemia, arterial hypertension, sedentary lifestyle, menarche, hormone treatment and atheroma deposits on carotid artery assessed by Doppler ultrasonography did not significantly differ between the two groups (data not shown). The right carotid-radial PWV did not significantly differ between the two groups, accounting for a similar arterial stiffness. However, patients with SSc had a significantly lower endothelium-dependent FMD of the brachial artery (Table 1).

Significant differences were observed between patients with SSc and control subjects regarding biological parameters such as white blood cell count, haemoglobin level and creatinine clearance. All of the values remained within the normal range. CRP level was slightly higher in the patient group than in healthy control subjects (Additional file 1: Table S2).

Circulating cellular biomarkers of endothelial activation and injury in patients with SSc

Because EMPs and CECs reflect endothelial cell activation and injury, we aimed to investigate these markers in patients with SSc using standardised methods. The patients with SSc had significantly higher plasma levels of EMPs (93.5/μl, IQR 64.75–130.5) than control subjects (33/μl, IQR 21–46.5; $P < 0.0001$) (Fig. 1). Comparable levels of CECs were found in patients with SSc (2/ml of blood, IQR 1–8.5) and healthy control subjects (2.5/ml of blood, IQR 0–16.5).

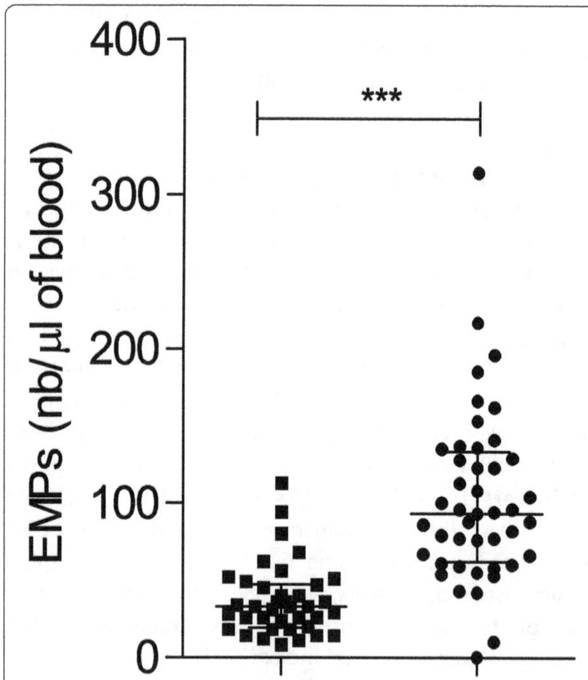

Fig. 1 Quantification of endothelial microparticles (EMPs) in the peripheral blood of healthy control subjects (HCs) and patients with systemic sclerosis (SSc). EMP numbers (nb) were defined as annexin V^+/$CD31^+CD41^-$ events and quantified by high-sensitivity flow cytometry using counting beads. *** $P < 0.0005$

Colony forming unit-endothelial cell generation in patients with SSc

The assessment of CFU-ECs established by culture of MNCs from patients with SSc and healthy control subjects revealed higher numbers of colonies in patients with SSc (11 per 10^6 MNCs, IQR 3–20.25) than in healthy control subjects (3 per 10^6 MNCs, IQR 0.85–8; $P = 0.0032$) (Additional file 2: Figure S2).

Flow cytometric analysis of circulating $CD34^+$ progenitor cell subsets in patients with SSc

To cover most of the literature-reported phenotypes of EPCs and CACs, we enumerated various circulating $CD34^+$ cell populations, including total $CD34^+$ PCs, $CD34^+CD45^-$ EPCs and HPCs, $CD34^+CD45^+$ HPCs, immature $CD34^+CD45^+CD133^+$ PCs and $CD34^+CD45^+KDR^+$ PCs. We observed that patients with SSc had significantly higher numbers of total circulating $CD34^+$ PCs (2074.5/ml, IQR 1459.5–2578) than control subjects (1555/ml, IQR 1225–1960; $P = 0.0442$). The number of circulating HPCs did not differ significantly between patients with SSc and control subjects (1662/ml, IQR 1297.7–2134.2, versus 1485/ml, IQR 1117.5–1912.5; $P = 0.4247$) (Fig. 2a). Moreover, KDR^+ PCs (37/ml, IQR 5.5–100.5, versus 57.01/ml, IQR 27.5–96; $P = 0.243$) and $CD133^+$ PCs (1185/ml, IQR 827–1456, versus

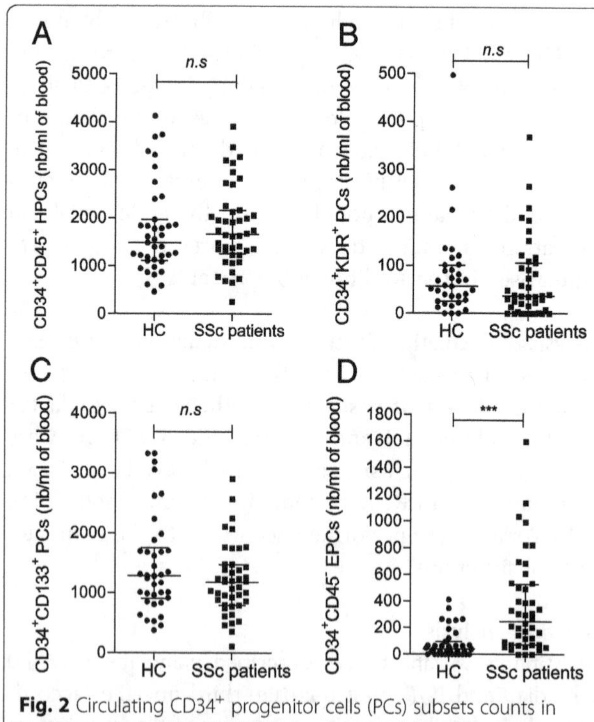

Fig. 2 Circulating $CD34^+$ progenitor cells (PCs) subsets counts in healthy control subjects (HC) and patients with systemic sclerosis (SSc). Number (nb) of (**a**) $CD34^+CD45^+$ haematopoietic progenitor cells (HPCs), (**b**) $CD34^+KDR^+$ PCs, (**c**) $CD34^+CD133^+$ PCs and (**d**) non-haematopoietic $CD34^+CD45^-$ endothelial PCs were determined by flow cytometric analysis. *** $P < 0.0005$. *n.s* Non-significant

1287/ml, IQR 929.71–1705.13; $P = 0.2463$) did not differ between the two groups (Fig. 2b and c). The number of circulating $CD34^{+}CD45^{-}$ EPCs was significantly higher in patients with SSc (247/ml, IQR 74.2–508.2, versus 40/ml, IQR 0–82.5; $P < 0.0001$) (Fig. 2d). No correlation was found between EMPs (marker of endothelial activation) and PC subsets (CFU-ECs, $CD34^{+}$ PCs and $CD34^{+}CD45^{-}$ EPCs) in patients with SSc.

Elevation of soluble endothelial biomarkers in patients with SSc

First, we investigated the circulating levels of the endothelial biomarkers VEGF, s-Fractalkine and endothelin-1 in patients with SSc and healthy control subjects. Median serum concentrations of these biomarkers were significantly elevated in patients with SSc compared with control subjects: VEGF (57 pg/ml, IQR 39–118, versus 42 pg/ml, IQR 26–78.7; $P = 0.0357$) (Fig. 3a), endothelin-1 (1.68 pg/ml, IQR 1.3–2.0, versus 1.2 pg/ml, IQR 1.0–1.3; $P < 0.0001$) (Fig. 3b) and s-Fractalkine (465.45 pg/ml, IQR 366.4–598.5, versus 186 pg/ml, IQR 140.5–268.0 pg/ml; $P < 0.0001$) (Fig. 3c). Next, we assessed whether these soluble biomarkers correlated with the aforementioned cellular biomarkers in patients with SSc. We observed a significant positive correlation between s-Fractalkine levels and $CD34^{+}CD45^{-}$ EPC numbers ($r_s = 0.35$, $P = 0.0166$) (Fig. 3d). No other correlation was noted in patients with SSc.

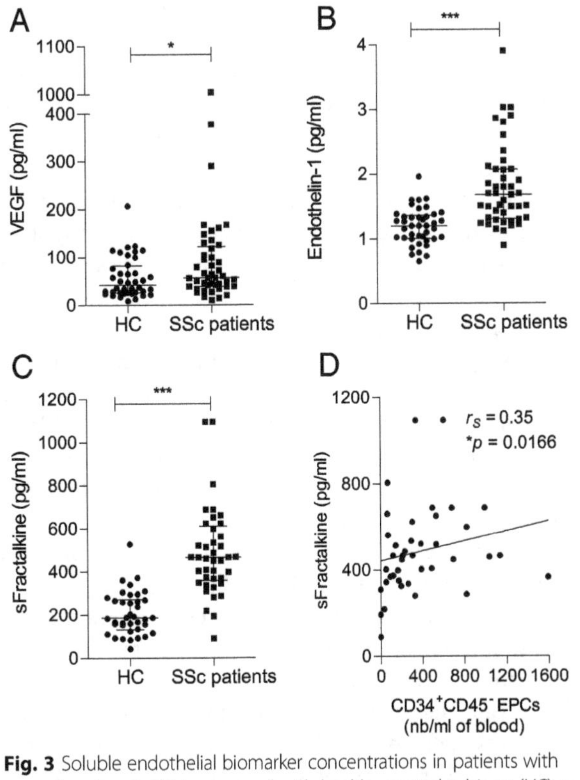

Fig. 3 Soluble endothelial biomarker concentrations in patients with systemic sclerosis (SSc) compared with healthy control subjects (HC). **a** Vascular endothelial growth factor (VEGF). **b** Endothelin-1. **c** Soluble fractalkine (s-Fractalkine). **d** Correlation between s-Fractalkine and $CD34^{+}CD45^{-}$ endothelial progenitor cell (EPC) counts (nb). Correlation was established using the non-parametric Spearman's correlation coefficient (r_s). * $P < 0.05$; *** $P < 0.0005$. *n.s* = non-significant

Association of endothelial biomarkers with SSc

The univariate analyses showed that the variables age, BMI, creatinine clearance and CRP, as well as the endothelial biomarkers EMPs, CFU-ECs, $CD34^{+}$ PCs, CD34 $^{+}CD45^{-}$ EPCs, VEGF, endothelin-1 and s-Fractalkine, were different between healthy control subjects and patients with SSc ($P < 0.05$) (Table 3).

In the multivariate model including all of these variables, EMPs, endothelin-1 and s-Fractalkine were independent markers associated with SSc (Table 4).

Because s-Fractalkine level and $CD34^{+}CD45^{-}$ EPC count were correlated, a multivariate model with the same variables except for s-Fractalkine was tested. In this model, EMPs ($P = 0.007$), endothelin-1 ($P = 0.001$) and $CD34^{+}CD45^{-}$ EPCs ($P = 0.025$) were independently associated with SSc (Additional file 1: Table S4).

Association of endothelial biomarkers with disease clinical characteristics and severity

We investigated whether each of the independent biomarkers associated with SSc (i.e., EMPs, $CD34^{+}CD45^{-}$ EPCs, endothelin-1 and s-Fractalkine) could be associated with the clinical characteristics of patients with SSc. The first level of analysis of the quantitative values of these biomarkers did not allow for identifying markers that discriminated the cutaneous subtype, disease duration, clinical characteristic and group of severity defined by the Medsger severity scale ($P > 0.05$ for all).

The CHAID algorithm allowed us to propose cut-off values for s-Fractalkine (486 pg/ml), $CD34^{+}CD45^{-}$ EPC level (395/ml) and endothelin-1 (1.26 ng/ml). According to this approach, values of EMPs could not be discriminated in a dichotomous manner.

The frequency of patients with more severe disease was higher in the group with s-Fractalkine concentrations above the cut-off value ($P = 0.041$). Patients belonging to this group also had decreased DLCO/VA and a higher frequency of pulmonary fibrosis (Table 5). Patients with lower FVC had $CD34^{+}CD45^{-}$ EPC numbers above the cut-off value ($P = 0.0282$). No significant difference was noted between patients with endothelin-1 levels less than or greater than the cut-off value.

Discussion

The non-invasive monitoring of endothelial alterations is a challenge for physicians to better assess the severity of the disease and to sustain the development of therapeutic approaches [45, 46]. Based on an integrative analysis of

Table 3 Circulating endothelial biomarkers studied in univariate analysis

	Patients with SSc	Control subjects	*P* value
Endothelial cellular markers			
EMPs, *n*/μl	93.5 [64.75–130.5]	33 [21– 46.5]	<0.0001***
CECs, *n*/ml	2 [1–8.5]	2.5 [0–16,5]	0.7677
PC subsets			
CFU-ECs, *n*/10^6 MNCs	11 [3–20.25]	3 [0.85–8]	0.0032**
$CD34^+$ PCs, *n*/ml	2074.5 [1459.5–2578]	1555 [1225–1960]	0.0442*
$CD34^+CD45^+$ PCs, *n*/ml	1662 [1297.7–2134.2]	1485 [1117.5–1912.5]	0.4247
KDR^+ PCs, *n*/ml	37 [5.5–100.5]	57.01 [27.5–96]	0.243
$CD133^+$ PCs, *n*/ml	1185 [827–1456]	1287 [929.71–1705.13]	0.2463
$CD34^+CD45^-$ EPCs, *n*/ml	247 [74.2–508.2]	40 [0–82.5]	<0.0001***
Soluble endothelial markers			
VEGF, pg/ml	57 [39–118]	42 [26–78.7]	0.0357*
Endothelin-1, pg/ml	1.68 [1.3–2.0]	1.2 [1.0–1.3]	<0.0001***
s-Fractalkine, pg/ml	465.45 [366.4–598.5]	186 [140.5–268.0]	<0.0001***

Abbreviations: EMP Endothelial microparticle, *CEC* Circulating endothelial cell, *CFU-EC* Colony-forming unit-endothelial cell, *EPC* Endothelial progenitor cell, *KDR* Kinas insert domain receptor, *PC* Progenitor cell, *VEGF* Vascular endothelial growth factor, *s-Fractalkine* Soluble fractalkine, *MNC* Mononuclear cell, *SSc* Systemic sclerosis * $P < 0.05$; 0.001 < **$P < 0.01$; *** $P < 0.0005$

endothelial biomarkers of damage and repair, this study identifies the mobilisation of $CD34^+CD45^-$ EPCs and high levels of s-Fractalkine as specific features of SSc-associated vascular activation and disease severity.

We confirmed the impaired endothelial function assessed by FMD in patients with SSc [2]. Consistent with a disrupted endothelial homeostasis [9], we confirmed that EMP release is increased in patients with SSc. The EMPs can promote or aggravate pre-existing vascular dysfunction in cardiovascular diseases [4] and have been shown to be deleterious via the induction of an oxidative burst in a murine model of SSc [47]. In the present study, EMP levels were not associated with disease severity. Researchers in other studies reported decreased levels of EMPs in SSc [48] or their association with lung and skin involvement, but they did not consider annexin V binding as a criterion to define EMPs [49]. Our observations indicate that the release of annexin V^+ EMPs primarily reflects the activated endothelial status. Such activation might not result in a significant insult of the endothelial monolayer, given that the release of EMPs was not associated with CEC elevation assessed by anti-CD146-based immunomagnetic separation. Indeed, this standardised assay has been shown to quantify mature endothelial cells that are detached from the endothelial monolayer as a consequence of pathological processes that disrupt its integrity [6]. Such a restricted definition criterion of CECs might explain discrepancies observed in other studies in which researchers used flow cytometric approaches to quantify CECs in patients with SSc [14].

Table 4 Multivariate logistic regression analysis for systemic sclerosis with robust estimator

Variables	OR (95% CI)	*P* value
EMPs	1.002 (1.000-1.004)	0.015
Endothelin-1	1.044 (1.009-1.082)	0.012
s-Fractalkine	92.388 (2.729-3127.533)	0.035

EMP Endothelial microparticle, *s-Fractalkine* Soluble fractalkine
Variables introduced into this multivariate model were selected after univariate analysis ($P < 0.2$). The final model was established after stepwise backward elimination of non-significant variables (i.e., age, body mass index, creatinine, C-reactive protein, colony-forming unit-endothelial cells, $CD34^+$ progenitor cells, $CD34^+CD45^-$ endothelial progenitor cells and vascular endothelial growth factor). Independent variables associated with systemic sclerosis with an adjusted $P < 0.05$ were conserved

We also present the first evidence that enhanced levels of circulating $CD34^+CD45^-$ EPCs occur in patients with SSc, whereas these cells were barely detectable in healthy control subjects. The association between $CD34^+CD45^-$ EPC levels and decreased FVC may suggest that these cells are mobilised as a response to lung involvement-induced hypoxia. In accordance with this hypothesis, patients with SSc exhibited high levels of VEGF, the main pro-angiogenic factor promoting the mobilisation of PCs from the bone marrow [11]. Interestingly, $CD34^+CD45^-$ EPC counts were increased, whereas all the haematopoietic lineage-related $CD34^+$ PC subsets defined by $CD45^{dim}$ expression and CD133 or KDR markers remained unchanged in the analysed cohort. These data may indicate defective mobilisation of the bone marrow-derived pool of these CACs, as reported by Kuwana et al. [13]. In line with this hypothesis, quantitative and qualitative alterations of this bone marrow pool of HPCs have been described in SSc [17]. Of note, our

Table 5 Clinical and laboratory data of patients with systemic sclerosis, depending on soluble fractalkine concentrations

	s-Fractalkine >486 pg/ml (*n* = 16)	s-Fractalkine <486 pg/ml (*n* = 25)	*P* value
Clinical features			
Age, years, median [IQR]	55.06 [50.94–72.84]	62.52 [52.8–71.33]	0.56
Duration, years, median [IQR]	5.5 [3–12.75]	8 [3–12.5]	0.8933
Pitting scars or skin ulcers, *n*	11/16	14/25	0.41
Pulmonary fibrosis, *n*	3/16	3/22	<0.0001***
FVC, %, median [IQR]	98.5[85.75–113.3]	95.9 [82–111.3]	0.558
DLCO/VA, %, median [IQR]	62 [53–76]	75 [63.5–81.45]	0.0445*
Oesophagus, *n*	13/16	13/25	0.0579
Telangiectasia, *n*	9/16	20/25	0.1030
mRSS, median [IQR]	11.5 [5.25–23]	10 [5–16]	0.6166
Pulmonary arterial pressure, mmHg, median [IQR]	27 [21.25–34]	25 [20–31]	0.32
Severity grades 0, 1 and 2, *n*	4/16	15/25	0.0284*
Severity grades 3 and 4, *n*	12/16	10/25	0.0284*
Laboratory findings			
Anti-topoisomerase I antibody, *n*	6/16	13/25	0.3638
Anti-centromere antibody, *n*	7/16	12/25	0.79

Abbreviations: DLCO Diffusing capacity of the lung for carbon monoxide, *CEC* Circulating endothelial cell, *FVC* Forced vital capacity, *mRSS* Modified Rodnan skin score, *VA* Alveolar volume, *s-Fractalkine* Soluble fractalkine
Qualitative variables are described using frequencies. Quantitative variables are described using median and IQR [first quartile–third quartile] * $P < 0.05$; *** $P < 0.0005$

flow cytometric analysis did not include the circulating cells co-expressing CD133, CD34 and KDR. Although this phenotype was initially proposed to identify the immature part of EPC populations, we failed to detect these cells in both healthy control subjects and patients with SSc (data not shown), as recently published [50].

The functional ability of the cells derived from mobilised $CD34^+CD45^-$ EPCs could not be analysed in the present study, because the clonogenic and angiogenic assays require large blood samples that are hardly obtainable from patients with SSc. Nevertheless, Avouac et al. observed that the number of late-outgrowth ECFCs derived in culture was not increased in patients with SSc in comparison with control subjects [16]. Along with our results, we can assume that the mobilisation of $CD34^+CD45^-$ EPCs may represent a quantitative response to activation that is not translated in the acquisition of progenitor-associated vascular regenerative potential.

In this study, the mobilisation of $CD34^+CD45^-$ EPCs occurred in a context of vascular inflammation, as revealed by the moderate elevation of CRP and CFU-ECs and the increase in endothelial activation biomarkers such as EMPs, endothelin-1 and s-Fractalkine. Furthermore, we established a positive correlation between the $CD34^+CD45^-$ EPC levels and the circulating levels of s-Fractalkine in patients with SSc. Animal models suggest that the fractalkine/CX3CR1 pathway is involved in the recruitment of EPCs to the ischaemic sites during stroke [51] and regulates progenitor-dependent endothelial repair during atherosclerosis [52]. Moreover, we have previously shown that membrane-bound fractalkine can play a role in controlling EPC homeostasis in the alloreactive environment of renal transplant [53]. The first evidence provided here of the interplay between s-Fractalkine and EPCs in the context of SSc may deserve further mechanistic investigation. In the present study, the SSc group exhibited reduced FMD values but similar arterial stiffness in comparison with the control group, suggesting that the alterations of the biological markers observed here were due to the SSc-related endothelial dysfunction rather than to atherosclerosis.

The limits of our exploratory study are inherent to a one-point biological assessment performed in a low number of patients with heterogeneous clinical phenotypes. Furthermore, the impact of long-standing therapies could not be appreciated. This could also account in part for the lack of association between endothelin-1 levels and disease severity, notably in patients treated with endothelin-1 receptor antagonists. s-Fractalkine was the only soluble marker found to be associated with disease severity in SSc in this study [30]. Such an observation is consistent with the involvement of the fractalkine/CX3CR1 pathway in the mechanisms linking the endothelial inflammation to the onset of fibrosis.

Conclusions

Our data identify a specific signature of inflammatory endothelial activation that encompasses high levels of EMPs, CFU-ECs, endothelin-1, VEGF and s-Fractalkine and links the levels of s-Fractalkine with the mobilisation of CD34$^+$CD45$^-$ EPCs. s-Fractalkine and CD34$^+$CD45$^-$ EPCs seem to be associated with lung involvement. Further studies are needed to determine the exact prognostic value of the combined assessment of s-Fractalkine and CD34$^+$CD45$^-$ EPCs in patients with SSc.

Additional files

Additional file 1: Table S1. Ongoing treatments in patients with SSc. **Table S2.** Biological characteristics of the study population. **Table S3.** Summary of the main immunophenotypic and functional characteristics of the investigated circulating progenitor cell subsets. **Table S4.** Multivariate logistic regression analysis for SSc with robust estimator. (DOCX 16 kb)

Additional file 2: Figure S1. Gating strategy of endothelial progenitor cells (EPCs) by flow cytometry. CD34$^+$CD45$^+$ haematopoietic progenitor cells (HPCs) and CD34$^+$CD45$^-$ EPCs were identified within 7-AAD-negative viable (**a**), CD34$^+$ cells (**b**), with CD45^{dim} or CD45$^-$ expression (**c**), and displaying forward scatter (FS)/side scatter (SS) characteristics corresponding to the lymphocyte cluster (**d**, **e**). Non-specific binding of CD34-PE antibody is checked on CD34$^+$CD45$^+$ (**f**) and CD34$^+$CD45$^-$ gate of each sample (**g**) by means of a control tube in which CD34-PE antibody is replaced by its isoclonic control. *LYMPH* Lymphocytes. **Figure S2.** CFU-EC count in the peripheral venous blood of healthy control subjects (HC) and patients with systemic sclerosis (SSc). Number (n) of CFU-ECs was determined after cell culture of MNCs. ** $P < 0.005$. (PDF 311 kb)

Abbreviations

7-AAD: 7-Aminoactinomycin D; APHM: Assistance Publique-Hôpitaux de Marseille; BMI: Body mass index; CAC: Circulating angiogenic cell; CEC: Circulating endothelial cell; CFU-EC: Colony-forming unit-endothelial cell; CHAID: Chi-square automatic interaction detection; CRP: C-reactive protein; CX3CL1: Chemokine (C-X3-C motif) ligand 1; CX3CR1: Chemokine (C-X3-C motif) receptor 1; DLCO: Diffusing capacity of the lung for carbon monoxide; ECFC: Endothelial colony-forming cell; EDTA: Ethylenediaminetetraacetic acid; ELISA: Enzyme-linked immunosorbent assay; EMP: Endothelial microparticle; EPC: Endothelial progenitor cell; FITC: Fluorescein isothiocyanate; FMD: Flow-mediated dilation; FSC: Forward scatter; FVC: Forced vital capacity; HC: Healthy control subject; HDL: High-density lipoprotein; HPC: Haematopoietic progenitor cell; IgG1: Immunoglobulin G1; KDR: Kinase insert domain receptor; LDL: Low-density lipoprotein; MNC: Mononuclear cell; mRSS: Modified Rodnan skin score; PBMC: Peripheral blood mononuclear cell; PC: Progenitor cell; PE: Phycoerythrin; PFP: Platelet-free plasma; PWV: Pulse wave velocity; s-Fractalkine: Soluble fractalkine; SSC: Side scatter; SSc: Systemic sclerosis; VA: alveolar volume; VEGF: Vascular endothelial growth factor

Acknowledgements

We thank Patricia Berenger and Evelyne Doria for technical support. We also thank the patients who were included in the study.

Funding

This study was supported by Assistance Publique-Hôpitaux de Marseille Appel d'Offre de Recherche Clinique (AORC) junior number 2011-A00095-35.

Authors' contributions

FS, BG, PR, NB and FDG designed the study. AB, JM, FS, PP and BG contributed to the analysis of the data and the editing of the manuscript. LA, SC and RL performed experiments and analysed data. DB and EJ performed statistical analysis. FC filled the case report forms of the systemic sclerosis patients and the healthy volunteers. NL, YF, PR, JRH, GK, PJW, FBG and PB included subjects and participated in the critical review of the manuscript. AB and JM equally contributed to this work. All authors read and approved the final manuscript.

Competing interests

The authors declare that they have no competing interests.

Author details

[1]Internal Medicine Department, Assistance Publique-Hôpitaux de Marseille (APHM), CHU Nord, 13015 Marseilles, France. [2]Haematology and Vascular Biology Laboratory, APHM, CHU Conception, 13005 Marseilles, France. [3]Vascular Research Centre of Marseille (VRCM) UMR-S1076, INSERM, Aix-Marseille Université, 13385 Marseilles, Cedex, France. [4]Culture and Cell Therapy Laboratory, CICBT 1409, APHM, CHU Conception, 13005 Marseilles, France. [5]Immunology Laboratory, APHM, CHU Conception, 13005 Marseilles, France. [6]Internal Medicine Department, APHM, CHU Conception, 13005 Marseilles, France. [7]Internal Medicine Department, APHM, CHU Timone, 13005 Marseilles, France. [8]Dermatology Department, APHM, CHU Nord, 13015 Marseilles, France. [9]Centre d'Investigation Clinique Centre de Pharmacologie Clinique et d'Evaluations Thérapeutiques, APHM, CHU Timone, CHU Nord, Marseille, France.

References

1. Sgonc R, Gruschwitz MS, Dietrich H, Recheis H, Gershwin ME, Wick G. Endothelial cell apoptosis is a primary pathogenetic event underlying skin lesions in avian and human scleroderma. J Clin Invest. 1996;98:785–92.
2. Rossi P, Granel B, Marziale D, Le Mée F, Francès Y. Endothelial function and hemodynamics in systemic sclerosis. Clin Physiol Funct Imaging. 2010;30:453–9.
3. Blann AD, Woywodt A, Bertolini F, Bull TM, Buyon JP, Clancy RM, et al. Circulating endothelial cells: biomarker of vascular disease. Thromb Haemost. 2005;93:228–35.
4. Chironi GN, Boulanger CM, Simon A, Dignat-George F, Freyssinet JM, Tedgui A. Endothelial microparticles in diseases. Cell Tissue Res. 2009;335:143–51.
5. Quilici J, Banzet N, Paule P, Meynard JB, Mutin M, Bonnet JL, et al. Circulating endothelial cell count as a diagnostic marker for non-ST-elevation acute coronary syndromes. Circulation. 2004;110:1586–91.
6. Mutin M, Canavy I, Blann A, Bory M, Sampol J, Dignat-George F. Direct evidence of endothelial injury in acute myocardial infarction and unstable angina by demonstration of circulating endothelial cells. Blood. 1999;93:2951–8.
7. Widemann A, Pasero C, Arnaud L, Poullin P, Loundou AD, Choukroun G, et al. Circulating endothelial cells and progenitors as prognostic factors during autoimmune thrombotic thrombocytopenic purpura: results of a prospective multicenter French study. J Thromb Haemost. 2014;12:1601–9.
8. Parker B, Al-Husain A, Pemberton P, Yates AP, Ho P, Gorodkin R, et al. Suppression of inflammation reduces endothelial microparticles in active systemic lupus erythematosus. Ann Rheum Dis. 2014;73:1144–50.
9. Guiducci S, Distler JHW, Jüngel A, Huscher D, Huber LC, Michel BA, et al. The relationship between plasma microparticles and disease manifestations in patients with systemic sclerosis. Arthritis Rheum. 2008;58:2845–53.
10. Asahara T, Murohara T, Sullivan A, Silver M, van der Zee R, Li T, et al. Isolation of putative progenitor endothelial cells for angiogenesis. Science. 1997;275:964–7.
11. Zaccone V, Flore R, Santoro L, De Matteis G, Giupponi B, Li Puma DD, et al. Focus on biological identity of endothelial progenitors cells. Eur Rev Med Pharmacol Sci. 2015;19:4047–63.
12. Attar A, Aghasadeghi K, Parsanezhad ME, Namavar Jahromi B, Habibagahi M. Absence of correlation between changes in the number of endothelial progenitor cell subsets. Korean Circ J. 2015;45:325–32.
13. Kuwana M, Okazaki Y, Yasuoka H, Kawakami Y, Ikeda Y. Defective vasculogenesis in systemic sclerosis. Lancet. 2004;364:603–10.
14. Del Papa N, Colombo G, Fracchiolla N, Moronetti LM, Ingegnoli F, Maglione W, et al. Circulating endothelial cells as a marker of ongoing vascular disease in systemic sclerosis. Arthritis Rheum. 2004;50:1296–304.
15. Allanore Y, Batteux F, Avouac J, Assous N, Weill B, Kahan A. Levels of circulating endothelial progenitor cells in systemic sclerosis. Clin Exp Rheumatol. 2007;25:60–6.
16. Avouac J, Juin F, Wipff J, Couraud PO, Chiocchia G, Kahan A, et al. Circulating endothelial progenitor cells in systemic sclerosis: association with disease severity. Ann Rheum Dis. 2008;67:1455–60.
17. Del Papa N, Quirici N, Soligo D, Scavullo C, Cortiana M, Borsotti C, et al. Bone marrow endothelial progenitors are defective in systemic sclerosis. Arthritis Rheum. 2006;54:2605–15.

18. Mok MY, Yiu KH, Wong CY, Qiuwaxi J, Lai WH, Wong WS, et al. Low circulating level of CD133$^+$KDR$^+$ cells in patients with systemic sclerosis. Clin Exp Rheumatol. 2010;28(5 Suppl 62):S19–25.
19. Nevskaya T, Bykovskaia S, Lyssuk E, Shakhov I, Zaprjagaeva M, Mach E, et al. Circulating endothelial progenitor cells in systemic sclerosis: relation to impaired angiogenesis and cardiovascular manifestations. Clin Exp Rheumatol. 2008;26:421–9.
20. Zhu S, Evans S, Yan B, Povsic TJ, Tapson V, Goldschmidt-Clermont PJ, et al. Transcriptional regulation of Bim by FOXO3a and Akt mediates scleroderma serum-induced apoptosis in endothelial progenitor cells. Circulation. 2008;118:2156–65.
21. Avouac J, Meune C, Ruiz B, Couraud PO, Uzan G, Boileau C, et al. Angiogenic biomarkers predict the occurrence of digital ulcers in systemic sclerosis. Ann Rheum Dis. 2012;71:394–9.
22. Distler JHW, Allanore Y, Avouac J, Giacomelli R, Guiducci S, Moritz F, et al. EULAR Scleroderma Trials and Research group statement and recommendations on endothelial precursor cells. Ann Rheum Dis. 2009; 68:163–8.
23. Brunasso AMG, Massone C. Update on the pathogenesis of scleroderma: focus on circulating progenitor cells. F1000Res. 2016;5:723. doi:10.12688/f1000research.7986.1.
24. Case J, Mead LE, Bessler WK, Prater D, White HA, Saadatzadeh MR, et al. Human CD34$^+$AC133$^+$VEGFR-2$^+$ cells are not endothelial progenitor cells but distinct, primitive hematopoietic progenitors. Exp Hematol. 2007;35:1109–18.
25. Hill JM, Zalos G, Halcox JPJ, Schenke WH, Waclawiw MA, Quyyumi AA, et al. Circulating endothelial progenitor cells, vascular function, and cardiovascular risk. N Engl J Med. 2003;348:593–600.
26. Padfield GJ, Tura O, Haeck MLA, Short A, Freyer E, Barclay GR, et al. Circulating endothelial progenitor cells are not affected by acute systemic inflammation. Am J Physiol Heart Circ Physiol. 2010;298:H2054–61.
27. Padfield GJ, Tura-Ceide O, Freyer E, Barclay GR, Turner M, Newby DE, et al. Endothelial progenitor cells, atheroma burden and clinical outcome in patients with coronary artery disease. Heart. 2013;99:791–8.
28. Padfield GJ, Tura-Ceide O, Freyer E, Barclay GR, Turner M, Newby DE, et al. Percutaneous coronary intervention causes a rapid but transient mobilisation of CD34$^+$CD45$^-$ cells. Open Heart. 2014;1:e000047.
29. Kahaleh MB. Endothelin, an endothelial-dependent vasoconstrictor in scleroderma. Enhanced production and profibrotic action. Arthritis Rheum. 1991;34:978–83.
30. Hasegawa M, Sato S, Echigo T, Hamaguchi Y, Yasui M, Takehara K. Up regulated expression of fractalkine/CX_3CL1 and CX_3CR1 in patients with systemic sclerosis. Ann Rheum Dis. 2005;64:21–8.
31. Channick RN, Simonneau G, Sitbon O, Robbins IM, Frost A, Tapson VF, et al. Effects of the dual endothelin-receptor antagonist bosentan in patients with pulmonary hypertension: a randomised placebo-controlled study. Lancet. 2001;358:1119–23.
32. Korn JH, Mayes M, Matucci Cerinic M, Rainisio M, Pope J, Hachulla E, et al. Digital ulcers in systemic sclerosis: prevention by treatment with bosentan, an oral endothelin receptor antagonist. Arthritis Rheum. 2004;50:3985–93.
33. Bazan JF, Bacon KB, Hardiman G, Wang W, Soo K, Rossi D, et al. A new class of membrane-bound chemokine with a CX3C motif. Nature. 1997;385:640–4.
34. Umehara H, Bloom ET, Okazaki T, Nagano Y, Yoshie O, Imai T. Fractalkine in vascular biology: from basic research to clinical disease. Arterioscler Thromb Vasc Biol. 2004;24:34–40.
35. Nishimura M, Umehara H, Nakayama T, Yoneda O, Hieshima K, Kakizaki M, et al. Dual functions of fractalkine/CX3C ligand 1 in trafficking of perforin $^+$/granzyme B$^+$ cytotoxic effector lymphocytes that are defined by CX3CR1 expression. J Immunol. 2002;168:6173–80.
36. Marasini B, Cossutta R, Selmi C, Pozzi MR, Gardinali M, Massarotti M, et al. Polymorphism of the fractalkine receptor CX3CR1 and systemic sclerosis-associated pulmonary arterial hypertension. Clin Dev Immunol. 2005;12:275–9.
37. Arai M, Ikawa Y, Chujo S, Hamaguchi Y, Ishida W, Shirasaki F, et al. Chemokine receptors CCR2 and CX3CR1 regulate skin fibrosis in the mouse model of cytokine-induced systemic sclerosis. J Dermatol Sci. 2013;69:250–8.
38. van den Hoogen F, Khanna D, Fransen J, Johnson SR, Baron M, Tyndall A, et al. 2013 classification criteria for systemic sclerosis: an American College of Rheumatology/European League against Rheumatism collaborative initiative. Arthritis Rheum. 2013;65:2737–47.
39. Medsger Jr TA, Silman AJ, Steen VD, Black CM, Akesson A, Bacon PA, et al. A disease severity scale for systemic sclerosis: development and testing. J Rheumatol. 1999;26:2159–67.
40. Lacroix R, Judicone C, Mooberry M, Boucekine M, Key NS, Dignat-George F, ISTH SSC Workshop. Standardization of pre-analytical variables in plasma microparticle determination: results of the International Society on Thrombosis and Haemostasis SSC Collaborative Workshop. J Thromb Haemost. 2013;11:1190–3.
41. Robert S, Lacroix R, Poncelet P, Harhouri K, Bouriche T, Judicone C, et al. High-sensitivity flow cytometry provides access to standardized measurement of small-size microparticles—brief report. Arterioscler Thromb Vasc Biol. 2012;32:1054–8.
42. Woywodt A, Blann AD, Kirsch T, Erdbruegger U, Banzet N, Haubitz M, et al. Isolation and enumeration of circulating endothelial cells by immunomagnetic isolation: proposal of a definition and a consensus protocol. J Thromb Haemost. 2006;4:671–7.
43. Smadja DM, Mauge L, Gaussem P, d'Audigier C, Israel-Biet D, Celermajer DS, et al. Treprostinil increases the number and angiogenic potential of endothelial progenitor cells in children with pulmonary hypertension. Angiogenesis. 2011;14:17–27.
44. Sutherland DR, Anderson L, Keeney M, Nayar R, Chin-Yee I. The ISHAGE guidelines for CD34$^+$ cell determination by flow cytometry. J Hematother. 1996;5:213–26.
45. Granel B, Daumas A, Jouve E, Harlé JR, Nguyen PS, Chabannon C, et al. Safety, tolerability and potential efficacy of injection of autologous adipose-derived stromal vascular fraction in the fingers of patients with systemic sclerosis: an open-label phase I trial. Ann Rheum Dis. 2015;74:2175–82.
46. Guillaume-Jugnot P, Daumas A, Magalon J, Jouve E, Nguyen PS, Truillet R, et al. Autologous adipose-derived stromal vascular fraction in patients with systemic sclerosis: 12-month follow-up. Rheumatology (Oxford). 2016;55:301–6.
47. Kavian N, Marut W, Servettaz A, Nicco C, Chéreau C, Lemaréchal H, et al. Pantethine prevents murine systemic sclerosis through the inhibition of microparticle shedding. Arthritis Rheumatol. 2015;67:1881–90.
48. Jung C, Drummer K, Oelzner P, Figulla HR, Boettcher J, Franz M, et al. The association between endothelial microparticles and inflammation in patients with systemic sclerosis and Raynaud's phenomenon as detected by functional imaging. Clin Hemorheol Microcirc. 2015;61:549–57.
49. Iversen LV, Ullman S, Østergaard O, Nielsen CT, Halberg P, Karlsmark T, et al. Cross-sectional study of soluble selectins, fractions of circulating microparticles and their relationship to lung and skin involvement in systemic sclerosis. BMC Musculoskelet Disord. 2015;16:191.
50. Lanuti P, Rotta G, Almici C, Avvisati G, Budillon A, Doretto P, et al. Endothelial progenitor cells, defined by the simultaneous surface expression of VEGFR2 and CD133, are not detectable in healthy peripheral and cord blood. Cytometry A. 2016;89:259–70.
51. Qin W, Li Z, Luo S, Wu R, Pei Z, Huang R. Exogenous fractalkine enhances proliferation of endothelial cells, promotes migration of endothelial progenitor cells and improves neurological deficits in a rat model of ischemic stroke. Neurosci Lett. 2014;569:80–4.
52. Herlea-Pana O, Yao L, Heuser-Baker J, Wang Q, Wang Q, Georgescu C, et al. Chemokine receptors CXCR2 and CX3CR1 differentially regulate functional responses of bone marrow endothelial progenitors during atherosclerotic plaque regression. Cardiovasc Res. 2015;106:324–37.
53. Todorova D, Sabatier F, Doria E, Lyonnet L, Vacher Coponat H, Robert S, et al. Fractalkine expression induces endothelial progenitor cell lysis by natural killer cells. PLoS One. 2011;6:e26663.

3

High sensitivity and negative predictive value of the DETECT algorithm for an early diagnosis of pulmonary arterial hypertension in systemic sclerosis

Alfredo Guillén-Del Castillo[1*], Eduardo L. Callejas-Moraga[1], Gabriela García[2], José F. Rodríguez-Palomares[2], Antonio Román[3], Cristina Berastegui[3], Manuel López-Meseguer[3], Enric Domingo[2], Vicente Fonollosa-Plá[1] and Carmen Pilar Simeón-Aznar[1]

Abstract

Background: Pulmonary arterial hypertension (PAH) is one of the most relevant causes of death in systemic sclerosis. The aims of this study were to analyse the recently published DETECT algorithm comparing it with European Society of Cardiology/European Respiratory Society (ESC/ERS) 2009 guidelines: as screening of PAH; (2) identifying median pulmonary arterial pressure (mPAP) ≥21 mmHg; and (3) determining any group of pulmonary hypertension (PH).

Methods: Eighty-three patients fulfilling LeRoy's systemic sclerosis diagnostic criteria with at least right heart catheterization were studied retrospectively. Clinical data, serological biomarkers, echocardiographic and hemodynamic features were collected. SPSS 20.0 was used for statistical analysis.

Results: According to right heart catheterization findings, 35 patients with PAH and 28 with no PH met the standards for DETECT algorithm analysis: 27.0% of patients presented with functional class III/IV. Applying DETECT, the sensitivity was 100%, specificity 42.9%, the positive predictive value 68.6% and the negative predictive value 100%, whereas employing the ESC/ERS guidelines these were 91.4%, 85.7%, 88.9% and 89.3%, respectively. There were no missed diagnoses of PAH using DETECT compared with three patients missed (8.5%) using ESC/ERS guidelines. The DETECT algorithm also showed greater sensitivity and negative predictive value to identify patients with mPAP ≥21 mmHg or with any type of PH.

Conclusions: The DETECT algorithm is confirmed as an excellent screening method due to its high sensitivity and negative predictive value, minimizing missed diagnosis of PAH. DETECT would be accurate either for early diagnosis of borderline mPAP or any group of PH.

Keywords: Systemic sclerosis, Pulmonary arterial hypertension, Echocardiography, Screening tools

* Correspondence: alguille@vhebron.net; alguillen@vhebron.net
[1]Department of Systemic Autoimmune Diseases, Hospital Universitari Vall d'Hebron, Universitat Autònoma de Barcelona, Passeig Vall d'Hebron 119-129, PC: 08035 Barcelona, Spain
Full list of author information is available at the end of the article

Background

Systemic sclerosis (SSc) is an autoimmune disease characterized by inflammation and autoimmunity, aberrant tissue reparation with excessive extracellular matrix deposition and altered vascular regeneration and endothelial injury [1, 2]. Pulmonary arterial hypertension (PAH) is one of the most severe complications in patients with SSc, in whom the prevalence is 10% as diagnosed by right heart catheterization (RHC) [3, 4]. PAH has a major negative impact on survival and has become one of the leading causes of SSc-related deaths [5–7]. The outcome of this disease unfortunately is poor, with a 51% survival rate at 5 years of diagnosis even after the introduction of potent vasodilatator agents [8]. Despite SSc being a well-known risk factor for developing PAH, there are still delays in diagnosing PAH and consequently more than 80% of patients present with World Health Organization (WHO) functional class III or IV at this point [8].

A French nationwide prospective multicentre study aimed to compare early PAH diagnosis using Doppler echocardiography prior to referral for RHC compared with routine clinical practice [9]. Later, the authors demonstrated prompt PAH identification in patients with lower functional classes of disease and subsequently a fourfold superior survival ratio [10]. The European Society of Cardiology and the European Respiratory Society (ESC/ERS) guidelines published in 2009 [11] recommended echocardiography in symptomatic patients. RHC was carried out if the tricuspid regurgitant velocity (TRV) was ≥3.4 m/s, TRV between 2.8-3.4 m/s with symptoms or TRV ≤2.8 m/s with symptoms plus additional echocardiographic variables suggestive of PH.

Recently, Coghlan et al. reported the first evidence-based algorithm for the screening of PAH in SSc (DETECT) [12]. The DETECT algorithm is a tool to identify patients with PAH in the asymptomatic stages, through the study of clinical variables, pulmonary function tests, immunological, biological, electrocardiographic and finally echocardiographic parameters. The authors demonstrated higher sensitivity of PAH detection than that achieved using the ESC/ERS 2009 guidelines.

The main aim of this study was to determine the value of the DETECT algorithm in a different population of patients with SSc from that studied in the original work and to compare it with the ESC/ERS 2009 guidelines. Other objectives were to ascertain the ability of DETECT to predict median pulmonary arterial pressure (mPAP) ≥21 mmHg or to predict patients with pulmonary hypertension (PH) versus patients with no PH.

Methods

Patients

Eighty-three patients with SSc who had undergone at least one RHC were studied retrospectively. The RHC was indicated due to suspicion of PAH after undergoing an annual complete pulmonary function test and annual echocardiography as routine monitoring of SSc. The reasons for carrying out the RHC in our population were the presence of right ventricular systolic pressure (RVSP) >36 mmHg plus a forced vital capacity/diffusing capacity for carbon monoxide (FVC/DLCO) ratio >1.6 in 35 patients, 34 patients had RVSP >36 mmHg, 8 patients had a FVC/DLCO ratio >1.6 and 6 patients suffered exclusively from progressive unexplained dyspnoea. All patients fulfilled LeRoy's SSc diagnostic criteria [13], and 80 patients also met the American College of Rheumatology/European League Against Rheumatism (ACR/EULAR) 2013 classification criteria [14]. The duration of disease was more than 3 years from the first non-Raynaud's phenomenon symptom in all cases. For validation of the DETECT algorithm, four patients were excluded as they presented with a FVC lower than the 40% predicted value, and another patient was excluded who did not meet the inclusion criteria due to DLCO ≥60%.

Comparisons of the DETECT algorithm and the ESC/ERS 2009 guidelines

Three different scenarios were conducted for the comparison of the DETECT algorithm with the ESC/ERS 2009 guidelines: First, 35 patients diagnosed with PAH and 28 with no PH after undergoing RHC were selected for the application of the DETECT algorithm (see Fig. 1). Second, these 63 patients were used to explore the capacity of both screening tests to identify mPAP ≥21 mmHg (both borderline mPAP and PAH). Third, with neither inclusion nor exclusion criteria 52 patients diagnosed with PH and 31 with no PH were selected to investigate the detection of any sort of PH.

Data collection

Data from the first available RHC of each patient were revised. PH was defined as mPAP ≥25 mmHg in RHC, and was classified in the following groups: WHO group 1 or PAH was defined if pulmonary artery wedge pressure (PAWP) was ≤15 mmHg and pulmonary vascular resistance (PVR) was >3 Wood units in RHC [15]; WHO group 2 or PH due to left heart disease, if PAWP was >15 mmHg; WHO group 3 or PH due to interstitial lung disease (ILD) if PAWP was ≤15 mmHg and predicted FVC <60% or if the extent of interstitial disease was identified as moderate-severe on high-resolution computed tomography (HRCT) [12]. Borderline mPAP (BoPAP) was considered if mPAP was between 21 and 24 mmHg, with PAWP ≤15 mmHg and if there was no ILD or the FVC was >60% [16].

Based on the extent of skin involvement, patients were divided into those with diffuse cutaneous SSc (dcSSc) if

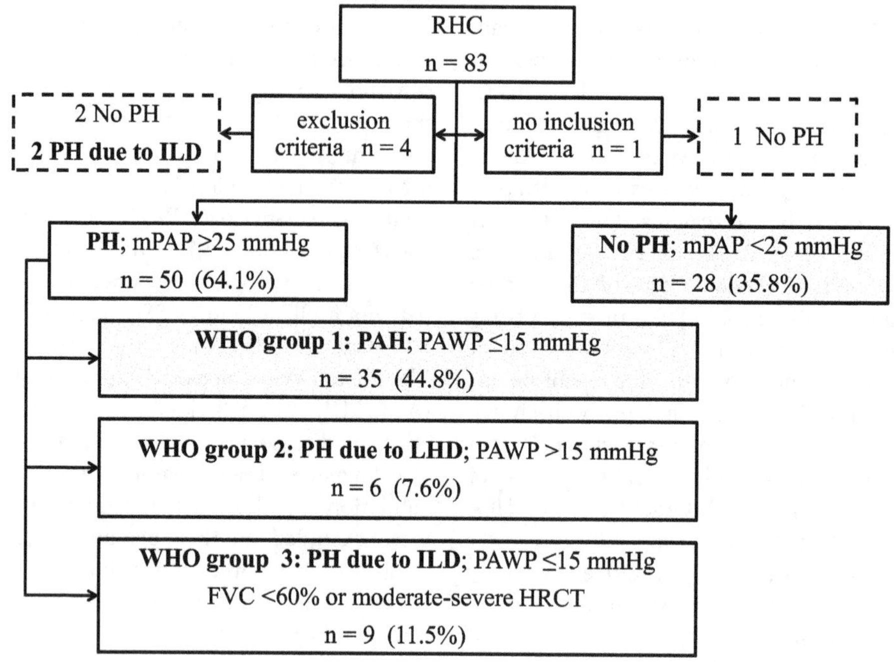

Fig. 1 Flow of patients in the study population. Eighty-three patients with systemic sclerosis had at least one right heart catherization (*RHC*), which was revised retrospectively. Four patients were excluded due to the exclusion criteria (all patients had forced vital capacity (*FVC*) <40%), and another patient was excluded due to not meeting the inclusion criteria, who had a diffusing capacity for carbon monoxide (DLCO) ≥60%. Patients with pulmonary arterial hypertension (*PAH*) and patients without pulmonary hypertension (*no PH*) ($n = 63$) were selected for the following studies: (1) validation of the DETECT algorithm for screening of PAH and (2) identification of patients with median pulmonary arterial pressure (mPAP) ≥21 mmHg and (3) determination of any group of PH (all patients ($n = 83$) were included in this study). *WHO* World Health Organization, *PAWP* pulmonary artery wedge pressure, *LHD* left heart disease, *ILD* interstitial lung disease, *HRCT* high-resolution computed tomography

thickening of the skin was distal and proximal to the elbows or knees, limited cutaneous SSc (lcSSc) if the affected skin did not exceed this limit proximally and sine scleroderma systemic sclerosis (ssSSc) if no skin thickening was present [17]. The disease onset was described as the date of the first symptom attributable to SSc, including Raynaud's phenomenon (RP), although the time from the first symptom excluding RP also was analysed. All data were collected at the time of RHC.

The presence of telangiectasias, past or current digital ulcers (DU) and past history of scleroderma renal crisis (SRC) was recorded. ILD was defined as radiological evidence of interstitial disease on HRCT. Cardiac involvement was defined as current or past history of pericardial effusion, left ventricular ejection fraction (LVEF) <50% and ischaemic heart disease with no cardiovascular risk factor or conduction abnormalities.

Antinuclear antibodies (ANA) were evaluated by indirect immunofluorescence (IIF) assay using HEp-cell line 2. Anticentromere antibodies (ACA) were described by IIF or commercial line blot assay to centromere proteins A and B (EUROLINE Systemic Sclerosis (Nucleoli) Profile (IgG), Euroimmun, Germany). Anti-topoisomerase I antibodies were determined by enzyme-linked immunosorbent assay.

Demographics, cardiovascular risk factors, anthropometrical data, complete pulmonary function test (PFT), 6-minute walking distance (6MWD), WHO-functional class, laboratory data including serum urate, N-terminal pro-brain natriuretic peptide (NT-proBNP) and right axis deviation in electrocardiography (ECG) were registered. Echocardiography included the determination of left ventricular ejection fraction (LVEF), right atrium (RA) area, tricuspid annular plane systolic excursion (TAPSE), tricuspid regurgitation velocity (TRV) and RVSP.

RHC details consisted of mPAP, PAWP, right atrial pressure (RAP), transpulmonary pressure gradient (TPG), cardiac output (CO), pulmonary vascular resistance (PVR), systemic vascular resistance (SVR), mixed venous oxygen saturation (SvO2) measured in pulmonary artery and arterial oxygen saturation (SaO2) measured in arterial blood gas analysis.

The application of the DETECT algorithm was conducted in two steps through the website PAH risk calculator (http://detect-pah.com) [18], the first step for referring the patient for echocardiography and the second for carrying out RHC [12]. The indication of RHC following ESC/ERS 2009 guidelines was considered if: (1) TRV was >3.4 m/s; or (2) TRV was >2.8 to ≤3.4 m/s, with symptoms (undue dyspnoea or fatigue, chest pain, near syncope or signs of right heart failure); or (3) TRV was ≤2.8 m/s, with symptoms and additional echocardiographic variables suggestive of PH.

Statistical analysis

Qualitative data were expressed as the mean and standard deviation (SD) after checking the data using the normal distribution test, and non-normally distributed qualitative variables were described as the median and interquartile range (IQR). To assess whether there were statistically significant differences, Student's *t* test or the Mann-Whitney *U* test were used according to the result of the normal distribution test. Categorical variables were analysed by the chi-square test and Fisher's exact test. The 95% confidence intervals (CIs) were calculated for sensitivity, specificity, positive predictive value (PPV) and negative predictive value (NPV). A *p* value <0.05 was considered significant. Statistical analysis was conducted using SPSS 20.0 for Windows (SPSS Inc., Chicago, IL, USA).

Results

Baseline characteristics

Comparing the indications for RHC in 83 patients, the proportions of patients diagnosed with PH were 24/35 patients (68.5%) with RVSP >36 mmHg plus FVC/DLCO ratio >1.6, 23/34 patients (67.6%) with RVSP >36 mmHg, 4/8 patients (50.0%) with FVC/DLCO ratio >1.6 and 1/6 patients (16.6%) with progressive unexplained dyspnoea. Two the four patients who were excluded had PH due to ILD. Following the RHC results in the 78 patients who fulfilled the inclusion criteria and did not meet the exclusion criteria, PH was identified in 50 patients (64.1%) and PH was ruled out in the other 28 subjects (35.8%), although 14 of them had BoPAP with mPAP between 21 and 24 mmHg (Fig. 1). According to PH classification, 35 patients (44.8%) were diagnosed with PAH, 6 (7.6%) had PH due to left heart disease and 9 (11.5%) had PH due to ILD. Sixty-three patients with PAH and without PH were selected for DETECT algorithm analysis.

The baseline characteristics of the selected patients with SSc are summarized in Table 1. There were 59 women and 4 men, the mean ± SD age at RHC was 62.4 ± 11.6 years. Based on skin involvement, lcSSc was the most frequent cutaneous subtype in 45 patients (71.4%), 10 patients (15.9%) had dcSSc and 8 patients (12.7%) had ssSSc. The mean time from the first SSc symptom including RP was 18.6 ± 12.3 years, while for the time from first non-RP it was 10.5 ± 8.9 years. Almost the whole study population ($n = 61$ (96.8%)) fulfilled the ACR/EULAR 2013 classification criteria. There were no statistical differences in the presence of telangiectasias, past or current DU, history of SRC, ILD or cardiac involvement, when comparing the two groups. Although there were no statistical differences in positivity to antinuclear antibodies or the observation of a nucleolar pattern in the indirect immunofluorescence, patients with PAH more often had ACA ($n = 23$, 65.7% vs $n = 11$, 39.3%, $p = 0.03$), but lower positivity against anti-topoisomerase I antibodies ($n = 3$, 8.6% vs $n = 9$, 32.1%, $p = 0.01$). Arterial hypertension was the most frequent cardiovascular risk factor in the whole group, being identified in 27 patients (42.9%), followed by dyslipidaemia in 15 patients (23.8%); however, there were no patients with diabetes mellitus. No statistical differences were identified in the anthropometrical variables. The patients with PAH received less immunosuppressant therapy than the control group, and less treatment with calcium channel blockers. However, there were no statistical differences in the use of specific vasodilator therapy, for which the indication was RP in all cases.

Regarding respiratory parameters, the PAH group had higher FVC percent predicted/DLCO percent predicted than controls (2.0 ± 0.7% vs 1.5 ± 0.4%, $p < 0.01$) and shorter 6MWD (232.8 ± 76.7 m vs 322.4 ± 105.0 m, $p = 0.01$) (Table 2). Advanced WHO functional classes III/IV were more common in patients with PAH ($n = 15$ (42.9%)), than in the group with no PH ($n = 2$ (7.1%)) ($p < 0.01$). There were higher NT-proBNP and serum urate levels and higher prevalence of right axis deviation on ECG in the PAH group. In relation to echocardiographic data, patients with PAH had a greater RA area; moreover, they presented with higher TRV and RVSP than patients with no PH. Therefore, there were statistically significant differences between PAH and without PH patients in seven out of eight variables considered in DETECT algorithm.

RHC in the PAH group was characterized by superior mean PAP (Table 3). Specifically, the median (IQR) of mPAP was 42.0 (33.0 – 50.0) mmHg in patients with PAH, while it was 20.5 (17.0 to 23.0) mmHg in the group with no PH ($p < 0.001$). Furthermore, TPG was increased in patients with PAH, but CO was lower in those patients. The PAH group had higher pulmonary vascular resistance, with lower SvO2 and SaO2 during the RHC, compared with the group with no PH.

Comparisons of the DETECT algorithm and the ESC/ERS 2009 guidelines

The DETECT algorithm steps are represented in Table 4. After step 1 of the algorithm 35 patients in the PAH group (100%) would have been referred to echocardiography compared to 24 in the group without PH (85.7%) ($p = 0.03$). Following the echocardiography results, RHC would have been recommended in all 35 patients in the PAH group (100%), while this was only the case in 16

Table 1 Demographic data and baseline characteristics

	All patients ($n = 63$)	PAH patients ($n = 35$)	No PH patients ($n = 28$)	*P* value
Female[a]	59 (93.7)	34 (97.1)	25 (89.3)	0.31
Age, years[b]	62.4 (±11.6)	64.4 (± 10.8)	59.9 (± 12.4)	0.13
DcSSc[a]	10 (15.9)	4 (11.4)	6 (21.4)	0.31
Time from first symptom, years[b]	18.6 (± 12.3)	19.6 (±11.2)	17.2 (± 13.7)	0.29
Time from first non-RP symptom, years[b]	10.5 (± 8.9)	9.7 (±9.4)	11.5 (± 8.2)	0.21
ACR/EULAR 2013 classification criteria[a]	61 (96.8)	34 (97.1)	27 (96.4)	1.0
Telangiectasias[a]	59 (93.7)	33 (94.3)	26 (92.9)	1.0
Digital ulcers[a]	35 (55.6)	20 (57.1)	15 (53.6)	0.77
Scleroderma renal crisis[a]	2 (3.2)	2 (5.7)	0 (0)	0.49
Interstitial lung disease[a]	32 (50.8)	19 (54.3)	12 (42.9)	0.45
Cardiac involvement[a]	26 (41.3)	17 (48.6)	9 (32.1)	0.18
Antinuclear antibodies[a]	62 (98.4)	34 (97.1)	28 (100)	1.0
ACA[a]	34 (54.0)	23 (65.7)	11 (39.3)	0.03
Anti-Scl-70[a]	12 (19.0)	3 (8.6)	9 (32.1)	0.01
Nucleolar IIF pattern[a]	4 (6.3)	3 (8.6)	1 (3.6)	0.62
Arterial hypertension[a]	27 (42.9)	14 (40)	13 (43.4)	0.60
Dyslipidaemia[a]	15 (23.8)	6 (17.1)	9 (32.1)	0.16
Diabetes mellitus[a]	0 (0)	0 (0)	0 (0)	NA
Immunosuppressant therapy[a]	25 (39.7)	8 (22.9)	17 (60.7)	<0.01
Prednisone[a]	19 (30.2)	7 (20.0)	12 (40.9)	0.04
Sodium mycophenolate[a]	7 (11.1)	1 (2.9)	6 (21.4)	0.03
Azathioprine	3 (4.8)	0 (0)	3 (10.7)	0.08
IV cyclophosphamide[a]	12 (19.0)	3 (8.6)	9 (32.1)	0.01
Calcium channel blocker[a]	33 (52.4)	14 (40.0)	19 (67.9)	0.02
Specific vasodilator therapy[a]	13 (20.6)	7 (20.0)	6 (21.4)	0.88
IV prostanoids[a]	1 (1.6)	1 (2.9)	0 (0)	1.0
ERA[a]	10 (15.9)	5 (14.3)	5 (17.9)	0.74
PDE5 I[a]	5 (7.9)	2 (5.7)	3 (10.7)	0.64

PAH pulmonary arterial hypertension, *PH* pulmonary hypertension, *dcSSc* diffuse cutaneous systemic sclerosis, *ACR/EULAR* American College of Rheumatology/ European League Against Rheumatism, *RP* Raynaud's phenomenon, *ACA* anticentromere antibodies, *IIF* indirect immunofluorescence, *NA* not applicable, *IV* intravenous, *ERA* endothelin receptor antagonist, *PDE5 I* phosphodiesterase type-5 inhibitor. [a]Data are shown as number (%) for categorical variables. [b]Data are shown as mean (± SD)

subjects (57.1%) in patients with no PH ($p < 0.001$). However, based on the ESC/ERS 2009 guidelines, 32 patients with PAH (91.4%) and 4 patients in the group without PH (14.3%) would have been referred for RHC. The RHC referral ratio was higher using DETECT than it was using the ESC/ERS guidelines. The main reasons for not referring these patients for RHC using the ESC/ERS 2009 guidelines would have been that 12 patients had TRV >2.8 to ≤3.4 m/s but with no symptoms, 5 patients presented with TRV ≤2.8 m/s with symptoms but with no additional echocardiographic signs of PH, and another 10 patients had TRV ≤2.8 m/s with no symptoms and no additional echocardiographic signs of PH. There would have been no missed diagnosis of PAH with DETECT, but using the ESC/ERS guidelines it would have reached 8.5% (Table 5). The sensitivity (95% CI) of the DETECT algorithm was 100% (90.1–100) compared to sensitivity of 91.4% (77.6–97.0) using the ESC/ERS 2009 guidelines. The specificity was lower with DETECT at 42.9% (26.5–60.9) whereas it was 85.7% (68.2–94.3) using the ESC/ERS 2009 guidelines. No statistical differences were found in PPV, which was 68.6% (55.0–79.7) using DETECT compared to 88.9% (74.7–95.6) using the ESC/ERS 2009 guidelines. However, NPV reached 100% (75.7–100) using the DETECT algorithm, while using the ESC/ERS 2009 guidelines it was 88.9% (71.9–96.1).

Table 2 Respiratory, laboratory and echocardiography data

	All patients ($n = 63$)	PAH patients ($n = 35$)	No PH patients ($n = 28$)	*P* value
Pulmonary function tests				
FVC, % predicted[b]	75.2 (± 16.4)	75.6 (± 15.5)	74.7 (± 17.8)	0.86
DLCO, % predicted[b]	46.3 (± 14.2)	41.5 (± 13.9)	51.0 (± 13.1)	0.01
FVC%/DLCO%[b]	1.8 (± 0.6)	2.0 (± 0.7)	1.5 (± 0.4)	<0.01
6MWD, m[b]	256.5 (± 92.5)	232.8 (± 76.7)	322.4 (± 105.0)	0.01
WHO functional class III/IV[a]	17 (27.0)	15 (42.9)	2 (7.1)	<0.01
Laboratory				
NT-proBNP, pg/mL[c]	198 (41 to 647)	1271 (580 to 3154)	87 (32 to 202)	<0.001
Serum urate, mg/dL[b]	5.6 (± 1.9)	6.8 (± 1.9)	4.6 (± 1.0)	<0.001
Right axis in ECG[a]	18 (28.6)	10 (28.6)	1 (3.6)	0.01
Echocardiography				
LVEF, %[c]	60.0 (59.0 to 65.0)	60.0 (58.5 to 65.0)	62.0 (59.7 to 65.0)	0.43
TAPSE, mm[b]	19.4 (± 3.9)	19.1 (± 4.6)	19.8 (± 3.0)	0.55
RA area, cm2[c]	16.0 (13.0 to 21.0)	17.0 (15.0 to 22.7)	14.0 (12.0 to 16.0)	<0.01
TRV, m/s[b]	3.5 (± 0.7)	4.0 (± 0.6)	2.8 (± 0.3)	<0.001
RVSP, mmHg[c]	59.5 (44.0 to 76.2)	73.0 (61.0 to 85.0)	44.0 (37.0 to 51.0)	<0.001

PAH pulmonary arterial hypertension, *PH* pulmonary hypertension, *FVC* forced vital capacity, *DLCO* diffusing capacity for carbon monoxide, *6MWD* 6-minute walking distance, *WHO* World Health Organization, *NT-proBNP* N-terminal pro-brain natriuretic peptide, *ECG* electrocardiography, *LVEF* left ventricular ejection fraction, *TAPSE* tricuspid annular plane systolic excursion, *RA* right atrium, *TRV* tricuspid regurgitant velocity, *RVSP* right ventricular systolic pressure. [a]Data are shown as number (%) for categorical variables. [b]Data are shown as mean (± SD). [c]Data are shown as median (IQR)

As a strategy to identify mPAP ≥21 mmHg (both BoPAP and PAH), the DETECT algorithm had superior sensitivity of 93.9% (83.5–97.9) and NPV of 75.0% (46.8–91.1) compared to ESC/ERS guidelines for which the sensitivity and NPV was 69.4% (55.5–80.5) and 44.4% (27.6–62.7), respectively. Furthermore, DETECT missed 6.1% of diagnoses of mPAP ≥21, whereas using the ESC/ERS 2009 guidelines the percentage was increased to 30.6%. In fact, analysing only patients with BoPAP, there were 3 out of 14 (21.1%) missed diagnoses using DETECT, whereas there were 12 out of 14 (85.7%) missed using the ESC/ERS 2009 guidelines. However, specificity and PPV were slightly lower using the DETECT algorithm, at 64.3% and 90.2% compared to 85.7% and 94.4%, respectively, using the ESC/ERS guidelines.

To investigate the capacity for the detection of any type of PH, the whole cohort of patients ($n = 83$) with a first RHC were studied, regardless of whether they met the inclusion or exclusion criteria for application of the DETECT algorithm: 1.9% of diagnoses of PH were missed using the DETECT algorithm compared with

Table 3 Haemodynamic characteristics on right heart catheterization

	All patients ($n = 63$)	PAH patients ($n = 35$)	No PH patients ($n = 28$)	*P* value
Mean PAP, mmHg[b]	31.0 (21.0 to 44.0)	42.0 (33.0 to 50.0)	20.5 (17.0 to 23.0)	<0.001
PAWP, mmHg[a]	9.6 (± 4.0)	9.7 (± 4.8)	9.5 (± 3.4)	0.90
RAP, mmHg[b]	5.0 (2.5 to 8.5)	5.0 (3.0 to 10.0)	4.5 (2.0 to 7.0)	0.14
TPG, mmHg[a]	20.0 (± 13.4)	31.4 (± 11.8)	10.6 (± 3.9)	<0.001
Cardiac output, L/min[b]	3.5 (2.9 to 4.5)	3.4 (2.8 to 4.0)	3.9 (2.9 to 5.1)	0.05
PVR, WU[a]	6.6 (± 4.8)	9.9 (± 4.6)	3.2 (± 1.6)	<0.001
SVR, WU[a]	26.9 (± 10.3)	28.6 (± 9.7)	25.2 (± 11.0)	0.42
SvO2, %[a]	66.3 (± 8.1)	61.8 (± 8.3)	71.0 (± 4,7)	<0.001
SaO2, %[a]	93.5 (± 4.0)	91.2 (± 3.7)	96.1 (± 2.5)	<0.001

PAH pulmonary arterial hypertension, *PH* pulmonary hypertension, *PAP* pulmonary artery pressure, *PAWP* pulmonary artery wedge pressure, *RAP* right atrial pressure, *TPG* transpulmonary pressure gradient, *PVR* pulmonary vascular resistance, *WU* Wood units, *SVR* systemic vascular resistance, *SvO2* mixed venous oxygen saturation, *SaO2* arterial oxygen saturation. [a]Data are shown as mean (± SD). [b]Data are shown as median (IQR)

Table 4 Comparisons of the DETECT algorithm and the ESC/ERS 2009 guidelines

	PAH vs no PH patients (*n* = 63)			Patients with mPAP ≥21 vs mPAP <21mmg (*n* = 63)			PH vs no PH patients (*n* = 83)		
	PAH (*n* = 35)	No PH (*n* = 28)	*P* value	mPAP ≥21 mmHg (*n* = 49)	mPAP <21mmg (*n* = 14)	*P* value	PH (*n* = 52)	No PH (*n* = 31)	*P* value
DETECT algorithm									
Score step 1[b]	330.0 (±25.3)	313.7 (±17.5)	<0.01	326.9 (±22.8)	308.6 (±20.8)	<0.01	327.9 (±23.6)	311.8 (±17.6)	<0.01
Indication of Echo[a]	35 (100)	24 (85.7)	0.03	49 (100)	10 (71.4)	<0.01	51 (98.1)	24 (77.4)	<0.01
Score step 2[b]	60.2 (±11.3)	37.3 (±8.4)	<0.001	54.7 (±13.3)	33.5 (±8.8)	<0.001	56.4 (±12.4)	36.5 (±8.4)	<0.001
RHC recommendation[a]	35 (100)	16 (57.1)	<0.001	46 (93.9)	5 (35.7)	<0.001	51 (98.1)	17 (54.8)	<0.001
ESC/ERS 2009 guidelines									
RHC recommendation[a]	32 (91.4)	4 (14.3)	<0.001	34 (69.4)	2 (14.3)	<0.001	42 (80.8)	4 (12.9)	<0.001

PAH pulmonary arterial hypertension, *PH* pulmonary hypertension, *mPAP* mean pulmonary artery pressure, *Echo* echocardiography, *RHC* right heart catheterization, *ESC/ERS* European Society of Cardiology and the European Respiratory Society. [a]Data are shown as number (%) for categorical variables. [b]Data are shown as mean (± SD)

19.2% missed using the ESC/ERS 2009 guidelines. Moreover, sensitivity and NPV were greater at 98.1% and 93.3% using the DETECT method, compared with 80.8% and 73.0%, respectively, using the ESC/ERS guidelines. Nevertheless, specificity and PPV were again slightly inferior at 45.2% and 75.0% when applying the DETECT algorithm, whereas the values were 87.1% and 91.3%, respectively, using in the ESC/ERS guidelines.

Discussion

The present retrospective study compared the application of the DETECT algorithm with the ESC/ERS 2009 guidelines in patients with PAH and patients without PH, who had undergone RHC. The DETECT programme had greater sensitivity, the RHC would have been recommended in all patients suffering from PAH, and also superior NPV compared to the ESC/ERS guidelines. Nevertheless, the ESC/ERS 2009 guidelines had higher specificity and PPV than the DETECT algorithm. Furthermore, the DETECT algorithm had higher percentage sensitivity and NPV both for the detection of patients with mPAP ≥21 and for patients with any type of PH, although specificity and PPV were lower.

For the application of the DETECT algorithm it is necessary to meet the inclusion criteria, so patients must present with a duration of SSc longer than 3 years from the first non-RP symptom and DLCO <60% predicted. This was to increase the specificity of the screening method, due to the fact that <10% of a cohort of 243 patients with SSc-PH have been found to present with DLCO >60% [19]. Furthermore, patients could not fulfil the exclusion criteria such as previous PH diagnosed by RHC, forced vital capacity (FVC) <40% or the involvement of left heart disease [12]. Nevertheless, DETECT does not establish the periodicity of an assessment by this method, it has not been evaluated over a monitoring period in a cohort of patients and its ability to predict mPAP ≥21 mmHg or any type of PH have not been explored. As a consequence of this work, the new ESC/ESR 2015 guidelines were recently published, which strengthen the recommendation for annual screening of PH in this set of patients with SSc and introduce the

Table 5 Observation of PAH detection programs

		RHC referral rate, %	Missed diagnoses, %	Sensitivity %	Specificity %	PPV %	NPV %
PAH vs no PH patients	DETECT algorithm (95% CI)	51/63, 80.9% -	0/35, 0% -	100% (90.1–100)	42.9% (26.5–60.9)	68.6% (55.0–79.7)	100% (75.7–100)
	ESC/ERS guidelines (95% CI)	36/63, 57.1% -	3/35, 8.5% -	91.4% (77.6–97.0)	85.7% (68.5–94.3)	88.9% (74.7–95.6)	88.9% (71.9–96.1)
Patients with mPAP ≥21 vs mPAP <21mmg	DETECT algorithm (95% CI)	51/63, 80.9% -	3/49, 6.1% -	93.9% (83.5–97.9)	64.3% (38.8–83.7)	90.2% (79.0–95.7)	75.0% (46.8–91.1)
	ESC/ERS guidelines (95% CI)	36/63, 57.1% -	15/49, 30.6% -	69.4% (55.5–80.5)	85.7% (60.1–96.0)	94.4% (81.9–98.5)	44.4% (27.6–62.7)
PH vs no PH patients	DETECT algorithm (95% CI)	68/83, 81.9% -	1/52, 1.9% -	98.1% (89.9–99.7)	45.2% (29.2–62.2)	75.0% (63.6–83.8)	93.3% (70.2–98.8)
	ESC/ERS guidelines (95% CI)	46/83, 55.4% -	10/52, 19.2% -	80.8% (68.1–89.2)	87.1% (71.1–94.9)	91.3% (79.7–96.6)	73.0% (57.0–84.6)

Data shown as number (%). *RHC* right heart catheterization, *PPV* positive predictive value, *NPV* negative positive value, *PAH* pulmonary arterial hypertension, *PH* pulmonary hypertension, *CI* confidence interval, *mPAP* mean pulmonary artery pressure, *ESC/ERS* European Society of Cardiology and the European Respiratory Society

DETECT algorithm as a valid method to be performed in this group of patients based on the evidence demonstrated [15].

Compared to the study of Coghlan et al., patients in our cohort had a surprisingly higher prevalence of telangiectasias and ACA antibodies. Almost 60% of patients with PAH presented with WHO functional class I or II and mild reduced 6MWD comparable to the detection cohorts of previous studies that have focused on early PAH diagnosis [10, 12]. This fact seems to reflect that patients in our study were referred promptly for RHC as a result of active and early suspicion of PAH during monitoring. In the present paper we describe similar sensitivity, specificity and NPV values, although with a higher RHC referral ratio and PPV using the DETECT algorithm than in the original work. However, regarding the application of ESC/ERS 2009 guidelines we report higher sensitivity, specificity and PPV values and a higher RHC referral ratio than Coghlan et al. This may be explained due to the fact that the main indication for performing RHC in our study was the presence of an abnormal echocardiographic result, suggesting the presence of PAH. Furthermore, the high RHC referral ratio may be justified because the study was conducted in a selected population of patients at high risk of PAH based on clinical, pulmonary function test and echocardiographic parameters.

Few groups have published on the application of the DETECT algorithm. Hao et al. analysed the DETECT algorithm in patients from the multicentre Australian Scleroderma Cohort Study (ASCS) along with the Australian Scleroderma Interest Group (ASIG) algorithm and the ESC/ERS 2009 guidelines [20, 21]. The authors found higher sensitivity and NPV using the DETECT or the ASIG algorithm than they did using the ESC/ERS guidelines, which we can confirm in our study. Surprisingly, the ASIG protocol had superior specificity to the DETECT algorithm and even to the ESC/ERS guidelines, which contrasts with the values of 48% and 69%, respectively, that were previously published [12]. The authors reported that nine patients did not meet the criterion of DLCO <60% or the criterion for disease duration, and this may explain the lower specificity of the DETECT algorithm [21]. Furthermore, the DETECT and ASIG screening methods had the highest sensitivity and specificity to identify both precapillary PH and any group of PH, results that we have corroborated in our work. In the present work the ASIG programme was not analysed due to the fact that this method is not based on evidence and has not been well-validated in European cohorts.

Recently, a Czech scleroderma group designed a modified DETECT algorithm, in which a right ventricular outflow tract is evaluated instead of RA area [22]. Using this modified DETECT programme the RHC referral ratio was 41.4% compared to 24.1% using the ESC/ERS guidelines. Interestingly, although only 11/58 patients (18.9%) had undergone RHC, in patients who were recommended by the modified DETECT algorithm there were also other types of PH diagnosed, such as PH due to left heart disease and PH due to ILD. Therefore, this article suggests that the DETECT algorithm would be useful for recommending RHC for diagnosing other types of PH according to the WHO classification.

Although there are some discrepancies on the prognostic role of BoPAP, a study has been recently published evidencing a higher risk of mortality and hospitalization in US veteran patients with BoPAP (defined as 19–24 mmHg) [23]. Consequently, the study highlights the relevance of diagnosing BoPAP in selected groups of patients such as those with scleroderma. In a post-hoc analysis of the DETECT study, the authors demonstrated that patients with BoPAP had a higher FVC/DLCO rate, and higher TRV and NT-proBNP levels than in patients with normal mPAP [16]. Although the paper does not evaluate the application of DETECT in both groups of patients, it would support the increment of the specificity of this programme identified in our work when studying patients with mPAP ≥21 versus mPAP <21mmg, compared to the PAH versus no PH strategy. In the set of patients with SSc, identifying BoPAP in the first RHC was demonstrated as a high risk factor for developing PH, with a hazard ratio of 3.7 during follow up compared to patients with mPAP <21 mmHg [24]. In this line, in a multicentre prospective SSc cohort, the Pulmonary Hypertension Assessment and Recognition of Outcomes in Scleroderma (PHAROS) study group reported that 55% of patients with BoPAP progressed to PH, whereas in the group of patients with mPAP <21 mmHg this was 32%, over a mean 25.7-month period of monitoring [25]. Having established the relevance of identifying patients with SSc and BoPAP for close supervision, this is the first paper that demonstrates the accuracy of the DETECT algorithm in the identification of patients with mPAP ≥21.

The main limitation of the present study was the retrospective design. RHC was not performed in the whole cohort of patients with SSc, therefore some mild forms of PAH may have been undiagnosed. In the same line, although the periodicity of performing the screening methods is not well established, these were not carried out in the whole cohort, which may not reflect the real referral rate for RHC.

Conclusions

Pulmonary arterial hypertension in one of the leading causes of death in patients with SSc, and its early diagnosis has demonstrated increased survival rates. The present study supports the DETECT algorithm as an excellent screening method due to its high sensitivity and NPV, which minimizes the number of missed diagnoses of previous recommendations. Furthermore, our data suggest the DETECT algorithm is also accurate either for an early diagnosis of borderline mPAP, patients who are at highest risk of developing PAH, or the diagnosis of any type of PH.

Abbreviations

6MWD: 6-Minute walking distance; ACA: Anticentromere antibodies; ACR: American College of Rheumatology; ANA: Antinuclear antibodies; ASCS: Australian Scleroderma Cohort Study; ASIG: Australian Scleroderma Interest Group; BoPAP: Borderline median pulmonary arterial pressure; CI: Confidence interval; CO: Cardiac output; dcSSc: Diffuse cutaneous systemic sclerosis; DLCO: Diffusing capacity for carbon monoxide; DU: Digital ulcers; ECG: Electrocardiography; ERA: Endothelin receptor antagonist; ESC/ERS: European Society of Cardiology and the European Respiratory Society; EULAR: European League Against Rheumatism; FVC: Forced vital capacity; HR: Hazard ratio; HRCT: High-resolution computed tomography; IIF: Indirect immunofluorescence; ILD: Interstitial lung disease; IQR: Interquartile range; IV: Intravenous; lcSSc: limited cutaneous systemic sclerosis; LHD: Left heart disease; LVEF: Left ventricular ejection fraction; mPAP: Median pulmonary arterial pressure; NPV: Negative predictive value; NT-proBNP: N-terminal pro-brain natriuretic peptide; PAH: Pulmonary arterial hypertension; PAWP: Pulmonary artery wedge pressure; PDE5 I: Phosphodiesterase type-5 inhibitor; PFT: Pulmonary function test; PH: Pulmonary hypertension; PHAROS: Pulmonary Hypertension Assessment and Recognition of Outcomes in Scleroderma; PPV: Positive predictive value; PVR: Pulmonary vascular resistance; RA: Right atrium; RAP: Right atrial pressure; RHC: Right heart catheterization; RP: Raynaud's phenomenon; RVSP: Right ventricular systolic pressure; SaO2: Arterial oxygen saturation; SD: Standard deviation; SRC: Scleroderma renal crisis; SSc: Systemic sclerosis; ssSSc: Sine scleroderma systemic sclerosis; SvO2: Mixed venous oxygen saturation; SVR: Systemic vascular resistance; TAPSE: Tricuspid annular plane systolic excursion; TPG: Transpulmonary pressure gradient; TRV: Tricuspid regurgitant velocity; vs: Versus; WHO: World Health Organization; WU: Wood units

Acknowledgements

The authors thank the patients for their participation.

Funding

This work was funded by Instituto de Salud Carlos III, grant PI16/02088 co-financed by the European Regional Development Fund (ERDF). This work was supported by an educational unrestricted scholarship granted by Actelion Pharmaceuticals. AGDC was supported by the Contratos Predoctorales de Formación en Investigación (PFIS) grant from Instituto de Salud Carlos III (FI14/00643).

Authors' contributions

AGDC made substantial contributions to study conception and design, acquisition, analysis and interpretation of data, drafting the article and approval of the final manuscript. ELCM and GG made substantial contributions to study conception and design, analysis and interpretation of data, revising the manuscript critically for important intellectual content and approval of the final manuscript. JFRP, AR, CB, MLM, ED and VFP made substantial contributions to study conception and design, revising the manuscript critically for important intellectual content and approval of the final manuscript. CPSA made substantial contributions to study conception and design, interpretation of data, revising the manuscript critically for important intellectual content and approval of the final manuscript. AGDC and ELCM had full access to all of the data in the study and they both take responsibility for the integrity and accuracy of the data. Funders had no access to the data, were not involved in study design, acquisition, analysis or interpretation of data or writing the manuscript. All authors read and approved the final manuscript.

Competing interests

The authors declare that they have no competing interests.

Author details

[1]Department of Systemic Autoimmune Diseases, Hospital Universitari Vall d'Hebron, Universitat Autònoma de Barcelona, Passeig Vall d'Hebron 119-129, PC: 08035 Barcelona, Spain. [2]Department of Cardiology, Hospital Universitari Vall d'Hebron, Universitat Autònoma de Barcelona, Barcelona, Spain. [3]Department of Pneumology, Hospital Universitari Vall d'Hebron, Universitat Autònoma de Barcelona, Barcelona, Spain.

References

1. Denton CP, Ong VH. Targeted therapies for systemic sclerosis. Nat Rev Rheumatol. 2013;9:451–64.
2. Allanore Y, Simms R, Distler O, Trojanowska M, Pope J, Denton CP, et al. Systemic sclerosis. Nat Rev Dis Primers. 2015;1:15002.
3. Mukerjee D, St George D, Coleiro B, Knight C, Denton CP, Davar J, et al. Prevalence and outcome in systemic sclerosis associated pulmonary arterial hypertension: application of a registry approach. Ann Rheum Dis. 2003;62: 1088–93.
4. Avouac J, Airo P, Meune C, Beretta L, Dieude P, Caramaschi P, et al. Prevalence of pulmonary hypertension in systemic sclerosis in European Caucasians and meta analysis of 5 studies. J Rheumatol. 2010;37:2290–8.
5. Steen VD, Medsger TA. Changes in causes of death in systemic sclerosis, 1972-2002. Ann Rheum Dis. 2007;66:940–4.
6. Nihtyanova SI, Schreiber BE, Ong VH, Rosenberg D, Moinzadeh P, Coghlan JG, et al. Prediction of pulmonary complications and long-term survival in systemic sclerosis. Arthritis Rheumatol. 2014;66:1625–35.
7. Simeon-Aznar CP, Fonollosa-Pla V, Tolosa-Vilella C, Espinosa-Garriga G, Campillo-Grau M, Ramos-Casals M, et al. Registry of the Spanish Network for Systemic Sclerosis: survival, prognostic factors, and causes of death. Medicine (Baltimore). 2015;94:e1728.
8. Rubenfire M, Huffman MD, Krishnan S, Seibold JR, Schiopu E, McLaughlin W. Survival in systemic sclerosis with pulmonary arterial hypertension has not improved in the modern era. Chest. 2013;144:1282–90.
9. Hachulla E, Gressin V, Guillevin L, Carpentier P, Diot E, Sibilia J, et al. Early detection of pulmonary arterial hypertension in systemic sclerosis: a French nationwide prospective multicenter study. Arthritis Rheum. 2005; 52:3792–800.
10. Humbert M, Yaici A, de Groote P, Montani D, Sitbon O, Launay D, et al. Screening for pulmonary arterial hypertension in patients with systemic sclerosis: clinical characteristics at diagnosis and long-term survival. Arthritis Rheum. 2011;63:3522–30.
11. Galie N, Hoeper MM, Humbert M, Torbicki A, Vachiery JL, Barbera JA, et al. Guidelines for the diagnosis and treatment of pulmonary hypertension: the Task Force for the Diagnosis and Treatment of Pulmonary Hypertension of the European Society of Cardiology (ESC) and the European Respiratory Society (ERS), endorsed by the International Society of Heart and Lung Transplantation (ISHLT). Eur Heart J. 2009;30:2493–537.
12. Coghlan JG, Denton CP, Grunig E, Bonderman D, Distler O, Khanna D, et al. Evidence-based detection of pulmonary arterial hypertension in systemic sclerosis: the DETECT study. Ann Rheum Dis. 2014;73:1340–9.
13. LeRoy EC, Black C, Fleischmajer R, Jablonska S, Krieg T, Medsger Jr TA, et al. Scleroderma (systemic sclerosis): classification, subsets and pathogenesis. J Rheumatol. 1988;15:202–5.
14. van den Hoogen F, Khanna D, Fransen J, Johnson SR, Baron M, Tyndall A, et al. 2013 classification criteria for systemic sclerosis: an American College of Rheumatology/European League against Rheumatism collaborative initiative. Arthritis Rheum. 2013;65:2737–47.
15. Galie N, Humbert M, Vachiery JL, Gibbs S, Lang I, Torbicki A, et al. 2015 ESC/ERS Guidelines for the diagnosis and treatment of pulmonary hypertension: The Joint Task Force for the Diagnosis and Treatment of Pulmonary Hypertension of the European Society of Cardiology (ESC) and the European Respiratory Society (ERS): endorsed by: Association for European Paediatric and Congenital Cardiology (AEPC), International Society for Heart and Lung Transplantation (ISHLT). Eur Heart J. 2016;37:67–119.

16. Visovatti SH, Distler O, Coghlan JG, Denton CP, Grunig E, Bonderman D, et al. Borderline pulmonary arterial pressure in systemic sclerosis patients: a post-hoc analysis of the DETECT study. Arthritis Res Ther. 2014;16:493.
17. Simeon-Aznar CP, Tolosa-Vilella C, Gabarro-Julia L, Campillo-Grau M, Guillen Del Castillo A, Fonollosa-Pla V, et al. Systemic sclerosis sine scleroderma and limited cutaneous systemic sclerosis: similarities and differences. Clin Exp Rheumatol. 2014;32:S-33–40.
18. DETECT - DETECTion of PAH in SSC. http://detect-pah.com. Accessed 25 Apr 2016.
19. Schwaiger JP, Khanna D, Gerry Coghlan J. Screening patients with scleroderma for pulmonary arterial hypertension and implications for other at-risk populations. Eur Respir Rev. 2013;22:515–25.
20. Thakkar V, Stevens W, Prior D, Youssef P, Liew D, Gabbay E, et al. The inclusion of N-terminal pro-brain natriuretic peptide in a sensitive screening strategy for systemic sclerosis-related pulmonary arterial hypertension: a cohort study. Arthritis Res Ther. 2013;15:R193.
21. Hao Y, Thakkar V, Stevens W, Morrisroe K, Prior D, Rabusa C, et al. A comparison of the predictive accuracy of three screening models for pulmonary arterial hypertension in systemic sclerosis. Arthritis Res Ther. 2015;17:7.
22. Soukup T, Pudil R, Kubinova K, Hromadkova L, Dusek J, Tosovsky M, et al. Application of the DETECT algorithm for detection of risk of pulmonary arterial hypertension in systemic sclerosis: data from a Czech tertiary centre. Rheumatology (Oxford). 2016;55:109–14.
23. Maron BA, Hess E, Maddox TM, Opotowsky AR, Tedford RJ, Lahm T, et al. Association of borderline pulmonary hypertension with mortality and hospitalization in a large patient cohort: insights from the Veterans Affairs Clinical Assessment, Reporting, and Tracking Program. Circulation. 2016; 133:1240–8.
24. Valerio CJ, Schreiber BE, Handler CE, Denton CP, Coghlan JG. Borderline mean pulmonary artery pressure in patients with systemic sclerosis: transpulmonary gradient predicts risk of developing pulmonary hypertension. Arthritis Rheum. 2013;65:1074–84.
25. Bae S, Saggar R, Bolster MB, Chung L, Csuka ME, Derk C, et al. Baseline characteristics and follow-up in patients with normal haemodynamics versus borderline mean pulmonary arterial pressure in systemic sclerosis: results from the PHAROS registry. Ann Rheum Dis. 2012;71:1335–42.

4

Preliminary safety and efficacy profile of prucalopride in the treatment of systemic sclerosis (SSc)-related intestinal involvement: results from the open label cross-over PROGASS study

Barbara Vigone[1], Monica Caronni[1], Adriana Severino[1], Chiara Bellocchi[1], Anna Rita Baldassarri[2], Mirella Fraquelli[2], Gaia Montanelli[1], Alessandro Santaniello[1] and Lorenzo Beretta[1*]

Abstract

Background: Prokinetics are used to treat enteric dismotility symptoms in systemic sclerosis (SSc) patients, but they often lack adequate efficacy. The most effective prokinetics belonging to the serotonin (5-HT_4) receptor agonists class were withdrawn due to cardiac toxicity in relation to modest 5-HT_4 receptor affinity. Prucalopride is a high-affinity 5-HT_4 receptor agonist with no major cardiac issues, for which the efficacy in SSc has not yet been assessed.

Methods: Forty patients with self-reported mild to moderately severe enteric symptoms were enrolled in a cross-over 2 × 2 study. Subjects were randomized 1:1 to prucalopride 2 mg/day or no treatment for one month and vice versa after a 2-week washout period. Before and after each sequence the patients compiled the University of California Los Angeles gastrointestinal tract (UCLA GIT) 2.0 questionnaire and the numbers of complete intestinal movements were recorded. Oro-cecal transit time (OCTT) was evaluated by lactulose breath test in a subgroup of patients. Data were evaluated by mixed linear models corrected for the number of laxatives used during the study periods.

Results: There were 29 subjects who completed the study; 7 subjects withdrew due to side-effects and 4 subjects were not compliant with the study procedures. As compared to dummy treatment, prucalopride was associated with more intestinal evacuations ($p < 0.001$), improvement of UCLA GIT constipation (-0.672 ± 0.112 vs 0.086 ± 0.115; $p < 0.001$), reflux (-0.409 ± 0.094 vs 0.01 ± 0.096; $p < 0.005$) and bloating (-0.418 ± 0.088 vs -0.084 ± 0.09; $p = 0.01$) scores. Treatment was ranked moderately to more than moderately effective by 22 patients (72.4%). OCTT was significantly reduced during prucalopruide consumption (prucalopride: -20.1 ± 20.1 vs no treatment: 45.8 ± 21.3 minutes; treatment effect = -65.9 minutes; $p = 0.035$).

Conclusions: The safety profile of prucalopride in SSc is similar to what is known from the literature. In patients with mild to severe gastrointestinal problems, prucalopride may be effective in treating dismotility symptoms, increasing the number of complete bowel movements and improving bowel transit, reducing reflux disease and bloating.

Keywords: Systemic sclerosis, Intestinal involvement, Constipation, Serotonin agonist

* Correspondence: lorberimm@hotmail.com
[1]Scleroderma Unit, Referral Center for Systemic Autoimmune Diseases, Fondazione IRCCS Ca' Granda Ospedale Maggiore Policlinico di Milano, Via Pace 9, 20122 Milano, Italy
Full list of author information is available at the end of the article

Background

Systemic sclerosis (SSc) is an autoimmune disease characterized by widespread vasculopathy, immune system activation and fibrosis of the skin and of the internal organs [1]. The gastrointestinal tract (GIT) is frequently affected in SSc with up to 90% of patients presenting with upper or lower GIT involvement [2] as a consequence of motor disturbances [3–5] secondary to myenteric neuropathy, muscle atrophy and fibrosis [6]. The reduction of enteric propulsive forces leads to symptoms of enteric dismotility syndromes, such as constipation, bacterial overgrowth with bloating, diarrhea and malabsorption and, in the most severe cases, acute or chronic pseudo-obstruction may occur [7].

The treatment of SSc-related intestinal involvement is challenging and often limited to supportive measures [8]. The use of prokinetcs has been advocated to ameliorate dismotility symptoms in SSc patients, yet often with disappointing results, especially in those with more advanced disease. Among prokinetics, the ones with the most favorable therapeutic profile are those belonging to the serotonin (5-HT_4) receptor agonists class. As a prototypical representative of this class, cisapride has been shown to ameliorate gastric contractions and increase esophageal amplitude waves [9] and to reduce the colonic transit time in SSc patients [10]. Nonetheless, cisapride has been withdrawn from the global market due to safety concerns related to cardiac toxicity [11, 12]. These side-effects were linked to the lack of selectivity for the for the 5-HT_4 receptor and to the blockade of the human ether-a-go-go-related gene (hERG)-encoded K^+ channel. The consequences of this interaction are the prolongation of cardiac action potential repolarisation and, thus, QT interval, leading to a clinically significant arrhythmogenic potential [12, 13]. On the contrary, novel agonists that specifically interact with the 5-HT_4 receptor and possess GIT tissue-specific agonist activity, have a favorable cardiac profile and no major cardiac issues. Among those, prucalopride, a member of the benzofurancarboxamide agonists possesses markedly increased selectivity for the 5-HT_4 receptor as compared to cisapride (150 times vs <1, respectively) [14]. In vitro, high concentrations of prucalopride are equivalent to 5-HT in stimulating peristalsis [14] and in vivo, prucalopride dose-dependently stimulates high-amplitude clustered contractions in the proximal colon and inhibits contractile activity in the distal colon [15]. In humans, prucalopride has proved effective in treating chronic constipation unresponsive to laxatives, improving stool frequency, stool consistency, straining and quality of life [16–18]. Results of mechanistic studies in patients with idiopathic constipation suggest the usefulness of prucalopride in patients with an associated upper or generalized gastrointestinal motility disorder [18]. Prucalopride does not interact with hERG channels and in large placebo-controlled studies no differences in vital signs or electrocardiogram parameters have been observed between groups [16, 17, 19].

In relation to its safety and efficacy profile, the use of prucalopride has been postulated in SSc [2]; however, only one report describing two cases of SSc patients with GIT unresponsive to other prokinetics has been published so far [20]. To increase our knowledge about prucalopride and to evaluate its therapeutic potential in SSc, we conducted a randomized crossover trial in subjects with mild to severe constipation, providing evidence for a beneficial effect on enteric symptoms and health-related quality of life (HQoL).

Methods

Patients and study procedures

A cross-over 2 × 2 randomized controlled trial comparing prucalopride to no treatment was designed. Forty female subjects with SSc and chronic constipation were randomized 1:1 to receive prucalopride 2 mg/day or no treatment for one month and vice versa after a 2-week washout period, according to the ABBA design. Recruitment was limited to female subjects as prucalopride is not currently approved for the treatment of chronic constipation in men.

All the subjects fulfilled the American College of Rheumatology (ACR)/European League Against Rheumatism (EULAR) 2013 criteria for the classification of SSc [21], the Rome III criteria for functional constipation (Table 1a) [22] and had mild-to-severe subjective symptoms of constipation on a 5-point Likert scale (Table 1b) (minimum and maximum allowed score = 1 and 3, respectively) [23].

The number of complete spontaneous bowel movements (CSBMs) per month (4 weeks) and the proportion

Table 1 Scales and criteria used for patient selection

a. Rome III diagnostic criteria for functional constipation [22]

1. Must include* two or more of the following:
   - Straining during at least 25% of defecations
   - Lumpy or hard stools in at least 25% of defecations
   - Sensation of incomplete evacuation for at least 25% of defecations
   - Sensation of anorectal obstruction/blockage for at least 25% of defecations
   - Manual manoeuvres to facilitate at least 25% of defecations (e.g., digital evacuation, support of the pelvic floor)
   - Fewer than three defecations per week
2. Loose stools are rarely present without the use of laxatives
3. Insufficient criteria for irritable bowel syndrome

*criteria fulfilled for the last 3 months.

b. Likert scale for the subjective evaluation of constipation [23]

0. Absent
1. Mild
2. Moderate
3. Severe
4. Very severe

of patients reporting ≥3 defecations per week were used as study endpoints according to the European Medicines Agency (EMA) recommendations [24] and to previous registration trials [16, 17]. To this end, patients were given a diary and were instructed to record their daily CSBMs throughout the study periods [16, 17]. The use of bisacodyl 10 mg as laxative was allowed and the number of used tablets was recorded as well. Patients were not allowed to take any other laxatives or to perform enemas to treat constipation.

Additionally, before and after each treatment period the patients compiled the Italian version of the UCLA GIT 2.0 questionnaire [25], the 5-point Likert scale for constipation (Table 1a) and a modified 4-point Likert scale for gastroesophageal symptoms (0: no symptoms, no burning sensation; 1: mild symptoms, self-awareness of burning but well-tolerated; 2: moderate symptoms, initially incapacitating burning sensation that may impair normal activities, including rest; 3: severe symptoms, incapacitating burning sensation that impairs normal activities, including rest).

Finally, the patients globally evaluated the efficacy of treatment using a 5-point scale [26] (0: not at all effective; 1: a little effective; 2: moderately effective; 3: quite effective; 4: extremely effective).

None of the selected patients made use of laxatives the week before the initiation of the study procedures or was treated with systemic antibiotics the preceding month.

Explorative analysis of the OCTT

To evaluate the effect of prucalopride on the OCTT, patients were also given the possibility to perform a lactulose breath test (LBT) [27] at the beginning and at the end of each study period. The procedure was performed in accordance with accepted criteria [28] in fasting conditions, measuring H_2 breath concentration by Gastro + ™ Gastrolyzer® (Bedfont Scientific Ltd, Station Road, Harrietsham, Maidstone, Kent, ME17 1JA, UK) in basal conditions and every 10 minutes for at least 3 h after the administration of an oral loading dose of lactulose (10 g in 100 ml of water). The OCTT results were interpreted as previously described [28].

Statistical analysis

To compare treatment effects and to account for carry-over effects, mixed linear models were used, correcting the results for the number of laxatives used during the study periods [29]. Estimated marginal means corrected for the number of laxatives ± estimated standard errors (SE) are presented. For categorical variables, binary logistic multivariate models were used. To test the correct allocation into the study arms, the paired samples *t* test and the Fisher exact test were performed. Results of descriptive statistics, binary logistic regression, the *t* test and the Fisher test are presented as mean ± standard deviation (SD). Statistical analyses were performed using the SPSS 23.0 software (IBM Corp, Armonk NY, USA).

The sample size for the cross-over trial was determined based on a theoretical 66.6% increase in CSBMs in the treatment arm vs the non-treatment arm (20 vs 12 CSBMs/month) with a within-patients SD equal to 12 CSMBs. With these parameters, 40 patients were required to reject the null hypothesis of non-superiority (one-sided 0.05 alpha) with power = 0.9 (n = 30 required for power = 0.8). Calculations were performed using the sample size online calculator provided by the Massachusetts General Hospital's Biostatistics Center (http:// http://hedwig.mgh.harvard.edu/biostatistics/).

Results

Overall 29 participants completed all the study procedures (Fig. 1). Seven patients (17.5%) did not tolerate prucalopride due to side effects; the reported adverse events were: headache (three subjects), abdominal pain (two subjects), dizziness (one subject) and the sensation of feeling sick (one subject). In most cases (four out of seven) side effects were observed the first day of treatment and were considered severe enough to preclude the prosecution of the study, despite the proposal of mitigation strategies (i.e. use of pain killers); in the remaining cases attempts were made to go on with the treatment; however, this was discontinued within 1 week due to the persistence of side effects. Patients experiencing side effects were not clinically different from those who completed the study procedures in terms of disease duration, autoantibody profile or baseline self-reported measures of GIT disease severity (results not shown). Four patients were finally excluded from the analysis (10%) because not they were not compliant with the study procedures (badly or non-compiled diaries and self-efficacy forms including those completed during the non-treatment period, $n = 2$), because of inadequate drug intake ($n = 1$) or because the patient did not attend the assessment visit ($n = 1$).

The clinical and baseline characteristics of the remaining 29 study participants are reported in Table 2. Randomization was well-balanced with no statistical differences between arms, except for older age in participants who took the study drug first. Overall, 10 patients (34.5%) rated their constipation as "severe", 17 (58.6%) as "moderate" and 2 (6.9%) as "mild".

Prucalopride improves the number of CSBMs and ameliorates constipation in patients with SSc

During the treatment period, patients achieved more complete bowel movements than during the non-treatment period (Fig. 2). The number of patients reporting ≥3 defecations per week was 25 (86.2%) and 14 (48.3%) in the two

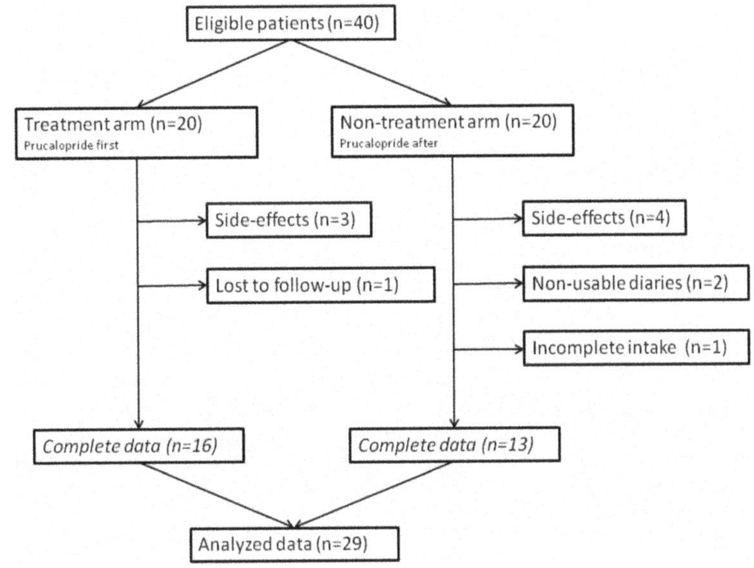

Fig. 1 Flow chart of patients included in the study

arms, respectively; these results were significant in binary logistic models that accounted for the use of laxatives and the randomization order ($p = 0.014$). In this model, patients receiving prucalopride were five times more likely to have ≥3 defecations per week than when they did not receive the study drug (odds ratio = 5.2, 95% confidence interval 1.39–19.2).

Treatment with prucalopride was associated with the improvement of constipation symptoms and of gastroesophageal reflux disease (GERD) as assessed both by Likert scales and by the specific UCLA GIT 2.0 subscales (Table 3); bloating was also significantly reduced by the treatment. The treatment effect on constipation could be rated as "much better" according to the minimally important differences in the UCLA GIT 2.0 questionnaire reported in [30]; the treatment effect on GERD

Table 2 Demographics and baseline clinical characteristics

Variable	Patients with SSc ($n = 29$)	Arm 1 (drug first, $n = 16$)	Arm 2 (drug after, $n = 13$)
Age, years	54.4 ± 10.5	59 ± 9.2	48.8 ± 9.5*
Disease duration, years	12.3 ± 8.7	13.7 ± 9.9	10.7 ± 7.1
lcSSc, *n* (%)	22 (75.8)	12 (75%)	10 (79.6)
Autoantibody, *n* (%)			
ANA	27 (93.1)	15 (93.7)	12 (92.7)
ACA	18 (62.1)	11 (68.8)	7 (53.8)
Topo I	9 (31)	4 (25)	5 (38.5)
Likert GERD (0–4)	2.24 ± 0.74	2.25 ± 0.68	2.23 ± 0.83
Likert constipation (0–4)	2.24 ± 0.64	2.44 ± 0.63	2 ± 0.58
UCLA GIT 2.0	0.99 ± 1.,28	1.23 ± 1.65	0.69 ± 0.49
UCLA GIT 2.0 constipation	1.27 ± 0.67	1.31 ± 0.68	1.21 ± 0.68
UCLA GIT 2.0 subscales			
Reflux	1.01 ± 0.69	1 ± 0.76	1.02 ± 0.63
Bloating	1.48 ± 0.9	1.5 ± 0.97	1.46 ± 0.85
Fecal soilage	0.51 ± 0.91	0.61 ± 1.02	0.38 ± 0.77
Diarrhea	0.22 ± 0.41	0.34 ± 0.47	0.08 ± 0.28
Social activities	0.72 ± 0.59	0.83 ± 0.68	0.59 ± 0.44
Emotional wellbeing	0.77 ± 0.78	0.86 ± 0.85	0.67 ± 0.71

Values expressed as mean ± standard deviation except where otherwise indicated. *SSc* systemic sclerosis, *lcSSc* limited cutaneous SSc, *ANA* antinuclear antibodies, *ACA* anticentromere antibodies, *Topo I* anti-Topomerase I antibodies, *GERD* gastroesophageal reflux disease, *UCLA GIT* University of California Los Angeles gastrointestinal tract questionnaire

*$p < 0.05$ vs Arm 1

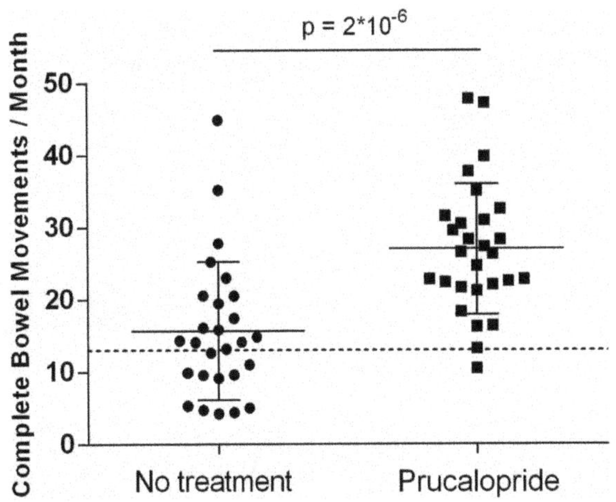

Fig. 2 Effect of prucalopride on defecation. Number of complete spontaneous bowel movements recorded by patients during the 1-month consumption of prucalopride 2 mg/day or the 1-month period without treatment. The plot represents the values adjusted for the mean of used laxatives. *Dashed lines* indicate the occurrence of ≥3 evacuations/week (12/month)

Table 3 Effect of treatment

Variable	Change with prucalopride[a]	Change without treatment[a]	Effect size[a]	Rating[b]	p
Likert GERD	-0.678 ± 0.108	-0.001 ± 0.114	-0.677	NA	$7.8*10^{-5}$
Likert constipation	-1.282 ± 0.155	0.135 ± 0.158	-1.417	NA	$2.01*10^{-7}$
UCLA GIT 2.0	-0.147 ± 0.061	0.021 ± 0.063	-0.168	Same	0.047
UCLA GIT 2.0 Constipation	-0.672 ± 0.112	0.086 ± 0.115	-0.758	Much better	$5.4*10^{-5}$
UCLA GIT 2.0 Subscales					
Reflux	-0.409 ± 0.094	0.01 ± 0.096	-0.419	Better	0.003
Bloating	-0.418 ± 0.088	-0.084 ± 0.09	-0.334	Better	0.011
Fecal soilage	-0.097 ± 0.133	0.074 ± 0.141	-0.171	Same	0.38
Diarrhea	0.367 ± 0.093	0.089 ± 0.097	0.277	Worse	0.053
Social activities	-0.106 ± 0.11	-0.006 ± 0.112	-0.1	Better	0.503
Emotional wellbeing	-0.214 ± 0.093	0.017 ± 0.093	-0.231	Same	0.051

Change in specific scales and scores used to evaluate gastro-intestinal involvement in the period after treatment (prucalopride) or in the no-treatment 4-week periods. Values presented as estimated marginal mean ± estimated standard error corrected for the number of laxatives. *GERD* gastroesophageal reflux disease, *UCLA GIT* University of California Los Angeles gastrointestinal tract questionnaire, *NA* not available. [a]Negative values indicate improvement. [b]Interpretation of treatment effect size according to [30]

and bloating could be rated as "somewhat better" (Table 3). Out of the 29 patients, 20 (69%) had changes in the UCLA GIT 2.0 constipation scores greater than the lower bound of the 95% confidence interval for marked responses [30]. Accordingly, prucalopride was ranked as moderately to extremely effective by 22 patients (72.4%) (extremely effective = 34.5%; quite effective = 37.9%; moderately effective = 20.7%; little effective = 6.9%). A reduction in the subjective grading of constipation was observed in patients in the active treatment arm, while at the end of the no-treatment period they mostly reported no change in the severity of constipation (Fig. 3).

OCTT is favorably influenced by prucalopride and correlates with the number of CSBMs

Sixteen patients participated in the LBT substudy and had complete LBT evaluations before and after the treatment/no treatment study periods. Baseline OCTT was 127 ± 70 minutes. One-month treatment with prucalopride led to a reduction in the OCTT that, on the contrary, increased in the no-treatment arm. Allowing for the order of treatment administration and the concurrent therapy with bisacodyl in the model, these differences were statistically significant in favor of the study drug (prucalopride: -20.1 ± 20.1 vs no-treatment: 45.8 ± 21.3 minutes; treatment effect = -65.9 minutes; $p = 0.035$). The change in the OCTT was an independent predictor of the number of complete bowel movements in a mixed model that accounted for the carry-over effect of the treatment and for the concurrent therapy with laxatives ($p = 0.011$) (direction of correlation: reduction in the OCTT, increase in the number of defecations). Similarly, changes in the perceived severity of constipation according to Likert scales directly correlated with changes in the OCTT ($p = 0.014$), yet there was no

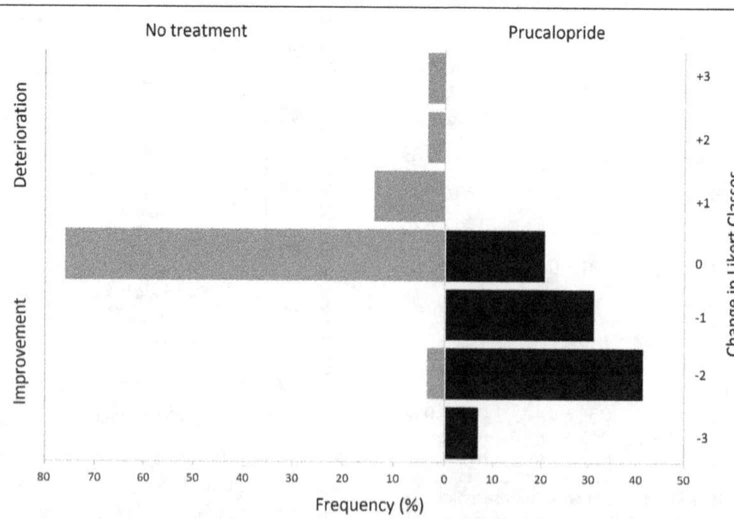

Fig. 3 Change in Likert scale for the evaluation of constipation. Change in the grading of the Likert scale for constipation at the end of the study periods. Negative values (*black bars*) indicate improvement; positive values (*gray bars*) indicate deterioration. Improvement was almost exclusively observed in patients in the active treatment arm

correlation with change in the UCLA GIT 2.0 constipation scores.

Discussion

The use of prokinetics has been advocated to treat enteric dismotility symptoms in SSc [8]; however, evidence in favor of this approach is lacking. In the EULAR recommendations for the treatment of SSc, the strength of the recommendation in favor of prokinetics is ranked as "C" due to the lack of proper controlled trials. The major source of evidence comes from studies on upper GIT disturbances treated with cisapride [8, 9], and there is just one report that this unselective 5-HT_4 receptor agonist may accelerate colonic transit in a small unselected case series of patients with SSc [10]. Safety issues related to this class of drugs that led to their marked withdrawal may have frustrated further attempts to study the potential of prokinetics in SSc-related enteric dismotility symptoms. However, it comes as a surprise that newer agents with no major cardiac issues have not been evaluated so far [12–14].

Our study clearly illustrates the beneficial effect of prucalopride in selected SSc patients with symptoms of constipation. In our work, we focused on patients with mild-to-severe colonic functional alterations, while we excluded patients with self-reported very severe dismotility symptoms. Indeed, in this subset of patients, prokinetics are likely to be ineffective due to end-stage fibrosis and the ablation of myenteric propulsive forces [6]. Despite these restrictions, constipation was quite severe in patients according to the average UCLA GIT 2.0 constipation scores [31] and to Likert scales, and considering the relevant number of cases (>50%) with fewer than three complete spontaneous bowel movements per week. All the aforementioned parameters used to evaluate the severity of constipation were positively affected by prucalopride. The UCLA GIT 2.0 constipation scores were markedly reduced after treatment, with an effect size that would classify the drug response as "much better" according to the minimally important differences of the UCLA GIT questionnaire [30]. Accordingly, about 70% of study participants ranked the efficacy of the treatment as very/extremely effective. Finally, the proportion of patients achieving ≥3 defecations per week, which is the threshold to define normal colonic function [21], was much higher in the treatment arm than in the non-treatment arm.

The improvement in colonic function that is observed after treatment with prucalopride is partially attributable to accelerated colonic transit times, as shown by the reduction in the OCTT in the LBT. These results are in accordance with a previous prucalopride study conducted in subjects with chronic constipation [32] according to the Rome III criteria [21], which we also used to select our patients. The correlation between the change in the subjective severity of constipation as measured by Likert scale (i.e. its improvement) or the increased number of defecations and an accelerated OCTT is also in accordance with the aforementioned work [32]. Of interest, in this report patients receiving placebo had increased OCTT and also in another report [33] dummy treatment was associated with a worsening of transit time. Therefore, the increase in OCTT we observed in the no-treatment arm is not surprising; however, we advise some caution in the interpretation of the results as the increase in OCTT in the no-treatment arm was a major contributor to the significance of results. Overall, considering the limited number of participants that completed this additional study procedure, OCTT results should be carefully gauged and considered mostly explorative.

Treatment with prucalopride was not only associated with an improvement in intestinal symptoms, including bloating, but also with a reduction in the subjective severity of GERD as assessed by the dedicated Likert scale and by the specific UCLA GIT 2.0 subscale. In a previous study prucalopride was shown to have no effect on the lower esophageal sphincter, esophageal motility or total reflux events; however, it was capable of improving acid clearance time and of increasing gastric emptying [34] contributing thus to the amelioration of GERD symptoms. These results are quite relevant considering that on average the severity of reflux in our population could be graded as severe to very severe in relation to the reflux UCLA GIT 2.0 subscale [31].

Despite its efficacy, treatment with prucalopride is characterized by a number of adverse events that precluded the prosecution of the treatment in 17.5% of patients. These figures are slightly worse, but substantially in accordance with previous phase III trials showing that discontinuation rates may be as high as 15% [17]. In relation to the study design, we cannot rule out the possibility that the large number of side effects we observed might somewhat be due to the open-label administration of the study drug. As in previous reports, in our study, many discontinuations were the consequence of adverse events that occurred on the first day of drug administration. Besides that, the increase in intestinal propulsive forces may promote defecation to such an extent that it may be perceived as diarrhoea, as indicated by the worsening of the specific UCLA GIT 2.0 subscale.

The major limitation of our study is the lack of a placebo arm, as patient-reported outcomes that constitute the core of our evaluation are largely subjective. This problem is partially addressed, yet incompletely circumvented by the OCTT substudy demonstrating the functional efficacy of prucalopride. Thus, the results of our research should be considered preliminary, yet our encouraging findings provide evidence and support for larger, controlled studies. Finally, our study does not address the question about the long-term efficacy of prucalopride and dose escalation to reduce side-effects and increase adherence to treatment.

Conclusions

Despite limitations linked to the nature of the study, prucalopride seems to be well-tolerated and effective in patients with SSc with mild to moderately severe constipation, favoring defecation, reducing bloating and ameliorating GERD. A careful evaluation of patients may be necessary to select those that may most benefit from this kind of treatment. Further larger and controlled studies may thus be warranted to address this issue and to assess the efficacy of prucalopride in a wider population of patients with scleroderma.

Abbreviations

5-HT_4: Serotonin; CSBMs: Complete spontaneous bowel movements; EULAR: European League Against Rheumatism; GERD: Gastroesophageal reflux disease; GIT: Gastrointestinal tract; LBT: Lactulose breath test; OCTT: Oro-cecal transit time; SD: Standard deviation; SSc: Systemic sclerosis

Acknowledgements

None.

Funding

This work was supported by Shire Pharmaceutical Development Ltd., Basingstoke, UK.

Authors' contributions

BV conducted the study procedures and drafted, reviewed and approved the manuscript; MC helped to conduct the study and reviewed and approved the manuscript; AS(1) helped to conducted the study and reviewed and approved the manuscript; CB helped to conduct the study and reviewed and approved the manuscript; ARB conducted the lactulose-breath test and reviewed and approved the manuscript; MF conducted the lactulose-breath test and reviewed and approved the manuscript; GM helped to conduct the study and reviewed and approved the manuscript; AS(2) helped to conducted the study and reviewed and approved the manuscript; LB designed the study, conducted the analyses and reviewed and approved the manuscript.

Competing interests

The authors declare that they have no competing interests.

Author details

[1]Scleroderma Unit, Referral Center for Systemic Autoimmune Diseases, Fondazione IRCCS Ca' Granda Ospedale Maggiore Policlinico di Milano, Via Pace 9, 20122 Milano, Italy. [2]Gastroenterology and Endoscopy Unit, Fondazione IRCCS Ca' Granda Ospedale Maggiore Policlinico di Milano, Via Francesco Sforza 35, Milano, Italy.

References

1. Gabrielli A, Avvedimento EV, Krieg T. Scleroderma. N Engl J Med. 2009;360:1989–2003.
2. Ebert EC. Gastric and enteric involvement in progressive systemic sclerosis. J Clin Gastroenterol. 2008;42:5–12.
3. Marie I, Levesque H, Ducrotté P, Denis P, Benichou J, Hellot MF, et al. Manometry of the upper intestinal tract in patients with systemic sclerosis: a prospective study. Arthritis Rheum. 1998;41:1874–83.
4. Henry MA, Harbermann MC, Rocha OM. Esophageal motor disturbances in progressive systemic sclerosis. Dis Esophagus. 1999;12:51–3.
5. McNearney TA, Sallam HS, Hunnicutt SE, Doshi D, Wollaston DE, Mayes MD, et al. Gastric slow waves, gastrointestinal symptoms and peptides in systemic sclerosis patients. Neurogastroenterol Motil. 2009;21:1269–e120.
6. Sjogren RW. Gastrointestinal motility disorders in scleroderma. Arthritis Rheum. 1994;37:1265–82.
7. Lindberg G, Törnblom H, Iwarzon M, Nyberg B, Martin JE, Veress B. Full-thickness biopsy findings in chronic intestinal pseudo-obstruction and enteric dysmotility. Gut. 2009;58:1084–90.
8. Kowal-Bielecka O, Fransen J, Avouac J, Becker M, Kulak A, Allanore Y, Distler O, Clements P, Cutolo M, Czirjak L, Damjanov N, Del Galdo F, Denton CP, Distler JHW, Foeldvari I, Figelstone K, Frerix M, Furst DE, Guiducci S, Hunzelmann N, Khanna D, Matucci-Cerinic M, Herrick AL, van den Hoogen F, van Laar JM, Riemekasten G, Silver R, Smith V, Sulli A, Tarner I, Tyndall A, Welling J, Wigley F, Valentini G, Walker UA, Zulian F, Müller-Ladner U; EUSTAR Coauthors. Update of EULAR recommendations for the treatment of systemic sclerosis. Ann Rheum Dis. 2016. doi:10.1136/annrheumdis-2016-209909. [Epub ahead of print] PubMed PMID: 27941129.
9. Kahan A, Chaussade S, Gaudric M, Freitag B, Amor B, Menkes CJ, et al. The effect of cisapride on gastro-oesophageal dysfunction in systemic sclerosis: a controlled manometric study. Br J Clin Pharmacol. 1991;31:683–7.
10. Wang SJ, Lan JL, Lan JL, Chen DY, Chen YH, Hsieh TY, et al. Effects of cisapride on colonic transit in patients with progressive systemic sclerosis. Clin Rheumatol. 2002;21:271–4.
11. Henney JE. From the Food and Drug Administration. JAMA. 2000;283:1131.
12. Keller GA, Di Girolamo G. Prokinetic agents and QT prolongation: a familiar scene with new actors. Curr Drug Saf. 2010;5:73–8.
13. Tack J, Camilleri M, Chang L, Chey WD, Galligan JJ, Lacy BE, et al. Systematic review: cardiovascular safety profile of 5-HT(4) agonists developed for gastrointestinal disorders. Aliment Pharmacol Ther. 2012;35:745–67.
14. Briejer MR, Bosmans JP, Van Daele P, Jurzak M, Heylen L, Leysen JE, et al. The in vitro pharmacological profile of prucalopride, a novel enterokinetic compound. Eur J Pharmacol. 2001;423:71–83.
15. Briejer MR, Prins NH, Schuurkes JA. Effects of the enterokinetic prucalopride (R093877) on colonic motility in fasted dogs. Neurogastroenterol Motil. 2001;13:465–72.
16. Camilleri M, Kerstens R, Rykx A, Vandeplassche L. A placebo-controlled trial of prucalopride for severe chronic constipation. N Engl J Med. 2008;358:2344–54.
17. Tack J, Camilleri M, Dubois D, Vandeplassche L, Joseph A, Kerstens R. Association between health-related quality of life and symptoms in patients with chronic constipation: an integrated analysis of three phase 3 trials of prucalopride. Neurogastroenterol Motil. 2015;27:397–405.
18. Coremans G. Prucalopride: the evidence for its use in the treatment of chronic constipation. Core Evid. 2008;3:45–54.
19. Mendzelevski B, Ausma J, Chanter DO, Robinson P, Kerstens R, Vandeplassche L, et al. Assessment of the cardiac safety of prucalopride in healthy volunteers: a randomized, double-blind, placebo- and positive-controlled thorough QT study. Br J Clin Pharmacol. 2012;73:203–9.
20. Boeckxstaens GE, Bartelsman JF, Lauwers L, Tytgat GN. Treatment of GI dysmotility in scleroderma with the new enterokinetic agent prucalopride. Am J Gastroenterol. 2002;97:194–7.
21. van den Hoogen F, Khanna D, Fransen J, Johnson SR, Baron M, Tyndall A, et al. 2013 classification criteria for systemic sclerosis: an American College of Rheumatology/European League Against Rheumatism collaborative initiative. Ann Rheum Dis. 2013;72:1747–55.
22. Longstreth GF, Thompson WG, Chey WD, Houghton LA, Mearin F, Spiller RC. Functional bowel disorders. Gastroenterology. 2006;130:1480–91.
23. McCrea GL, Miaskowski C, Stotts NA, Macera L, Hart SA, Varma MG. Review article: self-report measures to evaluate constipation. Aliment Pharmacol Ther. 2008;27:638–48.

24. European Medicines Agency (EMA), Committee for Medicinal Products for Human Use (CHMP): Guideline on the evaluation of medicinal products for the treatment of chronic constipation. Available at: http://www.ema.europa.eu/docs/en_GB/document_library/Scientific_guideline/2015/09/WC500193391.pdf. Accessed 12 June 2017.
25. Gualtierotti R, Ingegnoli F, Two R, Meroni PL, Khanna D, Adorni G, et al. Reliability and validity of the Italian version of the UCLA Scleroderma Clinical Trial Consortium Gastrointestinal Tract Instrument in patients with systemic sclerosis. Clin Exp Rheumatol. 2015;33:S55–60.
26. Yiannakou Y, Piessevaux H, Bouchoucha M, Schiefke I, Filip R, Gabalec L, et al. A randomized, double-blind, placebo-controlled, phase 3 trial to evaluate the efficacy, safety, and tolerability of prucalopride in men with chronic constipation. Am J Gastroenterol. 2015;110:741–8.
27. Jorge JM, Wexner SD, Ehrenpreis ED. The lactulose hydrogen breath test as a measure of orocaecal transit time. Eur J Surg. 1994;160:409–16.
28. Gasbarrini A, Corazza GR, Gasbarrini G, Montalto M, Di Stefano M, Basilisco G, et al. Methodology and indications of H2-breath testing in gastrointestinal diseases: the Rome Consensus Conference. Aliment Pharmacol Ther. 2009;29:1–49.
29. Wellek S, Blettner M. On the proper use of the crossover design in clinical trials: part 18 of a series on evaluation of scientific publications. Dtsch Arztebl Int. 2012;109:276–81.
30. Khanna D, Furst DE, Maranian P, Seibold JR, Impens A, Mayes MD, et al. Minimally important differences of the UCLA Scleroderma Clinical Trial Consortium Gastrointestinal Tract Instrument. J Rheumatol. 2011;38:1920–4.
31. Khanna D, Nagaraja V, Gladue H, Chey W, Pimentel M, Frech T. Measuring response in the gastrointestinal tract in systemic sclerosis. Curr Opin Rheumatol. 2013;25:700–6.
32. Emmanuel A, Cools M, Vandeplassche L, Kerstens R. Prucalopride improves bowel function and colonic transit time in patients with chronic constipation: an integrated analysis. Am J Gastroenterol. 2014;109:887–94.
33. Malpeli A, González S, Vicentin D, Apás A, González HF. Randomised, double-blind and placebo-controlled study of the effect of a synbiotic dairy product on orocecal transit time in healthy adult women. Nutr Hosp. 2012;27:1314–9.
34. Kessing BF, Smout AJ, Bennink RJ, Kraaijpoel N, Oors JM, Bredenoord AJ. Prucalopride decreases esophageal acid exposure and accelerates gastric emptying in healthy subjects. Neurogastroenterol Motil. 2014;26:1079–86.

5

The cumulative number of micro-haemorrhages and micro-thromboses in nailfold videocapillaroscopy is a good indicator of disease activity in systemic sclerosis: a validation study of the NEMO score

Romina Andracco[1], Rosaria Irace[2], Eleonora Zaccara[1], Serena Vettori[2], Wanda Maglione[1], Antonella Riccardi[2], Francesca Pignataro[1], Roberta Ferrara[2], Domenico Sambataro[1], Gianluca Sambataro[1], Claudio Vitali[3], Gabriele Valentini[2] and Nicoletta Del Papa[1*]

Abstract

Background: Some abnormalities in nailfold videocapillaroscopy (NVC), such as the presence of micro-haemorrhages (MHEs), micro-thromboses (MTs), giant capillaries (GCs) and reduction in the number of capillaries (nCs), suggest a disease activity (DA) phase in systemic sclerosis (SSc). In a previous paper, we showed that the number of micro-haemorrhages and micro-thromboses (the so-called NEMO score) was the NVC feature more closely associated with DA. The present study was aimed at validating the NEMO score as a measure of DA in patients with SSc.

Methods: Two cohorts of 122 and 97 patients with SSc who were referred to two different rheumatology units, one in Milan and one in Naples, respectively, constituted the validation cohorts. The NEMO score, the total number of GCs and the mean nCs per digit were the parameters defined in each patient by eight-finger NVC. An expert operator analysed the NVCs in each of the participating units. The European Scleroderma Study Group (ESSG) index was used to define the DA level in each patient at the time of NVC examination.

Results: The NEMO score was the NVC parameter more strictly correlated with the ESSG score in both the Milan and Naples cohorts ($p < 0.0001$), and it was the only one among the NVC variables that gave a significant contribution in a logistic model where the ESSG score represented the dependent variable. ROC curve analysis confirmed that the NEMO score had the best performance in measuring DA. The AUC of the NEMO score was significantly greater than the AUCs obtained by plotting the sensitivity and specificity of the number of GCs and the mean nCs ($p < 0.0001$ in all cases). The NEMO score values that showed the best sensitivity-specificity balance in capturing patients with a relevant DA level were slightly higher in the Naples cohort than in the Milan cohort.

Conclusions: This study confirms that the presence of a certain number of MHEs and MTs in NVC may be considered a strong warning signal of a current phase of DA in patients with SSc.

Keywords: Systemic sclerosis, Nailfold videocapillaroscopy, Disease activity

* Correspondence: nicoletta.delpapa@asst-pini-cto.it
[1]UOC Day Hospital of Rheumatology, Department of Rheumatology, ASST G. Pini-CTO, Milan, Italy
Full list of author information is available at the end of the article

Background

Nailfold videocapillaroscopy (NVC) is commonly considered as a feasible method that allows observation and follow-up, in an easily accessible capillary bed, of the micro-vascular changes that characterise the course of systemic sclerosis (SSc) [1]. Some peculiar NVC abnormalities, namely dilated capillaries and avascular areas, have been defined as closely associated with SSc, and consequently these NVC changes have been included as a separate item in the 2013 classification criteria for this disorder [2]. Furthermore, different NVC pictures have been described as potentially predictive of specific disease evolution and some disease-related manifestations [3, 4]. Finally, different NVC aspects have been proposed as being characteristic of the different phases of the disease. Therefore, early, active and late NVC patterns have been carefully described [1]. It has been suggested that the presence of numerous ectasic and giant capillaries (GCs), micro-haemorrhages (MHEs) and micro-thrombosis (MT), and the reduced number of capillaries (nCs) within scattered avascular areas characterise the active pattern [5, 6].

In a previous study, we investigated which of the abnormalities defining the active NVC pattern was more strictly predictive of disease activity (DA) [7]. To do that, we used the proposed and validated European Scleroderma Study Group (ESSG) index as the gold standard for defining DA [8, 9]. We finally demonstrated that the cumulative number of micro-haemorrhages and micro-thromboses (the so-called NEMO score), and to a lesser extent the number of GCs, were positively correlated with the ESSG index [7].

Following this preliminary cross-sectional study that indicates how computing the NEMO score may be a feasible, inexpensive, non-invasive method of measuring the level of DA in patients with SSc, we decided to carry out a second study to validate this new NVC parameter. The present study was performed in two cohorts of patients. The first one was prospectively collected in the centre where the preliminary study was carried out (internal validation cohort), and the second one was retrospectively analysed in a different centre (external validation cohort). The aim of the present study is to confirm the validity of the NEMO score as a measure of DA in SSc when different observers from those who took part in the previous study were asked to measure this NVC parameter. Furthermore, the validity of the NEMO score has been verified by comparing NVC data collected from prospectively enrolled patients in Milan with those derived from the retrospective analysis of stored NVC images of patients from a completely different cohort (Naples).

Methods

Patients

The validation cohorts were constituted of a cumulative number of 219 patients. All enrolled patients met the American College of Rheumatology/European League Against Rheumatism (ACR/EULAR) classification criteria for SSc [2], and they were also sub-classified as having limited cutaneous systemic sclerosis (lcSSc) or diffuse cutaneous systemic sclerosis (dcSSc) following the LeRoy et al. criteria [10]. Exclusion criteria were concomitant conditions that may potentially cause additional microvascular changes, such as diabetes, smoking and onychophagic habitus; presence of anti-phospholipid antibodies; and pregnancy. Current treatment with beta-blockers was also an exclusion criterion because it is well known that this drug may cause or exacerbate Raynaud's phenomenon (RP).

At the time of study enrolment, 52 of the 219 patients were receiving treatment with infusions of intravenous prostanoids (45 with monthly iloprost and 7 with weekly alprostadil), and 16 were taking bosentan. It was decided for ethical reasons to continue the vasodilatory treatments for the prospectively enrolled patients in Milan. Furthermore, all of the patients were receiving stable treatment with low-dose acetylsalicylic acid and calcium channel blockers.

One hundred twenty-two patients with SSc who were referred to the rheumatic disease unit of the Gaetano Pini Institute of Milan formed the prospectively collected internal validation cohort. It was preliminarily established to consecutively include around half the patients with inactive disease (ESSG score <3 and a similar proportion of patients with active disease [ESSG score ≥3]). This cohort did not include any patient who had been recruited for the previous study [7].

Ninety-seven patients with SSc who were referred to the rheumatology unit of the 2nd University of Naples formed the external validation cohort. These patients and their NVC images were randomly selected from the database on the condition that about one-third of them should have an ESSG score ≥3.

Clinical work-up and assessment of disease activity

The ESSG index was taken as the reference tool (gold standard) for DA assessment. This is a composite scoring system that includes a number of clinical, laboratory and instrument items [8, 9]. According to the ESSG indications, a score ≥3.5 is considered to have good sensitivity and specificity in characterising patients with a high DA level, and a cut-off value of 3.0 [8, 9] also allows capture of patients with a moderate level of DA. The clinical data needed for the ESSG score definition were to be collected within the same month as the NVC examination.

Experienced physicians other than those who performed the NVC were in charge of calculating the modified Rodnan skin score (mRSS). It is well known that the mRSS is a valid and reliable method of assessing skin involvement in SSc and is also closely related to the skin histological features [11–13].

Nailfold videocapillaroscopy

RA in Milan and RI in Naples were the two investigators responsible for performing and revising the NVC examinations of all the patients in their own centres. Because it is well known that inter-observer reliability is commonly unsatisfactory in medical imaging evaluations, including NVC [14], and because the level of agreement can be improved, even between expert observers, by establishing more precise criteria in pre-study consensus meetings [14, 15], the investigators of the two participating centres entrusted with the task of analysing the NVC images took part in a meeting in Milan before the beginning of the study. During this meeting, these investigators established the precise methodology with which to perform the NVC examination and then performed a pre-test for inter-observer reliability using a series of stored NVC pictures obtained from 30 patients.

The same video capillaroscope with a × 200 magnification lens was used in both centres to examine the nailfold capillaries of all fingers of both hands, excluding thumbs, of each patient. Each digit was positioned in such a way that the capillaroscopic light was 90 degrees incident on the centre of the nailfold. Four consecutive 1-mm fields, for a total extension of 4 mm in the middle of the nailfold, were examined. The derived digital images were stored and analysed using dedicated software (VideoCap; Scalar Co. Ltd., Tokyo, Japan).

For each patient, the following NVC parameters were considered, and the related scores were computed:

1. The NEMO score was calculated by counting the total number of MHEs and MTs observed in the images obtained from the eight fingers of both hands of each patient and defined as the NEMO score. A score of 1 was given to each separate MHE and MT, independently of its size.
2. The GC score was calculated as the total number of GCs found in the eight examined digits. A GC was defined as dilated capillaries with a maximum diameter over 50 μm [16].
3. The nC score was derived by calculating the mean nCs per digit, considering all the NVC fields examined in each finger. The capillary count had to include normal, slightly dilated and ectasic capillaries. The ectasic capillaries were the largely dilated ones, but with a maximum diameter ≤50 μm.

Examples of NVC pictures showing an example of a GC and dilated capillaries are shown in Fig. 1a and b. Figure 1c and d show NVC pictures with a high and low number of MHEs and MTs. The respective NEMO and ESSG scores are also reported.

Statistical methods

Statistical analysis was performed according to standard procedures using IBM SPSS® Statistics version 21 software (IBM, Armonk, NY, USA) and the MedCalc software package, 2014 version (MedCalc® Inc., Ostend, Belgium). Non-parametric tests were used to perform the statistical analysis of the different NVC variables and ESSG scores for DA. This was decided because all the considered NVC variables showed that they did not have a normal distribution (Shapiro-Wilk test, $p < 0.05$ in all the cases). Logistic regression models were built to test the contribution of defined values of NEMO, GC and nC scores in predicting the presence of DA according to the predefined ESSG cut-off value ≥3.

ROC curves were constructed, and the AUC was calculated by plotting the sensitivity and specificity values of the NEMO, GC and nC scores in correctly classifying patients with defined levels of DA. The Hanley-McNeil test was applied to verify the presence of a significant difference between the AUCs obtained by the analysis of different NVC items.

Cohen's *k* statistics were applied to evaluate the inter-observer level of agreement in the pre-test study on the assessment of NVC abnormalities. No correction of the statistical results was made for the presence of missing values, because there were no missing data in our database. Bonferroni's correction for multiple comparisons was also applied when indicated.

Ethical rules

This study was conducted according to the Helsinki declaration and approved by the ethics committee of the Azienda Socio Sanitaria Territoriale Lombardia Centro Specialistico Ortopedico Traumatologico Gaetano Pini of Milan and the 2nd University of Naples, where the study was carried out and where all the study patients included in the two cohorts were recruited. Written informed consent was obtained from all of the enrolled patients.

Results

The level of agreement between the observers from the two participating centres, which was assessed in the pre-test assay, was good for the NEMO score and number of GCs ($k = 0.75$ and 0.68, respectively) and moderate ($k = 0.56$) when the mean nC value was computed. The internal validation cohort included 122 patients with SSc, of whom 60 and 62 had the

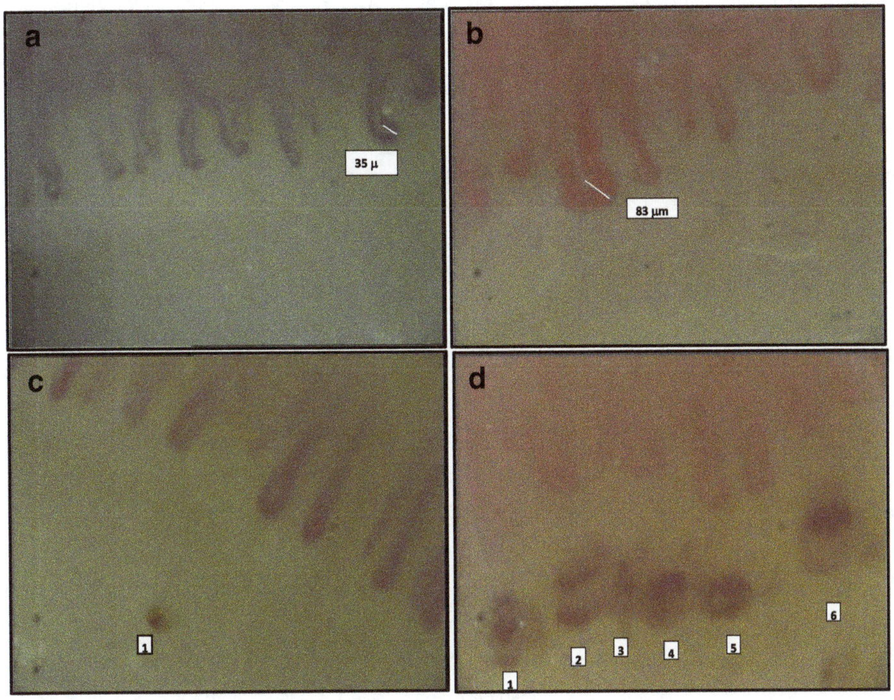

Fig. 1 Different nailfold videocapillaroscopic (NVC) features observed in our patients with systemic sclerosis. **a** and **b** A series of dilated capillaries. **a** None of the observed capillaries reaches the limit of 50 μm and so were not defined as giant capillaries (GCs), the larger one having a diameter of 35 μm. **b** One of these capillaries has a diameter of 83 μm, so it can be classified as a GC. **c** An NVC picture where one deposit of hemosiderin (*1*) indicating a previous micro-haemorrhage is present distal to the capillaries aligned in the cuticle. Multiple micro-thromboses are evident in the largely dilated capillaries, and a hemosiderin deposit can be observed distally in the right side of (**d**), just distal to capillary *6*. In (**c**) and (**d**), the number of micro-haemorrhages and micro-thromboses scores were 2 and 49, and the European Scleroderma Study Group index scores were 1 and 7, respectively

limited cutaneous and the diffuse cutaneous variants of SSc, respectively. Ninety-seven patients, of whom 72 and 25 were classified as having lcSSc and dcSSc, respectively, made up the external validation cohort. The main demographic, clinical and serological features of the two populations were separately analysed and compiled and are reported in Table 1. The disease duration appears to be lower in the Milan cohort than in the Naples cohort, but this difference did not reach statistical significance ($p = 0.06$).

It is worth noting that anti-centromere antibodies (ACAs) were largely predominant in the Naples cohort and that anti-Scl-70 antibodies more frequently found in the Milan cohort. This is a largely expected result when one considers the different prevalence of lcSSc and dcSSc in the two cohorts (Table 1). Of course, the composition of the two cohorts in terms of clinical subsetting may also be responsible for the different prevalence of some specific clinical features we found in the Milan cohort compared with the Naples cohort (Table 1). Furthermore, these differences can also be ascribed to the fact that patients with active disease (i.e., patients with an ESSG score ≥3) were more prevalent in the Milan cohort than in the Naples cohort (Table 1).

Despite the fact that patients with more active disease and a greater number of patients with dcSSc were present in the Milan cohort, there were no differences in either the ESSG or NEMO scores between the two cohorts ($p = 0.2$ and 0.08, respectively). The distribution of values of the NEMO score was slightly different, however. The highest NEMO score values were recorded in the Milan cohort, whereas values <7 points were found in 40% and 28% of patients in the Milan and Naples cohorts, respectively. Moreover, no differences in the NEMO and ESSG score values were observed, when we considered all the patients of the two cohorts together, between patients with lcSSc and dcSSc with ACAs and anti-Scl-70 antibodies.

In both cohorts, we found that a very strong correlation existed between the NEMO and ESSG scores. A weaker correlation was also present between the ESSG score and the number of GCs in both cohorts, whilst the mean nC score did not correlate with the ESSG score in the Milan cohort and was negatively correlated with the DA score in the Naples cohort (*see* Table 2). Both NEMO and ESSG score values showed a significant negative correlation with disease duration in the Milan cohort (Spearman's $r = -0.38$ and -0.35, respectively;

Table 1 Main demographic data and clinical and laboratory features composing the European Scleroderma Study Group index among patients enrolled in both the internal (Milan) and external (Naples) cohorts

	Milan cohort	Naples cohort	All patients
Number of patients	122	97	219
Male/female ratio	8/114	9/88	17/202
Median age, years (range)	52 (17–82)	55 (19–79)	54 (17–82)
Median disease duration, years (range)	4 (0–28)	6 (0–36)	5 (0–36)
lcSSc/dcSSc	60/62	72/25	132/87
Autoantibodies			
ACAs	57	53	110
Anti-Scl-70	58	22	80
Others	7	22	29
ESSG index ≥3, *n* (%)	57 (46.8)	30 (30.9)	87 (39.7)
ESSG index ≥3.5, *n* (%)	49 (40.2)	20 (20.6)	69 (31.5)
Mean mRSS (range)	5.9 (0–22)	3.4 (0–23)	4.6 (0–23)
Scleroderma, *n* (%)	74 (60.7)	17 (17.5)	91 (41.5)
Change in skin involvement[a], *n* (%)	35 (28.7)	23 (23.7)	58 (26.4)
Ulcers, *n* (%)	34 (27.9)	11 (11.3)	45 (20.5)
Change in vascular features[a,b], *n* (%)	56 (46.7)	19 (19.5)	75 (34.2)
Arthritis, *n* (%)	30 (24.6)	7 (7.2)	37 (16.8)
DLCO <80%, *n* (%)	86 (71.3)	85 (87.6)	171 (78)
Change in cardiopulmonary features[a,c], *n* (%)	25 (20.5)	19 (19.5)	44 (20)
ESR >30 mm/h, *n* (%)	33 (27)	35 (36)	68 (31.1)
Low complement, *n* (%)	15 (12.3)	13 (13.4)	28 (12.7)

Abbreviations: ACAs Anti-centromere antibodies, *DLCO* Diffusing capacity of the lung for carbon monoxide, *ESR* Erythrocyte sedimentation rate, *ESSG* European Scleroderma Study Group, *dcSSc* Diffuse cutaneous systemic sclerosis, *lcSSc* Limited cutaneous systemic sclerosis, *mRSS* Modified Rodnan skin score
Data are expressed as number of patients (percent), unless otherwise specified
[a]Difference with respect to previous observation
[b]Change in vascular features was defined as subjective feeling of worsening of vascular manifestations (namely Raynaud's phenomenon)
[c]Change in cardiopulmonary features was defined as subjective feeling of worsening of cardiopulmonary manifestations (namely dyspnoea)

$p < 0.0001$ in both cases). This kind of correlation was not confirmed in the Naples cohort. The same significant negative correlation between disease duration and both NEMO and ESSG scores was found when all the patients with dcSSc in the two cohorts were pooled together ($r = -0.39$, $p < 0.0002$, and $r = -0.40$, $p < 0.0001$, respectively). The same finding was not confirmed when all the patients of the two cohorts with lcSSc were analysed.

On the basis of these results, and considering that the aim of our study was simply to validate an NVC scoring system that could predict the presence of a certain degree of DA in all the patients with SSc independently of their clinical subset, we decided to build a logistic regression model in which only the NVC variables (i.e., the NEMO score, CG counts and mean nCs) were considered as independent variables, whereas the presence of an ESSG score ≥3 represented the dependent variable. Only the NEMO score had a significant predictive value for the presence of at least a moderate level of DA in the logistic model constructed for both the Milan and Naples cohorts (*see* Table 3).

ROC curves were built by plotting the sensitivity and specificity of the NEMO scores, the number of GCs and

Table 2 Correlation between capillaroscopic parameters and European Scleroderma Study Group index score for disease activity

	ESSG score vs NEMO score	ESSG score vs GC count	ESSG score vs capillary count
Milan cohort	$r = 0.69$, $p < 0.0001$	$r = 0.30$, $p < 0.001$	$r = 0.18$, $p =$ n.s.
Naples cohort	$r = 0.76$, $p < 0.0001$	$r = 0.39$, $p < 0.0005$	$r = -038$, $p < 0.0005$

Abbreviations: ESSG European Scleroderma Study Group index, *GC* Giant capillary, *NEMO* Number of micro-haemorrhages and micro-thromboses, *n.s.* Not significant
r = the correlation coefficient by Spearman's rank correlation. p Values were corrected for multiple comparisons by Bonferroni's method

Table 3 Logistic regression models where number of micro-haemorrhages and micro-thromboses score, giant capillary count and mean number of capillaries were tested as combined predictors of disease activity (European Scleroderma Study Group index score ≥3)

Cohort	Coefficient ± SE	*p* Value	Odds ratio (95% CI)
Milan cohort			
NEMO score	0.36 ± 0.07	<0.0001	1.43 (1.24–1.66)
GC count	−0.002 ± 0.05	0.96	0.99 (0.91–1.09)
Mean number of capillaries	0.14 ± 0 ± 0.01	0.16	1.15 (0.95–1.40)
Constant	−4.19		
Naples cohort			
NEMO score	0.51 ± 0.12	<0.0001	1.67 (1.32–2.11)
GC count	−0.15 ± 0.19	0.45	0.86 (0.59–1.26)
Mean number of capillaries	−0.33 ± 0.22	0.12	0.71 (0.47–1.10)
Constant	−2.90		

Abbreviations: GC Giant capillary, *NEMO* Number of micro-haemorrhages and micro-thromboses

mean nCs in correctly classifying patients with either ESSG scores ≥3 or ≥3.5 for both the Milan and Naples cohorts (Fig. 2).

In all cases, the AUC of the NEMO score was significant greater than those designed by plotting both the GC counts and mean nCs (always $p < 0.0001$). Conversely, no differences were found when we compared the AUC of GCs and mean nCs of both cohorts (*see* Fig. 2).

The best performance in terms of sensitivity/specificity ratio in predicting the different levels of DA was obtained in the Milan cohort when the NEMO scores were ≥8 for an ESSG score ≥3. In the Naples cohort, these results differed slightly because the best performance in predicting an ESSG score ≥3 was observed with a NEMO score ≥11 (Table 4). The possibility that these differences could be related to the different ratios of patients with lcSSc and dcSSc in the two cohorts (*see* Table 1) being taken into account. However, there were no differences in the NEMO score between the patients with lcSSc and dcSSc in both cohorts when they were separately analysed and considered as a whole.

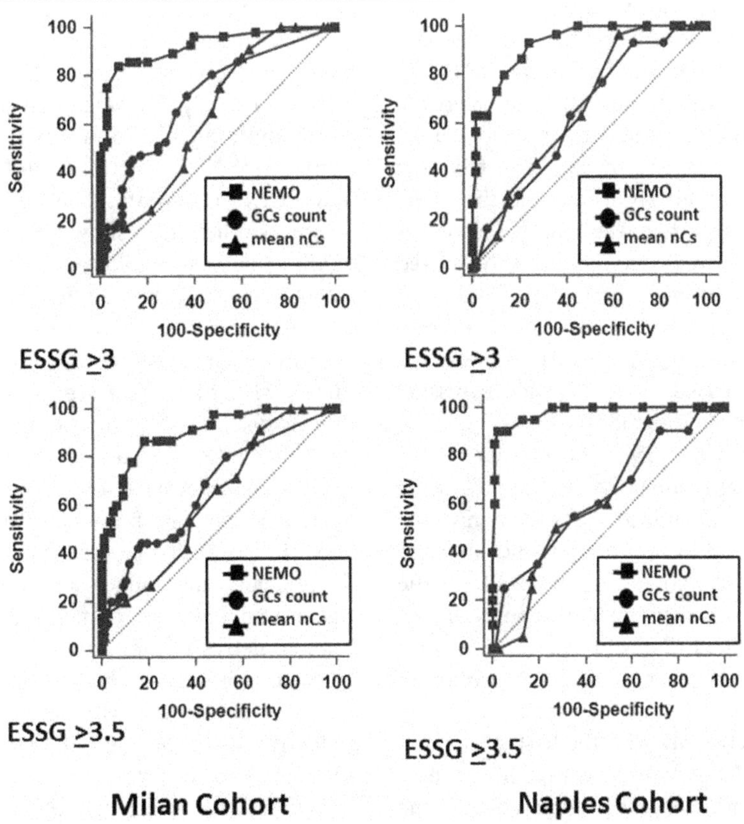

Fig. 2 ROC curves built by plotting the sensitivity and specificity values of the number of micro-haemorrhages and micro-thromboses (NEMO) score (*squares*), giant capillary (GC) count (*circles*), and mean number of capillaries (nCs; *triangles*) in correctly classifying patients with either European Scleroderma Study Group (ESSG) index scores ≥3 or ≥3.5 are shown for both the Milan (*left*) and Naples (*right*) cohorts. In both cohorts, the AUC of the NEMO score was always significantly greater than the AUCs designed by plotting both the GC counts and the mean nCs ($p < 0.0001$). Conversely, no differences were found when we compared the AUC of the GC and capillary counts of both cohorts

Table 4 Number of micro-haemorrhages and micro-thromboses scores having best performance in terms of sensitivity/specificity ratio in predicting different degrees of disease activity according European Scleroderma Study Group index score cut-off values

Cohort	Score cut-off values	
Milan cohort	NEMO score ≥8 for ESSG score ≥3	NEMO score ≥9 for ESSG score ≥3.5
	Sensitivity 86.0 (95% CI 74.2–93.7) Specificity 87.7 (95% CI 77.2–94.5)	Sensitivity 86.7 (95% CI 73.2–94.9) Specificity 81.8 (95% CI 71.4–89.7)
Naples cohort	NEMO score ≥11 for ESSG score ≥3	NEMO score ≥15 for ESSG score ≥3.5
	Sensitivity 80.0 (95% CI 61.4–92.3) Specificity 86.6 (95% CI 76.0–93.7)	Sensitivity 90.0 (95% CI 68.3–98.8) Specificity 97.4 (95% CI 90.9–99.7)

ESSG European Scleroderma Study Group, *NEMO* Number of micro-haemorrhages and micro-thromboses

Discussion

In this study, we confirmed that the presence of a given NEMO score is highly indicative of an active phase of SSc. Even the presence of a sufficient number GCs may suggest the presence of DA, although the correlation is stronger for the former NVC abnormality.

The present results may contribute to validating our previous study confirming that a defined level of NEMO score could represent a warning signal that may alert the physician to the possibility that the patient under observation may be in an active phase of SSc. The fact that the correlation between the NEMO score and the ESSG scale also remains strong when the NEMO score is derived by different observers on the basis of stored images and images directly taken of real patients reinforces the validity of this new NVC parameter as a measure of DA. In a previous paper, we also proposed a modified NEMO score based on a logistic regression model where GCs also made a significant contribution to identifying patients with active SSc. The present results did not confirm this, because after constructing the same logistic model in both examined cohorts, only the presence of MHEs and MTs appeared to be effective in capturing patients with active SSc (Table 3). In the previous study, however, the performance in terms of accuracy of the modified NEMO score was not significantly different from that of a simple count of MHEs and MTs (the NEMO score).

The levels of the NEMO score with the best sensitivity/specificity ratio in identifying patients with active disease were slightly different in the two cohorts. However, if one considers this score as a feasible, non-invasive and relatively inexpensive method of suspecting a phase of DA in SSc, this difference actually can be considered marginal. This concept seems to be reinforced by the fact that a NEMO score ≥8 has sensitivity in capturing active patients of 86.0% in the Milan cohort and 96.7% in the Naples cohort, albeit with an expected difference in specificity (87.7% and 69.2% in the Milan and Naples cohorts, respectively).

Besides the known existence of a certain inter-rater variability in NVC evaluation between observers [14], the reasons why the NEMO score demonstrated different performance in the two cohorts in measuring DA remains purely speculative at the moment. This result does not appear to be related to existing differences in the levels of the ESSG score, the prevalence of different disease subsets and their associated serological markers between the cohorts in Milan and Naples. The fact that both ESSG and NEMO scores were closely related to disease duration in the Milan cohort but not in the Naples cohort can be ascribed to the higher prevalence of patients with dcSSc in the Milan cohort. A confirmation of this comes from the evidence that similar negative correlations were also found in the totality of the patients with dcSSc, but not in that of the patients with lcSSc, when the two cohorts were pooled together. The lcSSc and dcSSc variants certainly have differences in their pathological mechanisms, clinical expression and disease course. It is well known dcSSc can be a more aggressive condition where active phases are commonly more concentrated in the early phase of the disease [10, 17]. However, to our knowledge, no specific longitudinal studies have been performed so far comparing NVC pictures and their evolution over time in two different subsets of SSc.

Some studies have shown that the clinical expression of SSc may vary in different geographical areas [18, 19]. RP, including RP related to SSc, may have a different presentation pattern in terms of the number and severity of episodes in relation to seasonal changes and local climate [18–20]. There are no specific surveys demonstrating that the NVC patterns may change in populations that differ because of ethnic origin or geographic localization. However, climate is certainly different in Milan and Naples, particularly for the lower temperatures in winter in Milan, which has a Continental climate, and the longer summer season, with usually higher temperatures, that characterises Naples, around 800 kilometres farther south. How these climatic differences may influence the NVC pattern and the natural course of SSc in the patients referred to the two rheumatologic units in the present study is a completely unknown issue at present.

NVC is a feasible technique widely used in the diagnostic approach [1] and in disease monitoring for patients with SSc [4]. A relevant prognostic value has also been ascribed to NVC, and different NVC patterns have been defined as being predictive of a worse outcome [21]. Finally, different NVC features have been proposed as characteristic of the early, active and late phases of disease [1, 6]. In particular, the features that define the active disease phase are the presence of MHEs and GCs together with an initial loss of capillaries.

It is not absolutely surprising that MHEs and MTs were the NVC abnormalities more closely related to DA when one considers the present knowledge on the small vessel vasculopathy of SSc. SSc is commonly defined as a disease of the micro-vascular bed of the skin compartment, but potentially involving the small vessels of internal organs. The endothelial involvement is believed to be the first step of the pathological process in SSc, whereas homing of mononuclear inflammatory cells in the interstitium, activation of myofibroblast and fibroblast lineage, together with the consequent fibrotic changes, could be considered as the following evolutionary changes [22, 23]. The typical response to the initial micro-vascular damage and capillary loss in SSc is the compensatory dilation of remaining capillary loops, sometimes with the appearance of formation of GCs. In late disease, enlarged capillaries are much less frequently found, whereas an evident capillary loss and the appearance of vascular areas are the most typical NVC features.

In progressive disease, the destiny of enlarged capillaries is thrombotic obliteration followed by extravasation [24, 25]. When these phenomena are synchronous, several extravasations with hemosiderin deposits aligned in the cuticle distal from capillary areas can be observed by NVC.

Koenig et al. [26] described the appearance of dilated capillaries as an early event, whereas loss of capillaries and telangiectases were observed later. This is partially in contrast with our findings, suggesting that GCs may appear early together with the other enlarged capillaries. However, it has been reported that the observation of enormous GCs in the late phase of the disorder is not a rare finding [25]. This NVC feature may correspond to the stable telangiectases that can often be observed in the skin of patients with late SSc. Of course, some differences between Koenig's survey and the present study can be largely explained by the different structure of the two studies. The first one was a longitudinal study aimed at investigating NVC changes during the evolution from isolated RP to overt SSc [26]. The present one is a cross-sectional study aimed at understanding which of the NVC features can be more indicative of an active phase of the disease in patients with already defined SSc. Therefore, the terms *early* and *late* may not have equal meaning because of the differences in the design of the two studies.

The finding that the presence of a given amount of MHEs and MTs (more closely than that of GCs) predicts that the DA phases in SSc may simply indicate that these abnormalities could represent the NVC aspects corresponding to the evolution of microvascular involvement in the active phases of the disease. It is self-evident that DA in SSc is characterised and conditioned by a large number of other, more complex and still poorly understood pathological mechanisms [21, 22].

The present study confirms that the NEMO score can be considered a feasible and valid method of identifying patients with SSc who may cross a phase of DA. Of course, this kind of suspicion should be confirmed by an accurate clinical and instrumental work-up of the observed patient. Nevertheless, NEMO score assessment might help the clinician in measuring DA when other items are not available. In this respect, a longitudinal study where the NEMO score and level of DA may be contemporaneously measured along the disease course in a large series of patients is certainly needed to definitively confirm the utility of such a simple NVC scoring system, not only as a steady-state scoring system of DA but also as a reliable transition index to be applied in the follow-up of patients with SSc.

The comparison between the internal and external validation cohorts examined in the study may suggest that the NVC abnormalities could be influenced by some environmental factors, and consequently the NEMO score levels that can identify active patients should be verified at all centres. EULAR Scleroderma Trials and Research Group investigators recently identified and validated a new activity index that performs better than the previous ESSG activity index used in this study and in the previous one [27]. A study has just been set up in our centres to investigate the relationships between the NEMO score and the revised activity index.

Conclusions

The present study confirms that the presence of a certain NEMO score in NVC may be considered as an indirect measure of a current phase of DA in patients with SSc. Even the presence of a sufficient number GCs may suggest the presence of DA, although the correlation is stronger for the former NVC abnormality. These results contribute to validating our previous study by demonstrating that the presence of a defined number of MHs and MTs (the so-called NEMO score) could represent a warning signal that may alert the physician to the possibility that the patient under observation may be in an active phase of SSc.

Abbreviations

ACA: Anti-centromere antibodies; ACR/EULAR: American College of Rheumatology/European League Against Rheumatism; DA: Disease activity; dcSSc: Diffuse cutaneous systemic sclerosis; DLCO: Diffusing capacity of the lung for carbon monoxide; ESR: Erythrocyte sedimentation rate; ESSG: European Scleroderma Study Group; GC: Giant capillary; lcSSc: Limited cutaneous systemic sclerosis; MHE: Micro-haemorrhage; mRSS: Modified Rodnan skin score; MT: Micro-thrombosis; nC: Number of capillaries; NEMO: Number of micro-haemorrhages and micro-thromboses; NVC: Nailfold videocapillaroscopy; RP: Raynaud's phenomenon; SSc: Systemic sclerosis

Acknowledgements

Not applicable.

Funding
No funding was received for this study.

Authors' contributions
RA and RI made substantial contributions to acquisition of capillaroscopic data. EZ, SV, WM, AR, FP, RF, and NDP made substantial contributions to acquisition of clinical data. DS and GS contributed to study conception and design. RA, RI, CV, NDP, and GV made substantial intellectual contributions to study conception and data interpretation, and they helped draft and revise the manuscript for important intellectual content. RA, RI, EZ, SV, WM, AR, FP, RF, DS, GS, CV, NDP, and GV agree to be accountable for all aspects of the work in ensuring that questions related to the accuracy or integrity of any part of the work are appropriately investigated and resolved. RA, RI, EZ, SV, WM, AR, FP, RF, DS, GS, CV, NDP, and GV read and approved the final manuscript.

Authors' information
RA, RI, EZ, WM, AR, FP, RF, DS, GS, CV, NDP, and GV hold MD degrees; SV holds MD and PhD degrees.

Competing interests
The authors declare that they have no competing interests.

Author details
[1]UOC Day Hospital of Rheumatology, Department of Rheumatology, ASST G. Pini-CTO, Milan, Italy. [2]Rheumatology Unit, Department of Internal Medicine, 2nd University of Naples, Naples, Italy. [3]Section of Rheumatology, Villa San Giuseppe, Istituto Santo Stefano, Como, Italy.

References

1. Cutolo M, Pizzorni C, Secchi ME, Sulli A. Capillaroscopy. Best Pract Res Clin Rheumatol. 2008;22:1093–108.
2. Van den Hoogen F, Khanna D, Fransen J, Johnson SR, Baron M, Tyndall A, et al. 2013 Classification criteria for systemic sclerosis: an American College of Rheumatology/European League Against Rheumatism Collaborative Initiative. Arthritis Rheumatol. 2013;65:2737–47.
3. Ingegnoli F, Boracchi P, Gualtierotti R, Lubatti C, Meani L, Zahalkova L, et al. Prognostic model based on nailfold capillaroscopy for identifying Raynaud's phenomenon patients at high risk for the development of a scleroderma spectrum disorder. Arthritis Rheumatol. 2008;58:2174–82.
4. Sulli A, Secchi ME, Pizzorni C, Cutolo M. Scoring the nailfold microvascular changes during the capillaroscopic analysis in systemic sclerosis patients. Ann Rheum Dis. 2008;67:885–7.
5. Corrado A, Carpagnano GE, Gaudio A, Foschino-Barbaro MP, Cantatore FP. Nailfold capillaroscopic findings in systemic sclerosis related lung fibrosis and in idiopathic lung fibrosis. Joint Bone Spine. 2010;77:570–4.
6. Cutolo M, Sulli A, Pizzorni C, Accardo S. Nailfold videocapillaroscopy assessment of microvascular damage in systemic sclerosis. J Rheumatol. 2000;27:155–60.
7. Sambataro D, Sambataro G, Zaccara E, Maglione W, Polosa R, Afeltra AMV, et al. Nailfold videocapillaroscopy micro-haemorrhage and giant capillary counting as an accurate approach for a steady state definition of disease activity in systemic sclerosis. Arthritis Res Ther. 2014;16:462.
8. Valentini G, Della Rossa A, Bombardieri S, Bencivelli W, Silman AJ, D'Angelo S, et al. European multicentre study to define disease activity criteria for systemic sclerosis. II. Identification of disease activity variables and development of preliminary activity indexes. Ann Rheum Dis. 2001;60:592–8.
9. Valentini G, Bencivelli W, Bombardieri S, D'Angelo S, Della Rossa A, Silman AJ, et al. European multicentre study to define disease activity criteria for systemic sclerosis. III. Assessment of the construct validity of the preliminary activity criteria. Ann Rheum Dis. 2003;62:901–3.
10. LeRoy EC, Black C, Fleischmajer R, Jablonska S, Krieg T, Medsger Jr TA, et al. Scleroderma (systemic sclerosis): classification, subset and pathogenesis. J Rheumatol. 1988;15:202–5.
11. Cutolo M, Sulli A, Smith V. How to perform and interpret capillaroscopy. Best Pract Res Clin Rheumatol. 2013;27:237–48.
12. Clements PJ, Lachenbrunch PA, Seibold JR, Zee B, Steen VD, Brennan P, et al. Skin thickness score in systemic sclerosis: an assessment of interobserver variability in 3 independent studies. J Rheumatol. 1993;20:1892–6.
13. Furst DE, Clements PJ, Steen VD, Medsger Jr TA, Masi AT, D'Angelo WA, et al. The modified Rodnan skin score is an accurate reflection of skin biopsy thickness in systemic sclerosis. J Rheumatol. 1998;25:84–8.
14. Smith V, Beeckman S, Herrich AL, Decuman S, Deschepper E, De Keyser F, et al. An EULAR study group pilot study on reliability of simple capillaroscopic definitions to describe capillary morphology in rheumatic diseases. Rheumatology (Oxford). 2016;55:883–90.
15. Oudkerk SF, de Jong PA, Attrach M, Luijkx T, Buckens CF, Mali WPTM, et al. Diagnosis of diffuse idiopathic skeletal hyperostosis with chest computed tomography: inter-observer agreement. Eur Radiol. 2017;27:188–94.
16. Olski TM, Hunzelmann N, Krieg T. The skin in systemic scleroderma. In: Sarzi-Puttini P, Doria A, Girolomoni G, Kuhn A, editors. Handbook of autoimmune diseases. Volume 5: The skin in systemic autoimmune diseases. London: Elsevier; 2006. p. 119–33.
17. Domsic RT, Rodriguez-Reyna T, Lucas M, Fertig N, Medsger Jr TA. Skin thickness progression rate: a predictor of mortality and early internal organ involvement in diffuse scleroderma. Ann Rheum Dis. 2011;70:104–9.
18. Walker UA, Tyndall A, Czirják L, Denton CP, Farge-Bancel D, Kowal-Bielecka O, et al. Geographical variation of disease manifestations in systemic sclerosis: a report. Ann Rheum Dis. 2009;68:856–62.
19. Watson HR, Robb R, Belcher G, Belch JJ. Seasonal variation of Raynaud's phenomenon secondary to systemic sclerosis. J Rheumatol. 1999;26:1734–7.
20. Maricq HR, Carpentier PH, Weinrich MC, Keil JE, Palesch Y, Biro C, et al. Geographic variation in the prevalence of Raynaud's phenomenon: a 5 region comparison. J Rheumatol. 1997;24:879–89.
21. Zufferey P, Depairon M, Chamot AM, Monti M. Prognostic significance of nailfold capillary microscopy in patients with Raynaud's phenomenon and scleroderma pattern abnormalities: a six-year follow-up study. Clin Rheumatol. 1992;11:536–41.
22. Kahaleh B. The microvascular endothelium in scleroderma. Rheumatology (Oxford). 2008;47:14–5.
23. Gabrielli A, Avvendimento EV, Krieg T. Scleroderma. N Engl J Med. 2009;360: 1989–2003.
24. Grassi W, Del Medico P. Microbleeding and capillary thrombosis. In: Grassi W, Del Medico P, editors. Atlas of capillaroscopy. Milan, Italy: EDRA Medical Publishing & New Media; 2004. p. 122–30.
25. Wong ML, Highton J, Palmer DG. Sequential nailfold capillary microscopy in scleroderma related disorders. Ann Rheum Dis. 1988;47:53–61.
26. Koenig M, Joyal F, Fritzler MJ, Roussin A, Abrahamowicz M, Boire G, et al. Autoantibodies and microvascular damage are independent predictive factors for the progression of Raynaud's phenomenon to systemic sclerosis: a twenty-year prospective of 586 patients with validation of proposed criteria for early systemic sclerosis. Arthritis Rheum. 2008;58:3902–12.
27. Valentini G, Iudici M, Walker UA, Jaeger VK, Baron M, Carreira P, et al. The European Scleroderma Trials and Research group (EUSTAR) task force for the development of revised activity criteria for systemic sclerosis: derivation and validation of a preliminarily revised EUSTAR activity index. Ann Rheum Dis. 2016;76:270–6.

6

Anti-connective tissue growth factor (CTGF/CCN2) monoclonal antibody attenuates skin fibrosis in mice models of systemic sclerosis

Katsunari Makino[1], Tomoko Makino[1], Lukasz Stawski[1], Kenneth E. Lipson[2], Andrew Leask[3] and Maria Trojanowska[1*]

Abstract

Background: Systemic sclerosis (SSc) is characterized by fibrosis of the skin and internal organs. Although the involvement of connective tissue growth factor (CTGF/CCN2) has been well-documented in SSc fibrosis, the therapeutic potential of targeting CTGF in SSc has not been fully investigated. Our aim was to examine the therapeutic potential of CTGF blockade in a preclinical model of SSc using two approaches: smooth muscle cell fibroblast-specific deletion of CTGF (CTGF knockout (KO)) or a human anti-CTGF monoclonal antibody, FG-3019.

Methods: Angiotensin II (Ang II) was administered for 14 days by subcutaneous osmotic pump to CTGF KO or C57BL/6 J mice. FG-3019 was administered intraperitoneally three times per week for 2 weeks. Skin fibrosis was evaluated by histology and hydroxyproline assay. Immunohistochemistry staining was used for alpha smooth muscle actin (αSMA), platelet-derived growth factor receptor β (PDGFRβ), pSmad2, CD45, von Willebrand factor (vWF), and immunofluorescence staining was utilized for procollagen and Fsp1.

Results: Ang II-induced skin fibrosis was mitigated in both CTGF KO and FG-3019-treated mice. The blockade of CTGF reduced the number of cells expressing PDGFRβ, procollagen, αSMA, pSmad2, CD45, and Fsp1 in the dermis. In addition, inhibition of CTGF attenuated vascular injury as measured by the presence of vWF-positive cells.

Conclusions: Our data indicate that inhibition of CTGF signaling presents an attractive therapeutic approach in SSc.

Keywords: Angiotensin II, CTGF/CCN2, FG-3019, Fibrosis, Skin, Systemic sclerosis

Background

Systemic sclerosis (SSc) is a multisystem connective tissue disorder that typically results in fibrosis of the skin and internal organs [1]. SSc is characterized by autoimmunity, inflammation, and widespread microvascular injury, leading to the activation of fibroblasts and excessive accumulation of extracellular matrix (ECM) proteins; however, the causes and the pathogenesis of this disease are not yet fully explained [2]. Accumulation of ECM proteins restricts normal function of the affected tissues and organs leading to high morbidity and mortality. Despite significant improvements in the management of SSc, effective disease modifying therapies are not yet available.

Connective tissue growth factor (CTGF, also known as CCN2), a member of the CCN family of matricellular proteins, is widely known as a hallmark of fibrosis in multiple tissues, including skin, heart, lung, liver, and kidney [3, 4]. A key study in support of the essential role of CTGF in fibrosis was published by Takehara and colleagues who showed that subcutaneous injection of transforming growth factor (TGF)-β and CTGF led to sustained fibrosis, while either factor alone failed to do so [5]. Further support was provided by a recent study that showed that fibroblast-specific ablation of CTGF inhibited development of dermal fibrosis in the bleomycin injection model [6]. The role of CTGF in fibrosis

* Correspondence: trojanme@bu.edu
[1]Arthritis Center, Boston University School of Medicine, 72 East Concord Street, E-5, Boston, MA 02118, USA
Full list of author information is available at the end of the article

may not be limited to its function as a co-factor of TGF-β, but CTGF may also regulate other aspects of the fibrogenic process, consistent with its multifunctional nature [7, 8]. Accordingly, it has been suggested that CTGF may contribute to myofibroblast recruitment during bleomycin-induced skin fibrosis [6]. Transgenic mice overexpressing CTGF develop skin fibrosis and microvascular abnormalities [9], and loss of CTGF results in a reduction of bleomycin-induced skin fibrosis [6].

Accumulating reports show that CTGF is highly expressed in SSc [10]. Elevated levels of CTGF have been identified in fibrotic skin and serum from patients with SSc, and have been correlated with the severity of skin and lung fibrosis [11, 12]. Elevated CTGF protein expression has been observed in fibroblasts in affected skin in SSc [13]. Furthermore, N-terminal cleavage products of CTGF have been identified in interstitial fluid in the skin of patients with SSc [14].

Given the key role of CTGF in the development of skin fibrosis in SSc, the goal of this study was to evaluate the efficacy of FG-3019 as a potential therapeutic agent for SSc using a murine model of angiotensin II (Ang II)-induced skin fibrosis [15–17]. FG-3019 is a fully human monoclonal antibody specific for CTGF [18]. Clinically, FG-3019 is being evaluated for treatment of idiopathic pulmonary fibrosis, pancreatic cancer, and Duchenne muscular dystrophy [19–21]. In parallel studies, we employed mice with smooth muscle cell fibroblast-specific deletion of CTGF to assess the contribution of CTGF to the process of skin fibrosis in the Ang II model [6]. Together, these studies showed that FG-3019 was comparable to genetic CTGF deletion in attenuating skin fibrosis. The results of this study support the use of FG-3019 as therapy for skin fibrosis.

Methods

Reagents

A fully human IgG1kappa monoclonal antibody recognizing domain 2 of human and rodent CTGF (FG-3019) and whole human IgG control antibody were obtained from Fibrogen (San Francisco, CA, USA).

Mice

Smooth muscle cell fibroblast-specific CTGF knockout (KO) mice were generated as described [6]. In brief, mice with CTGF flanked by loxP sites were crossed with mice containing a Cre recombinase gene located downstream of a collagen α2 (I) promoter enhancer that confers fibroblast-specific gene expression. The expression of Cre is dependent on the presence of tamoxifen. Tamoxifen was diluted in corn oil to 10 mg/ml. Three-week-old mice were given intraperitoneal injections of the tamoxifen suspension (100 μl of 10 mg/ml) over 10 days. Three weeks later, the mice were used for further studies. We used mice homozygous for CTGF gene flanked by loxP sites and heterozygous for Cre as CTGF KO mice. Littermate mice homozygous for loxP-flanked CTGF that were wild for Cre (non Cre) were used as control mice. C57BL/6 J mice for FG-3019 injection were purchased from the Jackson Laboratory (Bar Harbor, ME, USA). All mice experiments were performed in accordance with the National Institutes of Health and institutional guidelines for animal care, and approved by the Committee on the Ethics of Animal Experiments of the Boston University (Protocol AN-15037).

Cell culture and immunoblotting

Mouse dermal fibroblasts were obtained from skin from the backs of male CTGF KO and control littermate mice. Fibroblasts between the third and fifth sub passages were used for experiments. Mouse dermal fibroblasts were lysed and subjected to immunoblotting, as described previously [22]. Primary antibodies used were (1:1000): CTGF from Santa Cruz Biotechnology (Dallas, TX, USA) and β-actin from Sigma (St. Louis, MO, USA).

Ang II-induced dermal fibrosis

Alzet osmotic miniature pumps (Model 1002, DURECT, Cupertino, CA, USA) delivering Ang II (EMD Millipore, Billerica, MA, USA) at a rate of 1000 ng/kg/min (pressor dose) or PBS, were implanted subcutaneously on the back of 8-week-old mice, as described previously [17]. After 2 weeks, mice were euthanized and the skin surrounding the pump outlet was collected. FG-3019 (25 mg/kg) or control IgG (25 mg/kg) was administered intraperitoneally three times per week for 2 weeks, after the osmotic pump was installed.

Histologic assessment

Mice skin samples were paraffin-embedded, and sections (5 μm in thickness) were stained with hematoxylin and eosin (HE). Dermal thickness was evaluated by measuring the distance between the epidermal-dermal junction and the dermal-fat junction in HE sections. Skin trichrome staining was performed by Masson's trichrome stain kit (Polysciences, Warrington, PA, USA). The αSMA positive cells were counted in five random high-power fields using a light microscope. The mean score was used for analysis. The von Willebrand factor (vWF) staining intensity for immunohistochemical assessment was scored semi-quantitatively. The staining intensity (1: negative or weak staining, 2: moderate staining, and 3: strong staining) was evaluated in six randomly selected fields in the subcutaneous area. Then a semi-quantitative score per sample was generated by calculating the average of the six intensity scores per sample.

Hydroxyproline assay

Collagen deposition was determined by measuring total hydroxyproline content in 8-mm skin punch biopsies obtained from PBS and Ang II infusion sites as described previously [16]. Briefly, the skin samples were hydrolyzed with 6 M sodium hydroxide at 120 °C for 16 h. The hydrolysate was then oxidized with oxidation buffer (one part 7% chloramine T and four parts acetate citrate buffer) for 4 minutes at room temperature. Ehrlich's aldehyde reagent was added to each sample, and the chromophore was developed by incubating the samples at 60 °C for 25 minutes. Absorbance of each sample was read at 560 nm using a spectrophotometer. Results were expressed as relative hydroxyproline content. A standard curve was performed for all hydroxyproline measurements using known quantities of hydroxyproline.

Immunohistochemical assessment

For single antibody staining, formalin-fixed, paraffin-embedded 5-μm skin tissue sections were de-paraffinized and rehydrated through a graded series of ethanol. Antigens were retrieved by incubation with a proteinase K solution (EMD Millipore, Billerica, MA, USA) for 5 minutes. Blocking was done by 2.5% normal horse serum for 1 h. Tissue sections were then incubated with primary antibody to αSMA (1:100, Novus Biologicals, Littleton, CO, USA), PDGFRβ (1:50, Cell Signaling Technology, Danvers, MA, USA), rat anti-mouse CD45 Ab (1:100, BD Pharmingen, San Diego, CA, USA), phospho-Smad2 (Ser465/467) Ab (1:100, Cell Signaling), or vWF (1:1000, DAKO, Santa Clara, CA, USA) at 4 °C for 16 h. Next, sections were incubated with ImmPress horseradish peroxidase (HRP) anti-rabbit IgG (Vector Laboratories, Burlingame, CA, USA) for 30 minutes. The color was developed using 3,3-diaminobenzidine (DAB) substrate (DAKO). Immunohistochemical images were collected using a microscope (BH-2; Olympus, Center Valley, PA, USA).

Immunofluorescence staining

Staining was performed on 5-μm paraffin sections or cryosections. Slides were blocked with a blocking solution (3% BSA, and 0.2% Triton X-100 in PBS) for 2 h.

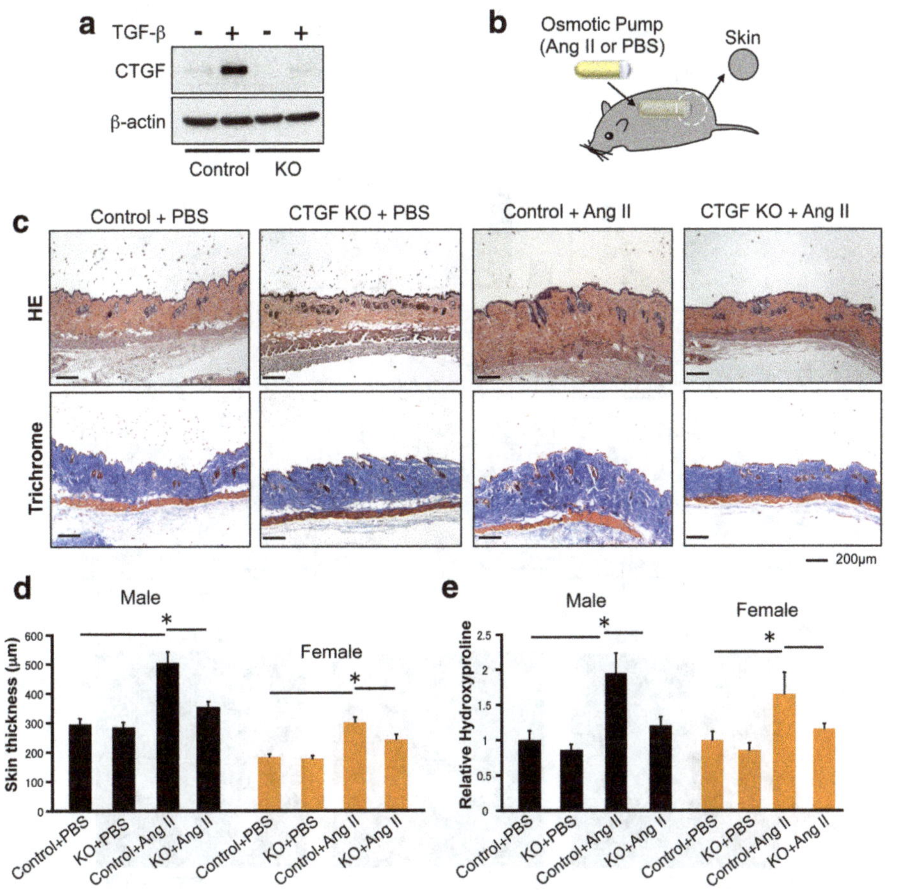

Fig. 1 Fibroblast-specific connective tissue growth factor (*CTGF*) knockout inhibits angiotensin II (*Ang II*)-induced skin fibrosis. **a** Mice skin fibroblasts from CTGF knockout (*CTGF KO*) and control mice were treated for 24 h with transforming growth factor beta 1 (*TGF-β1*) (2.5 ng/ml). Cell lysates were subjected to immunoblotting. **b** Skin fibrosis in mice was induced by Ang II administered via subcutaneously installed osmotic pumps. After 2 weeks, the skin surrounding the pump outlet was collected. **c** Mice skin sections were stained with HE and trichrome. *Scale bar* 200 μm. **d** Dermal thickness is summarized. **e** Collagen contents were measured by hydroxyproline assay. Values are normalized relative to the PBS control group. Each graph represents mean ± SD; n = 3 per group; *$P < 0.05$

Then, tissue sections were incubated at 4 °C overnight with primary antibodies: procollagen (*COL1A1* propeptide, 1:50, Thermo Fisher Scientific) for the cryosections and rabbit anti-mouse FSP1 (1:100, Abcam, Cambridge, MA, USA) for the paraffin sections. Secondary antibodies conjugated with Alexa 594 (Thermo Fisher Scientific) were used. Coverslips were mounted by using Vectashield with 4′,6-diamidino-2-phenylindole (DAPI) (Vector Laboratories, Burlingame, CA, USA). Fluorescence images were recorded with FV10i fluorescence microscope (Olympus, Tokyo, Japan).

Statistical analysis

Values are presented as means ± standard deviation (SD). One-way analysis of variance with Tukey-Kramer test was used to determine significant differences between more than two groups. Analyses were performed with Statcel software (OMS, Tokorozawa, Japan). Significance was defined as $P < 0.05$.

Results

Fibroblast-specific deletion of CTGF alleviates Ang II-induced skin fibrosis

To evaluate the therapeutic effects of CTGF blockade in the in vivo model of SSc, we used a mouse model of Ang II-induced skin fibrosis [17]. Ang II-induced skin fibrosis is accompanied by diverse pathogenic mechanisms, including collagen accumulation, CTGF upregulation, myofibroblast accumulation, endothelial cell injury, inflammation, and fibrosis [15–17]. In an initial experiment, we examined the

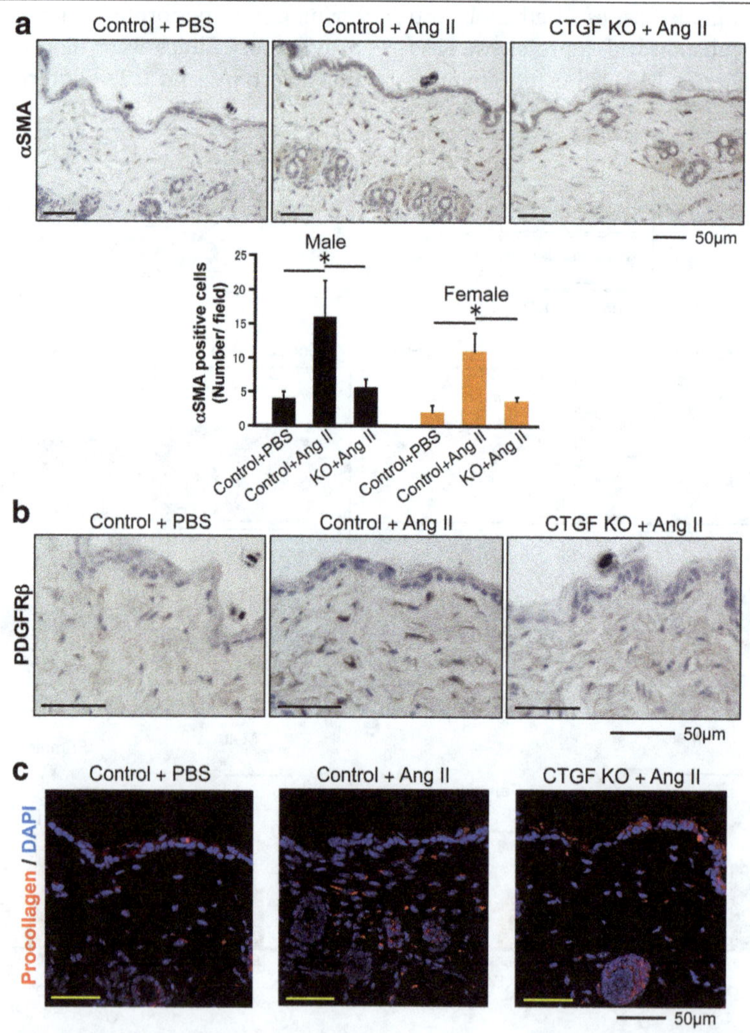

Fig. 2 Fibroblast-specific connective tissue growth factor knockout (*CTGF KO*) reduces alpha smooth muscle actin (α*SMA*)-positive cells number. **a** Skin sections were stained with anti-αSMA antibody. Representative images are shown. The αSMA-positive cells were counted in five random high-power fields using a light microscope. The mean score was used for analysis. Each graph represents mean ± SD. **b** Skin sections were stained with anti-platelet-derived growth factor receptor β (*PDGFR*β) antibody. Representative images are shown. **c** Immunofluorescent staining was performed on cryosections using procollagen antibody. Representative images are shown. *Scale bar* 50 μm; n = 3 per group; *$P < 0.05$. *DAPI* 4′,6-diamidino-2-phenylindole

contribution of CTGF to Ang II-induced skin fibrosis using mice with smooth muscle cell fibroblast-specific deletion of CTGF (CTGF KO mice). We observed >80% reduction in CTGF protein levels in skin fibroblasts cultured from CTGF KO mice when compared to control mice (Fig. 1a).

Because gender differences have been shown to affect pathogenic features, including the severity of fibrosis in SSc [23], we used both male and female mice in our experiments. CTGF KO and control male and female mice were then subjected to Ang II-induced skin fibrosis. Ang II or PBS was administered by subcutaneous osmotic pump, and the skin surrounding the pump outlet was collected on day 14 (Fig. 1b). In control mice, Ang II increased dermal thickness and the hydroxyproline content of lesional skin (Fig. 1c–e). Both male and female mice responded similarly to Ang II treatment. In contrast, male and female CTGF KO mice were resistant to the Ang II-induced changes (Fig. 1c–e). We next compared the number of αSMA-positive cells in the upper dermis of CTGF KO and control mice. The number of αSMA-positive cells in the upper dermis of CTGF KO mice challenged with Ang II was significantly decreased compared with control mice (Fig. 2a). Likewise, the number of PDGFRβ and procollagen positive cells were decreased in those mice (Fig. 2b and c). Collectively, these results indicated that CTGF is required for Ang II-induced skin fibrosis.

FG-3019 attenuates Ang II-induced skin fibrosis

We next investigated the effects of FG-3019 on Ang II-induced skin fibrosis. Ang II or PBS was administered by subcutaneous osmotic pump and FG-3019 (25 mg/kg) or control IgG (25 mg/kg) was administered intraperitoneally three times per week for 2 weeks. The skin surrounding the pump outlet was collected on day 14 (Fig. 3a). Treatment with FG-3019 significantly reduced dermal thickness and collagen content in skin from the backs of Ang II-challenged mice in both male and female animals (Fig. 3b and c). FG-3019 significantly decreased the number of αSMA-positive cells in the upper dermis of mice challenged with Ang II (Fig. 4a). FG-3019 also reduced PDGFRβ and procollagen expression in the upper dermis of mice challenged with Ang II (Fig. 4b and c). We only used male mice in subsequent experiments because we did not notice any apparent differences in responses to Ang II or the blockade of CTGF in male and female mice.

Inhibition of CTGF ameliorates activation of TGF-β signaling in Ang II-induced skin fibrosis

We have previously shown activation of the TGF-β signaling pathway in the skin of mice challenged with Ang II [17]. As reported, Ang II induced a significant increase in pSmad2-positive cells distributed throughout the dermis. However, the number of pSmad2-positive cells was

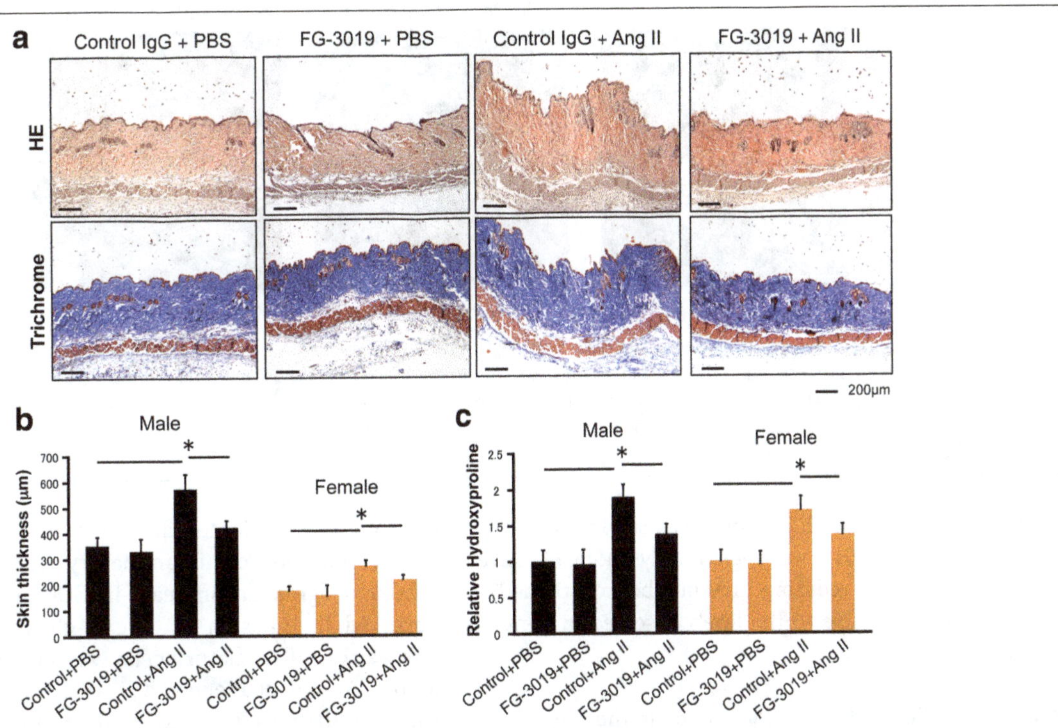

Fig. 3 FG-3019 ameliorates angiotensin II (*Ang II*)-induced skin fibrosis. **a** Mice skin sections were stained with HE and trichrome. *Scale bar* 200 μm. **b** Dermal thickness is summarized. **c** Collagen contents were measured by hydroxyproline assay. Values are normalized relative to the PBS control group. Each graph represents mean ± SD; n = 4 per group; *$P < 0.05$

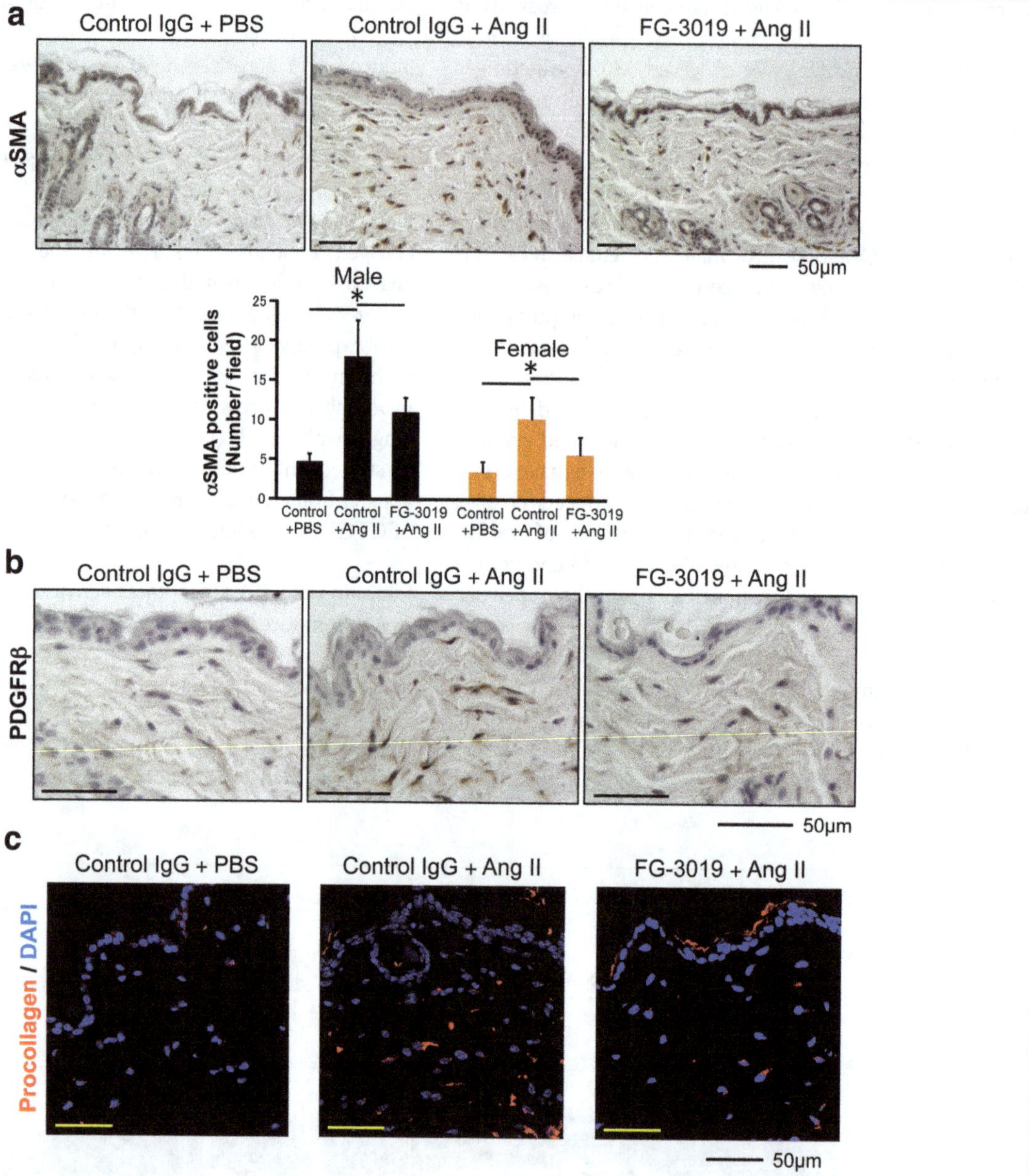

Fig. 4 FG-3019 reduces alpha smooth muscle actin (*αSMA*)-positive cell numbers. **a** Skin sections were stained with anti-αSMA antibody. Representative images are shown. The αSMA-positive cells were counted in five random high-power fields using a light microscope. The mean score was used for analysis. Each graph represents mean ± SD. **b** Skin sections were stained with anti-platelet-derived growth factor receptor β (*PDGFRβ*) antibody. Representative images are shown. **c** Immunofluorescent staining was performed on cryosections using procollagen antibody. Representative images are shown. *Scale bar* 50 μm; n = 4 per group; $^*P < 0.05$. *DAPI* 4′,6-diamidino-2-phenylindole

markedly reduced in CTGF KO mice (Fig. 5a). Interestingly, treatment with FG-3019 was significantly more effective than CTGF KO in reducing the number of pSmad2-positive cells comparable to the levels observed in control mice (Fig. 5b).

Inhibition of CTGF reduces inflammation in the skin of Ang II treated mice

Ang II-induced skin fibrosis is accompanied by the increased presence of inflammatory cells in the dermis [17]. We next evaluated the effect of CTGF blockade on the recruitment of inflammatory cells. As shown in Fig. 6a, a significant increase in CD45-positive cells was observed in the skin of Ang II-challenged mice. The number of inflammatory cells was significantly reduced in the Ang II-challenged CTGF KO mice. Treatment with FG-3019 was somewhat more efficient in reducing the number of CD45-positive cells; however, the difference between the two treatments was not statistically significant (Fig. 6b).

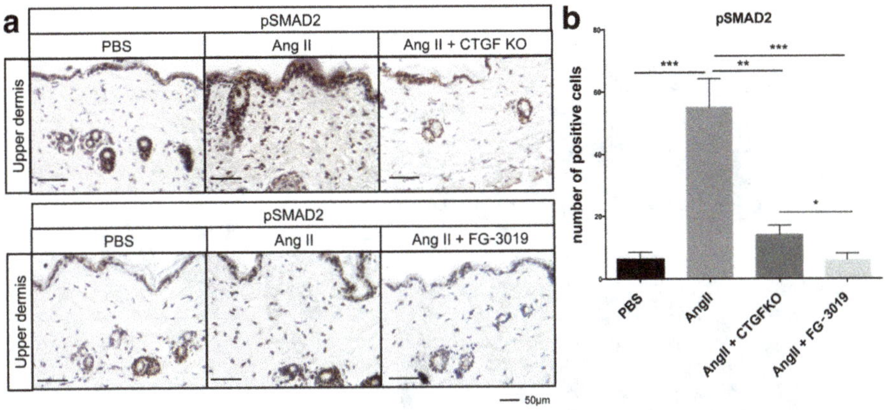

Fig. 5 Blockade of connective tissue growth factor (*CTGF*) reduces the number of pSmad-positive cells. **a** Representative results of immunostaining for pSmad2. *Scale bar* 50 μm. **b** The pSmad2-positive cells were counted in five random high-power fields using a light microscope. The mean score was used for analysis. Each graph represents mean ± SD; $^{*}P < 0.05$, $^{**}P < 0.01$, $^{***}P < 0.001$. *Ang II* angiotensin II, *KO* knockout

We have previously shown that the Ang II model of skin fibrosis is characterized by the infiltration of fibrocytes ($CD45^{+}/FSP1^{+}$ double-positive cells) [17]. Consistent with these findings, immunofluorescent staining showed numerous FSP1-positive cells in the dermis of Ang II-infused mice, while inhibition of CTGF significantly reduced their number (Fig. 7a and b). Both treatments similarly reduced fibrocyte infiltration.

Inhibition of CTGF reduces vascular damage in Ang II-induced skin fibrosis

Vascular damage is one of the key events in the pathogenesis of SSc. Mice challenged with Ang II develop prominent vascular injury [16]. We next examined whether inhibition of CTGF reduced vascular injury in this model. To evaluate the vascular injury, we used immunohistochemical staining of vWF, a widely used injury marker known to be elevated in SSc [24]. Consistent with the previous study [16], increased vWF staining was present in the dermal vessels of Ang II mice compared with the PBS control (Fig. 8a and b). The staining intensities were reduced in both CTGF KO and FG-3019-treated mice (Fig. 8a and b). Scoring of the staining intensity in the subcutaneous vessels and the representative images of each score (score 1–3) are shown in Fig. 8c. Although the intensity of vWF staining was significantly reduced in both CTGF KO and FG-3019-treated mice (Fig. 8d and e), the effect was more pronounced in CTGF KO mice.

Discussion

Currently, there are only limited treatment options for patients with SSc. Recent studies have provided evidence of an important role of CTGF in the development of organ fibrosis, including the skin [25]. Blockade of CTGF using the human anti-CTGF antibody, FG-3019,

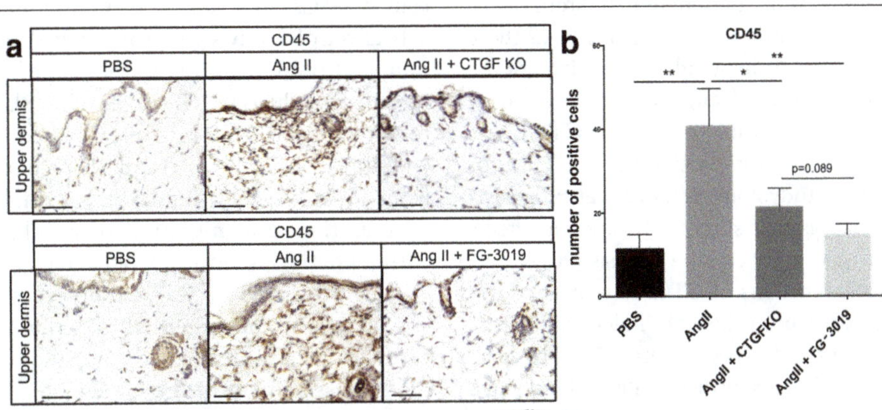

Fig. 6 Blockade of connective tissue growth factor (*CTGF*) reduces the number of CD45-positive cells. **a** Representative results of immunostaining for CD45. *Scale bar* 50 μm. The CD45-positive cells were counted in five random high-power fields using a light microscope. The mean score was used for analysis. Each graph represents mean ± SD; $^{*}P < 0.05$, $^{**}P < 0.01$. *Ang II* angiotensin II, *KO* knockout

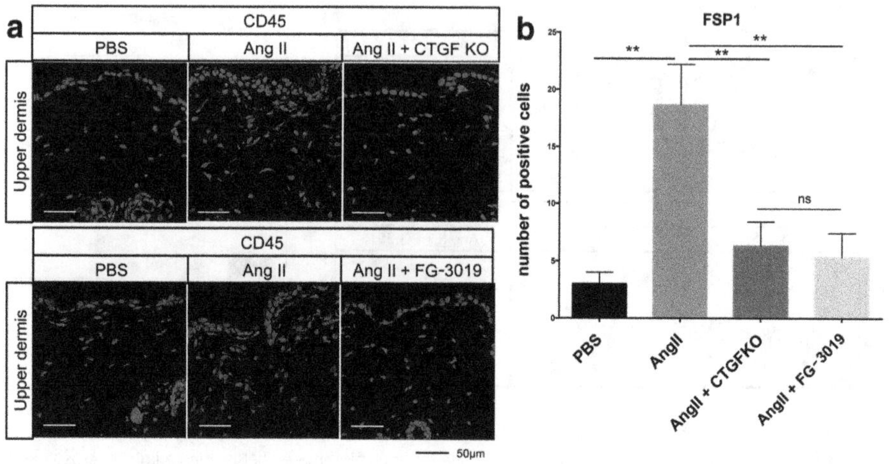

Fig. 7 Blockade of connective tissue growth factor (*CTGF*) reduces the number of Fsp1 positive cells. **a** Representative results of immunostaining for Fsp1. *Scale bar* 50 µm. **b** The Fsp1-positive cells were counted in five random high-power fields using a fluorescent microscope. The mean score was used for analysis. Each graph represents mean ± SD; *$P < 0.05$, **$P < 0.01$. *Ang II* angiotensin II, *KO* knockout

effectively prevented the development of skin fibrosis in response to Ang II challenge. The anti-fibrotic effect of FG-3019 was comparable to the genetic deletion of CTGF in collagen-producing cells. In addition, both treatments were very effective in reducing inflammation and lessening the damaging effects of Ang II on skin microvasculature.

The current study supports the findings of Liu et al. [6] who demonstrated the essential role of CTGF in bleomycin-induced fibrosis. In both studies, deletion of CTGF from fibroblasts and smooth muscle cells/pericytes prevented increased collagen deposition and myofibroblast accumulation in the skin. In addition, we also showed that blockade of CTGF significantly reduced the number of PDGFRβ-positive cells in the fibrotic lesion. Although the origin of these PDGFRβ collagen-producing cells in this model is not known, these cells may represent the expansion of local fibroblasts. Alternatively, they could originate from pericytes or mesenchymal stem cells. The role of CTGF in recruitment and expansion of these cells is not clear at present. Side by side comparison of the anti-fibrotic effects of FG-3019 and genetic deletion of CTGF showed that antibody directed against CTGF was comparable to CTGF deletion in blocking the CTGF profibrotic function in this study. Our results are also consistent with previous findings that showed therapeutic effects of FG-3019 in bleomycin-induced lung fibrosis [26].

Although profibrotic functions of CTGF are most widely recognized, CTGF has also been shown to induce inflammatory response in various cell types in vitro [7]. The proinflammatory role of CTGF was further confirmed in in vivo models of pancreatic and renal inflammation [27, 28]. In our model of Ang II-induced fibrosis, which is also characterized by increased inflammation, blockade of CTGF almost completely abrogated infiltration of inflammatory cells, including fibrocytes. Interestingly, treatment with FG-3019 appeared to be more potent than genetic CTGF deletion in reducing infiltration of CD45-positive cells and pSmad2 cells. However, both treatments were similarly effective in reducing the number of fibrocytes. These findings are consistent with a recent report that showed an inhibitory effect of FG-3019 on acute and delayed immune responses in a model of radiation-induced pulmonary fibrosis [29], where the effect appears to be indirect via modulation of myofibroblast activation and chemokine secretion (K. Lipson, personal communication). Thus, in this study, it is conceivable that blockade of CTGF inhibits recruitment of inflammatory cells from the circulation either by preventing secretion of the pro-inflammatory chemokines/cytokines by the activated resident cells or by reducing vascular injury and vessel permeability.

Ang II has a detrimental effect on the vasculature by affecting both endothelial and vascular smooth muscle cells (vSMCs) [30]. CTGF plays an important role in the activation of vSMCs by promoting their growth, migration, and production of collagen. Furthermore, Ang II is known to induce CTGF in vSMCs [8]. It has also been reported that CTGF is overexpressed in microvascular endothelial cells in SSc and that conditioned medium from microvascular endothelial cells stimulates the proliferation and migration of fibroblasts in SSc [31]. Although the association between CTGF and cardiovascular diseases is well-documented [8, 32], less is known about the potential contribution of CTGF to vascular disease in SSc. In this study, we performed a limited assessment of the effects of CTGF blockade on vascular damage by measuring the vascular injury marker, vWF. We showed that inhibition of CTGF partially reduced vWF expression. The effect was more pronounced in the CTGF KO than in FG-3019-treated

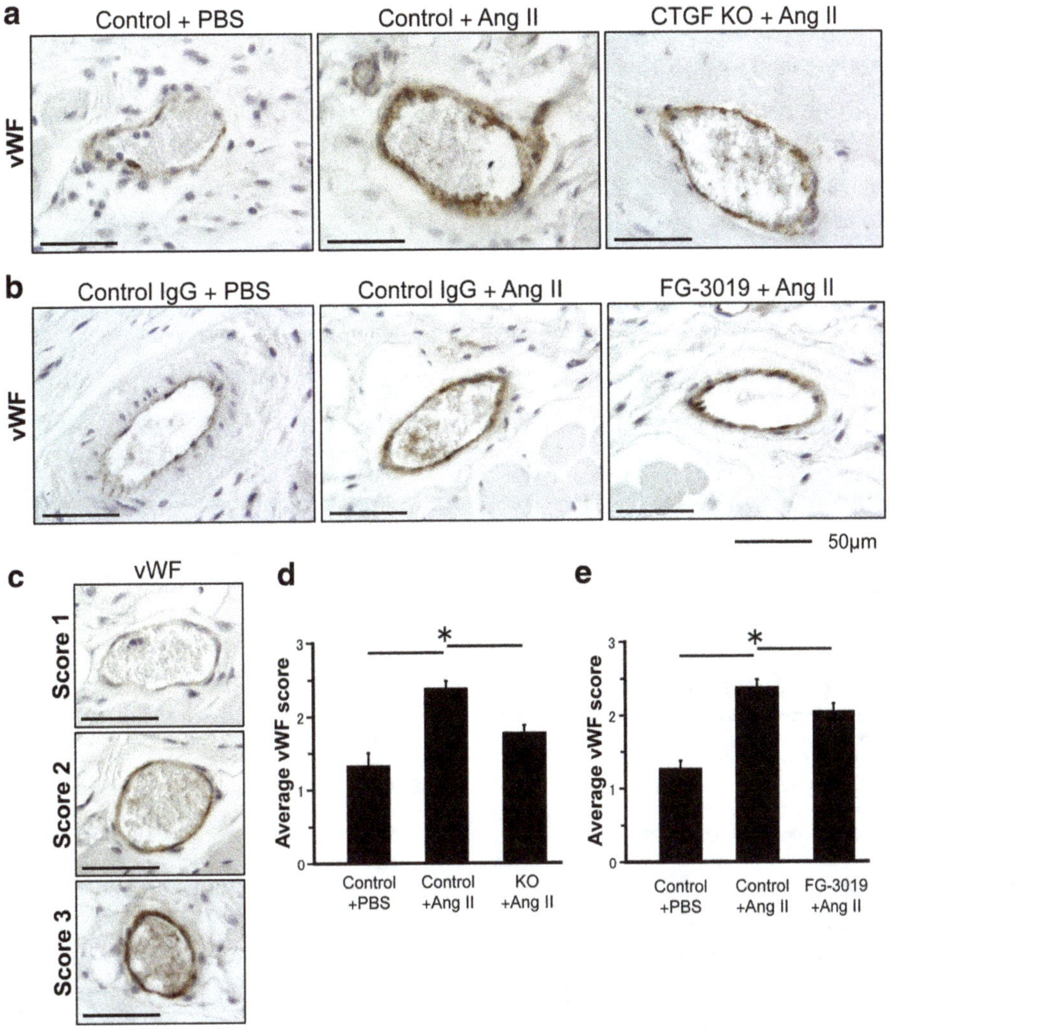

Fig. 8 Inhibition of connective tissue growth factor (*CTGF*) ameliorates vascular damage in angiotensin II (*Ang II*)-induced fibrotic skin. **a**, **b** Representative results of immunostaining for von Willebrand factor (*vWF*). *Scale bar* 50 μm. **c** Representative staining intensity (1: negative or weak staining, 2: moderate staining, and 3: strong staining). **d**, **e** Semi-quantitative vWF vascular staining scores. Each graph represents mean score ± SD; n = 3 per group; *$P < 0.05$. *KO* knockout

mice. Together, these data suggest that blockade of CTGF may have a beneficial effect on vascular injury. The limitation of this study is that it only assessed the preventive effect of FG-3019, and further studies are needed to evaluate whether FG-3019 is effective in reversing the established fibrosis. A phase II clinical trial evaluating FG-3019 as a treatment for idiopathic pulmonary fibrosis has recently been completed. Considering the anti-fibrotic effects of FG-3019 in the skin, our study strongly supports the testing of FG-3019 as a therapeutic agent for SSc dermal fibrosis.

Conclusions

We showed that FG-3019 is effective in reducing Ang II-induced inflammation and skin fibrosis in mice. FG-3019 also partially reduced the Ang II-induced vascular damage. This study supports the testing of FG-3019 as therapy for skin fibrosis in patients with SSc.

Abbreviations

Ang II: Angiotensin II; BSA: Bovine serum albumin; CTGF: Connective tissue growth factor; DAPI: 4′,6-Diamidino-2-phenylindole; ECM: Extracellular matrix; HE: Hematoxylin and eosin; KO: Knockout; PBS: Phosphate-buffered saline; PDGFRβ: Platelet-derived growth factor receptor β; SSc: Systemic sclerosis; vSMCs: vascular smooth muscle cells; vWF: von Willebrand factor; αSMA: Alpha smooth muscle actin

Acknowledgements

Not applicable.

Funding

This work was supported in part by the NIH NIAMS grant R01 AR44883 (MT).

Authors' contributions
KM and TM performed the research and wrote the manuscript. LS contributed to the experimental design and performed some experiments. AL contributed analytic tools. KL contributed reagents. MT was the principal investigator and was involved in conception and design of the study, data analysis, and manuscript writing. All authors read and approved the final manuscript.

Competing interests
K.E. Lipson is an employee of FibroGen, Inc. No other conflicts of interest exist for any of the authors other than K.E. Lipson.

Author details
[1]Arthritis Center, Boston University School of Medicine, 72 East Concord Street, E-5, Boston, MA 02118, USA. [2]FibroGen, Inc, San Francisco, CA, USA. [3]Departments of Dentistry and Physiology and Pharmacology, Schulich School of Medicine and Dentistry, University of Western Ontario, Dental Sciences Building, London, ON, Canada.

References

1. Allanore Y, Simms R, Distler O, Trojanowska M, Pope J, Denton CP, et al. Systemic sclerosis. Nat Rev Dis Primers. 2015;1:15002.
2. Lafyatis R. Transforming growth factor β–at the centre of systemic sclerosis. Nat Rev Rheumatol. 2014;10(12):706–19.
3. Leask A, Parapuram SK, Shi-Wen X, Abraham DJ. Connective tissue growth factor (CTGF, CCN2) gene regulation: a potent clinical bio-marker of fibroproliferative disease? J Cell Commun Signal. 2009;3(2):89–94.
4. Hall-Glenn F, Lyons KM. Roles for CCN2 in normal physiological processes. Cell Mol Life Sci. 2011;68(19):3209–17.
5. Mori T, Kawara S, Shinozaki M, Hayashi N, Kakinuma T, Igarashi A, et al. Role and interaction of connective tissue growth factor with transforming growth factor-β in persistent fibrosis: a mouse fibrosis model. J Cell Physiol. 1999;181(1):153–9.
6. Liu S, Shi-wen X, Abraham DJ, Leask A. CCN2 is required for bleomycin-induced skin fibrosis in mice. Arthritis Rheum. 2011;63(1):239–46.
7. Kular L, Pakradouni J, Kitabgi P, Laurent M, Martinerie C. The CCN family: a new class of inflammation modulators? Biochimie. 2011;93(3):377–88.
8. Ponticos M. Connective tissue growth factor (CCN2) in blood vessels. Vascul Pharmacol. 2013;58(3):189–93.
9. Sonnylal S, Shi-Wen X, Leoni P, Naff K, Van Pelt CS, Nakamura H, et al. Selective expression of connective tissue growth factor in fibroblasts in vivo promotes systemic tissue fibrosis. Arthritis Rheum. 2010;62(5):1523–32.
10. Rice LM, Ziemek J, Stratton EA, McLaughlin SR, Padilla CM, Mathes AL, et al. A longitudinal biomarker for the extent of skin disease in patients with diffuse cutaneous systemic sclerosis. Arthritis Rheumatol. 2015;67(11):3004–15.
11. Igarashi A, Nashiro K, Kikuchi K, Sato S, Ihn H, Fujimoto M, et al. Connective tissue growth factor gene expression in tissue sections from localized scleroderma, keloid, and other fibrotic skin disorders. J Invest Dermatol. 1996;106(4):729–33.
12. Sato S, Nagaoka T, Hasegawa M, Tamatani T, Nakanishi T, Takigawa M, et al. Serum levels of connective tissue growth factor are elevated in patients with systemic sclerosis: association with extent of skin sclerosis and severity of pulmonary fibrosis. J Rheumatol. 2000;27(1):149–54.
13. Holmes A, Abraham DJ, Chen Y, Denton C, Shi-wen X, Black CM, et al. Constitutive connective tissue growth factor expression in scleroderma fibroblasts is dependent on Sp1. J Biol Chem. 2003;278(43):41728–33.
14. Dziadzio M, Usinger W, Leask A, Abraham D, Black CM, Denton C, et al. N-terminal connective tissue growth factor is a marker of the fibrotic phenotype in scleroderma. QJM. 2005;98(7):485–92.
15. Makino K, Makino T, Stawski L, Mantero JC, Lafyatis R, Simms R, et al. Blockade of PDGF receptors by crenolanib has therapeutic effect in patient fibroblasts and in preclinical models of systemic sclerosis. J Invest Dermatol. 2017. doi: 10.1016/j.jid.2017.03.032
16. Stawski L, Haines P, Fine A, Rudnicka L, Trojanowska M. MMP-12 deficiency attenuates angiotensin II-induced vascular injury, M2 macrophage accumulation, and skin and heart fibrosis. PLoS One. 2014;9(10):e109763.
17. Stawski L, Han R, Bujor AM, Trojanowska M. Angiotensin II induces skin fibrosis: a novel mouse model of dermal fibrosis. Arthritis Res Ther. 2012;14(4):R194.
18. Brenner MC, Krzyzanski W, Chou JZ, Signore PE, Fung CK, Guzman D, et al. FG-3019, a human monoclonal antibody recognizing connective tissue growth factor, is subject to target-mediated drug disposition. Pharm Res. 2016;33(8):1833–49.
19. Raghu G, Scholand MB, de Andrade J, Lancaster L, Mageto Y, Goldin J, et al. FG-3019 anti-connective tissue growth factor monoclonal antibody: results of an open-label clinical trial in idiopathic pulmonary fibrosis. Eur Respir J. 2016;47(5):1481–91.
20. Neesse A, Frese KK, Bapiro TE, Nakagawa T, Sternlicht MD, Seeley TW, et al. CTGF antagonism with mAb FG-3019 enhances chemotherapy response without increasing drug delivery in murine ductal pancreas cancer. Proc Natl Acad Sci U S A. 2013;110(30):12325–30.
21. Morales MG, Gutierrez J, Cabello-Verrugio C, Cabrera D, Lipson KE, Goldschmeding R, et al. Reducing CTGF/CCN2 slows down mdx muscle dystrophy and improves cell therapy. Hum Mol Genet. 2013;22(24):4938–51.
22. Hattori T, Stawski L, Nakerakanti SS, Trojanowska M. Fli1 is a negative regulator of estrogen receptor α in dermal fibroblasts. J Invest Dermatol. 2011;131(7):1469–76.
23. Peoples C, Medsger TA, Lucas M, Rosario BL, Feghali-Bostwick CA. Gender differences in systemic sclerosis: relationship to clinical features, serologic status and outcomes. J scleroderma relat disord. 2016;1(2):204–12.
24. Springer TA. von Willebrand factor, Jedi knight of the bloodstream. Blood. 2014;124(9):1412–25.
25. Kubota S, Takigawa M. Cellular and molecular actions of CCN2/CTGF and its role under physiological and pathological conditions. Clin Sci (Lond). 2015;128(3):181–96.
26. Wang Q, Usinger W, Nichols B, Gray J, Xu L, Seeley TW, et al. Cooperative interaction of CTGF and TGF-β in animal models of fibrotic disease. Fibrogenesis Tissue Repair. 2011;4(1):4.
27. Charrier A, Chen R, Kemper S, Brigstock DR. Regulation of pancreatic inflammation by connective tissue growth factor (CTGF/CCN2). Immunology. 2014;141(4):564–76.
28. Sanchez-Lopez E, Rayego S, Rodrigues-Diez R, Rodriguez JS, Rodrigues-Diez R, Rodriguez-Vita J, et al. CTGF promotes inflammatory cell infiltration of the renal interstitium by activating NF-kappaB. J Am Soc Nephrol. 2009;20(7):1513–26.
29. Bickelhaupt S, Erbel C, Timke C, Wirkner U, Dadrich M, Flechsig P, et al. Effects of CTGF blockade on attenuation and reversal of radiation-induced pulmonary fibrosis. J Natl Cancer Inst. 2017;109(8):djw339.
30. Montezano AC, Nguyen Dinh Cat A, Rios FJ, Touyz RM. Angiotensin II and vascular injury. Curr Hypertens Rep. 2014;16(6):431.
31. Serrati S, Chilla A, Laurenzana A, Margheri F, Giannoni E, Magnelli L, et al. Systemic sclerosis endothelial cells recruit and activate dermal fibroblasts by induction of a connective tissue growth factor (CCN2)/transforming growth factor β-dependent mesenchymal-to-mesenchymal transition. Arthritis Rheum. 2013;65(1):258–69.
32. Alapati D, Rong M, Chen S, Hehre D, Rodriguez MM, Lipson KE, et al. Connective tissue growth factor antibody therapy attenuates hyperoxia-induced lung injury in neonatal rats. Am J Respir Cell Mol Biol. 2011;45(6):1169–77.

7

Factors associated with the 6-minute walk distance in patients with systemic sclerosis

Sébastien Sanges[1,2,3,4,5], Jonathan Giovannelli[1,2,3,4,5], Vincent Sobanski[1,2,3,4,5], Sandrine Morell-Dubois[3,4,5], Hélène Maillard[3,4,5], Marc Lambert[1,2,3,4,5], Céline Podevin[3,4], Nicolas Lamblin[6], Pascal De Groote[6], Jean-François Bervar[7], Thierry Perez[8], Régis Matran[8], Martine Rémy-Jardin[9], Pierre-Yves Hatron[1,2,3,4,5], Éric Hachulla[1,2,3,4,5] and David Launay[1,2,3,4,5*]

Abstract

Background: There is an ongoing debate regarding the relevance of the 6-minute walking distance (6MWD) in systemic sclerosis (SSc) assessment, widely used as a usual test in these patients as well as an outcome measure in clinical trials. In this work, we aimed to assess the associations between the 6MWD and various disease parameters in patients with SSc.

Methods: Consecutive patients followed in our SSc National Reference Centre were included in this cross-sectional study if they fulfilled the 2013 American College of Rheumatology/European League Against Rheumatism criteria for SSc. Data were systematically collected during a comprehensive standardized evaluation that included a 6-minute walk test, clinical assessment, biological results, pulmonary function tests, transthoracic echocardiography, composite scores (European Scleroderma Study Group Activity Index, Medsger severity score, Health Assessment Questionnaire–Disability Index (HAQ-DI)) and treatments.
Associations of the 6MWD with various disease parameters were assessed by linear regression in univariate and multivariate analyses.

Results: The study population comprised 298 patients (females 81%; mean age 58.2 ± 13.3 years; limited cutaneous SSc 82%; interstitial lung disease (ILD) 42%; pulmonary arterial hypertension (PAH) 6%). The 6MWD was significantly and independently associated with gender, age, body mass index, baseline heart rate (HR), HR variation during the test, PAH, history of arterial thrombosis and C-reactive protein levels, as well as with the HAQ-DI score in a sensitivity analysis. Muscle involvement, joint involvement and ILD were not independently associated with the 6MWD.

Conclusions: During SSc, the 6MWD is independently associated with initial HR and HR variation; with PAH but not ILD, suggesting that pulmonary vasculopathy may have a greater impact than parenchymal involvement on functional limitation; and with global markers of disease activity and patient disability. These results give clinicians further insight into how to interpret the 6MWD in the context of SSc.

Keywords: Systemic sclerosis, 6-minute walk test, Chronotropic incompetence, Exercise tolerance, Interstitial lung disease, Pulmonary hypertension

* Correspondence: david.launay@univ-lille2.fr
[1]University of Lille, INSERM U995, LIRIC—Lille Inflammation Research International Center, F-59000 Lille, France
[2]INSERM U995, F-59000 Lille, France
Full list of author information is available at the end of the article

Background

Systemic sclerosis (SSc) is a severe condition classified within the connective tissue disease spectrum [1]. Over the last decades, the respiratory complications of the disease, namely pulmonary hypertension (PH) and interstitial lung disease (ILD), have become the leading cause of mortality among SSc patients [2]. One of the most important objectives when managing SSc patients is therefore to detect these complications as early as possible, to properly assess their severity and to accurately follow up therapeutic efficacy.

Among the different tools available to evaluate SSc patients, the 6-minute walk test (6MWT) is simple, non-invasive, inexpensive and reproducible, and is frequently used in daily practice [3]. Initially developed to study exercise tolerance in aviation personnel [4], its use has since been translated to the field of cardiopulmonary diseases [5], such as chronic obstructive pulmonary disease (COPD), idiopathic pulmonary fibrosis (IPF) and idiopathic pulmonary arterial hypertension (PAH). In these mono-organ conditions, the 6-minute walk distance (6MWD) has proven to be an accurate reflection of disease severity with a prognostic significance [6–8].

However, conversely to these diseases, SSc is a systemic condition associated with various extrapulmonary features (skin fibrosis, musculoskeletal pain, heart involvement, anemia) and with significant disability that can confound the interpretation of the 6MWT. In this multi-organ setting, the assumption that the 6MWD is an adequate surrogate marker for the severity of cardiopulmonary complications is no longer straightforward, and this has led clinicians to wonder what is actually being measured during this test in SSc [9]. This is of crucial importance, since the 6MWD is used in daily practice to follow up SSc patients [3], and as an outcome measure in clinical trials for SSc-PAH [10–13] and ILD [14].

Several teams have tried to answer this question but their results are conflicting [15–30]. For instance, forced vital capacity (FVC) measured during pulmonary function tests (PFT) was significantly associated with the 6MWD in some studies [19, 21, 22, 25] but not in others [16, 18, 20, 28, 29]. Similarly, associations with musculoskeletal parameters have been observed inconsistently [21, 25, 26].

To address this issue, we performed a cross-sectional study and assessed the associations between the 6MWD and various disease characteristics in a large and well-phenotyped SSc patient population.

Methods

Patient selection

We designed a cross-sectional study and recruited consecutive patients over 18 years old followed in the National Referral Centre for Systemic Sclerosis of Lille from November 2014 to August 2016. They were included in the study if they fulfilled the 2013 ACR/EULAR classification criteria for SSc [31]. There was no exclusion criterion.

Data collection

Data were collected systematically by a physician in a standardized case-report form for all patients referred to our day-patient clinic. All of them underwent a comprehensive evaluation performed within the same day (except for transthoracic echocardiography (TTE) that could be performed up to 6 months before or after the 6MWT).

Patients underwent a non-encouraged 6MWT as recommended [32]. The total 6MWD (in absolute and relative values [33]), modified Borg score, peripheral oxygen saturation (SpO_2), blood pressure (BP) and heart rate (HR) were recorded at the beginning and the end of the test. Variations of (Δ) Borg score, SpO_2, BP and HR were defined as the difference between their final and initial values.

Other data collected included patient and SSc characteristics, clinical parameters (including modified Rodnan skin score (mRSS) and New York Heart Association (NYHA) functional class), biological results (including C-reactive protein (CRP), Nt-pro-BNP and creatinin kinase (CK) levels), TTE (including estimated systolic pulmonary artery pressure (sPAP) and left ventricle ejection fraction (LVEF)), PFT (including FVC, total lung capacity (TLC) and diffusing capacity of the lung for carbon monoxide (DLCO)), composite scores (European Scleroderma Study Group Activity Index (EScSG-AI) [34], Medsger severity score [35], Health Assessment Questionnaire—Disability Index (HAQ-DI) [36]) and treatments (for a complete list of collected data, see Additional file 1).

Statistical analyses

Characteristics of the population were described using the mean ± standard deviation (SD) for quantitative variables, and number (percentage) for qualitative variables.

In order to study the associations between the 6MWD (in absolute value) as the dependent variable and the various explanatory variables, in a first step we conducted univariate analyses using linear regressions. Results were expressed using nonadjusted coefficients (95% confidence interval (CI)) expressed in meters. To better identify relevant explanatory variables, linear regressions were then adjusted on the main potential confounding factors (gender, age, body mass index (BMI), disease duration, smoking history and SSc subtype).

As a second step, we built a multivariate linear regression model using the following strategy. Firstly, we included a priori the six potential confounding variables already described. Secondly, we made a first selection of variables based on univariate analyses ($p < 0.10$). Thirdly, we ensured that among these variables, those of interest were present (i.e., the complications identified a priori as being able to influence the 6MWD: in particular PAH, ILD, joint and muscle symptoms, heart involvement using the left ventricle ejection fraction). Fourthly, we excluded the variables that mediated the relationship between the 6MWD and organ involvements (e.g., symptoms of dyspnea for PAH or ILD), so as not to attenuate the regression coefficients related to organ involvement variables. We also excluded collinear variables and composite scores. Fifthly, we ensured that the number of variables included in the model was consistent with the number of patients (i.e., close to one variable per 10 patients). Finally, we tested several potential interactions: between PAH or ILD and joint symptoms, muscle symptoms, smoking history or SSc subtype; and between ΔHR, initial HR and chronotropic drugs. None of the interactions tested was significant. Additionally, the HAQ-DI score was included in a separate regression model as a sensitivity analysis. Coefficients (95% CI) were expressed in meters. Regression diagnostics were performed.

All statistical analyses were performed using R software, version 3.2.5 [37]. The threshold for statistical significance was set to $p < 0.05$.

Results

Patient characteristics

Overall, the study population comprised 298 patients (Table 1). Most of them were middle-aged females (sex ratio male/female 0.23; mean age 58.2 ± 13.3 years) with limited cutaneous SSc (82.2%) associated with anti-centromere antibodies (56.0%). ILD (41.1%) and digital ulcers (43.0%) were the most frequent complications of the disease, while PAH (5.9%) and renal crisis (0.4%) remained rare. Patients were mainly staged in NYHA class I or II (78.7%) and displayed no major PFT alterations (mean FVC 103.5 ± 21.8%; mean DLCO 70.0 ± 19.7%). Musculoskeletal complaints included joint (42.2%) and muscle symptoms (19.2%), with mostly normal muscle enzymes (mean CK levels 93 ± 59.5 IU).

During the 6MWT, patients walked a mean distance of 438.3 ± 108.1 m (81.6 ± 17.8% of the predicted value), decreased their SpO_2 by a mean of 0.58 ± 2.72% and increased their HR by a mean of 10.4 ± 11.2 bpm. The mean Borg score was 0.4 ± 1.1 at the beginning of the test and rose to 2.5 ± 2.2 at the end.

Associations with the 6-minute walk distance: nonadjusted and adjusted analyses

Univariate analyses revealed several associations between the 6MWD and the collected parameters (Table 2). To better identify relevant explanatory variables, these analyses were then adjusted on several potential confounding factors (gender, age, BMI, disease duration, smoking history and SSc subtype).

Regarding general patient and SSc characteristics, the 6MWD was associated with gender ($p < 10^{-3}$), age ($p < 10^{-6}$) and BMI ($p < 10^{-6}$) both before and after adjustment. Associations were observed with smoking habits and disease duration in nonadjusted analysis, but did not remain significant after adjustment. Although we found no association with cutaneous subtype, immunological profile or capillaroscopic anomalies in nonadjusted analysis, adjustment on confounding variables revealed a significant association of the 6MWD with the cutaneous subtype ($p = 0.008$).

Regarding cardiopulmonary parameters, the 6MWD was significantly associated with PAH ($p < 10^{-6}$), ILD ($p = 0.02$) and history of cardiovascular events (venous thrombosis $p = 0.001$; arterial thrombosis $p < 10^{-3}$) in nonadjusted analysis. Association with ILD was no longer significant after adjustment ($p = 0.08$). We also found significant associations of the 6WMD with NYHA functional class ($p < 10^{-6}$), elevated Nt-pro-BNP levels ($p < 10^{-6}$), echocardiographic markers of PH (estimated sPAP $p < 10^{-3}$; right atrium area $p = 0.01$) and left-heart dysfunction (LVEF $p = 0.03$), and PFT results (TLC $p = 0.007$; DLCO $p < 10^{-3}$) in nonadjusted analysis. These associations remained significant after adjustment.

Other cardiopulmonary parameters measured during the 6MWT also displayed significant associations with the total distance, especially initial HR ($p < 10^{-3}$) and ΔHR ($p < 10^{-3}$), both before and after adjustment. Significant associations with chronotropic drug intake were observed only in nonadjusted analysis.

Regarding extracardiopulmonary parameters, we observed an association with articular involvement (joint symptoms $p = 0.02$) that became nonsignificant after adjustment on confounding variables. Similarly, there was no association with markers of muscular (muscle symptoms $p = 0.08$; CK levels $p = 0.11$) and skin (mRSS $p = 0.74$; digital ulcers $p = 0.30$) involvements in nonadjusted analysis.

Regarding global indicators of disease activity and severity, the 6MWD was significantly associated with hemoglobin ($p < 10^{-3}$), CRP ($p < 10^{-3}$), EScSG-AI ($p = 0.001$) and Medsger severity scores ($p < 10^{-3}$), both before and after adjustment. We also found a markedly large association of the 6MWD with the HAQ-DI score ($p < 10^{-3}$) in both analyses.

Associations with the 6-minute walk distance: multivariate models

Based on the results of our nonadjusted and adjusted analyses, we built a multivariate model to determine the factors independently associated with the 6MWD (Table 3).

Table 1 Characteristics of the study population

	N	Value	
Demographic data			
Females, *n* (%)	298	242	(81.2)
Age at inclusion (years), mean (SD)	298	58.2	(13.3)
BMI (kg/m^2), mean (SD)	283	24.9	(5.3)
Smoking history, *n* (%)	297	119	(40.1)
Diagnosis of SSc			
SSc subtype			
lcSSc, *n* (%)	298	245	(82.2)
dcSSc, *n* (%)	298	53	(17.8)
Disease duration at inclusion			
Since diagnosis (years), mean (SD)	298	9.1	(8.1)
Since first non-Raynaud symptom (years), mean (SD)	244	9.9	(8.5)
Since Raynaud phenomenon onset (years), mean (SD)	279	15.6	(12.2)
Immunological profile			
Anti-centromere antibodies, *n* (%)	291	163	(56.0)
Anti-topoisomerase I antibodies, *n* (%)	291	57	(19.6)
Anti-RNA polymerase III antibodies, *n* (%)	291	7	(2.4)
Anti-RNP antibodies, *n* (%)	291	15	(5.2)
Nailfold capillaroscopy			
Specific organic microangiopathy, *n* (%)	109	98	(89.9)
History of organ involvement			
Interstitial lung disease			
No ILD, *n* (%)	270	159	(58.9)
Limited ILD, *n* (%)	270	82	(30.4)
Extensive ILD, *n* (%)	270	29	(10.7)
Pulmonary arterial hypertension, *n* (%)	286	17	(5.9)
Scleroderma renal crisis, *n* (%)	285	1	(0.4)
Digital ulcers (previously or at inclusion), *n* (%)	298	128	(43.0)
Acute venous thrombosis, *n* (%)	297	33	(11.1)
Acute arterial thrombosis, *n* (%)	297	39	(13.1)
Chronic cardiovascular disease, *n* (%)	296	21	(7.1)
Clinical evaluation at inclusion			
Modified Rodnan skin score, mean (SD)	297	4.96	(5.95)
Telangiectasia, *n* (%)	275	199	(72.4)
NYHA functional class			
Class I, *n* (%)	296	132	(44.6)
Class II, *n* (%)	296	101	(34.1)
Class III, *n* (%)	296	57	(19.3)
Class IV, *n* (%)	296	6	(2.0)
Cardiovascular symptoms, *n* (%)	298	24	(8.1)
Joint symptoms, *n* (%)	296	125	(42.2)
Muscle symptoms, *n* (%)	297	57	(19.2)
6-minute walk test			
Total distance (m), mean (SD)	298	438.3	(108.1)
Total distance (% predicted), mean (SD)	290	81.6	(17.8)
Initial SpO_2 (%), mean (SD)	280	98.1	(2.1)
Final SpO_2 (%), mean (SD)	275	97.5	(3.3)
ΔSpO_2 (%), mean (SD)	276	-0.58	(2.72)
Initial Borg score, mean (SD)	294	0.4	(1.1)
Final Borg score, mean (SD)	294	2.5	(2.2)
ΔBorg score, mean (SD)	293	2.1	(1.9)
Initial sBP (mmHg), mean (SD)	292	123.8	(16.6)
Final sBP (mmHg), mean (SD)	292	132.9	(18.2)
ΔsBP (mmHg), mean (SD)	291	9.2	(14.0)
Initial dBP (mmHg), mean (SD)	271	97.4	(3.4)
Final dBP (mmHg), mean (SD)	292	73.6	(10.0)
ΔdBP (mmHg), mean (SD)	291	0.95	(10.2)
Initial HR (bpm), mean (SD)	289	76.7	(12.3)
Final HR (bpm), mean (SD)	288	87.1	(15.9)
ΔHR (bpm), mean (SD)	288	10.4	(11.2)
Biological data			
Hemoglobin (g/dl), mean (SD)	291	13.4	(1.4)
ESR (mm/h), mean (SD)	258	14.8	(15.3)
CRP (mg/L), mean (SD)	293	4.0	(4.7)
Creatinin (mg/L), mean (SD)	294	8.0	(2.8)
Estimated GFR (ml/min/1.73 m^2), mean (SD)	294	89.1	(21.5)
Elevated Nt-pro-BNP, *n* (%)	290	43	(14.8)
CK (IU), mean (SD)	289	93	(59.5)
Ferritin (ng/ml), mean (SD)	268	105.5	(136.4)
Complement activation, *n* (%)	265	9	(3.4)
Transthoracic echocardiography			
Left ventricular ejection fraction (%), mean (SD)	250	62.8	(6.7)
Left ventricular diastolic dysfunction, *n* (%)	229	124	(54.2)
Valvular heart disease, *n* (%)	244	41	(16.8)
Peak TRV (m/s), mean (SD)	98	2.62	(0.54)
RA–RV pressure gradient (mmHg), mean (SD)	206	27.4	(13.4)
Estimated sPAP (mmHg), mean (SD)	194	31.5	(13.1)
RA area (cm^2), mean (SD)	139	15.0	(4.6)
IVC dilation and/or decreased IVC collapse, *n* (%)	210	16	(7.6)
Pericardial effusion, *n* (%)	230	5	(2.2)
Pulmonary function tests			
TLC (% predicted), mean (SD)	276	96.2	(16.4)
FVC (% predicted), mean (SD)	287	103.5	(21.8)
FEV1 (% predicted), mean (SD)	286	95.1	(21.8)
FEV1/FVC (%), mean (SD)	286	79.2	(10.7)
DLCO (% predicted), mean (SD)	285	70.0	(19.7)
KCO (% predicted), mean (SD)	278	80.9	(17.6)
Composite scores			
EScSG-AI score, mean (SD)	289	1.16	(1.2)
Medsger severity score, mean (SD)	228	4.17	(2.5)
HAQ-DI score, mean (SD)	223	0.61	(0.7)
Treatments			
Negative chronotropic drugs, *n* (%)	293	87	(29.7)
Positive chronotropic drugs, *n* (%)	293	10	(3.4)

BMI body mass index, *CK* creatin kinase, *CRP* C-reactive protein, *dBP* diastolic blood pressure, *dc* diffuse cutaneous, *DLCO* diffusing capacity of the lung for carbon monoxide, *EScSG-AI* European Scleroderma Study Group Activity Index, *ESR* erythrocyte sedimentation rate, *FEV1* forced expiratory volume during the first second, *FVC* forced vital capacity, *GFR* glomerular filtration rate, *HAQ-DI* Health Assessment Questionnaire—Disability Index, *HR* heart rate, *ILD* interstitial lung disease, *IU* international unit, *IVC* inferior vena cava, *KCO* diffusing coefficient for carbon monoxide, *lc* limited cutaneous, *NYHA* New York Heart Association, *RA* right atrium, *RV* right ventricle, *sBP* systolic blood pressure, *SD* standard deviation, *sPAP* systolic pulmonary arterial pressure, *SpO_2* peripheral oxygen saturation, *SSc* systemic sclerosis, *TLC* total lung capacity, *TRV* tricuspid regurgitation velocity, *Δ* variation of

Table 2 Nonadjusted and adjusted associations between 6MWD and SSc characteristics

	Nonadjusted			Adjusted*		
	β	(95% CI)	*p*	β	(95% CI)	*p*
Male (vs female)	52.7	(21.8; 83.6)	$<10^{-3}$	76.9	(46.4; 107.4)	$<10^{-3}$
Age (per 1-year increment)	−3.6	(−4.5; −2.8)	$<10^{-6}$	−3.9	(−4.8; −3.1)	$<10^{-6}$
Smoking history (vs no history)	31.8	(6.9; 56.7)	0.01	−11.2	(−34.9; 12.6)	0.36
BMI (per 1-kg/m² increment)	−4.1	(−6.4; −1.7)	$<10^{-3}$	−3.7	(−5.7; −1.6)	$<10^{-3}$
dcSSc (vs lcSSc)	−0.7	(−32.8; 31.5)	0.97	−40.2	(−69.7; −10.8)	0.008
Disease duration since diagnosis (per 1-year increment)	−1.8	(−3.3; −0.3)	0.02	0.7	(−0.8; 2.2)	0.38
Disease duration since first non-RP symptom (per 1-year increment)	−2.3	(−3.8; −0.7)	0.004	−0.7	(−2.3; 0.8)	0.33
Disease duration since RP onset (per 1-year increment)	−1.2	(−2.2; −0.2)	0.02	0.4	(−0.5; 1.4)	0.38
ACA (vs no ACA)	−23.4	(−48.1; 1.3)	0.06	−9.8	(−35.5; 16.0)	0.46
ATA (vs no ATA)	0.1	(−31.0; 31.3)	0.99	−2.4	(−31.5; 26.8)	0.87
ARA (vs no ARA)	47.2	(−33.2; 127.7)	0.25	14.7	(−61.6; 90.9)	0.71
Anti-RNP antibodies (vs no anti-RNP antibodies)	3.7	(−52.2; 59.5)	0.90	−22.3	(−71.0; 26.4)	0.37
Abnormal nailfold capillaroscopy (vs normal)	−18.1	(−86.7; 50.6)	0.61	−12.5	(−66.9; 41.8)	0.65
PAH (vs no PAH)	−131.8	(−183.2; −80.3)	$<10^{-6}$	−112.0	(−155.9; −68.2)	$<10^{-3}$
ILD (vs no ILD)			0.02			0.08
Limited ILD	16.4	(−13.0; 45.3)		14.2	(−13.8; 42.2)	
Extensive ILD	−52.3	(−95.6; −9.0)		−40.4	(−78.7; −2.1)	
DU (previously or at inclusion) (vs no DU)	13.2	(−11.6; 38.0)	0.30	−10.6	(−33.7; 12.6)	0.37
History of venous thrombosis (vs no history)	−65.0	(−103.4; −26.5)	0.001	−52.5	(−87.3; −17.6)	0.003
History of arterial thrombosis (vs no history)	−73.6	(−109.0; −38.1)	$<10^{-3}$	−43.5	(−76.4; −10.6)	0.01
History of cardiovascular disease (vs no history)	−103.8	(−150.2; −57.5)	$<10^{-3}$	−65.0	(−108.2; −21.8)	0.003
Modified Rodnan skin score (per 1-point increment)	−0.4	(−2.4; 1.7)	0.74	−0.9	(−3.1; 1.3)	0.42
Telangiectasia (vs no telangiectasia)	−12.4	(−41.0; 16.1)	0.39	13.4	(−12.6; 39.4)	0.31
NYHA functional class (vs class I)			$<10^{-6}$			$<10^{-6}$
NYHA class II	−76.1	(−100.1; −52.2)		−61.7	(−83.8; −39.6)	
NYHA class III	−132.1	(−160.8; −103.3)		−108.1	(−134.5; −81.7)	
NYHA class IV	−227.4	(−303.1; −151.7)		−216.0	(−281.6; −150.4	
Cardiovascular symptoms (vs no symptoms)	−49.8	(−94.6; −4.9)	0.03	−33.5	(−73.3; 6.2)	0.10
Joint symptoms (vs no symptoms)	−29.4	(−54.3; −4.6)	0.02	−5.8	(−28.4; 16.8)	0.61
Muscle symptoms (vs no symptoms)	−27.8	(−58.9; 3.4)	0.08	−16.1	(−44.0; 11.8)	0.26
Initial SpO_2 (per 1% increment)	14.9	(9.2; 20.7)	$<10^{-6}$	11.4	(6.3; 16.4)	$<10^{-3}$
Final SpO_2 (per 1% increment)	9.1	(5.5; 12.8)	$<10^{-3}$	7.2	(3.9; 10.4)	$<10^{-3}$
ΔSpO_2 (per 1% increment)	4.7	(0.0; 9.4)	0.05	3.7	(−0.3; 7.8)	0.07
Initial Borg score (per 1-point increment)	−22.5	(−33.3; −11.7)	$<10^{-3}$	−21.5	(−30.7; −12.3)	$<10^{-3}$
Final Borg score (per 1-point increment)	−17.7	(−23.0; −12.4)	$<10^{-6}$	−13.8	(−18.6; −8.9)	$<10^{-6}$
ΔBorg score (per 1-point increment)	−15.9	(−22.1; −9.6)	$<10^{-3}$	−10.4	(−16.3; −4.6)	$<10^{-3}$
Initial sBP (per 1-mmHg increment)	−1.0	(−1.7; −0.2)	0.01	0.4	(−0.3; 1.2)	0.26
Final sBP (per 1-mmHg increment)	−0.6	(−1.2; 0.1)	0.11	0.8	(0.1; 1.5)	0.02
ΔsBP (per 1-mmHg increment)	0.4	(−0.5; 1.3)	0.37	0.5	(−0.2; 1.3)	0.18
Initial dBP (per 1-mmHg increment)	9.1	(5.3; 12.8)	$<10^{-3}$	7.1	(3.9; 10.3)	$<10^{-3}$
Final dBP (per 1-mmHg increment)	0.5	(−0.7; 1.8)	0.42	0.1	(−1.0; 1.2)	0.91
ΔdBP (per 1-mmHg increment)	0.6	(−0.7; 1.8)	0.36	0.0	(−1.0; 1.1)	0.95

Table 2 Nonadjusted and adjusted associations between 6MWD and SSc characteristics *(Continued)*

	Nonadjusted			Adjusted*		
	β	(95% CI)	*p*	β	(95% CI)	*p*
Initial HR (per 1-bpm increment)	−1.9	(−2.9; −0.9)	$<10^{-3}$	−2.0	(−2.9; −1.2)	$<10^{-3}$
Final HR (per 1-bpm increment)	−0.1	(−0.9; 0.7)	0.86	0.1	(−0.6; 0.8)	0.85
ΔHR (per 1-bpm increment)	2.1	(1.0; 3.2)	$<10^{-3}$	2.5	(1.6; 3.5)	$<10^{-6}$
Hemoglobin (per 1-g/dl increment)	26.6	(18.0; 35.2)	$<10^{-6}$	19.9	(11.5; 28.2)	$<10^{-3}$
ESR (per 1-mm/h increment)	−2.3	(−3.1; −1.5)	$<10^{-6}$	−2.1	(−2.8; −1.3)	$<10^{-6}$
CRP (per 1-mg/L increment)	−5.8	(−8.4; −3.3)	$<10^{-3}$	−5.8	(−8.0; −3.5)	$<10^{-3}$
Creatinin (per 1-mg/L increment)	−3.6	(−8.0; 0.8)	0.11	−3.4	(−7.3; 0.5)	0.09
Estimated GFR (per 1-ml/min/1.73 m^2 increment)	1.1	(0.6; 1.7)	$<10^{-3}$	0.0	(−0.6; 0.5)	0.97
Elevated Nt-pro-BNP (vs normal Nt-pro-BNP)	−95.4	(−128.7; −62.1)	$<10^{-6}$	−66.5	(−98.4; −34.6)	$<10^{-3}$
CK (per 1-IU increment)	0.2	(0.0; 0.4)	0.11	0.2	(0.0; 0.3)	0.11
Ferritin (per 1-ng/ml increment)	0.0	(−0.1; 0.1)	0.55	0.0	(−0.1; 0.1)	0.84
Complement activation (vs no activation)	1.6	(−70.0; 73.3)	0.96	10.5	(−51.2; 72.1)	0.74
LVEF (per 1% increment)	2.1	(0.2; 4.1)	0.03	2.1	(0.4; 3.8)	0.02
LVDD (vs no LVDD)	−69.6	(−96.6; −42.7)	$<10^{-6}$	−17.1	(−45.6; 11.4)	0.24
Valvular heart disease (vs no valvular heart disease)	−22.5	(−59.3; 14.2)	0.23	26.2	(−7.5; 59.9)	0.13
Peak TRV (per 1-m/s increment)	−62.3	(−101.0; −23.6)	0.002	−33.2	(−67.4; 1.1)	0.06
RA–RV pressure gradient (per 1-mmHg increment)	−2.5	(−3.6; −1.5)	$<10^{-3}$	−1.8	(−2.8; −0.9)	$<10^{-3}$
Estimated sPAP (per 1-mmHg increment)	−2.5	(−3.6; −1.4)	$<10^{-3}$	−1.9	(−2.9; −0.9)	$<10^{-3}$
RA area (per 1-cm^2 increment)	−4.7	(−8.2; −1.2)	0.01	−4.6	(−8.4; −0.7)	0.02
Abnormal IVC (vs normal IVC)	−26.0	(−79.7; 27.6)	0.34	−22.5	(−68.9; 24.0)	0.34
Pericardial effusion (vs no pericardial effusion)	−57.4	(−154.7; 39.9)	0.25	−95.3	(−188.3; −2.2)	0.05
TLC (per 1% increment)	1.0	(0.3; 1.8)	0.007	1.1	(0.4; 1.8)	0.002
FVC (per 1% increment)	0.4	(−0.2; 0.9)	0.20	1.2	(0.7; 1.7)	$<10^{-3}$
FEV1 (per 1% increment)	0.3	(−0.3; 0.9)	0.29	1.0	(0.5; 1.5)	$<10^{-3}$
FEV1/FVC (per 1% increment)	0.8	(−0.3; 2.0)	0.16	−0.2	(−1.3; 0.9)	0.68
DLCO (per 1% increment)	1.4	(0.8; 2.0)	$<10^{-3}$	1.5	(1.0; 2.0)	$<10^{-6}$
KCO (per 1% increment)	0.7	(0.0; 1.5)	0.04	1.2	(0.6; 1.9)	$<10^{-3}$
EScSG-AI score (per 1-point increment)	−16.4	(−26.2; −6.5)	0.001	−14.6	(−23.5; −5.7)	0.001
Medsger severity score (per 1-point increment)	−10.8	(−16.3; −5.4)	$<10^{-3}$	−82.9	(−99.8; −66.0)	$<10^{-6}$
HAQ-DI score (per 1-point increment)	−104.6	(−122.0; −87.2)	$<10^{-6}$	−11.1	(−16.2; −6.1)	$<10^{-3}$
Positive chronotropic drug intake (vs no intake)	−68.4	(−136.5; −0.3)	0.05	−38.7	(−98.6; 21.1)	0.21
Negative chronotropic drug intake (vs no intake)	−48.1	(−74.7; −21.4)	$<10^{-3}$	−15.3	(−41.0; 10.5)	0.25

β coefficients expressed in meters
*Analyses adjusted on gender, age, BMI, disease duration, smoking history and SSc subtype
6MWD 6-minute walk distance, *ACA* anti-centromere antibodies, *ARA* anti-RNA polymerase III antibodies, *ATA* anti-topoisomerase I antibodies, *BMI* body mass index, *CI* confidence interval, *CK* creatin kinase, *CRP* C-reactive protein, *dBP* diastolic blood pressure, *dc* diffuse cutaneous, *DLCO* diffusing capacity of the lung for carbon monoxide, *DU* digital ulcers, *EScSG-AI* European Scleroderma Study Group Activity Index, *ESR* erythrocyte sedimentation rate, *FEV1* forced expiratory volume during the first second, *FVC* forced vital capacity, *GFR* glomerular filtration rate, *HAQ-DI* Health Assessment Questionnaire—Disability Index, *HR* heart rate, *ILD* interstitial lung disease, *IU* international unit, *IVC* inferior vena cava, *KCO* diffusing coefficient for carbon monoxide, *lc* limited cutaneous, *LVDD* left ventricular diastolic dysfunction, *LVEF* left ventricle ejection fraction, *NYHA* New York Heart Association, *PAH* pulmonary arterial hypertension, *RA* right atrium, *RP* Raynaud phenomenon, *RV* right ventricle, *sBP* systolic blood pressure, *sPAP* systolic pulmonary arterial pressure, *SpO$_2$* peripheral oxygen saturation, *SSc* systemic sclerosis, *TLC* total lung capacity, *TRV* tricuspid regurgitation velocity, *Δ* variation of

Parameters that were significantly and independently associated with 6MWD were gender (β = 58.9 (22.6; 95.2) m for men vs women, $p = 0.002$), age (β = −2.8 (−3.9; −1.7) m per 1-year increment, $p < 10^{-3}$), BMI (β = −2.7 (−5.1; −0.2) m per 1-kg/m^2 increment, $p = 0.03$), history of arterial thrombosis (β = −39.6 (−77.9; −1.4) m vs no history, $p = 0.04$), PAH (β = −79.2 (−129.7; −28.8) m vs no PAH, $p = 0.002$), CRP (β = −4.3 (−6.7; −1.9) m per 1-mg/L increment, $p < 10^{-3}$), initial HR (β = −1.1 (−2.2; −0.1) m per 1-bpm increment, $p = 0.03$) and ΔHR

Table 3 Multivariate regression model assessing the associations between 6MWD and SSc characteristics

	β	(95% CI)	*p*
Male (vs female)	58.9	(22.6; 95.2)	0.002
Age (per 1-year increment)	−2.8	(−3.9; −1.7)	$<10^{-3}$
Disease duration since diagnosis (per 1-year increment)	−0.7	(−2.5; 1.0)	0.42
BMI (per 1-kg/m^2 increment)	−2.7	(−5.1; −0.2)	0.03
Smoking history (vs no history)	−8.2	(−33.9; 17.5)	0.53
History of venous thrombosis (vs no history)	−10.8	(−48.6; 26.9)	0.57
History of arterial thrombosis (vs no history)	−39.6	(−77.9; −1.4)	0.04
dcSSc (vs lcSSc)	−22.7	(−57.6; 12.2)	0.20
PAH (vs no PAH)	−79.2	(−129.7; −28.8)	0.002
ILD (vs no ILD)			0.15
Limited ILD	22.0	(−6.9; 50.9)	
Extensive ILD	−14.7	(−55.8; 26.4)	
Joint symptoms (vs no symptoms)	−16.5	(−41.6; 8.6)	0.20
Muscle symptoms (vs no symptoms)	−7.5	(−40.6; 25.7)	0.66
Hemoglobin (per 1-g/dl increment)	9.2	(−0.8; 19.1)	0.07
CRP (per 1-mg/L increment)	−4.3	(−6.7; −1.9)	$<10^{-3}$
Estimated GFR (per 1-ml/min/1.73 m^2 increment)	0.2	(−0.4; 0.9)	0.46
Initial HR (per 1-bpm increment)	−1.1	(−2.2; −0.1)	0.03
ΔHR (per 1-bpm increment)	2.8	(1.8; 3.8)	$<10^{-6}$
LVEF (per 1% increment)	1.2	(−0.5; 2.9)	0.15
Positive chronotropic drug intake (vs no intake)	14.2	(−44.3; 72.6)	0.63
Negative chronotropic drug intake (vs no intake)	−25.3	(−52.3; 1.7)	0.07

$N = 192$. $R^2 = 0.59$, adjusted $R^2 = 0.54$
β coefficients expressed in meters
6MWD 6-minute walk distance, *BMI* body mass index, *CI* confidence interval, *CRP* C-reactive protein, *dc* diffuse cutaneous, *GFR* glomerular filtration rate, *HR* heart rate, *ILD* interstitial lung disease, *lc* limited cutaneous, *LVEF* left ventricle ejection fraction, *PAH* pulmonary arterial hypertension, *SSc* systemic sclerosis, *Δ* variation of

(β = 2.8 (1.8; 3.8) m per 1-bpm increment, $p < 10^{-6}$) (Fig. 1). This model accounted for 59% of the variance of the 6MWD.

A sensitivity analysis including the HAQ-DI score revealed its independent association with the 6MWD (β = −77.1 (−101.3; −53.0) m per 1-unit increment, $p < 10^{-6}$) (Additional file 2).

Discussion

In this cross-sectional study, we tried to identify the factors associated with the 6MWD in a large and fully characterized population of SSc patients. Our results can be summarized as follows: aside from demographic parameters, we observed significant and independent associations of the 6MWD with ΔHR and resting HR, with PAH and history of arterial thrombosis, and with CRP levels; we found no independent association of the 6MWD with ILD or musculoskeletal involvement; and in a sensitivity analysis, the HAQ-DI score was also independently associated with the 6MWD.

Although literature data are conflicting, the results of our univariate analyses mostly confirm findings from previous works, which observed associations of the 6MWD with age, BMI and cardiopulmonary parameters (especially PFT and TTE), but no major influence of musculoskeletal involvement [15–30]. Multivariate analyses from previous studies have also established age [16], gender [18], HAQ scores [21] and CRP [19] as independent factors associated with the 6MWD. Independent associations with dyspnea [16], initial and final SpO_2 [18], initial Borg score [18] and DLCO [21, 28] were also reported, but since our goal was to identify associations with specific organ involvements rather than their mediators, we chose not to include these variables in our multivariate model.

Association of the 6MWD with ΔHR

Association between the 6MWD and ΔHR has never been studied previously in SSc. Interestingly, similar findings were made in IPF [38] and PAH [39] patients, where the variation in HR was found to be an important

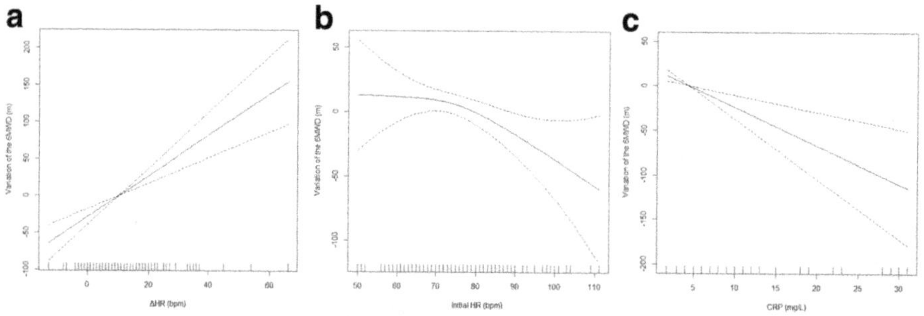

Fig. 1 Adjusted associations in a generalized additive model. Regression splines representing the adjusted associations in a generalized additive model between the 6-minute walk distance (6MWD) and (**a**) variation of heart rate (ΔHR) during the test, (**b**) initial heart rate (HR) at the beginning of the test and (**c**) C-reactive protein (CRP) levels. *y* axis corresponds to variation of 6MWD as a function of the explanatory variables. Dashed lines correspond to 95% CI of the spline

factor associated with the 6MWD as well as a valuable prognostic marker.

Interpretation of this result in the context of the 6MWT is challenging. On the one hand, the lower increase in HR observed in some SSc patients could simply indicate lower exercise intensity due to limited functional capacities or a lack of motivation [40]. On the other hand, it could also reflect an actual impairment of the chronotropic response to exercise. Chronotropic incompetence, defined as the inability to increase HR above 80% of its predicted peak value during a maximal exercise test, is a major cause of exercise intolerance in various cardiopulmonary diseases [40, 41]. It is a common finding in patients with heart diseases (sick sinus syndrome, atrial fibrillation, ischemic heart disease, chronic heart failure), neurological disorders (through autonomic dysfunction) or specific medication intakes (such as β-blockers and nondihydropyridine calcium-channel blockers) [40, 41].

Since the 6MWT is a submaximal exercise test, the diagnosis of chronotropic incompetence cannot be made here with certainty; and since detailed patient comorbidities are not available, the causes for the impaired chronotropic response in our population cannot be investigated fully. However, it is interesting to note that negative chronotropic drug intake was not independently associated with the 6MWD in our patients, making the hypothesis of a medication-induced chronotropic incompetence unlikely. Conversely, SSc is frequently associated with autonomic dysfunction [42] (especially in terms of HR regulation [43]) and with a specific myocardial disease [1], both of which could induce chronotropic incompetence.

Overall, this result suggests that an impaired chronotropic response could be an important factor associated with exercise intolerance in SSc. Interestingly, Someya et al. [44] showed in a previous work that the HR at the end of the 6MWT was higher in SSc patients than in controls to try and compensate for a decreased stroke volume. Thus, it seems reasonable to assume this compensation mechanism would be impaired in SSc patients with chronotropic incompetence, resulting in lower exercise capacities. In any case, this finding warrants further investigations, using maximal incremental exercise tests.

Association of the 6MWD with resting HR

Interestingly, we found that both ΔHR and resting HR are independently associated with the 6MWD. This result suggests that, during SSc, exercise capacities are conditioned not only by the patient's ability to increase his or her HR during exercise, but also by his or her baseline HR value.

Only two studies have so far tested the association of the 6MWD with resting HR in SSc and they yielded discrepant results [19, 29]. Our observation is supported by similar findings in patients with nonidiopathic PAH and chronic heart failure [39, 45].

Here again, interpretation of this result in the context of our study is difficult. Heart rate is tightly regulated by the autonomous system in order to adapt cardiac output to situations of stress or exercise [41]. Thus, the reduction of physical performance in SSc patients with increased resting HR could be suggestive of advanced autonomic dysfunction (loss of balance between sympathetic and vagal basal tones) and/or severe myocardial disease (compensating mechanism for a decreased resting stroke volume), as implied by our previous result. Alternatively, this could also indicate global deconditioning or performance anxiety.

Either way, further studies are needed to better appreciate the pathophysiological implications of this result.

Association of the 6MWD with PAH but not with ILD

Our multivariate analysis also revealed a significant and independent association of the 6MWD with PAH, but not with ILD. Interestingly, all previous studies that tested the relation between the 6MWD and PH consistently found a shorter walked distance in PH patients [21, 30] or an association with echocardiographic markers of PH [16, 19, 24, 29] (with only one exception [18]). Conversely, data regarding the influence of ILD on the 6MWD are more conflicting, with some studies observing shorter 6MWD in SSc-ILD patients [16, 30] and others reporting no significant difference [20, 21]. However, accurate comparison with previous works is challenging because of heterogeneity in design and population (notably in PH diagnosis, ILD definition and severity).

It is interesting to note that our result is in line with several data pleading for a predominant importance of pulmonary hemodynamic alterations over lung parenchymal involvement. In patients with IPF and PH, the 6MWD is significantly associated with hemodynamic parameters measured during right heart catheterization (RHC), but not with lung volumes assessed by spirometry [46]. In SSc-ILD patients, gas transfer alteration has a stronger prognostic value than lung volume reduction [47, 48].

However, if this result confirms that PAH contributes to impaired exercise capacities during SSc, we also observed in a previous work that the 6MWD correlated poorly with RHC parameters in SSc-PAH patients [49]. Taken together, these results suggest an impact of confounding extracardiopulmonary factors on the walked distance.

Association of the 6MWD with HAQ-DI score

Another interesting finding of our study is the strong association observed between the 6MWD and the HAQ-DI score.

Several teams have already reported similar results, both in univariate and multivariate regressions [21, 23]. Remarkably, in a previous work, Chow et al. [50] showed that the HAQ-DI score was not associated with parameters of cardiopulmonary severity in SSc patients with PAH. This implies that the patient perception of disability and functional limitation may not be entirely explained by the actual severity of the disease. Moreover, the 6MWD has been shown to be associated with scales of depression, anxiety and quality of life in several cardiorespiratory diseases [45, 51].

Overall, these results suggest that if the 6MWD is influenced to some extent by the objective severity of organ involvements, it is also greatly conditioned by the patient's subjective impression of disability and quality of life impairment.

Association of the 6MWD with CRP

An independent association between CRP levels and the 6WWD was observed in our population. A similar result was also found in previous work by Schoindre et al. [19] both in univariate and multivariate regressions, but not by Deuschle et al. [21]. Interestingly, CRP levels are associated with the EScSG-AI score, Medgser severity score and HAQ-DI score and with poorer prognosis in SSc patients [52]. In line with our prior results, this observation could suggest that the 6MWD also captures the overall disease activity and severity.

No major influence of the musculoskeletal involvement on the 6MWD

Contrary to a common idea [9], it is interesting to note that musculoskeletal involvement is not independently associated with the 6MWD in our population. However, we did not consider which sites were involved in patients with joint or muscle symptoms. Therefore, we could not test the association between the 6MWD and lower limb involvement, which could contribute to explain this negative result. The effect of joint and muscle symptoms has been suggested previously in univariate analyses [21, 25, 26] but has never been tested in multivariate regression. Interestingly, quadricipital strength and joint involvement have been found to correlate both with the 6MWD and with the HAQ-DI score in SSc patients [25, 26, 53], which suggests that this score may also account for the musculoskeletal-induced disability impacting on the 6MWD.

Our study draws strength from a large sample size and an important number of variables collected.

Our study also has some limitations. We did not perform incremental exercise testing to correlate the 6MWD with objective physiological parameters collected during effort. Similarly, we did not study autonomic dysfunction to help explain the results observed with HR variation and ΔHR.

In our multivariate regression, we chose to include only parameters relating to organ involvement (e.g., PAH and ILD) and exclude variables mediating them (e.g., NYHA class, PFT results and TTE data). Indeed, we believed that inserting the latter in our model could mask interesting associations of the 6MWD with organ involvement.

Conclusion

Our work showed that, aside from demographic parameters, ΔHR, resting HR, PAH, history of arterial thrombosis, CRP levels and HAQ-DI score are important factors associated with the 6MWD in SSc, while pulmonary interstitial and musculoskeletal involvements seem to have no major influence. This suggests that the 6MWD should be interpreted not only as a marker of cardiorespiratory severity, but also as a global assessment of disease activity and patient disability. Further studies are warranted to investigate the possibility of a chronotropic incompetence as a cause for exercise intolerance in SSc patients.

Abbreviations

6MWD: 6-minute walk distance; 6MWT: 6-minute walk test; ACR: American College of Rheumatology; BMI: Body mass index; BP: Blood pressure; CK: Creatinin kinase; COPD: Chronic obstructive pulmonary disease; CRP: C-reactive protein; DLCO: Diffusing capacity of the lung for carbon monoxide; EScSG-AI: European Scleroderma Study Group Activity Index; EULAR: European League Against Rheumatism; FVC: Forced vital capacity; HAQ-DI: Health Assessment Questionnaire—Disability Index; HR: Heart rate; ILD: Interstitial lung disease; IPF: Idiopathic pulmonary fibrosis; LVEF: Left ventricle ejection fraction; mRSS: Modified Rodnan skin score; NYHA: New York Heart Association; PAH: Pulmonary arterial hypertension; PFT: Pulmonary function tests; PH: Pulmonary hypertension; RHC: Right heart catheterization; sPAP: Systolic pulmonary artery pressure; SpO_2: Peripheral oxygen saturation; SSc: Systemic sclerosis; TLC: Total lung capacity; TTE: Transthoracic echocardiography; **Δ**: Variation of

Acknowledgements

None.

Authors' contributions

SS, VS and CP acquired patients' data. JG performed all statistical analyses. SS, JG and DL interpreted results and were major contributors in writing the manuscript. NL, PDG, J-FB, TP, RM and MR-J provided cardiorespiratory data and expertise. SM-D, HM, ML, P-YH and EH performed a critical reading of the manuscript. All authors read the final draft of the manuscript and approved its submitted version.

Funding

None.

Ethics approval and consent to participate

The study complied with the recommendations of the Helsinki declaration. French legislation on noninterventional studies does not require ethics committee approval for the use of de-identified data collected during patient care. As such, the need for an ethics committee approval was waived for this study by the *"Comité de Protection des Personnes"* (CPP).
The data were de-identified and complied with the requirements of the "Commission Nationale de l'Informatique et des Libertés" (CNIL), the organization responsible for ensuring the ethical use of data collected for scientific purposes in France. The CNIL approved the methods used to collect and analyze data from our patient database (approval #DC-2008-642). Written information was provided to each patient. French legislation on noninterventional studies requires collecting the nonopposition of patients but does not require written consent. As such, nonopposition was obtained from each patient included in the study for the use of their de-identified medical record data.

Competing interests

The authors declare that they have no competing interests.

Author details

[1]University of Lille, INSERM U995, LIRIC—Lille Inflammation Research International Center, F-59000 Lille, France. [2]INSERM U995, F-59000 Lille, France. [3]CHU Lille, Département de Médecine Interne et Immunologie Clinique, F-59000 Lille, France. [4]Centre National de Référence Maladies Systémiques et Auto-immunes Rares (Sclérodermie Systémique), F-59000 Lille, France. [5]Health Care Provider of the European Reference Network on Rare Connective Tissue and Musculoskeletal Diseases Network (ReCONNET), F-59000 Lille, France. [6]CHU Lille, Service de Cardiologie, F-59000 Lille, France. [7]CHU Lille, Service de Pneumologie, F-59000 Lille, France. [8]CHU Lille, Service d'Explorations Fonctionnelles Respiratoires, F-59000 Lille, France. [9]CHU Lille, Département d'Imagerie Thoracique, F-59000 Lille, France.

References

1. Hachulla E, Launay D. Diagnosis and classification of systemic sclerosis. Clin Rev Allergy Immunol. 2011;40:78–83.
2. Steen VD, Medsger TA. Changes in causes of death in systemic sclerosis, 1972-2002. Ann Rheum Dis. 2007;66:940–4.
3. Vandecasteele E, De Pauw M, De Keyser F, Decuman S, Deschepper E, Piette Y, et al. Six-minute walk test in systemic sclerosis: a systematic review and meta-analysis. Int J Cardiol. 2016;212:265–73.
4. Balke B. A simple field test for the assessment of physical fitness. Rep Civ Aeromed Res Inst US. 1963;6:1–8.
5. Holland AE, Spruit MA, Troosters T, Puhan MA, Pepin V, Saey D, et al. An official European Respiratory Society/American Thoracic Society Technical Standard: field walking tests in chronic respiratory disease. Eur Respir J. 2014;44:1428–46.
6. Miyamoto S, Nagaya N, Satoh T, Kyotani S, Sakamaki F, Fujita M, et al. Clinical correlates and prognostic significance of six-minute walk test in patients with primary pulmonary hypertension: comparison with cardiopulmonary exercise testing. Am J Respir Crit Care Med. 2000; 161:487–92.
7. Lederer DJ, Arcasoy SM, Wilt JS, D'Ovidio F, Sonett JR, Kawut SM. Six-minute-walk distance predicts waiting list survival in idiopathic pulmonary fibrosis. Am J Respir Crit Care Med. 2006;174:659–64.
8. Casanova C, Cote CG, Marin JM, de Torres JP, Aguirre-Jaime A, Mendez R, et al. The 6-min walking distance: long-term follow up in patients with COPD. Eur Respir J. 2007;29:535–40.
9. Impens AJ, Wangkaew S, Seibold JR. The 6-minute walk test in scleroderma—how measuring everything measures nothing. Rheumatol Oxf Engl. 2008;47 Suppl 5:v68–9.
10. Badesch DB, Tapson VF, McGoon MD, Brundage BH, Rubin LJ, Wigley FM, et al. Continuous intravenous epoprostenol for pulmonary hypertension due to the scleroderma spectrum of disease: a randomized, controlled trial. Ann Intern Med. 2000;132:425–34.
11. Rubin LJ, Badesch DB, Barst RJ, Galiè N, Black CM, Keogh A, et al. Bosentan therapy for pulmonary arterial hypertension. N Engl J Med. 2002;346:896–903.
12. Oudiz RJ, Schilz RJ, Barst RJ, Galié N, Rich S, Rubin LJ, et al. Treprostinil, a prostacyclin analogue, in pulmonary arterial hypertension associated with connective tissue disease. Chest. 2004;126:420–7.
13. Ahmadi-Simab K, Hellmich B, Gross WL. Bosentan for severe pulmonary arterial hypertension related to systemic sclerosis with interstitial lung disease. Eur J Clin Invest. 2006;36 Suppl 3:44–8.
14. Seibold JR, Denton CP, Furst DE, Guillevin L, Rubin LJ, Wells A, et al. Randomized, prospective, placebo-controlled trial of bosentan in interstitial lung disease secondary to systemic sclerosis. Arthritis Rheum. 2010;62:2101–8.
15. Buch MH, Denton CP, Furst DE, Guillevin L, Rubin LJ, Wells AU, et al. Submaximal exercise testing in the assessment of interstitial lung disease secondary to systemic sclerosis: reproducibility and correlations of the 6-min walk test. Ann Rheum Dis. 2007;66:169–73.
16. Villalba WO, Sampaio-Barros PD, Pereira MC, Cerqueira EM, Leme CA, Marques-Neto JF, et al. Six-minute walk test for the evaluation of pulmonary disease severity in scleroderma patients. Chest. 2007;131:217–22.
17. Ciurzyński M, Bienias P, Lichodziejewska B, Szewczyk A, Glińska-Wielochowska M, Jankowski K, et al. Assessment of left and right ventricular diastolic function in patients with systemic sclerosis. Kardiol Pol. 2008;66: 269–76. discussion 277–8.
18. Garin MC, Highland KB, Silver RM, Strange C. Limitations to the 6-minute walk test in interstitial lung disease and pulmonary hypertension in scleroderma. J Rheumatol. 2009;36:330–6.
19. Schoindre Y, Meune C, Dinh-Xuan AT, Avouac J, Kahan A, Allanore Y. Lack of specificity of the 6-minute walk test as an outcome measure for patients with systemic sclerosis. J Rheumatol. 2009;36:1481–5.
20. Akdogan A, Kaya EB, Sahin A, Okutucu S, Yakut E, Kalyoncu U, et al. Relationship between left ventricular diastolic dysfunction and six minute walk test in patients with systemic sclerosis. Int J Rheum Dis. 2011;14:379–83.
21. Deuschle K, Weinert K, Becker MO, Backhaus M, Huscher D, Riemekasten G. Six-minute walk distance as a marker for disability and complaints in patients with systemic sclerosis. Clin Exp Rheumatol. 2011;29:S53–9.
22. Wilsher M, Good N, Hopkins R, Young P, Milne D, Gibson A, et al. The six-minute walk test using forehead oximetry is reliable in the assessment of scleroderma lung disease. Respirology. 2012;17:647–52.

23. Chung L, Chen H, Khanna D, Steen VD. Dyspnea assessment and pulmonary hypertension in patients with systemic sclerosis: utility of the University of California, San Diego, Shortness of Breath Questionnaire. Arthritis Care Res. 2013;65:454–63.
24. Irzyk K, Bienias P, Kostrubiec M, Rymarczyk Z, Bartoszewicz Z, Siwicka M, et al. Six-minute walk test reflects neurohormonal activation and right ventricular function in systemic sclerosis patients. Clin Exp Rheumatol. 2013; 31:18–23.
25. Lima TRL, Guimarães FS, Silva LA, Silva DPG, Menezes SLS, Lopes AJ. Relationship between functional capacity, joint mobility and pulmonary function in patients with systemic sclerosis. J Bodyw Mov Ther. 2015;19:17–24.
26. Lima TRL, Guimarães FS, Carvalho MN, Sousa TLM, Menezes SLS, Lopes AJ. Lower limb muscle strength is associated with functional performance and quality of life in patients with systemic sclerosis. Braz J Phys Ther. 2015;19:129–36.
27. Rizzi M, Sarzi-Puttini P, Airoldi A, Antivalle M, Battellino M, Atzeni F. Performance capacity evaluated using the 6-minute walk test: 5-year results in patients with diffuse systemic sclerosis and initial interstitial lung disease. Clin Exp Rheumatol. 2015;33:S142–7.
28. Lopes AJ, Ferreira Ade S, Lima TRL, Menezes SLS, Guimarães FS. An explanatory model of functional exercise capacity in patients with systemic sclerosis: considerations for rehabilitation programs. J Phys Ther Sci. 2016;28:569–75.
29. Kusunose K, Yamada H, Nishio S, Hirata Y, Seno H, Saijo Y, et al. Echocardiographic Predictors for Worsening of Six-Minute Walk Distances in Patients With Systemic Sclerosis (Scleroderma). Am J Cardiol. 2017;120:315-21.
30. Vandecasteele E, Thevissen K, Melsens K, De Keyser F, De Pauw M, Deschepper E, et al. Six-minute walk test in or out in evaluation of systemic sclerosis patients? Clin Exp Rheumatol. 2017;35 Suppl 106(4):122-129.
31. van den Hoogen F, Khanna D, Fransen J, Johnson SR, Baron M, Tyndall A, et al. 2013 classification criteria for systemic sclerosis: an American College of Rheumatology/European League Against Rheumatism collaborative initiative. Ann Rheum Dis. 2013;72:1747–55.
32. ATS Committee on Proficiency Standards for Clinical Pulmonary Function Laboratories. ATS statement: guidelines for the six-minute walk test. Am J Respir Crit Care Med. 2002;166:111–7.
33. Enright PL, Sherill DL. Reference equations for the six-minute walk in healthy adults. Am J Respir Crit Care Med. 1998;158:1384–7.
34. Valentini G, Rossa AD, Bombardieri S, Bencivelli W, Silman AJ, D'Angelo S, et al. European multicentre study to define disease activity criteria for systemic sclerosis. II. Identification of disease activity variables and development of preliminary activity indexes. Ann Rheum Dis. 2001;60:592–8.
35. Medsger TA, Bombardieri S, Czirjak L, Scorza R, Rossa AD, Bencivelli W. Assessment of disease severity and prognosis in systemic sclerosis. Clin Exp Rheumatol. 2003;21:S42–6.
36. Fries JF, Spitz P, Kraines RG, Holman HR. Measurement of patient outcome in arthritis. Arthritis Rheum. 1980;23:137–45.
37. R Development Core Team. R: A language and environment for statistical computing. Vienna, Austria: R Foundation for Statistical Computing; 2008. http://www.R-project.org.
38. Holland AE, Hill CJ, Glaspole I, Goh N, Dowman L, McDonald CF. Impaired chronotropic response to 6-min walk test and reduced survival in interstitial lung disease. Respir Med. 2013;107:1066–72.
39. Provencher S, Chemla D, Hervé P, Sitbon O, Humbert M, Simonneau G. Heart rate responses during the 6-minute walk test in pulmonary arterial hypertension. Eur Respir J. 2006;27:114–20.
40. Lauer MS. Heart rate response in stress testing: clinical implications. ACC Curr J Rev. 2001;10:16–9.
41. Brubaker PH, Kitzman DW. Chronotropic incompetence: causes, consequences, and management. Circulation. 2011;123:1010–20.
42. Amaral TN, Peres FA, Lapa AT, Marques-Neto JF, Appenzeller S. Neurologic involvement in scleroderma: a systematic review. Semin Arthritis Rheum. 2013;43:335–47.
43. Bienias P, Ciurzyński M, Glińska-Wielochowska M, Szewczyk A, Korczak D, Kalińska-Bienias A, et al. Heart rate turbulence assessment in systemic sclerosis: the role for the detection of cardiac autonomic nervous system dysfunction. Rheumatol Oxf Engl. 2010;49:355–60.
44. Someya F, Mugii N, Oohata S. Factors relating to impaired stroke volume during the 6-minute walk test in patients with systemic sclerosis. Clin Exp Rheumatol. 2016;34 Suppl 100:152–6.
45. Ingle L, Rigby AS, Nabb S, Jones PK, Clark AL, Cleland JG. Clinical determinants of poor six-minute walk test performance in patients with left ventricular systolic dysfunction and no major structural heart disease. Eur J Heart Fail. 2006;8:321–5.
46. Minai OA, Santacruz JF, Alster JM, Budev MM, McCarthy K. Impact of pulmonary hemodynamics on 6-min walk test in idiopathic pulmonary fibrosis. Respir Med. 2012;106:1613–21.
47. Goh NS, Hoyles RK, Denton CP, Hansell DM, Renzoni EA, Maher TM, et al. Short term pulmonary function trends are predictive of mortality in interstitial lung disease associated with systemic sclerosis: pulmonary function trends in SSc-ILD. Arthritis Rheumatol. Arthritis Rheumatol. 2017; 69(8):1670-1678.
48. Le Gouellec N, Duhamel A, Perez T, Hachulla A-L, Sobanski V, Faivre J-B, et al. Predictors of lung function test severity and outcome in systemic sclerosis-associated interstitial lung disease. PLoS One. 2017;12:e0181692.
49. Sanges S, Launay D, Rhee RL, Sitbon O, Hachulla É, Mouthon L, et al. A prospective study of the 6 min walk test as a surrogate marker for haemodynamics in two independent cohorts of treatment-naïve systemic sclerosis-associated pulmonary arterial hypertension. Ann Rheum Dis. 2016; 75:1457–65.
50. Chow S, Pope JE, Mehta S. Lack of correlation of the health assessment questionnaire disability index with lung parameters in systemic sclerosis associated pulmonary arterial hypertension. Clin Exp Rheumatol. 2008;26:1012–7.
51. Spruit MA, Watkins ML, Edwards LD, Vestbo J, Calverley PMA, Pinto-Plata V, et al. Determinants of poor 6-min walking distance in patients with COPD: the ECLIPSE cohort. Respir Med. 2010;104:849–57.
52. Muangchan C, Harding S, Khimdas S, Bonner A. Canadian Scleroderma Research Group, Baron M, et al. Association of C-reactive protein with high disease activity in systemic sclerosis: results from the Canadian Scleroderma Research Group. Arthritis Care Res. 2012;64:1405–14.
53. Clements PJ, Wong WK, Hurwitz EL, Furst DE, Mayes M, White B, et al. Correlates of the disability index of the health assessment questionnaire: a measure of functional impairment in systemic sclerosis. Arthritis Rheum. 1999;42:2372–80.

Fli1-haploinsufficient dermal fibroblasts promote skin-localized transdifferentiation of Th2-like regulatory T cells

Ryosuke Saigusa[1], Yoshihide Asano[1*], Takashi Taniguchi[1], Megumi Hirabayashi[1], Kouki Nakamura[1], Shunsuke Miura[1], Takashi Yamashita[1], Takehiro Takahashi[1], Yohei Ichimura[1], Tetsuo Toyama[1], Ayumi Yoshizaki[1], Maria Trojanowska[2] and Shinichi Sato[1]

Abstract

Background: Friend leukemia virus integration 1 (Fli1) deficiency, a predisposing factor of systemic sclerosis (SSc), induces SSc-like phenotypes in various cell types. A recent study demonstrated the transdifferentiation of T helper type 2 cell (Th2)-like regulatory T cells (Tregs) in SSc lesional skin through interleukin (IL)-33 produced by fibroblasts. Therefore, we investigated the role of Fli1 deficiency in dermal fibroblast-mediated transdifferentiation of Tregs.

Methods: Cytokine expression was assessed in Tregs by flow cytometry and in skin samples and cultivated cells by immunostaining, immunoblotting, and/or qRT-PCR. Fli1 binding to the target gene promoters was examined by chromatin immunoprecipitation. Murine dermal fibroblasts and Tregs were cocultured with or without blocking antibodies against target cytokines.

Results: Th2- and Th17-like cell proportions in skin-homing Tregs were increased in bleomycin-treated *Fli1*$^{+/-}$ mice compared with bleomycin-treated wild-type mice, whereas Th1-, Th2-, and Th17-like cell proportions in splenic Tregs were comparable. *Fli1*$^{+/-}$ fibroblasts overproduced IL-33 and IL-6, in particular IL-33, and Fli1 occupied the *IL33* and *IL6* promoters in dermal fibroblasts. Importantly, the IL-4-producing cell proportion was significantly higher in wild-type Tregs cocultured with *Fli1*$^{+/-}$ fibroblasts than in those cocultured with wild-type fibroblasts, which were canceled by neutralizing anti-IL-33 antibody. Under the same coculture condition, an increased tendency of IL-17A-producing cell proportion, which was possibly mediated by IL-6, was evident.

Conclusions: Fli1 haploinsufficiency increases the proportions of Th2- and Th17-like Tregs in bleomycin-induced profibrotic skin conditions, in which IL-33-producing dermal fibroblasts contribute to Th2-like Treg transdifferentiation, suggesting a critical role of Fli1 deficiency in the interaction of dermal fibroblasts with immune cells in pathological skin fibrosis.

Keywords: Fli1, Fibroblasts, Regulatory T cells, IL-33, Systemic sclerosis

Background

Systemic sclerosis (SSc) is a multisystem autoimmune disease characterized by vasculopathy and fibrosis of the skin and certain internal organs. Although SSc pathogenesis has yet to be fully disclosed, the canonical wisdom is that dermal fibroblast activation is the final consequence of its sequential pathological processes, such as initial vascular injury due to autoimmune attack and subsequent chronic inflammation [1]. However, a recent study has demonstrated that activated fibroblasts regulate tissue-localized transdifferentiation of regulatory T cells (Tregs) into T helper type 2 cell (Th2)-like cells through IL-33 in SSc lesional skin [2], suggesting that activated dermal fibroblasts amplify an aberrant immune response characteristic of SSc. This notion provides new insight into the continuing discussion of the controversy of Tregs in SSc, with reports of decreased, increased, or equal proportions of Tregs in the blood of patients compared with healthy control subjects [3–6]. Although Treg transdifferentiation into Th1- and/or Th17-like cells has been reported in type 1

* Correspondence: yasano-tky@umin.ac.jp
[1]Department of Dermatology, University of Tokyo Graduate School of Medicine, 7-3-1 Hongo, Bunkyo-ku, Tokyo 113-8655, Japan
Full list of author information is available at the end of the article

diabetes [7], multiple sclerosis [8], and juvenile idiopathic arthritis [9], Treg transdifferentiation into Th2-like cells is documented exclusively in SSc so far, indicating that this pathological process is unique in this disease.

Friend leukemia virus integration 1 (Fli1) is a member of the Ets family of transcription factors, the deficiency of which is a potential predisposing factor of SSc [10]. Fli1 expression is suppressed in dermal fibroblasts, endothelial cells, and perivascular inflammatory cells in involved and noninvolved skin of patients with SSc [11]. Although the detailed mechanism explaining Fli1 down-regulation in SSc is still unknown, an epigenetic mechanism is reported at least in dermal fibroblasts [12]. According to a series of studies on *Fli1*-mutated mice and *FLI1* small interfering RNA-treated cultured cells, Fli1 deficiency promotes the induction of SSc-like phenotypes in dermal fibroblasts, dermal microvascular endothelial cells, and macrophages [13–16]. Most importantly, mice with simultaneous haploinsufficiency of the *Fli1* and *Klf5* genes, both of which are epigenetically suppressed in SSc dermal fibroblasts, spontaneously develop the three cardinal features of SSc, including immune abnormalities, vasculopathy, and tissue fibrosis [17]. These animal models are useful for obtaining a clue to understanding the role of certain cells and to elucidating the mechanisms of disease-modifying drugs in SSc [18, 19].

On the basis of this background, we investigated the role of Fli1 deficiency in fibroblast-mediated transdifferentiation of Tregs by using bleomycin (BLM)-treated *Fli1*$^{+/-}$ mice. The detailed molecular mechanism was further investigated by coculture experiments of Tregs with dermal fibroblasts.

Methods

A BLM-induced murine SSc model

BLM (200 μg, 02907278; Nippon Kayaku, Tokyo, Japan) dissolved in PBS or control PBS was injected subcutaneously into a single location on the back of 8-week-old female wild-type (WT) mice (C57BL/6) and *Fli1*$^{+/-}$ mice daily.

Flow cytometry

Mice were treated with BLM for 1 week. On the day after the final injection, lymphocytes from the spleen and the dermis of the lower back skin were obtained. Skin samples were incubated in 2 mg/ml dispase (383-02281; Wako Pure Chemical Industries, Osaka, Japan) and were separated into epidermis and dermis. Dermis was minced and then incubated with 2 mg/ml collagenase type 2 (CLS-2; Worthington Biochemical, Lakewood, NJ, USA) in Tyrode's solution for 60–90 minutes. The digested tissues were centrifuged, resuspended in PBS, and filtered through a 70-μm mesh. Single-cell suspensions were stained on ice with labeled monoclonal antibody. In the surface staining experiments, cells were stained with antibodies against CD4 (100526; BioLegend, San Diego, CA, USA). In intracellular cytokine staining, cells were stimulated with 10 ng/ml phorbol myristate acetate and 1 μg/ml ionomycin (10634; Sigma-Aldrich, St. Louis, MO, USA) in the presence of 1 mg/ml brefeldin A (420601; BioLegend) for 4 h. Cells were washed; stained for CD4; treated with fixative/permeabilization buffer (71-5775-40; eBioscience, San Diego, CA, USA); and then stained with anti-FoxP3 (71-5775-40; eBioscience), anti-IL-4 (554436; BD Biosciences, San Jose, CA, USA), anti-IL-13 (12-7133-41; eBioscience), anti-IL-17A (506919; BioLegend), and anti-interferon (IFN)-γ (505825; BioLegend) antibodies. Tregs were defined by CD4^{+}FoxP3^{+} cells. Cells were analyzed on a FACSVerse flow cytometer (BD Biosciences).

Immunohistochemistry

Immunohistochemistry with the Mouse on Mouse (M.O.M^{TM}) Elite Peroxidase Detection Kit (PK-2200; Vector Laboratories, Burlingame, CA, USA) was performed on formalin-fixed, paraffin-embedded skin sections using anti-IL-33 antibody (ab54384; Abcam, Cambridge, UK). To quantify the signal intensity of IL-33, color images were converted to grayscale, and then the brightness was measured in five different randomly selected fibroblasts and epidermal areas per specimen. These processes were analyzed using ImageJ software (National Institutes of Health, Bethesda, MD, USA), and the average values were compared.

Murine dermal fibroblast isolation

For isolation of murine fibroblasts, referring to a past report [20], we took the ears from mice and placed them in cell culture media. Then, collagenase (17100017; Thermo Fisher Scientific, Waltham, MA, USA) was added, and the ears were minced as much as possible with sterile scissors. After overnight incubation at 37 °C, the ears were further dissociated by vigorous pipetting. Cells were passed through a cell strainer to achieve a single-cell suspension and remove the remaining debris. Finally, the cells were pelleted by centrifugation, resuspended, and cultured until proliferated.

qRT-PCR

RNA isolation from cultivated cells and skin tissue, as well as qRT-PCR, was performed as described previously [21–23]. The sequences of primers were as follows: murine *Il33*-forward 5′-CAATCAGGCGACG GTGTGGATGG-3′, murine *Il33*-reverse 5′-TCCGGA GGCGAGACGTCACC-3′; murine *Il6*-forward 5′-GA TGGATGCTACCAAACTGGAT-3′, murine *Il6*-reverse 5′-CCAGGTAGCTATGGTACTCCAGA-3′; murine *Gapdh*-forward 5′-CGTGTTCCTACCCCCAATGT-3′, murine *Gapdh*-reverse 5′-TGTCATCATACTTGGCA GGTTTCT-3′.

Immunoblotting

Confluent quiescent fibroblasts were serum-starved for 24 h. Whole-cell lysates were prepared. Samples were subjected to sodium dodecyl sulfate-PAGE (NP0321; Life Technologies/Thermo Fisher Scientific, Carlsbad, CA, USA) and immunoblotting with anti-IL-33 antibody (ab54384; Abcam) and anti-β-actin antibody (sc-47778; Santa Cruz Biotechnology, Dallas, TX, USA). Bands were detected using enhanced chemiluminescence techniques (34080; Thermo Fisher Scientific, Rockford, IL, USA).

Chromatin immunoprecipitation assay

Human normal dermal fibroblasts were purchased from the American Type Culture Collection (PCS-201-010; Manassas, VA, USA) and used. The chromatin immunoprecipitation (ChIP) assay was conducted using the EpiQuik ChIP kit (P-2002-3; EpiGentek, Farmingdale, NY, USA) [17]. Putative Fli1 binding sites in the *IL33* and *IL6* promoters were predicted using Tfsitescan. The primers that amplify fragments of the *IL33* promoter (−1332 bp to approximately −1183 bp) and the *IL6* promoter (−1109 bp to approximately −944 bp) were as follows: *IL33* ChIP-forward 5′-TCAGCTGGGAGATGGGTAAG-3′; *IL33* ChIP-reverse 5′-ATAATCTATTCTCTCTGAAGCCTA-CAA-3′, *IL6* ChIP-forward 5′-GACACCATCCTGAG GGAAGA-3′; *IL6* ChIP-reverse 5′-TATCGC TCCCTCTCCCTGTA-3′. In some experiments, fibroblasts were treated with IL-1β (201-LB-005; R&D Systems, Minneapolis, MN, USA).

Cocultures

Murine dermal fibroblasts were prepared from WT and *Fli1*$^{+/-}$ mice and maintained as described previously [13]. Splenic Tregs were isolated from WT mice with a CD4$^+$CD25$^+$ Treg cell isolation kit (130-091-041; Miltenyi Biotec, Bergisch Gladbach, Germany) and cultured in RPMI 1640 medium supplemented with FCS. Murine dermal fibroblasts (1×10^5 cells) and CD4$^+$CD25$^+$ T cells (3×10^5 cells) were cocultured in 24-well plates for 2 days. Then, cells were analyzed on a FACSVerse flow cytometer. In some experiments, cocultured cells were treated with anti-mouse IL-33 antibody (M187-3; MBL, Nagoya, Japan) or antimouse IL-6 antibody (MAB406-SP; R&D Systems).

Statistical analysis

Statistical analysis was done with the Mann-Whitney *U* test to compare the distributions of two unmatched groups. Statistical significance was defined as a P value < 0.05.

Results

Th2- and Th17-like Tregs are increased in the skin of BLM-treated *Fli1*$^{+/-}$ mice

As an initial experiment, we employed BLM-treated mice because this murine model recapitulates inflammatory and fibrotic aspects of SSc [24]. In this model, inflammation and dermal fibrosis reach their peak at days 7 and 28 after BLM injection, respectively [25–28]. After confirming that BLM induces greater dermal fibrosis in *Fli1*$^{+/-}$ mice than in WT mice as previously reported [13], we collected skin samples and splenocytes at day 7 and evaluated the phenotypes of skin-homing and splenic Tregs by comparing the proportions of IFN-γ-, IL-4-, IL-13-, and IL-17A-producing cells among CD4$^+$FoxP3$^+$ cells. As shown in Fig. 1a, on one hand, BLM injection increased the proportions of IL-4-, IL-13-, and IL-17A-producing Tregs—namely, Th2- and Th17-like Tregs—in the skin of *Fli1*$^{+/-}$ mice compared with WT mice. On the other hand, the proportions of Th1-, Th2-, and Th17-like cells in splenic Tregs were comparable between BLM-treated *Fli1*$^{+/-}$ mice and BLM-treated WT mice (Fig. 1b; scatterplots also shown in Additional file 1: Figure S1). These results suggest that Fli1 haploinsufficiency promotes skin-localized transdifferentiation and/or skin infiltration of Th2- and Th17-like Tregs in BLM-treated mice.

IL-33 expression is higher in skin of BLM-treated *Fli1*$^{+/-}$ mice

Because IL-33 produced by dermal fibroblasts contributes to Th2-like Treg transdifferentiation in the lesional skin of patients with SSc [2], we next evaluated IL-33 expression in the skin of BLM-treated *Fli1*$^{+/-}$ mice. Of note, *Il33* messenger RNA (mRNA) expression was higher in the skin of BLM-treated *Fli1*$^{+/-}$ mice than in BLM-treated WT mice (Fig. 1c). To confirm the origin of BLM-induced IL-33 expression, we also carried out immunostaining with anti-IL-33 antibody. As shown in Fig. 1d and Additional file 2: Figure S2, the signal intensity of IL-33 in dermal fibroblasts was remarkably increased in BLM-treated *Fli1*$^{+/-}$ mice as compared with BLM-treated WT mice, whereas that in epidermal keratinocytes was comparable. When the staining was performed without anti-IL-33 antibody, no signals were detectable in the same skin sample from BLM-treated WT mice (Fig. 1e). Taken together, these results indicate that IL-33 produced by dermal fibroblasts may contribute to Th2-like Treg transdifferentiation in the skin of BLM-treated *Fli1*$^{+/-}$ mice.

Fli1 haploinsufficiency results in overexpression of IL-33 in dermal fibroblasts

To investigate the molecular mechanism underlying IL-33 overproduction in dermal fibroblasts of BLM-treated *Fli1*$^{+/-}$ mice, we first evaluated IL-33 expression levels in the skin of *Fli1*$^{+/-}$ and WT mice under a physiological condition. Of note, *Il33* mRNA levels were significantly elevated in the skin of *Fli1*$^{+/-}$ mice compared with WT mice (Fig. 2a). Furthermore, IL-33 expression was clearly elevated in dermal fibroblasts of *Fli1*$^{+/-}$ mice relative to

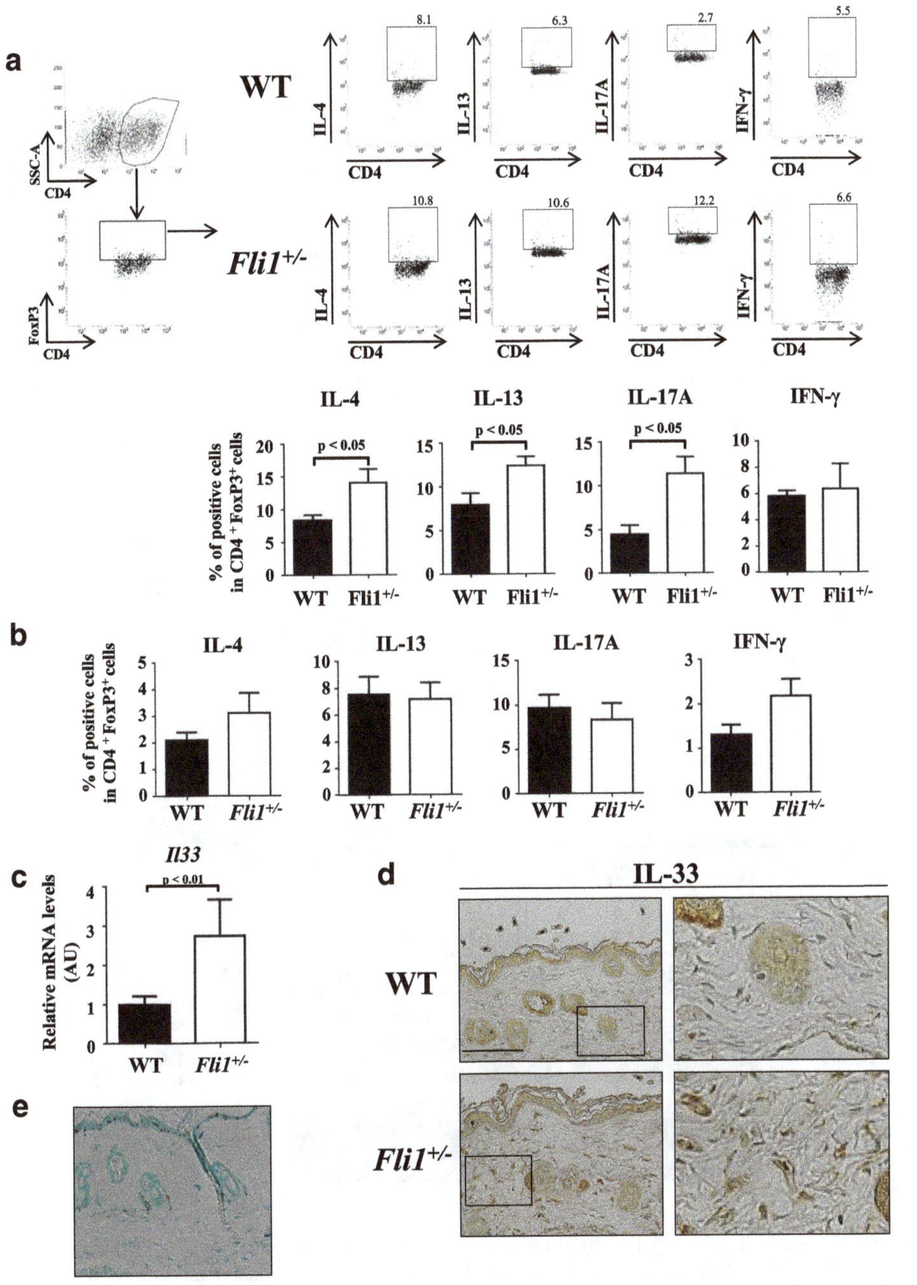

Fig. 1 Cytokine expression profiles of skin-homing and splenic regulatory T cells (Tregs) in bleomycin (BLM)-treated mice and interleukin (IL)-33 expression in the lesional skin of BLM-treated mice. **a** Evaluation of skin-homing Tregs from BLM-treated wild-type (WT) and *Fli1*$^{+/-}$ mice on IL-4, IL-13, IL17A, and IFN-γ expression by flow cytometry (*n* = 6). Gating strategy for identification of CD4$^+$FoxP3$^+$ Tregs is shown in the *leftmost panel.* **b** Evaluation of splenic Tregs from BLM-treated WT and *Fli1*$^{+/-}$ mice on IL-4, IL-17A, and IFN-γ expression by flow cytometry (*n* = 6). **c** qRT-PCR evaluation of *Il33* messenger RNA (mRNA) expression in the lesional skin of WT and *Fli1*$^{+/-}$ mice treated with BLM for 1 week (*n* = 10). **d** Representative images of staining for IL-33 in skin samples from WT and *Fli1*$^{+/-}$ mice treated with BLM for 1 week (original magnification ×400, scale bar = 50 μm). **e** The result of immunostaining without anti-IL-33 antibody in the skin of BLM-treated WT mice. Images of high-power field spotlighting dermal fibroblasts are in the *rightmost column*. Representative plots of one of five to eight individual animals from at least two separate experiments are shown in (**a**). In each graph, the relative value compared with the control group is expressed as mean ± SEM. *AU* Arbitrary units, *Fli1* Friend leukemia virus integration 1, *SSC-A* Side scatter area

those cells of WT mice while being comparable in epidermal keratinocytes (Fig. 2b and Additional file 2: Figure S2). Also, no nonspecific signals were confirmed by conducting staining without anti-IL-33 antibody (Fig. 2c). Importantly, the signal intensity of IL-33 in dermal fibroblasts was modestly but significantly elevated in BLM-treated *Fli1*$^{+/-}$ mice

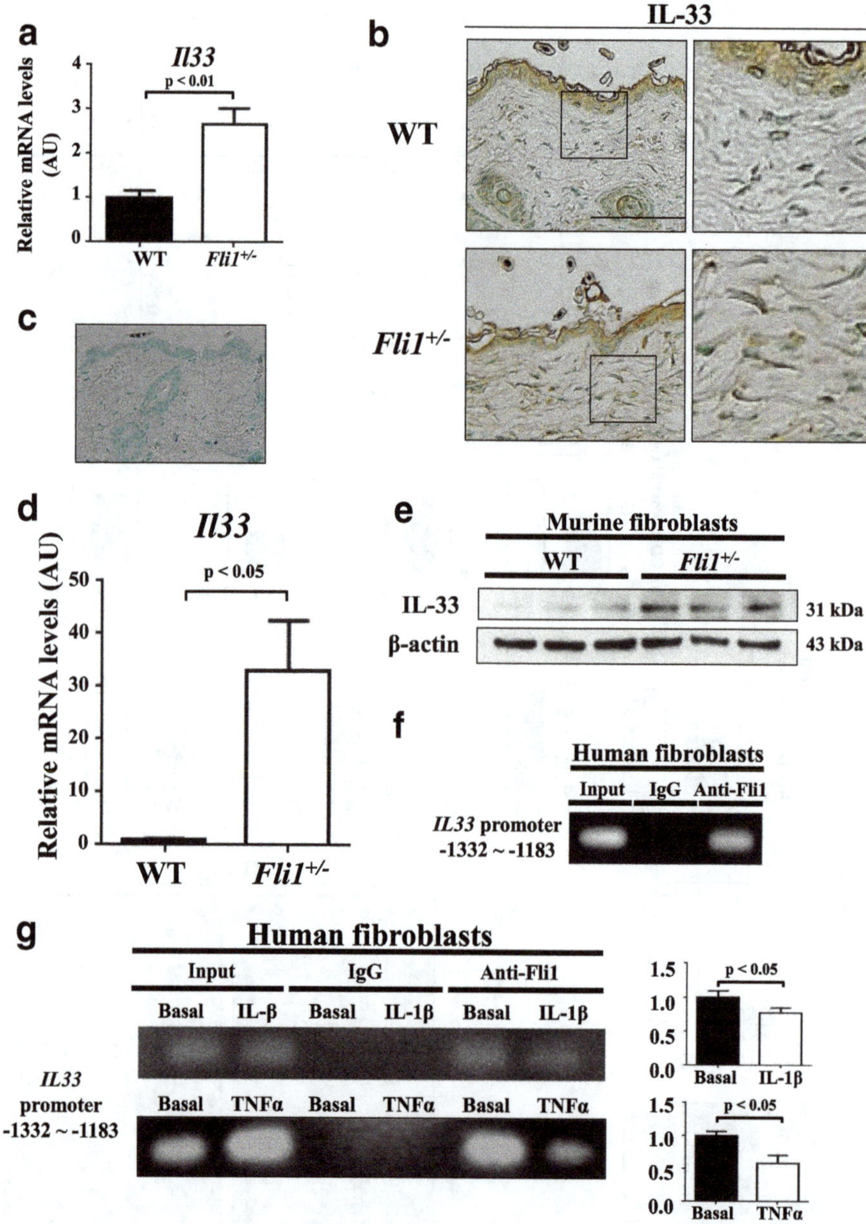

Fig. 2 Friend leukemia virus integration 1 (Fli1) regulates the expression of interleukin (IL)-33 in dermal fibroblasts. **a**, **b** Evaluation of IL-33 expression in skin from wild-type (WT) and *Fli1*$^{+/-}$ mice without any treatment by qRT-PCR (**a**, *n* = 10) and immunohistochemistry (**b**, *n* = 5; original magnification ×400, scale bar = 50 μm). High-power field images spotlighting dermal fibroblasts are in the *rightmost column*. **c** The result of immunostaining without anti-IL-33 antibody in the skin of WT mice under a physiological condition. **d**, **e** Evaluation of IL-33 expression in dermal fibroblasts isolated from WT and *Fli1*$^{+/-}$ mice by qRT-PCR (**d**, *n* = 10) and immunoblotting (**e**, *n* = 4). **f**, **g** Results of the chromatin immunoprecipitation assay regarding Fli1 occupation on the *IL33* promoter in human dermal fibroblasts without any treatment (**f**, *n* = 4) and those cells treated with IL-1β or tumor necrosis factor (TNF)-α for 24 h (**g**, *n* = 4). For **a** and **c**, messenger RNA (mRNA) levels of the *Il33* gene were normalized to those of the *Gapdh* gene. For **f**, the occupancy of the *Il33* promoter by Fli1 was quantified with qRT-PCR. For **b**, **d**, and **e**, representative results are shown. In each graph, the relative value compared with the control group is expressed as mean ± SEM. *AU* Arbitrary units, *IgG* Immunoglobulin G, *TNF-α* Tumor necrosis factor-α

compared with untreated *Fli1*$^{+/-}$ mice (Additional file 2: Figure S2). Supporting these in vivo findings, IL-33 expression was increased in *Fli1*$^{+/-}$ dermal fibroblasts at mRNA and protein levels compared with WT dermal fibroblasts in vitro (Fig. 2d and e; *see* Additional file 3: Figure S3 for an original file). These results indicate that *Fli1*$^{+/-}$ dermal fibroblasts produce excessive amounts of IL-33 even under a quiescent condition.

To further examine if Fli1 directly regulates the expression of IL-33, we conducted in vitro experiments with human dermal fibroblasts. The ChIP assay exhibited the binding of Fli1 to the *IL33* promoter (Fig. 2f), suggesting the direct regulation of IL-33 by Fli1. Given that IL-1β and tumor necrosis factor (TNF)-α induce the expression of IL-33 in dermal fibroblasts [29], we investigated whether these molecules affect the occupancy of Fli1 on the *IL33* promoter by performing ChIP analysis, showing that both of IL-1β and TNF-α induced the dissociation of Fli1 from the promoter (Fig. 2g). In aggregate, these results indicate that Fli1 directly regulates IL-33 expression as a potent repressor and that Fli1 deficiency possibly contributes to IL-33 production in SSc dermal fibroblasts.

Transdifferentiation of Tregs into Th2-like cells is promoted by *Fli1*$^{+/-}$ dermal fibroblasts through IL-33 in vitro

Because fibroblast-mediated transdifferentiation of Th2-like Tregs depends on IL-33 in SSc, we next assessed if the same scenario is applicable to Fli1 haploinsufficiency-dependent transdifferentiation of Th2-like Tregs in BLM-treated mice. To this end, we cocultured WT Tregs with dermal fibroblasts isolated from WT mice or *Fli1*$^{+/-}$ mice. The proportion of IL-4-producing cells was significantly higher and the proportion of IL-17A-producing cells tended to be higher in CD4^{+}FoxP3^{+} cells cocultured with *Fli1*$^{+/-}$ dermal fibroblasts than in those cells cocultured with WT fibroblasts, whereas no effect was seen on the proportion of IFN-γ-producing cells (Fig. 3a). On the basis of the data up to this point, Fli1 deficiency in dermal fibroblasts may induce IL-4-expressing Tregs, possibly through the key molecule IL-33. To address this issue, we cocultured these cells in the presence of neutralizing antibody for IL-33. As expected, this neutralizing antibody significantly attenuated the proportion of IL-4-producing cells, whereas it did not affect the proportions of IL-17A- and IFN-γ-producing cells in CD4^{+}FoxP3^{+} cells cocultured with *Fli1*$^{+/-}$ dermal fibroblasts (Fig. 3b). These results indicate that *Fli1*$^{+/-}$ dermal fibroblasts regulate the transdifferentiation of Th2-like Tregs at least partially through IL-33.

We also assessed whether *Fli1*$^{+/-}$ dermal fibroblasts promote the transdifferentiation of Th17-like Tregs, because a significant increase in the proportion of IL-17A-producing Tregs in the skin of BLM-treated *Fli1*$^{+/-}$ mice (Fig. 1a) and an increased tendency of IL-17A-producing cells in WT Tregs cocultured with *Fli1*$^{+/-}$ dermal fibroblasts (Fig. 3a) were evident. Because IL-6 is a key cytokine in the conversion of induced Tregs into Th17 cells [30, 31] and its mRNA expression is increased in the lesional skin of BLM-treated *Fli1*$^{+/-}$ mice compared with BLM-treated WT mice [13], we speculated that IL-6 produced by *Fli1*$^{+/-}$ dermal fibroblasts promotes the transdifferentiation of Th17-like Tregs. Consistent with this hypothesis, *Il6* mRNA expression was significantly higher in *Fli1*$^{+/-}$ dermal fibroblasts than in WT dermal fibroblasts (Fig. 4a, *left panel*). Also, IL-6 protein expression was elevated in cultured dermal fibroblasts from BLM-treated *Fli1*$^{+/-}$ mice compared with those from BLM-treated WT mice (Fig. 4a, *right panel; see* Additional file 3: Figure S3 for an original file). The ChIP analysis revealed the binding of Fli1 to the *IL6* promoter in human normal dermal fibroblasts, suggesting the direct regulation of IL-6 expression by Fli1 (Fig. 4b). More importantly, anti-IL-6 antibody tended to reduce the proportion of Th17-like cells in WT Tregs cocultured with *Fli1*$^{+/-}$ dermal fibroblasts (Fig. 4c). Taken together, these results indicate that Fli1 haploinsufficiency increases the proportion of Th17-like cells in skin-homing Tregs, possibly and partially through IL-6 produced by dermal fibroblasts.

Discussion

BLM-treated mice have been widely used as a useful model of SSc [32, 33]. On one hand, the benefit of this model is the highly reproducible induction of inflammation and tissue fibrosis similar to those of SSc. In addition, it can be used in various genetically manipulated mice to explore the relationship of targeted molecules with inflammatory and fibrotic pathways related to SSc development. On the other hand, the weak point of this model is the lack of persistent tissue fibrosis like that in SSc; namely, tissue fibrosis spontaneously improves within 3 months after ceasing BLM injection. We currently focused on the contribution of Fli1 haploinsufficiency to dermal fibroblast-dependent transdifferentiation of Tregs during the inflammatory phase of an SSc-like condition; therefore, we can say that BLM-treated mice would be suitable for addressing this issue. In our initial experiments, the proportions of Th2- and Th17-like cells in skin-homing Tregs were significantly increased in BLM-treated *Fli1*$^{+/-}$ mice compared with BLM-treated WT mice, which is consistent with our previous report demonstrating the increased expression of Th2 and Th17 cytokines in the lesional skin of BLM-treated mice [13]. Importantly, Th2-like Treg transdifferentiation was regulated at least partially by IL-33 overproduced by *Fli1*$^{+/-}$ dermal fibroblasts. In addition, IL-6 produced by *Fli1*$^{+/-}$ dermal fibroblasts seemed to be modestly involved in Th17-like Treg transdifferentiation. Because Fli1 occupied the *IL33* and *IL6* promoters, Fli1 haploinsufficiency is likely to directly enhance the production of IL-33 and IL-6 in dermal fibroblasts. These results indicate that Fli1 haploinsufficiency augments BLM-induced skin fibrosis by increasing the production of profibrotic Th2 cytokines and the induction of Th17 cytokine-mediated inflammation partially through the interaction of dermal fibroblasts and Tregs.

A critical contribution of Fli1 deficiency to the activation of dermal fibroblasts was initially proved on the basis of its impact on type I collagen expression. Fli1 binds to the *COL1A1* and *COL1A2* promoters [21, 34] and serves as a potent repressor of these genes in dermal

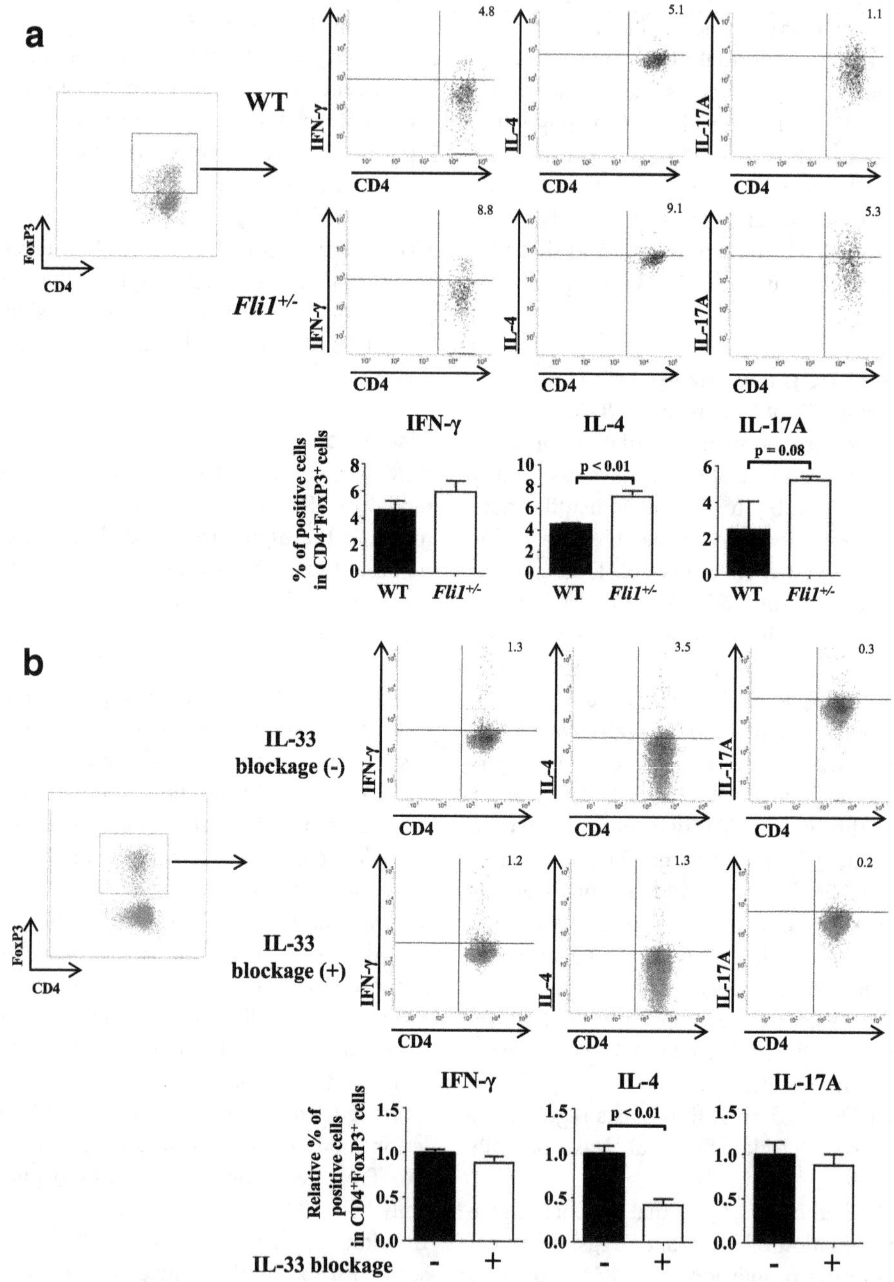

Fig. 3 T helper type 2 cell (Th2)-like regulatory T cells (Tregs) are induced by coculture with *Fli1*$^{+/-}$ dermal fibroblasts through interleukin (IL)-33. **a** Evaluation by flow cytometry of Th1-, Th2-, and Th17-like Treg induction by coculture with wild-type (WT) and *Fli1*$^{+/-}$ dermal fibroblasts (n = 6). **b** Evaluation by flow cytometry of the effect of IL-33-neutralizing antibody on Tregs cocultured with *Fli1*$^{+/-}$ dermal fibroblasts (n = 6). Representative plots of interferon (IFN)-γ-, IL-4-, and IL-17A-positive Tregs are shown in *right upper panels* of (**a**) and (**b**). Gating strategy for identification of CD4$^+$FoxP3$^+$ Tregs is shown in the *leftmost panels* of (**a**) and (**b**). In each graph, the relative value compared with the control group is expressed as mean ± SEM. *AU* Arbitrary units, *Fli1* Friend leukemia virus integration 1

fibroblasts [35]. The inverse correlation between Fli1 and type I collagen expression is clearly shown in *Fli1*$^{+/+}$, *Fli1*$^{+/-}$, and *Fli1*$^{-/-}$ murine embryonic fibroblasts [11]. In addition to type I collagen, Fli1 deficiency increases integrin $\alpha_v\beta_3$ and $\alpha_v\beta_5$ expression, establishing autocrine transforming growth factor (TGF)-β signaling in dermal fibroblasts [13]. Furthermore, Fli1 deficiency enhances progranulin production, which renders dermal fibroblasts resistant to the antifibrotic effect of TNF-α [36]. In the present study, we proposed a novel notion that Fli1 deficiency regulates skin-localized transdifferentiation of Th2-like Tregs through IL-33 and possibly that

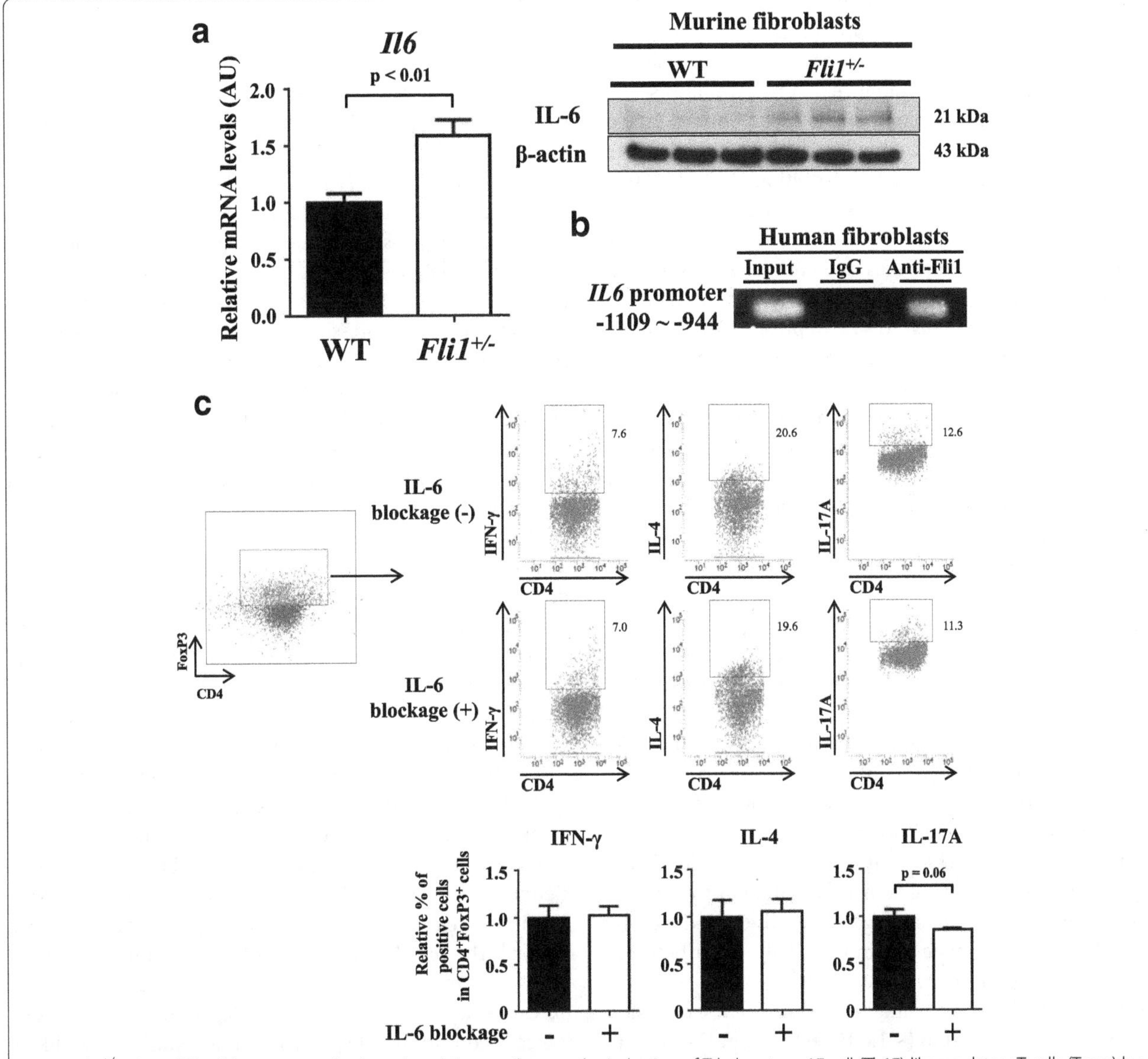

Fig. 4 *Fli1*$^{+/-}$ dermal fibroblasts may modestly and partially contribute to the induction of T helper type 17 cell (Th17)-like regulatory T cells (Tregs) by interleukin (IL)-6 production. **a** Evaluation of IL-6 expression in dermal fibroblasts isolated from wild-type (WT) and *Fli1*$^{+/-}$ mice (n = 10 for each group) by qRT-PCR (*left panel*) and in dermal fibroblasts isolated from bleomycin-treated WT and *Fli1*$^{+/-}$ mice (n = 3 for each group) by immunoblotting (*right panel*). **b** Results of the chromatin immunoprecipitation assay regarding Fli1 occupation on the *IL6* promoter with human dermal fibroblasts (n = 4). **c** Evaluation by flow cytometry of the effect of IL-6 neutralizing antibody on Tregs cocultured with *Fli1*$^{+/-}$ dermal fibroblasts (n = 6). Representative results of immunoblotting, agarose gel electrophoresis, and flow cytometry are shown for the *right panels* of **a** and **b** and the *right upper panel* of **c**, respectively. Gating strategy for identification of CD4^{+}FoxP3^{+} Tregs is shown in the *leftmost panel* of **c**. In each graph, the relative value compared with the control group is expressed as mean ± SEM. *AU* Arbitrary units, *Fli1* Friend leukemia virus integration 1, *IgG* Immunoglobulin G, *mRNA* Messenger RNA

of Th17-like Tregs through IL-6, both of which are produced by dermal fibroblasts. Considering that Fli1 deficiency promotes endothelial-to-mesenchymal transition and M2 macrophage differentiation [13], Fli1 deficiency integrates fibrosis-related gene programs toward the profibrotic condition in various types of cells.

Th2-skewed immune polarization has been implicated in the development of SSc-associated tissue fibrosis on the basis of clinical data. In the early stage of diffuse cutaneous systemic sclerosis (dcSSc), serum IL-6 and IL-10 levels are significantly elevated, whereas they are decreased to normal levels in the late stage of dcSSc characterized by the improvement of skin sclerosis [37]. IL-4 remains at normal levels in the early stage of dcSSc, but it is decreased along with the resolution of skin sclerosis. In contrast, serum IL-12 levels are decreased in the early stage of dcSSc, then they gradually increase in parallel with disease duration and finally reach significantly higher than levels normal controls in the late stage of dcSSc [38]. Thus, Th2-skewed immune polarization is quite evident in the early inflammatory phase of dcSSc. Because IL-4 and IL-13 have a profibrotic effect on dermal fibroblasts, such as the induction of type I collagen expression [39], the predominance of Th2 cytokines seems to be involved in the development of tissue fibrosis in SSc. Therefore, Th2-like Tregs may augment BLM-induced dermal fibrosis in *Fli1*$^{+/-}$ mice. In addition, Th2-like Tregs have the potential to induce SSc-like features in other types of cells under a Fli1-deficient condition. For instance, *Fli1*$^{+/-}$ macrophages preferentially differentiate into an M2 phenotype in response to IL-4 stimulation [13]. In endothelial cells, IL-4 suppresses VE-cadherin expression and reduces vascular integrity [40], which is a characteristic feature of SSc vasculopathy. Because Fli1 deficiency downregulates VE-cadherin expression [14], Th2-like Tregs further promote the induction of SSc-like vascular features in BLM-treated *Fli1*$^{+/-}$ mice. Also, *Fli1* $^{+/-}$ dermal fibroblasts overproduce progranulin, which suppresses the antifibrotic effect of TNF-α [36]. Therefore, dermal fibroblasts preferentially respond to the profibrotic stimuli in BLM-treated *Fli1*$^{+/-}$ mice. Thus, Th2-like Tregs possibly induced by IL-33-producing dermal fibroblasts coordinately amplify tissue fibrosis through the phenotypical alteration of various kinds of cells in BLM-treated *Fli1* $^{+/-}$ mice.

In contrast to a significant contribution of IL-33 to *Fli1* $^{+/-}$ dermal fibroblast-dependent Th2-like Treg transdifferentiation, there was just a trend toward the induction of Th17-like Tregs by coculture with *Fli1*$^{+/-}$ dermal fibroblasts and the suppression of *Fli1*$^{+/-}$ dermal fibroblast-dependent Th17-like Treg transdifferentiation by anti-IL-6 antibody. These results suggest that IL-6 produced by dermal fibroblasts modestly and partially contributes to Th17-like Treg transdifferentiation. Indeed, the fold induction of Fli1 haploinsufficiency-dependent expression was much smaller in IL-6 (~ 1.6 times) than in IL-33 (~ 33 times) in dermal fibroblasts. Taken together with the evidence that IL-6 is overproduced by a variety of cells under inflammatory conditions, including endothelial cells, keratinocytes, and inflammatory cells as well as dermal fibroblasts [41, 42], the contribution of dermal fibroblasts to the total amount of IL-6 expression seems to be relatively small in the lesional skin of BLM-treated *Fli1*$^{+/-}$ mice, suggesting a weak contribution of dermal fibroblasts to Th17-like Treg differentiation. However, we need to be aware that IL-6-dependent redifferentiation of Tregs into Th17 cells is dependent on IL-1 and TGF-β [43]. Given that IL-1β is upregulated in the lesional skin of BLM-treated *Fli1*$^{+/-}$ mice [13] and that integrin $\alpha_v\beta_3$ and $\alpha_v\beta_5$, which promote the release of active TGF-β from its latent form [44, 45], are upregulated in dermal fibroblasts of BLM-treated *Fli1*$^{+/-}$ mice [13], IL-6 seems to coordinately promote the differentiation of Th17-like Tregs together with IL-1β and TGF-β in the lesional skin of these mice. Therefore, the contribution of fibroblast-derived IL-6 to the development of Th17-like Tregs was likely underestimated in the coculture experiment. Another important point is that, in addition to skin-localized trans-differentiation of Th17-like Tregs, the increased infiltration of circulating Th17-like Tregs into the lesional skin may occur in BLM-treated *Fli1*$^{+/-}$ mice. Relevant to this hypothesis is our previous demonstration that Fli1 deficiency induces the expression of intercellular adhesion molecule-1 and glycosylation-dependent cell adhesion molecule-1, positive regulators for Th2 and Th17 cell infiltration, while suppressing the expression of E-selectin and P-selectin, positive regulators of Th1 cell infiltration [13, 46]. These previous data propose the possibility that the infiltration of circulating Th17-like Tregs into the lesional skin may be facilitated by altered expression of cell adhesion molecules in BLM-treated *Fli1*$^{+/-}$ mice. Further studies are required to clarify these points.

The contribution of IL-17A to the development of skin fibrosis has been well studied in BLM-treated mice. For instance, Th17 cell infiltration and IL-17A expression in the skin are increased and serum IL-17A levels correlate with the severity of skin fibrosis in this murine model [47]. Furthermore, loss of *Il17a*, but not *Ifnγ* and *Il4*, results in the reduction of BLM-induced skin fibrosis and IL-17A stimulation induces the expression of TGF-β and connective tissue growth factor in NIH3T6 fibroblasts [24]. Therefore, IL-17A serves as a potent profibrotic cytokine in skin fibrosis of BLM-treated mice. According to the present data, we speculate that Fli1 haploinsufficiency enhances Th17-like cell proportions in skin-homing Tregs, subsequently amplifying tissue fibrosis through the profibrotic effect of IL-17A on dermal fibroblasts. Given that *Fli1*$^{+/-}$ dermal fibroblasts produce excessive amounts of type I collagen under a physiological condition [11], Fli1 haploinsufficiency likely contributes to a feedforward relationship between dermal fibroblasts and Th17-like Tregs, which underlies extensive skin fibrosis.

In a recent study, MacDonald et al. [2] reported that the proportions of conventional Th17 cells in CD4$^+$FoxP3$^-$ T cells and Th17-like Tregs in CD4$^+$FoxP3$^+$ T cells are comparable in the skin of 36 patients with SSc (average disease duration 5.7 ± 1.1 years for dcSSc and 5.7 ± 1.8 years for limited cutaneous systemic sclerosis) and 20 healthy control subjects. In contrast, a significantly increased proportion of Th17-like Tregs in the skin of BLM-treated *Fli1*$^{+/-}$ mice was evident in the present study. This discrepancy seems to be plausible, considering that the activity and severity of profibrotic inflammation are quite variable in the lesional skin of individual patients with SSc owing to the diverse heterogeneity of this disease, even though patients with similar clinical backgrounds are selected. According to a couple of previous reports, the expression of Th17 cytokines is elevated in the lesional skin of patients with early SSc and positively correlates with the severity of skin sclerosis [25, 48–50]. The reproducibility of these results among several independent studies strongly indicates a critical role of Th17 cytokines in skin fibrosis of SSc. Taking into account the present data indicating that Fli1 haploinsufficiency increases the proportion of Th17-like Tregs under profibrotic inflammatory conditions, Th17-like Tregs are potentially involved in the development of skin fibrosis to variable degrees in individual SSc cases.

Conclusions

To our knowledge, this is the first report demonstrating that Fli1 haploinsufficiency increases Th2- and Th17-like Treg proportions in BLM-induced profibrotic skin condition, in which IL-33-producing dermal fibroblasts contribute to Th2-like Treg transdifferentiation. The present findings indicate that IL-33-dependent transdifferentiation of Th2-like Tregs in SSc lesional skin, a notion proposed by MacDonald et al. [2], is part of an Fli1 deficiency-dependent pathological process. Overall, these data further strengthen the importance of Fli1 deficiency in the developmental process of SSc and reinforce the notion that dermal fibroblast-dependent regulation of immune cell phenotypes is involved in the development of skin fibrosis in SSc.

Additional files

Additional file 1: Figure S1. Scatterplots of Fig. 1b. Scatterplots of the proportions of IL-4-, IL-13-, IL17A-, and IFN-γ-producing splenic Tregs from bleomycin (BLM)-treated wild-type and *Fli1*$^{+/-}$ mice ($n = 6$). (PDF 592 kb)

Additional file 2: Figure S2. Signal intensity of IL-33. Signal intensity of IL-33 was analyzed and summarized. To quantify signal intensity of IL-33, color images were converted to grayscale, and then the brightness was measured in five different randomly selected fibroblasts and epidermal areas per specimen. *WT* Wild-type mice; *Basal* Under physiological condition; *BLM* Bleomycin-treated. (PDF 57 kb)

Additional file 3: Figure S3. Original films of immunoblotting with molecular weight markers. Original films of Figs. 2e and 4a. Molecular weight markers are shown. (PDF 573 kb)

Abbreviations

AU: Arbitrary units; BLM: Bleomycin; ChIP: Chromatin immunoprecipitation; dcSSc: Diffuse cutaneous systemic sclerosis; Fli1: Friend leukemia virus integration 1; IFN: Interferon; IgG: Immunoglobulin G; IL: Interleukin; MFI: Mean fluorescence intensity; mRNA: Messenger RNA; Treg: Regulatory T cell; SSc: Systemic sclerosis; SSC-A: Side scatter area; TGF-β: Transforming growth factor-β; Th: T helper cell; TNF-α: Tumor necrosis factor-α; WT: Wild type

Acknowledgements

We thank Tamami Kaga, Yumi Hasegawa, Satoko Itakura, and Naoko Watanabe for technical assistance.

Funding

Funding for this work was provided as a project grant for research on intractable diseases from the Ministry of Health, Labour, and Welfare of Japan (16H05366).

Authors' contributions

RS and YA conceived of and designed the study. RS, KN, MH, SM, TY, TTan, YI, TTak, TToy, and AY acquired data. RS, YA, KN, MH, SM, TY, TTan, YI, TTak, TToy, AY, MT, and SS analyzed and interpreted data. YA, AY, and SS obtained funding. YA, MT, and SS supervised the study. All authors read and approved the final manuscript.

Competing interests

The authors declare that they have no competing interests.

Author details

[1]Department of Dermatology, University of Tokyo Graduate School of Medicine, 7-3-1 Hongo, Bunkyo-ku, Tokyo 113-8655, Japan. [2]Arthritis Center, Boston University School of Medicine, Boston, MA, USA.

References

1. Asano Y, Sato S. Vasculopathy in scleroderma. Semin Immunopathol. 2015;37(5):489–500.
2. MacDonald KG, Dawson NA, Huang Q, Dunne JV, Levings MK, Broady R. Regulatory T cells produce profibrotic cytokines in the skin of patients with systemic sclerosis. J Allergy Clin Immunol. 2015;135(4):946–55.e9.
3. Antiga E, Quaglino P, Bellandi S, Volpi W, Del Bianco E, Comessatti A, Osella-Abate S, De Simone C, Marzano A, Bernengo MG, et al. Regulatory T cells in the skin lesions and blood of patients with systemic sclerosis and morphoea. Br J Dermatol. 2010;162(5):1056–63.
4. Mathian A, Parizot C, Dorgham K, Trad S, Arnaud L, Larsen M, Miyara M, Hie M, Piette JC, Frances C, et al. Activated and resting regulatory T cell exhaustion concurs with high levels of interleukin-22 expression in systemic sclerosis lesions. Ann Rheum Dis. 2012;71(7):1227–34.
5. Slobodin G, Ahmad MS, Rosner I, Peri R, Rozenbaum M, Kessel A, Toubi E, Odeh M. Regulatory T cells ($CD4^+CD25^{bright}FoxP3^+$) expansion in systemic sclerosis correlates with disease activity and severity. Cell Immunol. 2010;261(2):77–80.
6. Klein S, Kretz CC, Ruland V, Stumpf C, Haust M, Hartschuh W, Hartmann M, Enk A, Suri-Payer E, Oberle N, et al. Reduction of regulatory T cells in skin lesions but not in peripheral blood of patients with systemic scleroderma. Ann Rheum Dis. 2011;70(8):1475–81.
7. McClymont SA, Putnam AL, Lee MR, Esensten JH, Liu W, Hulme MA, Hoffmuller U, Baron U, Olek S, Bluestone JA, et al. Plasticity of human regulatory T cells in healthy subjects and patients with type 1 diabetes. J Immunol. 2011;186(7):3918–26.
8. Kleinewietfeld M, Hafler DA. The plasticity of human Treg and Th17 cells and its role in autoimmunity. Semin Immunol. 2013;25(4):305–12.
9. Pesenacker AM, Bending D, Ursu S, Wu Q, Nistala K, Wedderburn LR. CD161 defines the subset of $FoxP3^+$ T cells capable of producing proinflammatory cytokines. Blood. 2013;121(14):2647–58.
10. Asano Y. Epigenetic suppression of Fli1, a potential predisposing factor in the pathogenesis of systemic sclerosis. Int J Biochem Cell Biol. 2015;67:86–91.
11. Wu KK. Analysis of protein-DNA binding by streptavidin-agarose pulldown. Methods Mol Biol. 2006;338:281–90.
12. Hasegawa M. Biomarkers in systemic sclerosis: their potential to predict clinical courses. J Dermatol. 2016;43(1):29–38.
13. Taniguchi T, Asano Y, Akamata K, Noda S, Takahashi T, Ichimura Y, Toyama T, Trojanowska M, Sato S. Fibrosis, vascular activation, and immune abnormalities resembling systemic sclerosis in bleomycin-treated Fli-1-haploinsufficient mice. Arthritis Rheum. 2015;67(2):517–26.
14. Asano Y, Stawski L, Hant F, Highland K, Silver R, Szalai G, Watson DK, Trojanowska M. Endothelial Fli1 deficiency impairs vascular homeostasis: a role in scleroderma vasculopathy. Am J Pathol. 2010;176(4):1983–98.
15. van Bon L, Affandi AJ, Broen J, Christmann RB, Marijnissen RJ, Stawski L, Farina GA, Stifano G, Mathes AL, Cossu M, et al. Proteome-wide analysis and CXCL4 as a biomarker in systemic sclerosis. N Engl J Med. 2014;370(5):433–43.
16. Romano E, Chora I, Manetti M, Mazzotta C, Rosa I, Bellando-Randone S, Blagojevic J, Soares R, Avouac J, Allanore Y, et al. Decreased expression of neuropilin-1 as a novel key factor contributing to peripheral microvasculopathy and defective angiogenesis in systemic sclerosis. Ann Rheum Dis. 2016;75(8):1541–9.

17. Noda S, Asano Y, Nishimura S, Taniguchi T, Fujiu K, Manabe I, Nakamura K, Yamashita T, Saigusa R, Akamata K, et al. Simultaneous downregulation of KLF5 and Fli1 is a key feature underlying systemic sclerosis. Nat Commun. 2014;5:5797.
18. Akamata K, Asano Y, Yamashita T, Noda S, Taniguchi T, Takahashi T, Ichimura Y, Toyama T, Trojanowska M, Sato S. Endothelin receptor blockade ameliorates vascular fragility in endothelial cell-specific Fli-1-knockout mice by increasing Fli-1 DNA binding ability. Arthritis Rheum. 2015;67(5):1335–44.
19. Saigusa R, Asano Y, Yamashita T, Taniguchi T, Takahashi T, Ichimura Y, Toyama T, Yoshizaki A, Miyagaki T, Sugaya M, et al. Fli1 deficiency contributes to the downregulation of endothelial protein C receptor in systemic sclerosis: a possible role in prothrombotic conditions. Br J Dermatol. 2016;174(2):338–47.
20. Moore CB, Allen IC. Primary ear fibroblast derivation from mice. Methods Mol Biol. 2013;1031:65–70.
21. Bouwens EA, Stavenuiter F, Mosnier LO. Mechanisms of anticoagulant and cytoprotective actions of the protein C pathway. J Thromb Haemost. 2013; 11(Suppl 1):242–53.
22. Pociask DA, Chen K, Choi SM, Oury TD, Steele C, Kolls JK. γδ T cells attenuate bleomycin-induced fibrosis through the production of CXCL10. Am J Pathol. 2011;178(3):1167–76.
23. Ichimura Y, Asano Y, Akamata K, Takahashi T, Noda S, Taniguchi T, Toyama T, Aozasa N, Sumida H, Kuwano Y, et al. Fli1 deficiency contributes to the suppression of endothelial CXCL5 expression in systemic sclerosis. Arch Dermatol Res. 2014;306(4):331–8.
24. Okamoto Y, Hasegawa M, Matsushita T, Hamaguchi Y, Huu DL, Iwakura Y, Fujimoto M, Takehara K. Potential roles of interleukin-17A in the development of skin fibrosis in mice. Arthritis Rheum. 2012;64(11):3726–35.
25. Radstake TR, van Bon L, Broen J, Hussiani A, Hesselstrand R, Wuttge DM, Deng Y, Simms R, Lubberts E, Lafyatis R. The pronounced Th17 profile in systemic sclerosis (SSc) together with intracellular expression of TGFβ and IFNγ distinguishes SSc phenotypes. PLoS One. 2009;4(6):e5903.
26. Yamamoto T, Takahashi Y, Takagawa S, Katayama I, Nishioka K. Animal model of sclerotic skin. II. Bleomycin induced scleroderma in genetically mast cell deficient WBB6F1-W/W(V) mice. J Rheumatol. 1999;26(12):2628–34.
27. Yamamoto T, Kuroda M, Nishioka K. Animal model of sclerotic skin. III: Histopathological comparison of bleomycin-induced scleroderma in various mice strains. Arch Dermatol Res. 2000;292(11):535–41.
28. Takagawa S, Lakos G, Mori Y, Yamamoto T, Nishioka K, Varga J. Sustained activation of fibroblast transforming growth factor-β/Smad signaling in a murine model of scleroderma. J Invest Dermatol. 2003;121(1):41–50.
29. Seltmann J, Werfel T, Wittmann M. Evidence for a regulatory loop between IFN-γ and IL-33 in skin inflammation. Exp Dermatol. 2013;22(2):102–7.
30. Bettelli E, Carrier Y, Gao W, Korn T, Strom TB, Oukka M, Weiner HL, Kuchroo VK. Reciprocal developmental pathways for the generation of pathogenic effector T_H17 and regulatory T cells. Nature. 2006;441(7090):235–8.
31. Xu L, Kitani A, Fuss I, Strober W. Cutting edge: regulatory T cells induce CD4 $^+$CD25$^-$Foxp3$^-$ T cells or are self-induced to become Th17 cells in the absence of exogenous TGF-β. J Immunol. 2007;178(11):6725–9.
32. Yamamoto T. Animal model of systemic sclerosis. J Dermatol. 2010;37(1):26–41.
33. Yamamoto T. The bleomycin-induced scleroderma model: what have we learned for scleroderma pathogenesis? Arch Dermatol Res. 2006;297(8):333–44.
34. Korn JH, Mayes M, Matucci Cerinic M, Rainisio M, Pope J, Hachulla E, Rich E, Carpentier P, Molitor J, Seibold JR, et al. Digital ulcers in systemic sclerosis: prevention by treatment with bosentan, an oral endothelin receptor antagonist. Arthritis Rheum. 2004;50(12):3985–93.
35. Czuwara-Ladykowska J, Shirasaki F, Jackers P, Watson DK, Trojanowska M. Fli-1 inhibits collagen type I production in dermal fibroblasts via an Sp1-dependent pathway. J Biol Chem. 2001;276(24):20839–48.
36. Ichimura Y, Asano Y, Akamata K, Noda S, Taniguchi T, Takahashi T, Toyama T, Tada Y, Sugaya M, Sato S, et al. Progranulin overproduction due to Fli-1 deficiency contributes to the resistance of dermal fibroblasts to tumor necrosis factor in systemic sclerosis. Arthritis Rheum. 2015;67(12):3245–55.
37. Sato S, Hasegawa M, Takehara K. Serum levels of interleukin-6 and interleukin-10 correlate with total skin thickness score in patients with systemic sclerosis. J Dermatol Sci. 2001;27(2):140–6.
38. Matsushita T, Hasegawa M, Hamaguchi Y, Takehara K, Sato S. Longitudinal analysis of serum cytokine concentrations in systemic sclerosis: association of interleukin 12 elevation with spontaneous regression of skin sclerosis. J Rheumatol. 2006;33(2):275–84.
39. Bhogal RK, Bona CA. Regulatory effect of extracellular signal-regulated kinases (ERK) on type I collagen synthesis in human dermal fibroblasts stimulated by IL-4 and IL-13. Int Rev Immunol. 2008;27(6):472–96.
40. Chalubinski M, Wojdan K, Luczak E, Gorzelak P, Borowiec M, Gajewski A, Rudnicka K, Chmiela M, Broncel M. IL-33 and IL-4 impair barrier functions of human vascular endothelium via different mechanisms. Vasc Pharmacol. 2015;73:57–63.
41. Khan K, Xu S, Nihtyanova S, Derrett-Smith E, Abraham D, Denton CP, Ong VH. Clinical and pathological significance of interleukin 6 overexpression in systemic sclerosis. Ann Rheum Dis. 2012;71(7):1235–42.
42. Desallais L, Avouac J, Frechet M, Elhai M, Ratsimandresy R, Montes M, Mouhsine H, Do H, Zagury JF, Allanore Y. Targeting IL-6 by both passive or active immunization strategies prevents bleomycin-induced skin fibrosis. Arthritis Res Ther. 2014;16(4):R157.
43. Yang XO, Nurieva R, Martinez GJ, Kang HS, Chung Y, Pappu BP, Shah B, Chang SH, Schluns KS, Watowich SS, et al. Molecular antagonism and plasticity of regulatory and inflammatory T cell programs. Immunity. 2008;29(1):44–56.
44. Asano Y, Ihn H, Yamane K, Jinnin M, Mimura Y, Tamaki K. Increased expression of integrin $\alpha_v\beta_3$ contributes to the establishment of autocrine TGF-β signaling in scleroderma fibroblasts. J Immunol. 2005;175(11):7708–18.
45. Asano Y, Ihn H, Yamane K, Jinnin M, Mimura Y, Tamaki K. Involvement of $\alpha_v\beta_5$ integrin-mediated activation of latent transforming growth factor β1 in autocrine transforming growth factor β signaling in systemic sclerosis fibroblasts. Arthritis Rheum. 2005;52(9):2897–905.
46. Yoshizaki A, Yanaba K, Iwata Y, Komura K, Ogawa A, Akiyama Y, Muroi E, Hara T, Ogawa F, Takenaka M, et al. Cell adhesion molecules regulate fibrotic process via Th1/Th2/Th17 cell balance in a bleomycin-induced scleroderma model. J Immunol. 2010;185(4):2502–15.
47. Lei L, Zhao C, Qin F, He ZY, Wang X, Zhong XN. Th17 cells and IL-17 promote the skin and lung inflammation and fibrosis process in a bleomycin-induced murine model of systemic sclerosis. Clin Exp Rheumatol. 2016;34(5 Suppl 100):14–22.
48. Zhou Y, Hou W, Xu K, Han D, Jiang C, Mou K, Li Y, Meng L, Lu S. The elevated expression of Th17-related cytokines and receptors is associated with skin lesion severity in early systemic sclerosis. Hum Immunol. 2015;76(1):22–9.
49. Yang X, Yang J, Xing X, Wan L, Li M. Increased frequency of Th17 cells in systemic sclerosis is related to disease activity and collagen overproduction. Arthritis Res Ther. 2014;16(1):R4.
50. Murata M, Fujimoto M, Matsushita T, Hamaguchi Y, Hasegawa M, Takehara K, Komura K, Sato S. Clinical association of serum interleukin-17 levels in systemic sclerosis: is systemic sclerosis a Th17 disease? J Dermatol Sci. 2008;50(3):240–2.

9

Blockade of TGF-β/Smad signaling by the small compound HPH-15 ameliorates experimental skin fibrosis

Vu Huy Luong[1], Takenao Chino[1], Noritaka Oyama[1], Takashi Matsushita[2], Yoko Sasaki[3], Dai Ogura[3], Shin-ichiro Niwa[3], Tanima Biswas[4], Akiyuki Hamasaki[4], Mikako Fujita[5], Yoshinari Okamoto[4], Masami Otsuka[4], Hironobu Ihn[6] and Minoru Hasegawa[1*]

Abstract

Background: Transforming growth factor-β (TGF-β)/Smad signaling is well known to play a critical role in the pathogenesis of systemic sclerosis (SSc). We previously developed an artificial molecule, the histidine-pyridine-histidine ligand derivative HPH-15, which may have an antifibrotic effect. The purpose of the present study was to clarify the effects of this drug in human skin fibroblasts and in a preclinical model of SSc.

Methods: The effects of HPH-15 on expression of extracellular matrix components and TGF-β signaling in human dermal fibroblasts were analyzed. The antifibrotic properties of HPH-15 and its mechanisms were also examined in a bleomycin-induced skin fibrosis mouse model.

Results: HPH-15 suppressed the TGF-β-induced phosphorylation of Smad3 and inhibited the expression of collagen I, fibronectin 1, connective tissue growth factor, and α-smooth muscle actin induced by TGF-β in cultured human skin fibroblasts. In the bleomycin-induced skin fibrosis model, oral administration of HPH-15 protected against the development of skin fibrosis and ameliorated established skin fibrosis. Additionally, HPH-15 suppressed the phosphorylation of Smad3 in various cells, including macrophages in the bleomycin-injected skin. Further, in the treated mice, dermal infiltration of proinflammatory macrophages ($CD11b^{+}Ly6C^{hi}$) and M2 profibrotic macrophages ($CD11b^{+}CD204^{+}$ or $CD11b^{+}CD206^{+}$) was significantly decreased during the early and late stages, respectively. HPH-15 treatment resulted in decreased messenger RNA (mRNA) expression of the M2 macrophage markers arginase 1 and *Ym-1* in the skin, whereas it inversely augmented expression of Friend leukemia integration 1 and Krüppel-like factor 5 mRNAs, the transcription factors that repress collagen synthesis. No apparent adverse effects of HPH-15 were found during the treatment.

Conclusions: HPH-15 may inhibit skin fibrosis by inhibiting the phosphorylation of Smad3 in dermal fibroblasts and possibly in macrophages. Our results demonstrate several positive qualities of HPH-15, including oral bioavailability, a good safety profile, and therapeutic effectiveness. Thus, this TGF-β/Smad inhibitor is a potential candidate therapeutic for SSc clinical trials.

Keywords: Systemic sclerosis, HPH-15, TGF-β, Macrophage, Fibroblast

* Correspondence: minoruha@u-fukui.ac.jp
[1]Department of Dermatology, Division of Medicine, Faculty of Medical Sciences, University of Fukui, Fukui, Japan
Full list of author information is available at the end of the article

Background

Systemic sclerosis (SSc), or scleroderma, is a systemic autoimmune disease of unknown etiology characterized by early inflammation and vascular injury followed by fibrosis of the skin and visceral organs [1, 2]. Excessive deposition of collagen and other extracellular matrix (ECM) components in the affected organs is the pathophysiological hallmark of SSc. Activated fibroblasts and α-smooth muscle actin (α-SMA)-positive myofibroblasts are largely responsible for excessive matrix synthesis and tissue deposition [3]. Fibroblast activation and myofibroblast transformation result from a complex series of events initiated by a number of profibrotic molecules, including transforming growth factor-β (TGF-β); connective tissue growth factor (CTGF); platelet-derived growth factor; interleukin (IL)-4, IL-6, and IL-13; and endothelin-1.

One set of the main inducers and producers of these mediators is macrophages. Mouse circulating monocytes can be divided into Ly6C^{hi} (classical or inflammatory monocytes) and Ly6C^{lo} (nonclassical or anti-inflammatory monocytes) [4]. After infiltrating the tissue, these monocytes can differentiate into macrophages in response to various stimuli dependent on the tissue microenvironment. The differentiated macrophages can be classified as classically activated inflammatory macrophages (M1) and alternatively activated tissue profibrotic macrophages (M2) [5]. M2 macrophages can induce and/or maintain tissue fibrosis by producing profibrotic cytokines, including IL-4, IL-13, and TGF-β. Among these, TGF-β is considered one of the most potent inducers of fibroblast activation and tissue fibrosis [6–8]. Binding of TGF-β to its cell surface receptors triggers intracellular signal transduction of Smad-dependent or Smad-independent pathways. In the Smad-dependent pathway, activation of TGF-β receptor type I leads to phosphorylation of Smad2 and Smad3, allowing these molecules to complex with Smad4 and translocate from the cytoplasm into the nucleus, where they bind to a consensus Smad-binding element within the 5′-flanking region of the targeted genes (or DNA). Upon binding to this element, activated Smad proteins recruit transcriptional cofactors to the targeted DNA, resulting in transcription of several key fibrotic genes, such as those encoding collagens and fibronectin [8, 9]. Sustained activation of TGF-β/Smad3 signaling has been detected in the skin fibroblasts of a bleomycin-induced SSc model, one of the most popular SSc models [10], and targeted disruption of this pathway inhibits bleomycin-induced skin fibrosis [11]. In addition, blockade of TGF-β signaling has been shown to reduce the development of skin fibrosis in several other experimental models [12–15]. However, molecular-based approaches targeting the TGF-β cascade have not been established for the treatment of patients with SSc. For this reason, we sought to identify novel therapeutic modalities for SSc. We previously reported a series of symmetrically substituted 2,6-pyridine derivatives, histidine-pyridine-histidine ligand (HPH), possessing varied biological activities dependent on the structure of the 2,6-substituents. These activities include antitumor activity [16, 17], inhibition of zinc finger proteins [18], and inhibition of nuclear factor-κB [19]. Among these, HPH-15, which was formerly named HPH-8, is an HPH derivative that has *S-tert*-butylcysteamine substituents (Additional file 1: Figure S1). We previously reported that HPH-15 has antiviral activities against herpes simplex virus 1, although the exact mechanism remains unknown [20]. In a preliminary study, we found novel antifibrotic activity of HPH-15 in several cell lines (Ogura D and Niwa S 2017, unpublished data).

In this study, we demonstrated that HPH-15 has antifibrotic effects in both a mouse model and cultured human dermal fibroblasts. Our findings indicate that HPH-15 inhibits fibrosis, at least partially, by antagonizing the phosphorylation of Smad3 in skin fibroblasts. Interestingly, HPH-15 reduces the infiltration of both inflammatory and profibrotic macrophages in bleomycin-injected skin.

Methods

Cell culture

Normal human dermal fibroblasts derived from neonatal foreskin were purchased (Kurabo Industries, Osaka, Japan) and grown in DMEM (Nacalai Tesque, Kyoto, Japan) containing 10% FBS, 100 U/ml penicillin, and 100 μg/ml streptomycin (Nacalai Tesque) at 37 °C in a humidified 5% CO_2 atmosphere. When cells reached ~ 70% confluency, they were starved in DMEM containing 0.1% FBS for 24 h and then pretreated with 0.05% dimethyl sulfoxide (DMSO) as a control or various concentrations of DMSO-diluted HPH-15. One hour later, cells were stimulated with 10 ng/ml human recombinant TGF-β1 (PeproTech, Rocky Hill, NJ, USA) and were used for the indicated experiments. All experiments used fibroblasts of passages between 8 and 13.

Animal studies

Female C57BL/6 mice ages 8–10 weeks (CLEA Japan, Tokyo, Japan) were used in two different animal trials for skin fibrosis according to a previous study with minor modification [21]. The preventive model (n = 4–6) was performed by daily subcutaneous injections of bleomycin (1 mg/ml in saline) into the shaved back of the mice (150 μl), concurrent with daily oral gavage of HPH-15 (100 mg/kg in sterilized olive oil) or vehicle alone (sterilized olive oil) for 1, 2, 3, or 4 weeks. Subcutaneous injections of 0.9% NaCl served as a control. In the curative model (n = 5), either bleomycin or saline was administered on alternate days for 6 weeks. Two weeks after the first injection, mice were given a daily dose of HPH-15 (100 mg/kg) or vehicle for the remaining 4 weeks. The HPH-15 doses were optimized on the basis of sequential pilot experiments (data not shown).

Histologic analysis

Mouse skin was fixed in 10% formalin and then embedded in paraffin. Sections (6 μm in thickness) were subjected to H&E and Masson's trichrome staining. For evaluation of skin fibrosis, dermal thickness was defined computationally as the thickness of the skin from the top of the granular layers to the junction between the dermis and subcutaneous fat [22] in five distinct fields at an equal magnification (×40) using a light microscope, and results were expressed as mean ± SEM. Collagen deposition was quantified on Masson's trichrome-stained sections as the ratio of blue-stained area to total stained area using Photoshop Elements version 12 software (Adobe Systems, San Jose, CA, USA).

Sircol Soluble Collagen Assay

Collagen deposition and fibrosis were quantified as total soluble collagen using the Sircol Soluble Collagen Assay (Biocolor, Carrickfergus, UK). Briefly, full-thickness 4-mm punch biopsy samples of mouse back skin (n = 5–6) were homogenized in acid-pepsin solution (0.5 M acetic acid containing 1 mg/ml pepsin) for 48 h at 4 °C. After centrifugation, 1 ml of Sircol dye reagent was added to 100 μl of supernatant and incubated for 30 minutes. After the suspension was removed, droplets were dissolved in 1 ml of Sircol alkali reagent, and relative absorbance was measured at 555 nm.

Western blot analysis

Total protein was extracted from human dermal fibroblasts using a total protein extraction kit (101Bio, Mountain View, CA, USA). Protein concentration was assessed using a spectrophotometer and a bicinchoninic acid protein assay kit (TaKaRa Bio, Shiga, Japan). Equal amounts of protein from each sample (40 μg) were subjected to SDS-PAGE on a Mini-PROTEAN TGX Precast gel and transferred to a nitrocellulose membrane (Bio-Rad Laboratories, Hercules, CA, USA). The blotted membrane was blocked for 30 minutes at room temperature with 5% skim milk/Tris-buffered saline with Tween 20 (TBS-T), followed by incubation with antiphosphorylated Smad3, anti-Smad3 (Cell Signaling Technology, Danvers, MA, USA), anti-collagen type I, alpha 2 (Col1a2; Abcam, Cambridge, UK), anti-fibronectin 1 (anti-FN1) (LSBio, Seattle, WA, USA), anti-CTGF (Santa Cruz Biotechnology, Dallas, TX, USA), or anti-glyceraldehyde 3-phosphate dehydrogenase (anti-GAPDH) (Thermo Fisher Scientific, Waltham, MA, USA) antibodies overnight at 4 °C. After being washed with TBS-T three times, the membrane was incubated for 1 h at room temperature with horseradish peroxidase-conjugated secondary antibody. The membrane was exposed to an enhanced chemiluminescence reagent, Chemi-Lumi One Super solution (Nacalai Tesque). Protein bands were quantified using ImageQuant TL software (version 7.0; GE Healthcare Life Sciences, Pittsburgh, PA, USA) and normalized against the loading control, GAPDH.

Immunofluorescence staining of cultured mouse fibroblasts

After stimulation with recombinant TGF-β1 for 2 h (for detecting p-Smad3) or 24 h (for detecting α-SMA), cells were washed twice in ice-cold PBS. Then cells were fixed for 10 minutes at room temperature in 100% ethanol or 4% paraformaldehyde phosphate buffer for staining of p-Smad3 or α-SMA, respectively. Next, cells were permeabilized with 0.1% Triton X-100 in PBS for 3 minutes. Cells were blocked with 2% FBS for 30 minutes, incubated with anti-p-Smad3 antibody (1:50 in 2% FBS; Cell Signaling Technology) or anti-α-SMA antibody (1:300 in 2% FBS; Abcam) for 60 minutes at room temperature, and then with Alexa Fluor 488-conjugated goat antirabbit antibody for 40 minutes. Coverslips were mounted by using VECTASHIELD mounting medium with 4′,6-diamidino-2-phenylindole (DAPI) (Vector Laboratories, Burlingame, CA, USA).

Immunohistochemical staining of mouse skin

Sections (6 μm in thickness) from paraffin-embedded mouse skin were incubated for 120 minutes at room temperature with monoclonal antibodies (mAbs) to CD3 (1:200; Nichirei Biosciences, Tokyo, Japan), F4/80 (1:1600; Abcam), and p-Smad3 (1:50; Santa Cruz Biotechnology), then with peroxidase-labeled secondary antibody (Nichirei Biosciences), followed by color development with the aminoethylcarbazole system (Nichirei Biosciences). $CD3^+$ cells, $F4/80^+$ cells, and p-Smad3-positive cells were counted under a high-power microscopic field (the Hall section for $CD3^+$ cells and distinct fields for the $F4/80^+$ cells and p-Smad3-positive cells). Each section was examined independently by two investigators (TC and NO) in a blinded manner.

Immunofluorescence staining of mouse skin

The 4-μm cryosections from bleomycin-injected mouse skin were incubated at 4 °C overnight with the primary antibodies p-Smad3 (1:50; Santa Cruz Biotechnology) and F4/80 (1:200; Abcam). Antibodies conjugated with Alexa Fluor 488 or Alexa Fluor 594 (Thermo Fisher Scientific) were used as secondary antibodies of p-Smad3 or F4/80, respectively. Coverslips were mounted by using

VECTASHIELD mounting medium with DAPI (Vector Laboratories).

Preparation of skin cell suspension

A 2 × 2.5-cm piece of depilated back skin was minced and then digested in 7 ml of RPMI 1640 medium containing 10% FBS and 2 mg/ml crude collagenase (Sigma-Aldrich, St. Louis, MO, USA), 1.5 mg/ml hyaluronidase (Sigma-Aldrich), and 0.03 mg/ml DNase I (Roche Applied Science, Indianapolis, IN, USA) at 37 °C for 90 minutes [23]. Samples were passed through a 70-μm Falcon cell strainer (Fisher Scientific/BD Biosciences, Pittsburgh, PA, USA) to obtain single-cell suspensions. After centrifugation at 1500 rpm for 5 minutes, the cell pellet was resuspended in a 70% Percoll solution (GE Healthcare Life Sciences) and then overlaid with a 37% Percoll solution, followed by centrifugation at 1800 rpm for 20 minutes. The cells were aspirated from the Percoll interface and passed through a 70-μm Falcon cell strainer. The harvested cells were washed with ice-cold PBS and used for flow cytometric analysis.

Flow cytometry

mAbs against the following mouse antigens were used: Alexa Fluor 488-conjugated anti-CD45, allophycocyanin (APC)-conjugated anti-Ly6G, Pacific Blue-conjugated anti-CD11b, peridinin-chlorophyll-conjugated anti-Ly6C, phycoerythrin-cyanine 7-conjugated anti-CD206 (all from BioLegend, San Diego, CA, USA), and APC-conjugated anti-CD204 (R&D Systems, Minneapolis, MN, USA). To distinguish dead cells from live cells, the LIVE/DEAD Fixable Aqua Dead Cell Stain Kit (Thermo Fisher Scientific) was used.

The single-cell suspensions obtained as described above were stained for 20 minutes at 4 °C using the indicated mAbs at predetermined optimal concentrations for six-color immunofluorescence analysis. Stained samples were analyzed using the FACSCanto II system (BD Biosciences, San Jose, CA, USA). Data were analyzed using FlowJo software version 7 (FlowJo, Ashland, OR, USA).

RT-PCR

Total RNA was isolated from the skin or cultured fibroblasts using RNeasy spin columns (Qiagen, Valencia, CA, USA) and digested with DNase I (Qiagen) to remove chromosomal DNA. Total RNA was reverse-transcribed to a complementary DNA using a reverse transcription system with random hexamers (TaKaRa Bio). Real-time RT-PCR was performed using the StepOnePlus Real-Time PCR System (Thermo Fisher Scientific). All data were normalized against *GAPDH* messenger RNA (mRNA) and quantified as relative expression.

Statistical analysis

All data are shown as the mean ± SEM and were analyzed using Prism software version 7 (GraphPad Software, La Jolla, CA, USA). The significance of differences between samples was determined by Student's two-tailed *t* test. *p* Values ≤ 0.05 were considered statistically significant.

Results

HPH-15 inhibits TGF-β-induced fibrotic responses in cultured human dermal fibroblasts

Fibroblasts are the main source of collagen and other ECM components in fibrotic skin. We first examined the biological effects of HPH-15 on in vitro ECM synthesis (relevant to the fibroblastic activity) using human dermal fibroblasts. As shown in Fig. 1a, recombinant TGF-β1 stimulated baseline expression of *Col1a2* and *FN1* mRNAs by 24 h of treatment. A 1-h pretreatment with 3 or 10 μM of HPH-15 significantly suppressed the TGF-β1-dependent induction of both mRNAs, although 1 μM HPH-15 had no effect. The suppression reached a sustained maximal level with 3 μM HPH-15. Moreover, the TGF-β1-dependent increase of *Col1a2* mRNA was decreased almost to the steady-state level at this dose.

Therefore, we confirmed the effect of 3 μM HPH-15 for protein expression of Col1a2, FN1, and CTGF, a representative TGF-β1-responsive profibrotic mediator, using Western blotting (Fig. 1b and c). TGF-β1-induced protein expression of Col1a2, FN1, and CTGF on human dermal fibroblasts was significantly inhibited by HPH-15 treatment. Additionally, immunofluorescent cell staining demonstrated that preincubation with HPH-15 inhibited the TGF-β1-induced α-SMA expression on dermal fibroblasts (Fig. 1d). The administration of HPH-15 did not significantly affect the expression of these proteins in the unstimulated fibroblasts. These data suggest that pretreatment with HPH-15 efficiently inhibits the fibrogenic activity induced by TGF-β1 in dermal fibroblasts.

HPH-15 antagonizes phosphorylation of Smad3 in cultured human dermal fibroblasts

The Smad signaling pathways mediate the transcriptional regulation of genes induced by TGF-β superfamily members. To investigate the antifibrotic effects of HPH-15 on the Smad-dependent pathway, we evaluated the expression of p-Smad3 in TGF-β1-treated human dermal fibroblasts.

Western blot assays demonstrated that HPH-15 significantly attenuates the TGF-β1-induced phosphorylation of Smad3 without affecting total Smad expression in cultured human fibroblasts (Fig. 2a). Immunocytochemistry revealed that preincubation with HPH-15 efficiently abrogated the TGF-β1-dependent increase of Smad3 phosphorylation in cultured human dermal

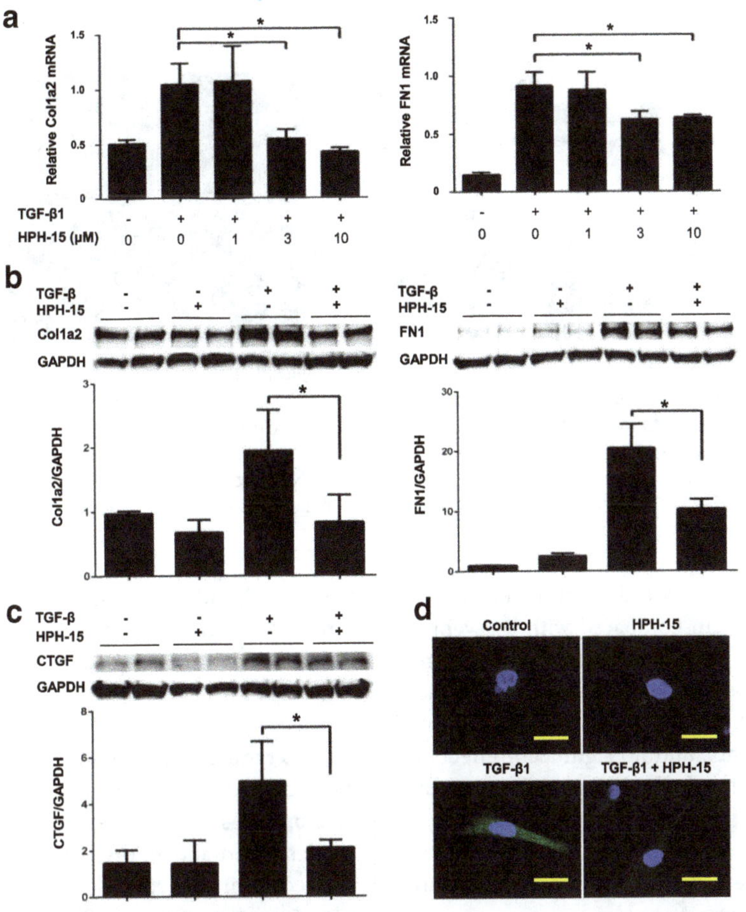

Fig. 1 The antifibrotic role of the histidine-pyridine-histidine ligand derivative HPH-15 in cultured human dermal fibroblasts stimulated with transforming growth factor-β1 (TGF-β1). Normal human dermal fibroblasts were pretreated with dimethyl sulfoxide (DMSO) or various concentrations of DMSO-diluted HPH-15 for 1 h. Then, cells were stimulated with 10 ng/ml human TGF-β1 for the next 24 h. **a** Messenger RNA (mRNA) expression of collagen type I, alpha 2 (*Col1a2*), and fibronectin 1 (*FN1*) in fibroblasts was measured by real-time RT-PCR. $n = 3$ per group. **b–d** HPH-15 at a dose of 3 μM was used on the basis of results shown in (**a**). **b** and **c** Total cell lysates were subjected to Western blotting of Col1a2, FN1, and connective tissue growth factor (CTGF). $n = 4$ per group. Values are normalized relative to control. **d** Normal human fibroblasts were stained with α-smooth muscle actin by immunofluorescent staining, and representative pictures are shown. Scale bar = 30 μm. $n = 3$ per group. All values represent mean ± SEM. * $p \leq 0.05$. *GAPDH* Glyceraldehyde 3-phosphate dehydrogenase

fibroblasts (Fig. 2b). HPH-15 did not significantly affect the phosphorylation of Smad3 in human dermal fibroblasts not stimulated with TGF-β1.

HPH-15 ameliorates bleomycin-induced skin fibrosis in mice

Using a bleomycin-induced skin fibrosis mouse model, we attempted to examine the in vivo antifibrotic effects of HPH-15 at two different treatment onsets, one in a preventive model (ongoing) and the other in a curative model (postonset). In the preventive experiment, the local bleomycin injection and oral HPH-15 were coadministered daily for 4 weeks. Histology of the bleomycin-injected skin sites revealed a marked decrease in the dermal thickness (89% decrease) and collagen deposition compared with mice coadministered sterilized olive oil as a control (Fig. 3a and b). In addition, the soluble collagen fraction in the bleomycin-injected skin was significantly reduced following the co-administration of HPH-15 (Fig. 3c). HPH-15 treatment did not affect the dermal thickness in the saline-injected skin (Fig. 3a and b). These data suggest that the coadministration of HPH-15 can counteract the fibrogenic activity of bleomycin in vivo.

To evaluate the effects of HPH-15 on established fibrosis, bleomycin or a saline control was administered to mice every other day. Two weeks after the first injection of bleomycin, significant skin fibrosis was detected (Additional file 2: Figure S2). At this point, mice were given a daily dose of HPH-15 or vehicle control for the remaining 4 weeks while the bleomycin injection was continued on alternate days. Treatment with HPH-15

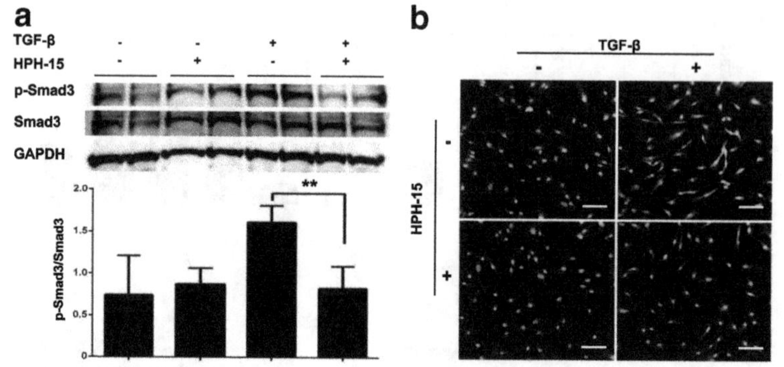

Fig. 2 The histidine-pyridine-histidine ligand derivative HPH-15 antagonizes the phosphorylation of Smad3 in cultured human dermal fibroblasts. **a** and **b** Normal human fibroblasts were pretreated with dimethyl sulfoxide (DMSO) or DMSO-diluted HPH-15 (3 μM) for 1 h. Then, cells were stimulated with 10 ng/ml human transforming growth factor-β1 (TGF-β1) for the next 3 h. **a** Phosphorylation of Smad3 in the cultured human dermal fibroblasts was assessed by Western blot analysis. $n = 4$ per group. Values are normalized relative to control. All values represent mean ± SEM. ** $p \leq 0.01$. **b** Human fibroblasts were immunostained for p-Smad3 (*green*). Nuclei (*blue*) was stained with 4′,6-diamidino-2-phenylindole. Scale bar = 100 μm. $n = 3$ per group. *GAPDH* Glyceraldehyde 3-phosphate dehydrogenase

resulted in significantly decreased dermal thickness (71% decrease) in the lesional skin compared with the vehicle-treated mice. Moreover, the Masson's trichrome-stained area was significantly reduced in the HPH-15-treated mice (Fig. 3d and e). HPH-15 was well tolerated throughout all experiments, and no significant effects on body weight loss (Additional file 3: Figure S3) or other signs of toxicity were noted.

HPH-15 inhibits inflammatory cell infiltration during early stage of bleomycin injection

It is known that injection of bleomycin induces an early and transient inflammatory response in the dermis. Among the infiltrating cells, macrophages are the most prominent [10]. Consistent with this, local injection of bleomycin, but not control saline, induced the infiltration of F4/80-positive macrophages into the middle dermis at day 14 (Fig. 4a). This increased infiltration of macrophages was significantly blocked by concurrent administration of HPH-15 ($p < 0.05$). Similar inhibitory effects of HPH-15 were observed on the local infiltration of CD3-positive T lymphocytes in bleomycin-treated skin (Fig. 4b). These results show the in vivo preventive effects of HPH-15 during the early inflammatory response of bleomycin-induced skin fibrosis.

HPH-15 suppresses phosphorylation of Smad3 in various cells, including macrophages, in bleomycin-injected skin

In bleomycin-injected mouse skin, immunohistochemical staining revealed a downregulated expression of p-Smad3 in the epidermis, dermis, and subcutaneous tissues of HPH-15-treated mice. The number of p-Smad3-positive cells in the dermis and subcutaneous tissues (suggestive of fibroblasts and leukocytes) was significantly decreased in the HPH-15-treated mice compared with control mice (Fig. 4c). In addition, immunofluorescence staining indicated that most infiltrating p-Smad3-positive cells were F4/80-positive macrophages in the bleomycin-injected skin (Fig. 4d).

HPH-15 reduces infiltration of inflammatory $CD11b^{+}Ly6C^{hi}$ monocytes during early-stage fibrosis and profibrotic M2 macrophages during late-stage fibrosis

As described above, the main infiltrating cell population in bleomycin-injected skin is macrophages (Fig. 4). To further investigate the effects of HPH-15 on subsets of macrophages, we isolated leukocytes from lesional skin at two different time points—the inflammatory stage (day 7) and the fibrotic stage (day 21)—and stained for monocyte/macrophage surface markers. The infiltration of $CD11b^{+}Ly6C^{hi}$ monocytes was remarkably increased after 7 days of bleomycin injections. Moreover, HPH-15 treatment significantly decreased the percentage of $CD11b^{+}Ly6C^{hi}$ monocytes in the skin (Fig. 5b).

M2 macrophages are well known to play a central role in the pathologic fibrotic response [24]. Therefore, we next evaluated the impact of HPH-15 on the M2 macrophage population using the M2 macrophage cell surface markers CD204 and CD206. On day 21, mice treated with bleomycin exhibited an increase in the proportion of $CD11b^{+}CD204^{+}$ and $CD11b^{+}CD206^{+}$ cells in the skin. HPH-15 administration significantly reduced these subsets (Fig. 5c) as well as the expression of *Arg1* and *Ym1* mRNAs, established markers of M2 macrophages, in the skin lesions of bleomycin-treated mice (Fig. 6a).

HPH-15 restores mRNA expression of Fli1 and KLF5 in bleomycin-injected skin

Friend leukemia integration 1 (Fli1) and Krüppel-like factor 5 (KLF5) are transcription factors that repress

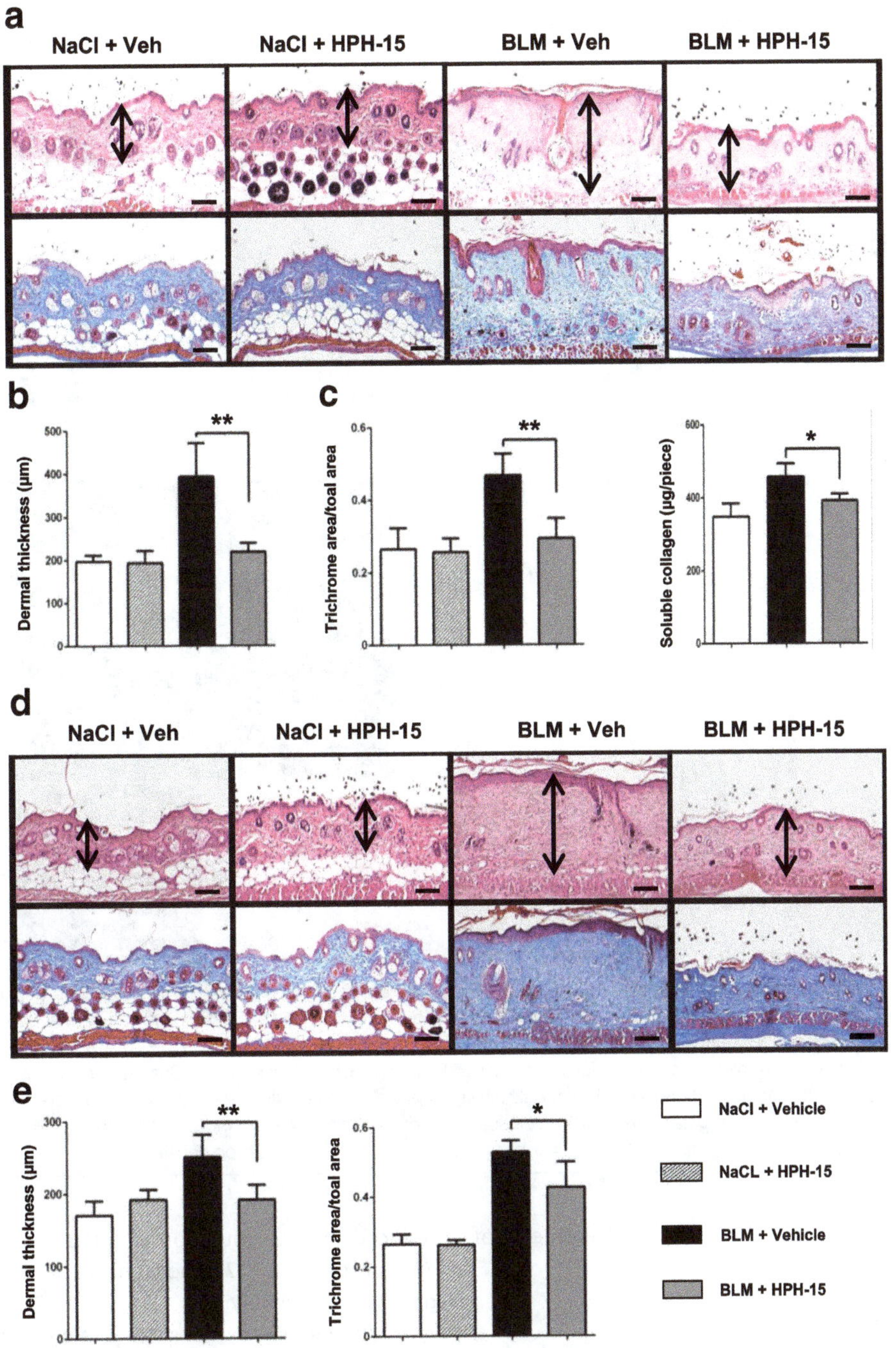

Fig. 3 Histidine-pyridine-histidine ligand derivative HPH-15 treatment ameliorates bleomycin (BLM)-induced skin fibrosis in mice. The antifibrotic effects of HPH-15 were analyzed at the endpoint of the preventive model (**a–c**) and curative model (**d** and **e**). The preventive model was performed by daily subcutaneous injections of BLM into the back skin of the mice concurrently with daily oral gavage of HPH-15 or vehicle (sterilized olive oil) for 4 weeks. In the curative model, BLM was administered on alternate days for 6 weeks. Two weeks after the first injection, mice were given a daily dose of HPH-15 or vehicle for the remaining 4 weeks. Representative images of H&E-stained (*upper pictures*) and Masson's trichrome-stained (*lower pictures*) tissue. Arrows indicate dermal thickness. Scale bar = 100 μm. Skin fibrosis was compared by determining dermal thickness, ratio of trichrome area/total area, and soluble collagen content. All values represent mean ± SEM; $n = 4$–6 per group. * $p \leq 0.05$; ** $p \leq 0.01$

expression of the collagen gene [25, 26]. Researchers in previous studies reported decreased mRNA levels of these transcription factors in murine skin fibrosis models [27]. We found that bleomycin injection caused remarkably decreased mRNA expression of *Fli1* and *KLF5*, and, as we expected, expression of *Fli1* and *KLF5* mRNAs

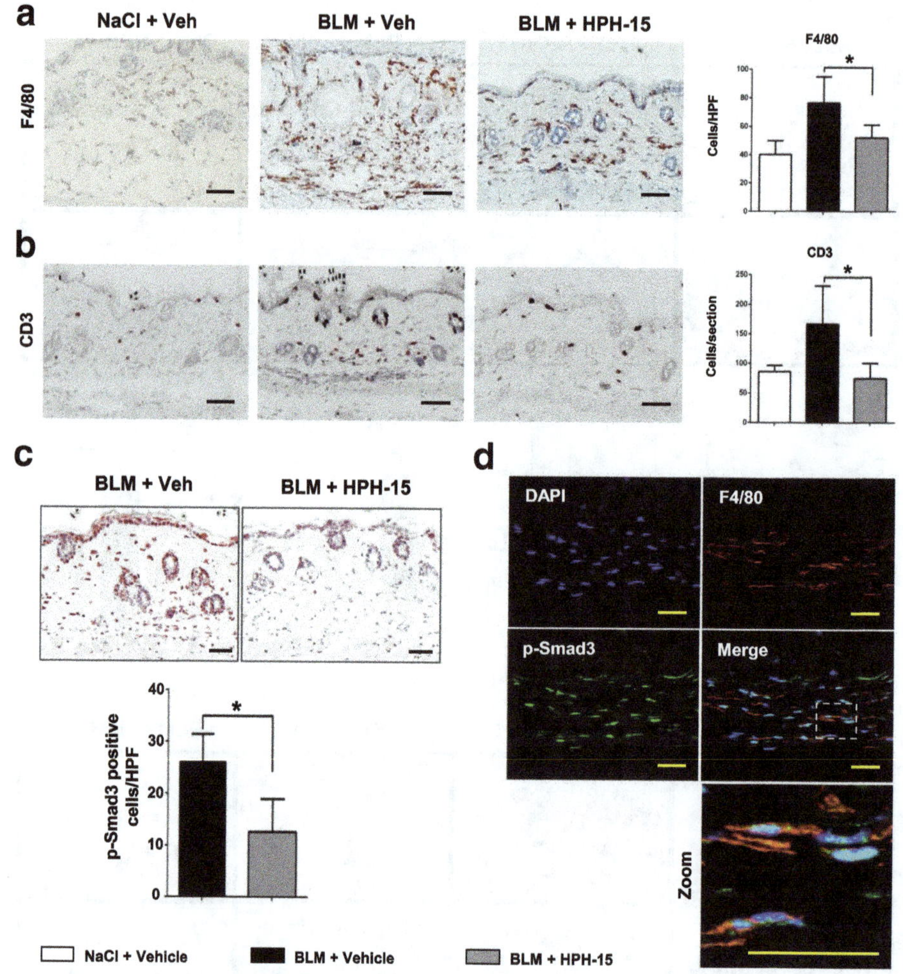

Fig. 4 The histidine-pyridine-histidine ligand derivative HPH-15 inhibits leukocyte infiltration and suppresses Smad3 phosphorylation in bleomycin (BLM)-injected skin. **a–d** Back skin samples of mice treated with HPH-15 or vehicle were harvested after 14 days of daily BLM injections. Skin sections were incubated with anti-F4/80 antibody (**a**) and anti-CD3 antibody (**b**). Representative images are shown on the *left*. Scale bar = 50 μm. Quantitative analysis is shown in the bar graph on the *right*. **c** Skin sections were stained for p-Smad3. Scale bar = 50 μm. Quantitative analysis of p-Smad3-positive cells in the dermis is shown in the bar graph. **d** Cryosections of the skin were subjected to immunofluorescent staining for 4′,6-diamidino-2-phenylindole (DAPI) (nuclear, *blue*), p-Smad3 (nuclear, *green*), and F4/80 (cell surface, *red*). Dashed box inset indicates the location of zoomed image. Scale bar = 30 μm. All values represent mean ± SEM; n = 5 per group. * $p \leq 0.05$. *HPF* High-power field

were significantly recovered by HPH-15 treatment of bleomycin-injected mice (Fig. 6b).

Discussion

We developed an orally active agent, HPH-15, and investigated its effects on fibrosis both in vivo and in vitro. HPH-15 disrupted the phosphorylation of Smad3 in human skin fibroblasts stimulated with TGF-β and effectively inhibited the expression of α-SMA, Col1a2, FN1, and CTGF. Furthermore, HPH-15 not only prevented skin fibrosis but also was effective against established skin fibrosis in the bleomycin-induced model. Treatment with HPH-15 inhibited the phosphorylation of Smad3 in keratinocytes, fibroblasts, and leukocytes (most of them being macrophages) in fibrotic skin and reduced the accumulation of inflammatory macrophages and profibrotic M2 macrophages in the early and late phases, respectively.

We previously synthesized a series of pyridine-based symmetrical molecules. Among these, HPH-15 showed promise as an antifibrotic agent in our preliminary cellular experiments (Ogura D and Niwa S 2017, unpublished data). In the present study, we confirmed that HPH-15 blocks Smad3 phosphorylation in human skin fibroblasts stimulated with TGF-β1. Furthermore, HPH-15 suppresses the TGF-β1-dependent expression of α-SMA, ECM components, and CTGF, a representative TGF-β1-responsive mediator, on human skin fibroblasts. These findings suggest that HPH-15 inhibits skin fibrosis via suppression of TGF-β/Smad signaling of fibroblasts.

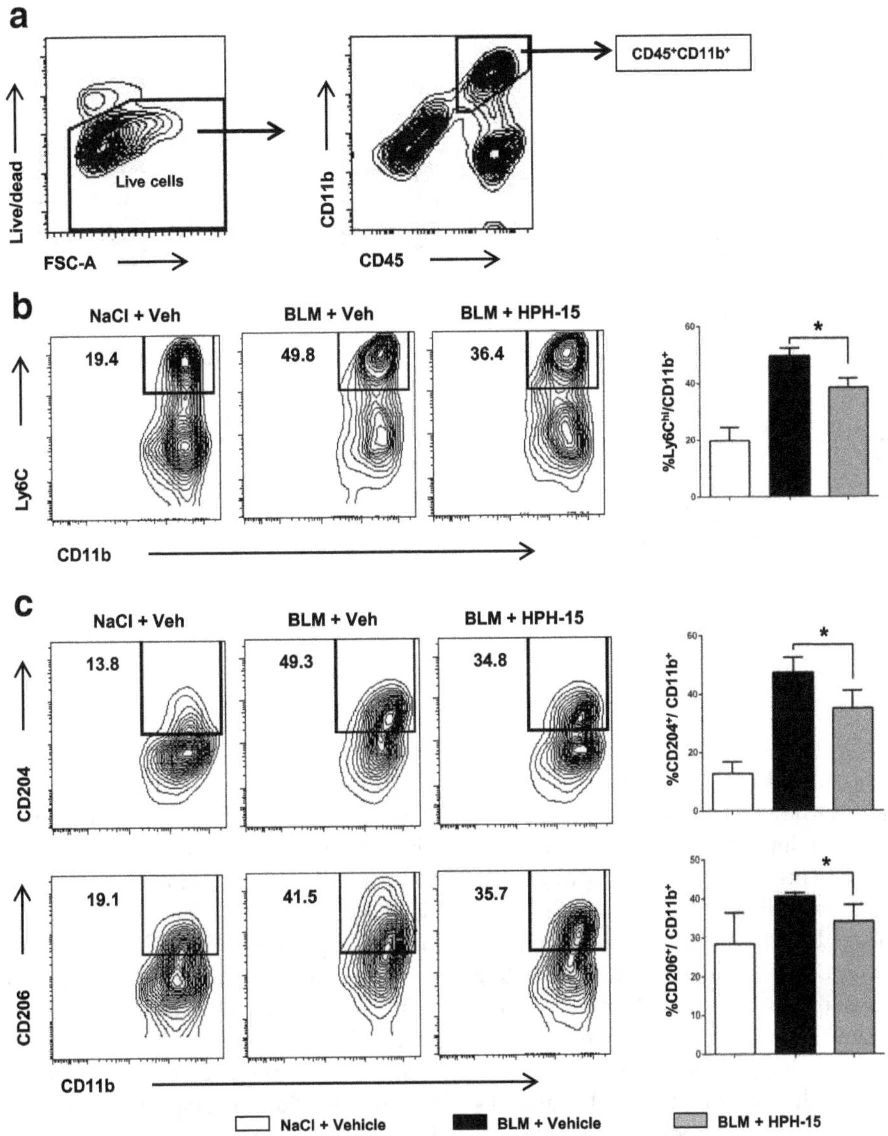

Fig. 5 The histidine-pyridine-histidine ligand derivative HPH-15 reduces the infiltration of inflammatory $CD11b^{+}Ly6C^{hi}$ monocytes in the early stage of fibrosis and profibrotic M2 macrophages during the late stage. Skin samples from normal, vehicle-treated, and HPH-15-treated mice were harvested 7 or 21 days after bleomycin (BLM) injection. **a** $CD45^{+}CD11b^{+}$ cells were gated for analysis of the subsets of macrophages. Representative images (*left*) and bar graphs (*right*) of $Ly6C^{hi}$ macrophages on day 7 (**b**) and $CD204^{+}$ and $CD206^{+}$ M2 macrophages on day 21 (**c**) analyzed by flow cytometry. All values represent mean ± SEM; $n = 3$ per group. * $p \leq 0.05$. *FSC-A* Forward scatter area

Recently, fresolimumab, a human immunoglobulin G4κ mAb that neutralizes all three TGF-β isoforms, was used in an open-label trial in patients with early diffuse SSc [28]. Interestingly, fresolimumab exhibited a tendency to decrease expression of macrophage/monocyte-associated genes in the skin. In our mouse experiments, macrophage accumulation was inhibited by HPH-15 in a manner similar to that of the antihuman TGF-β mAb. Although TGF-β is well known for its anti-inflammatory functions, it can also directly induce monocyte migration in vitro [29]. Furthermore, recombinant TGF-β injection induces macrophage infiltration in addition to fibrosis in mouse skin [30]. Although mice with the stiff skin syndrome mutation, a genetic mouse model of SSc, show the presence of increased proinflammatory cells, including plasmacytoid dendritic cells, T-helper cells, and plasma cells in the skin, TGF-β-neutralizing antibody inhibited the inflammation and reversed the established skin fibrosis [31]. Therefore, blockade of TGF-β signaling may directly inhibit the early inflammation that leads to fibrosis.

The presence of immunocyte infiltrate is usually detected in the skin of patients with early SSc [32]. Similar inflammatory cell infiltration is also found in the

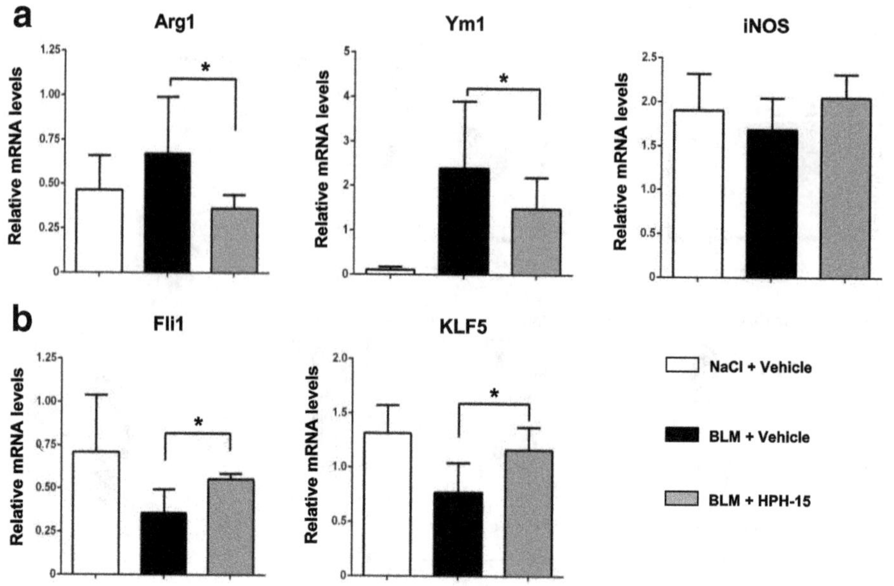

Fig. 6 The effect of the histidine-pyridine-histidine ligand HPH-15 on the messenger RNA (mRNA) expression of macrophage markers and transcription factors. Skin samples from normal, vehicle-treated, and HPH-15-treated mice were harvested 14 days after bleomycin (BLM) injection. Total RNA was extracted, and expression of arginase 1 (*Arg1*), *Ym1*, inducible NO synthase (*iNOS*) (**a**), Friend leukemia integration 1 (*Fli1*), and Krüppel-like factor 5 (*KLF5*) (**b**) mRNAs were quantitatively analyzed by real-time RT-PCR. Each sample was repeated in duplicate. All values represent mean ± SEM; $n = 4$–5 per group. * $p \leq 0.05$

skin of the bleomycin-induced skin fibrosis model [33, 34]. Macrophages are an important source of fibrotic cytokines, including TGF-β, and have been considered to play a central role in the pathogenesis of fibrotic disorders, including SSc [35, 36]. Specifically, M2 macrophages have been implicated as critical mediators in various tissue fibrosis models, including bleomycin-induced skin fibrosis [5, 24, 37]. Importantly, gene expression analysis demonstrated augmentation of the M2 macrophage signature in the skin of patients with SSc, which was suppressed by anti-IL-6R mAb (tocilizumab) therapy associated with an improvement of fibrosis [38]. In bleomycin-injected skin, the majority of immune cells were macrophages, and HPH-15 markedly inhibited this accumulation. In addition, most p-Smad3-positive infiltrating cells were F4/80-positive macrophages in the bleomycin-injected skin, and those cells were dramatically decreased by HPH-15 treatment. Therefore, HPH-15 may directly affect macrophages in addition to fibroblasts in bleomycin-injected fibrotic skin.

Circulating monocytes can be classified into Ly6C^{hi} and Ly6C^{low} monocytes [4]. Ly6C^{hi} or inflammatory monocytes respond to inflammatory signals and leave the circulation by extravasation, whereas Ly6C^{low} monocytes patrol the luminal side of the vasculature [39, 40]. Recent studies demonstrated that Ly6C^{hi} inflammatory monocytes are increased in the tissues of mouse models, including lung fibrosis and unilateral ureteral obstruction-induced fibrosis, during the progressive fibrotic phase [41, 42]. Depending on the specific cytokines to which they are exposed, tissue Ly6C^{hi} macrophages will polarize into inflammatory macrophages or downregulate Ly6C and polarize cells into tissue-remodeling/profibrotic (M2) macrophages [4, 39, 43]. In our experiments, following 7 days of bleomycin injections, there was a remarkable increase in the Ly6C^{hi} macrophage population in the skin, an effect that was significantly inhibited by administration of HPH-15. During the fibrotic stage (day 21), HPH-15 treatment inhibited the expansion of the M2 macrophage population and specifically caused a reduction of the CD11b^{+}CD204^{+} and CD11b^{+}CD206^{+} subsets. Although it would be ideal to compare numbers of infiltrating Ly6C^{hi} and M2 macrophages rather than just their frequencies, this proved to be technically difficult owing to the challenge of cell isolation from the skin. However, considering the immunohistochemical findings regarding total macrophages, the effect of HPH-15 on the reduction of these macrophage subsets is likely dramatic. Furthermore, HPH-15 inhibited expression of arginase 1 and *Ym1* mRNAs, markers of M2 macrophages, in bleomycin-treated skin. M2 macrophages likely appear during the fibrotic stage, either via differentiation of newly recruited infiltrating macrophages or by in situ transition of previously differentiated infiltrating M1 macrophages or Ly6C^{hi} inflammatory macrophages in the presence of Th2 cytokines such as IL-4 [24, 42, 44].

Additionally, a recent study demonstrated that TGF-β skews macrophage polarization toward an M2-like phenotype in human THP-1 macrophages [45]. Interestingly, TGF-β1/Smad3 signaling was critical for the transition of bone marrow-derived macrophages into collagen-producing myofibroblasts in a renal fibrosis mouse model of unilateral ureteric obstruction [46]. In that study, the macrophage myofibroblast transition was induced more predominantly in M2 macrophages.

In our study, the prevalence of Ly6C^{hi} monocytes was remarkably decreased in the skin of wild-type mice following bleomycin injection (from 49.6% on day 7 to 21.3% on day 21). Inversely, CD206^{+} M2 macrophages increased from 18.2% on day 7 to 40.5% on day 21 (Additional file 4: Figure S4). Although the detailed mechanisms regarding how HPH-15 reduces M2 macrophages in the skin remain unknown, the reduction of Ly6C^{hi} inflammatory macrophages during the inflammatory stage by HPH-15 treatment may partially explain this effect. In addition, inhibition of TGF-β function by HPH-15 might attenuate M2-polarized differentiation. Further studies are needed to confirm whether HPH-15 or the blockade of TGF-β/Smad signaling via other mechanisms inhibits the differentiation of Ly6C^{hi} macrophages into M2 macrophages.

Fli1 and KLF5 are transcription factors that repress collagen gene expression. The expression of both Fli1 and KLF5 were found to be decreased in SSc dermal fibroblasts [27, 47]. Importantly, heterozygous deficiency of both Fli1 and KLF5 results in the development of all three features of SSc, including autoimmunity, vasculopathy, and fibrosis [27]. More severe skin fibrosis and increased numbers of M2 macrophages were detected in Fli1-haploinsufficient mice by bleomycin injection [48]. Interestingly, Fli1 deficiency in epithelial cells spontaneously induces the fibrosis of skin, esophagus, and lungs as well as autoimmunity [49]. Consistent with these recent findings, our study demonstrates that *Fli1* and *KLF5* are downregulated in bleomycin-injected skin compared with normal skin. Moreover, these transcription factors were recovered with a concomitant amelioration of skin fibrosis in HPH-15-treated mice.

TGF-β has been considered to play a pivotal role in initiating and sustaining the fibrotic process in SSc, a function that is mediated via both canonical (Smad-dependent) and noncanonical (Smad-independent) pathways [2]. Fibroblasts from patients with SSc show constitutive Smad2/3 phosphorylation and nuclear localization, and various levels of abnormal Smad signaling have been detected. Therefore, targeting TGF-β/Smad signaling is an attractive strategy for treatment of SSc. Our data in vivo and in vitro showed that HPH-15 inhibits the phosphorylation of Smad3 protein in human dermal fibroblasts. The inhibition of Smad3 phosphorylation, thereby interfering with its binding to Smad-binding elements, likely results in the reduction of transcription of fibrotic genes such as *Col1a2* and *FN1*, as seen in cultured fibroblasts. Additionally, our limited data suggest that HPH-15 suppresses the Smad3 phosphorylation of dermal macrophages in bleomycin-injected skin.

Several points remain unclear, and future studies are required to address these. First, the effective concentration of HPH-15 should be improved if possible, such as by application of a drug delivery system or through structural optimization of HPH-15 before a clinical trial is conducted. Second, the effect of HPH-15 was investigated in only one mouse model of SSc. It has been suggested that the antifibrotic effects of specific molecules for SSc trials should be confirmed in at least two complementary animal models of SSc [50]. Therefore, further studies using other SSc models are required to clarify the utility of HPH-15. Third, the detailed mechanism of action of HPH-15, especially for macrophages and keratinocytes, should be determined in addition to fibroblasts.

Conclusions

Our study shows that HPH-15 inhibits TGF-β/Smad signaling and fibrogenic activity of human skin fibroblasts in vitro and attenuates skin inflammation and subsequent fibrosis in a mouse model of SSc. Because the findings of this early preclinical study demonstrate several advantages of HPH-15, including the fact that it is an orally active agent with an excellent safety profile, HPH-15 shows potential as a candidate for SSc clinical trials.

Additional files

Additional file 1: Figure S1. The molecular structure of HPH-15. (PDF 7 kb)

Additional file 2: Figure S2. HPH-15 treatment did not affect the growing of the mice. The body weight changes of mice treated with vehicle or HPH-15 were assessed every 3 days. All values represent mean ± SEM; $n = 5$ in each group. (PDF 6 kb)

Additional file 3: Figure S3. Every-other-day injection of bleomycin for 2 weeks induced significant skin fibrosis. Back skin of NaCl- or bleomycin-injected mice was harvested on day 14 and stained with H&E. Scale bar = 100 μm. $n = 3$ in each group. (PDF 80 kb)

Additional file 4: Figure S4. The inverse proportional change of Ly6C^{hi} macrophages and CD206^{+} M2 macrophages from the inflammation stage (day 7) to the fibrotic stage (day 21). The single-cell suspension obtained from the back skin of bleomycin-injected C57BL/6 mice on day 7 and day 21 was stained with the mAbs against CD45, CD11b, Ly6C, and CD206. Stained samples were analyzed using the FACSCanto II system. Data were analyzed using FlowJo software version 7. All values represent mean ± SEM. $n = 3$ at each time point. ** $p \leq 0.01$. (PDF 49 kb)

Abbreviations

APC: Allophycocyanin; Arg1: Arginase 1; BLM: Bleomycin; Col1a2: Collagen type I, alpha 2; CTGF: Connective tissue growth factor; DAPI: 4',6-Diamidino-2-phenylindole; DMSO: Dimethyl sulfoxide; ECM: Extracellular matrix; Fli1: Friend leukemia integration 1; FN1: Fibronectin 1; FSC-A: Forward scatter area; GAPDH: Glyceraldehyde 3-phosphate dehydrogenase; HPF: High-power field; HPH: Histidine-pyridine-histidine ligand; IL: Interleukin; iNOS: Inducible NO synthase; KLF5: Krüppel-like factor 5; mAb: Monoclonal antibody; mRNA: Messenger RNA; SSc: Systemic sclerosis; TBS-T: Tris-buffered saline with Tween 20; TGF-β: Transforming growth factor-β; α-SMA: α-Smooth muscle actin

Acknowledgements
We thank Yuka Nakayama for her technical assistance and Prof. Doanh Le Huu for his helpful discussion. We also thank Profs. Makoto Orisaka and Yoshio Yoshida for technical support during the histochemical analysis.

Funding
This work was supported by grants from KAKENHI (number 15 K09763 [to MH), the Japan Intractable Diseases Research Foundation (to MH), and Sumitomo Mitsui Trust Bank (to VHL). The funders had no role in the study design, data collection and analysis, decision to publish, or preparation of the manuscript.

Authors' contributions
VHL, SN, MO, HI, and MH designed the study. TC and NO participated in the study design. YS, DO, SN, TB, AH, MF, YO, and MO were responsible for the preparation of the original compound HPH-15. VHL and TC conducted the data acquisition. TM helped with data acquisition. VHL, TC, NO, and MH contributed to the data analysis and interpretation. VHL, NO, and MH drafted the manuscript. TC, TM, and MO assisted with drafting of the manuscript. All authors read and approved the final manuscript.

Competing interests
The authors declare that they have no competing interests.

Author details
[1]Department of Dermatology, Division of Medicine, Faculty of Medical Sciences, University of Fukui, Fukui, Japan. [2]Department of Dermatology, Faculty of Medicine, Institute of Medical, Pharmaceutical and Health Sciences, Kanazawa University, Kanazawa, Japan. [3]Link Genomics, Inc., Tokyo, Japan. [4]Department of Bioorganic Medicinal Chemistry, Kumamoto University, Kumamoto, Japan. [5]Research Institute for Drug Discovery, Kumamoto University, Kumamoto, Japan. [6]Department of Dermatology and Plastic Surgery, Faculty of Life Sciences, Kumamoto University, Kumamoto, Japan.

References

1. Allanore Y, Simms R, Distler O, Trojanowska M, Pope J, Denton CP, Varga J. Systemic sclerosis. Nat Rev Dis Primers. 2015;1:15002.
2. Bhattacharyya S, Wei J, Varga J. Understanding fibrosis in systemic sclerosis: shifting paradigms, emerging opportunities. Nat Rev Rheumatol. 2011;8(1):42–54.
3. Rosenbloom J, Castro SV, Jimenez SA. Narrative review: fibrotic diseases: cellular and molecular mechanisms and novel therapies. Ann Intern Med. 2010;152(3):159–66.
4. Yona S, Jung S. Monocytes: subsets, origins, fates and functions. Curr Opin Hematol. 2010;17(1):53–9.
5. Mosser DM, Edwards JP. Exploring the full spectrum of macrophage activation. Nat Rev Immunol. 2008;8(12):958–69.
6. Roberts AB, Heine UI, Flanders KC, Sporn MB. Transforming growth factor-β: major role in regulation of extracellular matrix. Ann N Y Acad Sci. 1990;580:225–32.
7. Lafyatis R. Transforming growth factor β at the centre of systemic sclerosis. Nat Rev Rheumatol. 2014;10(12):706–19.
8. Liu Q, Chu H, Ma Y, Wu T, Qian F, Ren X, Tu W, Zhou X, Jin L, Wu W, et al. Salvianolic acid B attenuates experimental pulmonary fibrosis through inhibition of the TGF-β signaling pathway. Sci Rep. 2016;6:27610.
9. Feng XH, Derynck R. Specificity and versatility in TGF-β signaling through Smads. Annu Rev Cell Dev Biol. 2005;21:659–93.
10. Takagawa S, Lakos G, Mori Y, Yamamoto T, Nishioka K, Varga J. Sustained activation of fibroblast transforming growth factor-β/Smad signaling in a murine model of scleroderma. J Invest Dermatol. 2003;121(1):41–50.
11. Lakos G, Takagawa S, Chen SJ, Ferreira AM, Han G, Masuda K, Wang XJ, DiPietro LA, Varga J. Targeted disruption of TGF-β/Smad3 signaling modulates skin fibrosis in a mouse model of scleroderma. Am J Pathol. 2004;165(1):203–17.
12. Hasegawa M, Matsushita Y, Horikawa M, Higashi K, Tomigahara Y, Kaneko H, Shirasaki F, Fujimoto M, Takehara K, Sato S. A novel inhibitor of Smad-dependent transcriptional activation suppresses tissue fibrosis in mouse models of systemic sclerosis. Arthritis Rheum. 2009;60(11):3465–75.
13. Distler JH, Jungel A, Huber LC, Schulze-Horsel U, Zwerina J, Gay RE, Michel BA, Hauser T, Schett G, Gay S, et al. Imatinib mesylate reduces production of extracellular matrix and prevents development of experimental dermal fibrosis. Arthritis Rheum. 2007;56(1):311–22.
14. Wei J, Zhu H, Komura K, Lord G, Tomcik M, Wang W, Doniparthi S, Tamaki Z, Hinchcliff M, Distler JH, et al. A synthetic PPAR-γ agonist triterpenoid ameliorates experimental fibrosis: PPAR-γ-independent suppression of fibrotic responses. Ann Rheum Dis. 2014;73(2):446–54.
15. Ruzehaji N, Frantz C, Ponsoye M, Avouac J, Pezet S, Guilbert T, Luccarini JM, Broqua P, Junien JL, Allanore Y. Pan PPAR agonist IVA337 is effective in prevention and treatment of experimental skin fibrosis. Ann Rheum Dis. 2016;75(12):2175–83.
16. Ali TF, Iwamaru K, Ciftci HI, Koga R, Matsumoto M, Oba Y, Kurosaki H, Fujita M, Okamoto Y, Umezawa K, et al. Novel metal chelating molecules with anticancer activity: striking effect of the imidazole substitution of the histidine-pyridine-histidine system. Bioorg Med Chem. 2015;23(17):5476–82.
17. Hamasaki A, Naka H, Tamanoi F, Umezawa K, Otsuka M. A novel metal-chelating inhibitor of protein farnesyltransferase. Bioorg Med Chem Lett. 2003;13(9):1523–6.
18. Radwan MO, Sonoda S, Ejima T, Tanaka A, Koga R, Okamoto Y, Fujita M, Otsuka M. Zinc-mediated binding of a low-molecular-weight stabilizer of the host anti-viral factor apolipoprotein B mRNA-editing enzyme, catalytic polypeptide-like 3G. Bioorg Med Chem. 2016;24(18):4398–405.
19. Kanemaru Y, Momiki Y, Matsuura S, Horikawa T, Gohda J, Inoue J, Okamoto Y, Fujita M, Otsuka M. An artificial copper complex incorporating a cell-penetrating peptide inhibits nuclear factor-k B (NF-κB) activation. Chem Pharm Bull. 2011;59(12):1555–8.
20. Hosono T, Yokomizo K, Hamasaki A, Okamoto Y, Okawara T, Otsuka M, Mukai R, Suzuki K. Antiviral activities against herpes simplex virus type 1 by HPH derivatives and their structure-activity relationships. Bioorg Med Chem Lett. 2008;18(1):371–4.
21. Huang J, Beyer C, Palumbo-Zerr K, Zhang Y, Ramming A, Distler A, Gelse K, Distler O, Schett G, Wollin L, et al. Nintedanib inhibits fibroblast activation and ameliorates fibrosis in preclinical models of systemic sclerosis. Ann Rheum Dis. 2016;75(5):883–90.
22. Tanaka C, Fujimoto M, Hamaguchi Y, Sato S, Takehara K, Hasegawa M. Inducible costimulator ligand regulates bleomycin-induced lung and skin fibrosis in a mouse model independently of the inducible costimulator/inducible costimulator ligand pathway. Arthritis Rheum. 2010;62(6):1723–32.
23. Huu DL, Matsushita T, Jin G, Hamaguchi Y, Hasegawa M, Takehara K, Fujimoto M. FTY720 ameliorates murine sclerodermatous chronic graft-versus-host disease by promoting expansion of splenic regulatory cells and inhibiting immune cell infiltration into skin. Arthritis Rheum. 2013;65(6):1624–35.
24. Wermuth PJ, Jimenez SA. The significance of macrophage polarization subtypes for animal models of tissue fibrosis and human fibrotic diseases. Clin Transl Med. 2015;4:2.
25. Asano Y, Bujor AM, Trojanowska M. The impact of Fli1 deficiency on the pathogenesis of systemic sclerosis. J Dermatol Sci. 2010;59(3):153–62.
26. Dong JT, Chen C. Essential role of KLF5 transcription factor in cell proliferation and differentiation and its implications for human diseases. Cell Mol Life Sci. 2009;66(16):2691–706.
27. Noda S, Asano Y, Nishimura S, Taniguchi T, Fujiu K, Manabe I, Nakamura K, Yamashita T, Saigusa R, Akamata K, et al. Simultaneous downregulation of KLF5 and Fli1 is a key feature underlying systemic sclerosis. Nat Commun. 2014;5:5797.
28. Rice LM, Padilla CM, McLaughlin SR, Mathes A, Ziemek J, Goummih S, Nakerakanti S, York M, Farina G, Whitfield ML, et al. Fresolimumab treatment decreases biomarkers and improves clinical symptoms in systemic sclerosis patients. J Clin Invest. 2015;125(7):2795–807.
29. Wahl SM, Hunt DA, Wakefield LM, McCartney-Francis N, Wahl LM, Roberts AB,

Sporn MB. Transforming growth factor type β induces monocyte chemotaxis and growth factor production. Proc Natl Acad Sci U S A. 1987;84(16):5788–92.

30. Arai M, Ikawa Y, Chujo S, Hamaguchi Y, Ishida W, Shirasaki F, Hasegawa M, Mukaida N, Fujimoto M, Takehara K. Chemokine receptors CCR2 and CX3CR1 regulate skin fibrosis in the mouse model of cytokine-induced systemic sclerosis. J Dermatol Sci. 2013;69(3):250–8.
31. Gerber EE, Gallo EM, Fontana SC, Davis EC, Wigley FM, Huso DL, Dietz HC. Integrin-modulating therapy prevents fibrosis and autoimmunity in mouse models of scleroderma. Nature. 2013;503(7474):126–30.
32. Fleischmajer R, Perlish JS, Reeves JR. Cellular infiltrates in scleroderma skin. Arthritis Rheum. 1977;20(4):975–84.
33. Yoshizaki A, Iwata Y, Komura K, Ogawa F, Hara T, Muroi E, Takenaka M, Shimizu K, Hasegawa M, Fujimoto M, et al. CD19 regulates skin and lung fibrosis via Toll-like receptor signaling in a model of bleomycin-induced scleroderma. Am J Pathol. 2008;172(6):1650–63.
34. Yoshizaki A, Yanaba K, Yoshizaki A, Iwata Y, Komura K, Ogawa F, Takenaka M, Shimizu K, Asano Y, Hasegawa M, et al. Treatment with rapamycin prevents fibrosis in tight-skin and bleomycin-induced mouse models of systemic sclerosis. Arthritis Rheum. 2010;62(8):2476–87.
35. Katsumoto TR, Whitfield ML, Connolly MK. The pathogenesis of systemic sclerosis. Annu Rev Pathol. 2011;6:509–37.
36. Wynn TA, Barron L. Macrophages: master regulators of inflammation and fibrosis. Semin Liver Dis. 2010;30(3):245–57.
37. Maier C, Ramming A, Bergmann C, Weinkam R, Kittan N, Schett G, Distler JHW, Beyer C. Inhibition of phosphodiesterase 4 (PDE4) reduces dermal fibrosis by interfering with the release of interleukin-6 from M2 macrophages. Ann Rheum Dis. 2017;76(6):1133–41.
38. Khanna D, Denton CP, Jahreis A, van Laar JM, Frech TM, Anderson ME, Baron M, Chung L, Fierlbeck G, Lakshminarayanan S, et al. Safety and efficacy of subcutaneous tocilizumab in adults with systemic sclerosis (faSScinate): a phase 2, randomised, controlled trial. Lancet. 2016;387(10038):2630–40.
39. Tacke F, Randolph GJ. Migratory fate and differentiation of blood monocyte subsets. Immunobiology. 2006;211(6–8):609–18.
40. Carlin LM, Stamatiades EG, Auffray C, Hanna RN, Glover L, Vizcay-Barrena G, Hedrick CC, Cook HT, Diebold S, Geissmann F. *Nr4a1*-dependent Ly6C^{low} monocytes monitor endothelial cells and orchestrate their disposal. Cell. 2013;153(2):362–75.
41. Gibbons MA, MacKinnon AC, Ramachandran P, Dhaliwal K, Duffin R, Phythian-Adams AT, van Rooijen N, Haslett C, Howie SE, Simpson AJ, et al. Ly6Chi monocytes direct alternatively activated profibrotic macrophage regulation of lung fibrosis. Am J Respir Crit Care Med. 2011;184(5):569–81.
42. Peng X, Zhang J, Xiao Z, Dong Y, Du J. CX3CL1–CX3CR1 interaction increases the population of Ly6C^{-}CX3CR1^{hi} macrophages contributing to unilateral ureteral obstruction-induced fibrosis. J Immunol. 2015;195(6):2797–805.
43. Lenzo JC, Turner AL, Cook AD, Vlahos R, Anderson GP, Reynolds EC, Hamilton JA. Control of macrophage lineage populations by CSF-1 receptor and GM-CSF in homeostasis and inflammation. Immunol Cell Biol. 2012;90(4):429–40.
44. Terry RL, Miller SD. Molecular control of monocyte development. Cell Immunol. 2014;291(1–2):16–21.
45. Zhang F, Wang H, Wang X, Jiang G, Liu H, Zhang G, Wang H, Fang R, Bu X, Cai S, et al. TGF-β induces M2-like macrophage polarization via SNAIL-mediated suppression of a pro-inflammatory phenotype. Oncotarget. 2016; 7(32):52294–306.
46. Wang S, Meng XM, Ng YY, Ma FY, Zhou S, Zhang Y, Yang C, Huang XR, Xiao J, Wang YY, et al. TGF-β/Smad3 signalling regulates the transition of bone marrow-derived macrophages into myofibroblasts during tissue fibrosis. Oncotarget. 2016;7(8):8809–22.
47. Wang Y, Fan PS, Kahaleh B. Association between enhanced type I collagen expression and epigenetic repression of the *FLI1* gene in scleroderma fibroblasts. Arthritis Rheum. 2006;54(7):2271–9.
48. Taniguchi T, Asano Y, Akamata K, Noda S, Takahashi T, Ichimura Y, Toyama T, Trojanowska M, Sato S. Fibrosis, vascular activation, and immune abnormalities resembling systemic sclerosis in bleomycin-treated Fli-1-haploinsufficient mice. Arthritis Rheumatol. 2015;67(2):517–26.
49. Takahashi T, Asano Y, Sugawara K, Yamashita T, Nakamura K, Saigusa R, Ichimura Y, Toyama T, Taniguchi T, Akamata K, et al. Epithelial Fli1 deficiency drives systemic autoimmunity and fibrosis: possible roles in scleroderma. J Exp Med. 2017;214(4):1129–51.
50. Distler JH, Distler O. Criteria to select molecular targets for anti-fibrotic therapy. Rheumatology (Oxford). 2008;47(Suppl 5):v12–3.

10

Changes in plasma CXCL4 levels are associated with improvements in lung function in patients receiving immunosuppressive therapy for systemic sclerosis-related interstitial lung disease

Elizabeth R. Volkmann[1*], Donald P. Tashkin[1], Michael D. Roth[1], Philip J. Clements[1], Dinesh Khanna[2], Daniel E. Furst[1], Maureen Mayes[3], Julio Charles[3], Chi-Hong Tseng[1], Robert M. Elashoff[4] and Shervin Assassi[3]

Abstract

Background: Increased circulatory levels of the chemokine CXCL4 have been associated with the presence of interstitial lung disease (ILD) in an observational study of patients with systemic sclerosis (SSc). The purpose of the present study was to evaluate the relationship between baseline CXCL4 level and extent of ILD in the context of a randomized controlled trial and to determine whether changes in CXCL4 levels in response to immunosuppression are associated with future progression of SSc-ILD.

Methods: A total of 142 SSc-ILD patients from Scleroderma Lung Study (SLS) II were randomized in a double-blind, parallel-arm trial, to receive mycophenolate (MMF) for 2 years or oral cyclophosphamide (CYC) for 1 year followed by 1 year of placebo. Plasma CXCL4 levels were measured at baseline, 12 months, and 24 months in SLS II participants ($N = 136$) and at a single time point in healthy controls ($N = 67$). A mixed-effects model evaluated the relationship between change in CXCL4 levels and SSc-ILD progression. The primary outcome was the course of the forced vital capacity.

Results: Baseline CXCL4 levels were significantly higher in SSc-ILD patients compared with healthy controls (2699 ± 1489 ng/ml vs 2233 ± 1351 ng/ml (mean ± SD); $P = 0.019$). However, no significant correlations were identified between CXCL4 levels and extent of ILD at baseline, as measured by the forced vital capacity, diffusing capacity of carbon monoxide, or radiographic extent of ILD. Plasma CXCL4 decreased significantly from baseline to 12 months in all patients (CYC: $P < 0.001$; MMF: $P = 0.006$) with no between-treatment differences (CYC vs MMF). Patients with the largest decline in CXCL4 levels during the first 12 months had an improved course of forced vital capacity %-predicted from 12 to 24 months ($P = 0.040$), even after adjusting for baseline disease severity and treatment arm assignment.

(Continued on next page)

* Correspondence: evolkmann@mednet.ucla.edu
[1]Department of Medicine, University of California, David Geffen School of Medicine, Los Angeles, CA, USA
Full list of author information is available at the end of the article

(Continued from previous page)

Conclusions: Levels of CXCL4 were higher in patients with SSc-ILD compared with controls and decreased in all patients treated with immunosuppressive therapy. While CXCL4 levels were not correlated with extent of ILD at baseline, changes in CXCL4 at 12 months predicted future progression of SSc-ILD from 12 to 24 months. These findings suggest that intermediate-term changes in CXCL4 may have predictive significance for long-term progression of SSc-ILD in patients receiving immunosuppressive therapy.

Keywords: Systemic sclerosis, Pulmonary fibrosis, Chemokines, Immunosuppression

Background

Although interstitial lung disease (ILD) occurs in the majority of patients with systemic sclerosis (SSc) and is also the leading cause of death in SSc [1], ILD progression rates vary considerably in this patient population [2].

Identifying specific factors that may predict response to immunosuppression is central to improving our ability to determine which SSc patients may derive the greatest benefit from ILD-targeted therapy. While numerous studies have examined baseline factors that are associated with ILD progression [3–9], relatively few studies have examined whether these factors are associated with a positive response to immunosuppression. In the Scleroderma Lung Study (SLS) I (comparing cyclophosphamide (CYC) with placebo), the severity of reticular infiltrates on baseline high-resolution computed tomography (HRCT) was associated with improved responsiveness to CYC therapy [10]. However, to our knowledge, no studies have examined responsiveness to therapy with mycophenolate (MMF) in SSc-ILD.

Biomarkers may have clinical application for predicting response to immunosuppression in patients with SSc-ILD. Several studies have identified potential circulating biomarkers associated with accelerated SSc-ILD progression, including interleukin (IL)-6 [11], C-reactive protein (CRP) [12], monocyte chemoattractant protein-1 (MCP-1) [13], CC chemokine ligand 18 (CCL18) [14, 15], and CXCL4 [16]. However, these markers have not been consistently shown to predict relevant clinical outcomes across a variety of treatments and SSc populations. Furthermore, all of the studies assessing the aforementioned candidate biomarkers were observational by design and consequently included patients who exhibited diverse phenotypic expressions of SSc, received a variety of immunosuppressant therapies, and were followed for varying periods of time [11–16].

Of these potential biomarkers, the chemokine, CXCL4, may play an important role in perpetuating profibrotic activity in the SSc-ILD disease state. An observational study found that CXCL4 levels were higher in SSc patients with ILD compared with those without ILD in a discovery cohort, as well as in two independent replication cohorts [16]. In a subgroup of patients from this study ($N = 79$), SSc patients with high baseline CXCL4 levels had accelerated progression of ILD as measured by a decline in the diffusing capacity for carbon monoxide (DLCO) [16]. Notably, this study also found that CXCL4 levels were remarkably higher in SSc patients compared with healthy controls (270-fold higher) [16].

The present study aimed to evaluate whether the chemokine CXCL4 is associated with the extent of ILD in a well-characterized cohort of SSc patients, all of whom had clinically significant ILD. Unlike previous studies of this nature, the present study analyzed CXCL4 at multiple time points in concert with the simultaneous collection of extensive clinical, physiologic, and radiographic data. A secondary aim was to determine whether changes in CXCL4 levels can predict improvements in lung function in patients receiving MMF or CYC in the setting of a randomized controlled clinical trial (RCT).

Methods

Study participants

Participants in the SLS II trial ($N = 142$) were all adults, aged 18–75 years, who exhibited either limited or diffuse cutaneous SSc [17] and active ILD as demonstrated by restrictive ventilatory impairment (forced vital capacity (FVC) <80% but ≥45% predicted), exertional dyspnea (Grade ≥2 on the Magnitude of Task component of the Mahler Baseline Dyspnea Index (BDI)) [18], and the presence of any ground glass opacity (GGO; hazy opacity through which normal lung markings can be discerned) on HRCT. Key exclusion criteria included pulmonary hypertension; clinically significant abnormalities on HRCT not attributable to SSc; and smoking within the past 6 months or evidence of significant airflow obstruction. Complete details of the SLS II population have been reported previously [19].

Healthy control participants were independently recruited at the University of Texas, Houston, and matched for age, ethnicity, and gender to SLS II participants in a 1:2 ratio.

SLS II study design

Enrolled patients were randomly (1:1 block) assigned in a double-blind, parallel-arm manner to receive either oral CYC for 1 year followed by 1 year of placebo or MMF for 2 years. SLS II was a superiority study conducted at 14 university hospitals throughout the USA (for the list of sites see Ethics approval and consent to participate) and recruited patients between November 2009 and January 2013. For complete details of the SLS II protocol, please see the supplementary Web appendix accompanying the main SLS manuscript [19]. There were no significant changes in the protocol involving the design, outcomes, treatment, or eligibility criteria during the trial. Baseline measurements included the following physiological variables: spirometry (FVC and forced expired volume in 1 second (FEV_1)), lung volumes (functional residual capacity (FRC), residual volume (RV), and total lung capacity (TLC) by whole-body plethysmography or helium dilution), hemoglobin-adjusted single-breath DLCO, and the ratio of DLCO to alveolar volume (DL/VA). The FVC (primary SLS II endpoint) and DLCO (secondary SLS II endpoint) were measured every 3 months, and the TLC was measured every 6 months during the trial. HRCT thoracic imaging was obtained at baseline and at 24 months and a computer-aided design (CAD) scoring system was employed to provide quantitative measures of different patterns of ILD as described previously [19, 20]. The Quantitative ILD (QILD) score was the sum of all abnormally classified scores, including scores for quantitative lung fibrosis (QLF, linear reticular markings), GGO, and honeycomb changes (clustered air-filled cysts with dense walls). Scores were calculated as the percentage of voxels for both the whole lung (WL), including both lungs, and for the lobe of maximal involvement (LM).

CXCL4 measurement

SLS II plasma samples were collected at the baseline, 12-month, and 24-month study visits and were immediately processed on-site on the day of collection, stored at −70 °C, and shipped on dry ice to the central repository at the University of Texas, Houston. Samples from healthy controls collected at the University of Texas, Houston, were handled in the same manner except that no shipping was required. Validated, commercially available ELISA kits (Human CXCL4/PF4 Quantikine Kit; R&D Systems) were used to assess CXCL4 levels. All assays were performed in duplicate and the coefficient of variance was <20%. Technicians performing the assays were blinded to the study arm assignment. CXCL4 data were logarithmically transformed to correct for data skewness.

Statistical analysis

Baseline characteristics

Summary statistics were generated for baseline characteristics. A two-sample t test was used to compare continuous variables and a chi-square test was used to compare categorical variables. Pearson correlations were performed to examine the relationship between CXCL4 levels and baseline measures of extent of ILD, as measured by the FVC, DLCO, QILD, and QLF, as well as the relationship between baseline CXCL4 levels and platelet counts.

Relationship between change in CXCL4 and progression of SSc-ILD

To determine whether a change in plasma CXCL4 might correlate with or predict the progression of SSc-ILD, we first plotted the course of measured plasma CXCL4, by treatment arm, from baseline to 24 months and determined the corresponding magnitude of change for individual subjects from baseline to 12 and 24 months. Pearson correlations were initially performed to examine the relationship between the change in CXCL4 levels from baseline to 12 months and the absolute change for the primary outcome (FVC %-predicted) and key secondary outcomes (DLCO %-predicted and HRCT measures of the extent of ILD).

Following these initial analyses, a mixed-effects model was generated, the outcome of which was the course of FVC %-predicted measured in 3-month increments from 12 to 24 months (primary outcome). The model included the following covariates: change in CXCL4 from baseline to 12 months, baseline FVC %-predicted, baseline extent of quantitative fibrosis/ILD, treatment arm, and a time trend. The covariate of baseline extent of quantitative fibrosis/ILD was defined as the first principal component from a principal component analysis of the following variables: QILD-LM, QILD-WL, QLF-LM, and QLF-WL.

All tests were two-sided, and all analyses were performed using SAS 9.2 (SAS Institute, Inc., Cary, NC, USA).

Results

Baseline characteristics

At baseline, there were no significant differences in any of the demographic or key disease-defining characteristics of SLS II participants assigned to MMF vs CYC (Table 1). Baseline CXCL4 levels (ng/ml) were higher in SLS II participants ($N = 136$) compared with healthy controls ($N = 67$) (SSc: mean 2699 (SD 1489), median 2480 (IR 1585, 3889); controls: mean 2233 (SD 1351),

Table 1 Baseline characteristics of SLS II participants with CXCL4 measurements at baseline

Characteristic	Cyclophosphamide N		Mycophenolate N	
Age (years)	71	52.3 ± 9.5	65	52.6 ± 10.0
Female sex (% of patients)	71	77.5	65	69.2
Duration of scleroderma (years)	70	2.5 ± 1.8	63	2.7 ± 1.7
% Limited/% diffuse	71	45.1/54.9	65	36.9/63.1
FVC (%-predicted)	71	66.2 ± 9.9	65	66.6 ± 8.2
FEV1:FVC (%-predicted)	71	83.5 ± 5.6	65	81.8 ± 5.7
TLC (%-predicted)	71	65.4 ± 12.1	65	66.5 ± 10.2
DLCO (%-predicted)[a]	71	53.8 ± 14.2	65	54.4 ± 11.3
DL/VA (%-predicted)	71	61.0 ± 13.7	65	60.9 ± 11.8
Mahler Dyspnea Index (focal score)	67	7.0 ± 2.3	61	7.3 ± 2.1
Skin-thickening score (mRSS)[b]				
All patients	71		65	
Mean		14.1 ± 10.8		15.2 ± 10.1
Range		2–46		1–41
Patients with dcSSc	39		41	
Mean		20.7 ± 9.9		20.7 ± 8.6
Range		3–46		4–41
Patients with lcSSc	32		24	
Mean		6.1 ± 4.3		5.9 ± 3.4
Range		2–18		1–14
HAQ disability index (0–3)[c]	71	0.7 ± 0.7	65	0.7 ± 0.6
QLF-WL	69	9.1 ± 7.0	62	8.2 ± 6.9
QLF-LM	69	23.2 ± 19.2	62	22.5 ± 19.9
QILD-WL	69	32.1 ± 14.2	62	27.2 ± 13.6
QILD-LM	69	53.2 ± 19.3	62	49.8 ± 21.0
Auto-antibody (% positive in patients tested)				
ANA	70	94.3	62	96.8
Topoisomerase-1	70	45.7	62	46.2
RNA polymerase III	70	11.4	62	14.5
Centromere	70	2.9	62	1.6
Th\to	67	7.5	60	5.0

Values are mean ± standard deviation, unless otherwise noted
[a]Adjusted for hemoglobin
[b]Scores for skin thickening (mRSS) can range from 0 to 51, with higher scores indicating more severe thickening
[c]Scores for HAQ Disability Index can range from 1 to 3, with higher numbers indicating greater disability
FVC forced vital capacity, *FEV*$_1$ forced expired volume in 1 second, *TLC* total lung capacity, *DLCO* diffusing capacity of the lung for carbon monoxide, *DL/VA* ratio of DLCO to alveolar volume, *mRSS* modified Rodnan skin score, *dcScc* diffuse cutaneous systemic sclerosis, *lcSSc* limited or cutaneous systemic sclerosis, *HAQ* Health Assessment Questionnaire, *QLF* quantitative extent of lung fibrosis on high-resolution chest computed tomography, *QILD* quantitative extent of total interstitial lung disease (including fibrosis, honeycomb, and ground glass opacity), *WL* whole lung, *LM* lobe of maximal involvement
ANA Anti-nuclear antibody, *Th/To* Th/To ribonucleoprotein antibody

median 1720 (IR 1224, 2874); $P = 0.019$) (Fig. 1). There were no significant differences in baseline CXCL4 levels between treatment arms, between limited or diffuse SSc patients, between men and women, or between ethnicities (all $P \geq 0.2$). There were also no significant correlations between baseline CXCL4 and age, or disease duration, as measured by the onset of the first Raynaud's phenomenon symptom ($r = -0.10$, $P = 0.24$), or as measured by the onset of the first non-Raynaud's phenomenon symptom attributable to SSc ($r = 0.040$, $P = 0.64$). Similarly, among the healthy controls there were no significant differences in CXCL4 levels between men and women or between ethnicities, and nor was there any correlation between CXCL4 levels and age.

CXCL4 correlations

At baseline there were no significant correlations between plasma CXCL4 levels and any of the physiologic or radiographic measures of extent or severity of SSc-ILD (Table 2). There were also no significant correlations between plasma CXCL4 and extent of SSc-ILD at 12 or 24 months (data not shown).

There was no significant correlation between baseline CXCL4 and baseline mRSS among all participants ($r = 0.10$; $P = 0.24$), or among patients with diffuse cutaneous sclerosis ($N = 80$; $r = 0.059$; $P = 0.60$).

At baseline, CXCL4 levels demonstrated a weak but significant correlation with the platelet count ($r = 0.320$, $P < 0.001$).

Plasma levels of CXCL4 levels decrease in response to immunosuppression

Among the 136 patients with baseline plasma CXCL4 levels measured, 103 patients had 12-month CXCL4

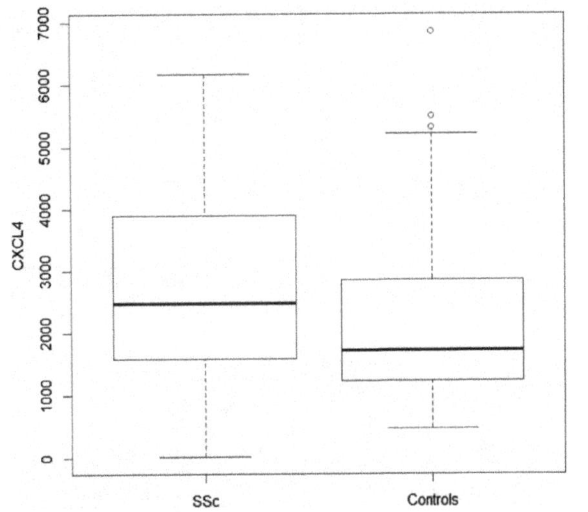

Fig. 1 Plasma CXCL4 levels (ng/ml) were significantly higher in SSc-ILD patients ($N = 136$) compared with healthy controls matched for age, gender, and ethnicity ($N = 67$), $P = 0.019$. *SSc* systemic sclerosis

Table 2 Baseline CXCL4 levels are not correlated with extent of ILD in SLS II subjects

Surrogate ILD measurements	Pearson correlation (*r*)	*P* value
TLC% predicted	0.123	0.154
FVC% predicted	0.089	0.304
DLCO% predicted	0.082	0.345
QLF-LM	−0.027	0.763
QILD-LM	−0.063	0.473
QLF-WL	−0.034	0.703
QILD-WL	−0.022	0.799

Values are mean ± standard deviation, unless otherwise noted
ILD interstitial lung disease, *SLS* Scleroderma Lung Study, *FVC* forced vital capacity, *TLC* total lung capacity, *DLCO* diffusing capacity of the lung for carbon monoxide, *QLF* quantitative extent of lung fibrosis on high-resolution chest computed tomography, *QILD* quantitative extent of total interstitial lung disease (including fibrosis, honeycomb, and ground glass opacity), *WL* whole lung, *LM* lobe of maximal involvement

measurements (CYC = 50; MMF = 53), and 86 patients had 24-month CXCL4 measurements (CYC = 41; MMF = 45) (Fig. 2). CXCL4 levels were measured in all patients who returned for the follow-up study visits at 12 and 24 months.

The majority of patients in both treatment arms experienced a decrease in CXCL4 levels from baseline to 12 months (CYC: 76% (37/49); MMF: 67% (35/52)) and from baseline to 24 months (CYC: 70% (28/40); MMF: 68% (30/44)). Plasma CXCL4 levels declined significantly in the CYC and MMF arms ($P < 0.001$ and $P = 0.006$, respectively). Similarly, CXCL4 levels showed a significant decrease from baseline to 24 months in the CYC and MMF arms ($P < 0.001$ and $P = 0.011$, respectively). Although participants in the CYC arm experienced numerically larger decreases in CXCL4 levels, there was no statistically significant difference in the change in CXCL4 levels between treatment arms from baseline to 12 months ($P = 0.120$) or from baseline to 24 months ($P = 0.380$) (Fig. 3). While CXCL4 levels slightly increased from 12 to 24 months in the CYC arm (during the placebo phase), CXCL4 levels continued to decline from 12 to 24 months in the MMF arm.

Changes in plasma levels of CXCL4 levels may predict improved course of FVC

As reported previously [19], the course of the FVC in SLS II improved significantly from baseline to 24 months in both the CYC and MMF treatment arms, with no between-treatment difference. Of note, FVC measurements were obtained in 51 and 59 participants at 12 months and in 50 and 53 participants at 24 months for the CYC and MMF arms, respectively. When changes in the plasma CXCL4 levels at 12 months were correlated with changes in the FVC (bivariate analysis), there was a trend for a negative correlation between the change in CXCL4 from baseline to 12 months and the change in FVC from baseline to 18 months ($r = -0.203$; $P = 0.063$), 21 months ($r = -0.212$; $P = 0.062$), and 24 months ($r = -0.182$; $P = 0.082$), but not at 12 months ($r = -0.070$; $P = 0.499$) or 15 months ($r = -0.048$; $P = 0.662$).

There were no significant correlations between the change from baseline in CXCL4 at 12 months and the change from baseline in DLCO at 12, 15, 18, 21, or 24 months (all $P > 0.3$). There was also no significant correlation between the change from baseline in CXCL4 at 12 months and the change from baseline in QLF-LM/WL or QILD-LM/WL at 24 months (all $P > 0.4$).

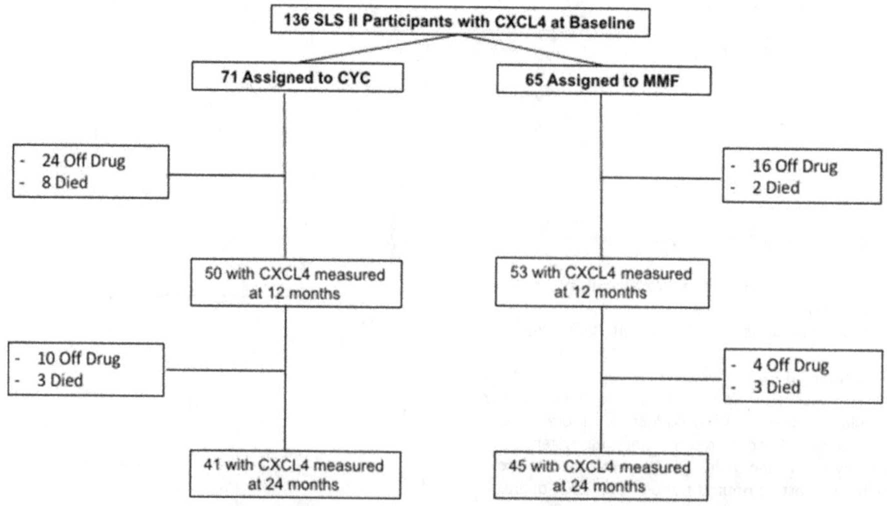

Fig. 2 Disposition of SLS II study participants with regard to CXCL4 measurement during the 24-month trial. FVC measurements were obtained in 51 and 59 participants at 12 months and in 50 and 53 participants at 24 months for the CYC and MMF arms, respectively. *CYC* cyclophosphamide, *MMF* mycophenolate, *SLS* Scleroderma Lung Study

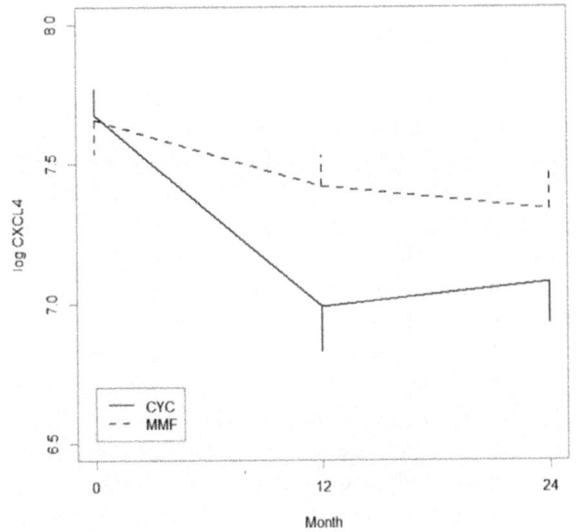

Fig. 3 CXCL4 levels decreased significantly in response to immunosuppression in each treatment arm from baseline to 12 months (CYC: $P < 0.001$; MMF: $P = 0.006$) and from baseline to 24 months (CYC: $P < 0.001$; MMF: $P = 0.011$). There was no between-treatment difference in the reduction in CXCL4 from baseline to 12 months or from baseline to 24 months. *CYC* cyclophosphamide, *MMF* mycophenolate

To further explore the relationship between the change in CXCL4 and the course of the FVC, a mixed-effects model was generated and the results demonstrated that the change in CXCL4 from baseline to 12 months was associated with the course of the FVC (as a continuous variable) from 12 to 24 months (estimate −1.232; 95% CI −2.405, −0.060; $P = 0.040$), after controlling for treatment arm assignment, a time trend, baseline quantitative extent of ILD/fibrosis, and baseline FVC. A similar statistical approach was used in the analysis of the primary and secondary outcomes in SLS II [19]. The results demonstrated that every 1-unit decrease in the log CXCL4 level was associated with a 1.23% increase in the FVC. In other words, patients who experienced the greatest decline in CXCL4 levels during the first 12 months of the study had an improved course of FVC from 12 to 24 months (Table 3).

Given the significant correlation between CXCL4 levels and platelet count at baseline, baseline platelet count was added to the mixed-effects model. Adding baseline platelet count to the model did not affect the significant relationship between change in CXCL4 levels and the outcome variable. However, the baseline platelet count was not independently associated with the course of the FVC ($P = 0.163$), and for this reason this variable was not included in the final model.

Because not all patients had CXCL4 measurements at 12 months, the final model included 97 patients with SSc-ILD. Notably, there were no significant differences

Table 3 Multivariable analysis examining the relationship between change in CXCL4 from baseline to 12 months and the course of FVC from 12 to 24 months ($N = 97$)

Baseline covariate	Estimate	95% CI	*P* value
ΔCXCL4	−1.232	−2.405, −0.060	0.040
Baseline FVC	0.972	0.807, 1.138	<0.0001
Baseline QILD/QLF[a]	0.297	−0.496, 1.089	0.464
Treatment arm	−0.361	−3.182, 2.460	0.802

[a]Defined as the first principal component from a principal component analysis of the following variables: QILD-LM, QILD-WL, QLF-LM, and QLF-WL
FVC forced vital capacity, *CI* confidence interval, *QLF* quantitative extent of lung fibrosis on high-resolution chest computed tomography, *QILD* quantitative extent of total interstitial lung disease (including fibrosis, honeycomb, and ground glass opacity), *WL* whole lung, *LM* lobe of maximal involvement

in baseline characteristics (i.e., age, gender, diffuse/limited, FVC, DLCO, MRSS, QILD-WL/LM, QLF-WL/LM) between the 97 patients included in the final mixed-effects model and the 39 patients who were not included.

Discussion

In a well-characterized cohort of patients with SSc-ILD, CXCL4 levels decreased significantly in response to immunosuppressive therapy with both CYC and MMF. Furthermore, a greater change in CXCL4 from baseline to 12 months led to improvements in SSc-ILD at 24 months as measured by the FVC %-predicted. These findings suggest that intermediate-term changes in CXCL4 may have predictive significance for long-term progression of SSc-ILD in patients receiving immunosuppressive therapy.

These findings are consistent with the purported pathobiological role of CXCL4 in moderating fibrotic and inflammatory processes. In addition to the previously reported association with various dimensions of SSc [16], CXCL4 levels have also been elevated in liver fibrosis [21] and in patients with antiphospholipid syndrome [22]. In a recent study, CXCL4 blocked the induction of the anti-inflammatory enzyme heme oxygenase-1. Furthermore, the product of heme oxygenase enzymatic activity, bilirubin, showed an inverse correlation with CXCL4 levels in plasma samples of SSc patients [23]. While our understanding of the role of CXCL4 in the development of SSc-ILD is evolving, the present manuscript provides further support for its role in the pathogenesis of SSc.

This study further sheds light on plausible biological mediators/targets of the two immunosuppressant agents under study (i.e. MMF and CYC). Although CXCL4 levels were not correlated with any of the baseline surrogate markers of ILD severity, CXCL4 levels significantly declined in both treatment arms in response to immunosuppression. Furthermore, the decline in CXCL4 paralleled the improvements appreciated in the course of the FVC over 24 months as reported in the main SLS II manuscript [19]. Although there was no significant difference in the degree to which CXCL4 decreased between treatment arms, the sample size may have limited our ability to detect a difference because CXCL4 levels appeared to decrease to a greater extent in the CYC arm compared with the MMF arm within the first 12 months of treatment (Fig. 3). Interestingly, CXCL4 levels declined most dramatically during the first 12 months of therapy in both study arms. The patients assigned to CYC received placebo in the second year, which may explain the slight upward trend in CXCL4 levels during the second year of the study. However, the CXCL4 levels did not return to those observed at the baseline visit after 2 years in the CYC arm. This finding may in part be related to the use of alternate therapy during the latter period. Of the 15 subjects in SLS II who withdrew from or failed treatment but returned for final study outcome measures, 12 indicated that they were switched to potentially disease-modifying therapy (MMF, intravenous CYC, rituximab, tocilizumab, intravenous immunoglobulin, or azathioprine) and these alternative therapies may have influenced the results [19]. In the MMF arm, CXCL4 levels continued to decline during the second year of the study, likely related to continuous use of immunosuppression in this arm.

Interestingly, we did not observe significant correlations between baseline CXCL4 levels and extent of ILD as measured by the FVC, DLCO, TLC, or extent of quantitative radiographic fibrosis at baseline, 12 months, or 24 months. While a prior study [16] demonstrated that patients with high CXCL4 were more likely to have fibrosis on HRCT, this prior observational study included SSc patients both with and without ILD and at varying disease stages. By contrast, the present study only included patients with ILD at a relatively early stage of disease (mean disease duration of 2.6 years from the onset of the first non-Raynaud's symptom attributable to SSc), nearly all of whom already had evidence of fibrosis on HRCT [19]. Our findings suggest that CXCL4 may be a more useful predictive biomarker for response to immunosuppression in patients with early SSc-ILD. Whether CXCL4 correlates with severity of ILD at later stages of SSc remains uncertain. Furthermore, because our cohort did not evaluate SSc patients without ILD, we could not assess whether CXCL4 levels can distinguish SSc patients with and without ILD.

We did observe a significant but weak correlation between CXCL4 levels and platelet levels. However, the platelet level did not demonstrate predictive significance for FVC progression in the mixed-effects model. Importantly, precautions were taken to limit platelet activation, which can significantly affect CXCL4 levels, including using strict caution to minimize venostasis during the blood draw with butterfly needles and immediately centrifuging the specimens. Of note, the prior study in this area [16] did not assess platelet levels.

Consistent with the work of van Bon et al. [16], we observed an increase in plasma CXCL4 levels in SSc-ILD patients compared with healthy controls. However, the magnitude of this difference was strikingly smaller in the present study (1.6-fold increase in our study vs 277-fold increase in the previous study). The observed difference in CXCL4 levels between SSc-ILD patients and healthy controls in the present report is consistent with the reported fold increases of other cytokines and chemokines in SSc plasma samples [12, 24]. While several possible explanations for this disparity exist, we note that we used a different ELISA assay in the present study than in the previous study (R&D Systems/Quantikine in the present study vs R&D Systems/DuoSet in the previous study). The assay we utilized has been fully validated for the measurement of CXCL4 in complex fluids such as serum and plasma [25].

There are notable strengths of the present study. First, this is the first study to measure CXCL4 levels at multiple time points in patients with early, symptomatic SSc-ILD. Second, our initial measurement of CXCL4 occurred prior to the initiation of immunosuppressive therapy for SSc-ILD; thus, the reported baseline levels of CXCL4 are likely closely related to the underlying disease state without any interference from disease-modifying therapies (patients were ineligible for SLS II if they had received CYC or MMF for >8 weeks ever in the past, or they had received intravenous CYC more than twice ever in the past, or were taking CYC/MMF/any medication with potential disease-modifying activity within 30 days of randomization). Third, unlike prior observational studies in this field, this cohort had uniform follow-up measurements with likely less missing data. Fourth, our analyses controlled for treatment assignment. Finally, this study was conducted at 14 centers and included patients from varying ethnic backgrounds, thereby increasing the generalizability of our findings.

The results of the present study should be interpreted within the context of certain limitations. Namely, although we attempted to control for treatment group, some patients in the SLS II cohort initiated alternate therapy for SSc-ILD during the course of the trial. Given the relatively small number of patients who switched therapies and the observation that there was no difference in the change in CXCL4 between the two treatment groups, it is unlikely that the use of alternate therapies would alter the outcomes of the present analyses. Another shortcoming was that only patients who returned for a 12-month and 24-month visit provided blood samples. The missing CXCL4 data reduce the statistical power of the analysis and may yield biased estimates.

Future studies may consider measuring CXCL4 at even earlier time points as a means of determining treatment response prior to 1 year. While we report that the change in CXCL4 at 1 year was associated with improved SSc-ILD progression at 2 years, additional studies would be useful to determine whether changes in CXCL4 at earlier time points might have similar predictive value. If the latter were found, it might be useful from a clinical standpoint to determine whether a patient is responding to a particular therapy at 3 or 6 months, to avoid the unfruitful continuation of an ineffective therapy.

Conclusions

While CXCL4 was not associated with extent of SSc-ILD at baseline, this chemokine decreased significantly in response to immunosuppressive therapy. Moreover, the change in CXCL4 levels was associated with future progression of SSc-ILD. Although the exact role of CXCL4 in the pathobiology of SSc-ILD is uncertain, these findings support the potential predictive capability of this chemokine for determining response to immunosuppressive therapy.

Abbreviations

CAD: Computer-aided design; CCL18: CC chemokine ligand 18; CRP: C-reactive protein; CYC: Cyclophosphamide; DL/VA: Ratio of DLCO to alveolar volume; DLCO: Diffusing capacity for carbon monoxide; FEV_1: Forced expired volume in 1 second; FRC: Functional residual capacity; FVC: Forced vital capacity; GGO: Ground glass opacity; HAQ: Health Assessment Questionnaire; HRCT: High-resolution chest computed tomography; IL: Interleukin; ILD: Interstitial lung disease; LM: Lobe of maximal involvement; MCP-1: Monocyte chemoattractant protein-1; MMF: Mycophenolate; mRSS: Modified Rodnan skin score; QILD: Quantitative extent of total interstitial lung disease (including fibrosis, honeycomb, and ground glass opacity); QLF: Quantitative extent of lung fibrosis on HRCT; RV: Residual volume; SLS: Scleroderma Lung Study; SSc: Systemic sclerosis; TLC: Total lung capacity; WL: Whole lung

Acknowledgements

The authors thank the patients for their participation in SLS II.

Funding

This work was supported by grants from the NHLBI/NIH: R01 HL089758 (DPT) and R01 HL089901 (RME), NIH/NIAMS K23AR061436 (SA), Rheumatology Research Foundation (SA), NIH/NIAMS K24 AR063120 (DK), and the Scleroderma Foundation (ERV). The study drug (MMF) and matching placebo were supplied at no charge through Drug Supply Grant # CEL539 from Hoffmann-La Roche/ Genentech.

Authors' contributions

ERV made substantial contributions to study conception and design, as well as analysis and interpretation of data, drafting the article, and approval of the final manuscript. DPT, MDR, PPC, DK, DEF, and MM made substantial contributions to study conception and design, revising the manuscript critically for important intellectual content, and approval of the final manuscript. JC and C-HT made substantial contributions to the analysis and interpretation of data, revising the manuscript critically for important intellectual content, and approval of the final manuscript. RME and SA made substantial contributions to study conception and design, the analysis and interpretation of data, revising the manuscript critically for important intellectual content, and approval of the final manuscript.

Competing interests

No nonfinancial conflicts of interest exist for any of the authors. Financial conflicts of interest are as follows.

ERV, PPC, RME, C-HT, and JC all report nothing to disclose.

DPT reports personal fees from EMD Serono, and nonfinancial support from Genentech, during the conduct of the study.

MDR reports nonfinancial support from Hoffmann-La Roche/Genentech, during the conduct of the study.

DEF reports grant/research support from AbbVie, Actelion, Amgen, BMS, Gilead, GSK, Novartis, Pfizer, Roche/Genentech, and UCB, and consultant work with AbbVie, Amgen, BMS, Cytori, Janssen, Gilead, GSK, NIH, Novartis, Pfizer, Roche/Genentech, UCB Speaker's Bureau (CME ONLY) AbbVie, Actelion, and UCB during the course of the study.

DK reports personal fees from Bayer, grants from Bristol-Myer Squibb, personal fees from Cytori, personal fees from EMD Serono (Merck), personal fees from Forward, grants and personal fees from Genentech/Roche (InterMune), and personal fees from Lycera during the course of the study.

MM reports grants from InterMune, grants from Roche/Genentech, grants from Bayer, grants from University of Michigan, grants from Boehringer-Ingelheim, grants from DOD, grants from Corbus, and grants from Cytori during the course of the study.

SA reports grants and personal fees from Boehringer Ingelheim, grants from Genentech, grants and personal fees from Biogen Idec, and grants from Bayer HealthCare during the course of the study.

Author details

[1]Department of Medicine, University of California, David Geffen School of Medicine, Los Angeles, CA, USA. [2]Department of Medicine, University of Michigan Medical School, Ann Arbor, MI, USA. [3]Department of Medicine, University of Texas Health Science Center at Houston, Houston, TX, USA. [4]Department of Biomathematics, University of California, Los Angeles, CA, USA.

References

1. Tyndall AJ, Bannert B, Vonk M, et al. Causes and risk factors for death in systemic sclerosis: a study from the EULAR Scleroderma Trials and Research (EUSTAR) database. Ann Rheum Dis. 2010;69:1809–15.
2. Wells AU. Interstitial lung disease in systemic sclerosis. Press Med. 2014;43: e329–43.
3. Morgan C, Knight C, Lunt M, et al. Predictors of end stage lung disease in a cohort of patients with scleroderma. Ann Rheum Dis. 2003;62:146–50.
4. Plastiras SC, Karadimitrakis SP, Ziakas PD, et al. Scleroderma lung: initial forced vital capacity as predictor of pulmonary function decline. Arthritis Rheum. 2006;55:598–602.
5. Nihtyanova SI, Schreiber BE, Ong VH, et al. Prediction of pulmonary complications and long-term survival in systemic sclerosis. Arthritis Rheumatol. 2014;66:1625–35.
6. Steen VD, Medsger Jr TA. Severe organ involvement in systemic sclerosis with diffuse scleroderma. Arthritis Rheum. 2000;43:2437–44.
7. Goh NSL, Desai SR, Veeraraghaven S, et al. Interstitial lung disease in systemic sclerosis. A simple staging system. Am J Respir Crit Care Med. 2008;177:1248–54.
8. Moore OA, Goh N, Corte T, et al. Extent of disease on high-resolution compute tomography lung is a predictor of decline and mortality in systemic sclerosis-related interstitial lung disease. Rheumatology (Oxford). 2013;165:378–81.
9. Assassi S, Sharif R, Lasky RE, et al. GENISOS Study Group. Arthritis Res Ther. 2010;12:R166.
10. Roth MD, Tseng CH, Clements PJ, et al. Predicting treatment outcomes and responder subsets in scleroderma-related interstitial lung disease. Arthritis Rheum. 2011;63:2797–808.
11. De Lauretis A, Sestini P, Pantelidis P, et al. Serum interleukin 6 is predictive of early functional decline and mortality in interstitial lung disease associated with systemic sclerosis. J Rheumatol. 2013;40:435–46.
12. Liu X, Mayes MD, Pedroza C, et al. Does C-reactive protein predict the long-term progression of interstitial lung disease and survival in patients with early systemic sclerosis? Arthritis Care Res. 2013;65:1375–80.

13. Wu M, Pedroza C, Salazar G, et al. Plasma MCP-1 and IL-10 levels predict long-term progression of interstitial lung disease in patients with early systemic sclerosis. Arthritis Rheum. 2013;65:S742.
14. Tiev KP, Hua-Huy T, Kettaneh A, et al. Serum CC chemokine ligand-18 predicts lung disease worsening in systemic sclerosis. Eur Respir. 2011;38:1355–60.
15. Schupp J, Becker M, Günther J, et al. Serum CCL18 is predictive for lung disease progression and mortality in systemic sclerosis. Eur Respir J. 2014;43:1530–2.
16. van Bon L, Affandi AJ, Broen J, et al. Proteome-wide analysis and CXCL4 as a biomarker in systemic sclerosis. N Engl J Med. 2014;370:433–43.
17. Masi T. Subcommittee for Scleroderma Criteria of the American Rheumatism Association Diagnostic and Therapeutic Criteria Committee. Preliminary criteria for the classification of systemic sclerosis (scleroderma). Arthritis Rheumatol. 1980;23:581–90.
18. Mahler DA, Weinberg DH, Wells CK, et al. The measurement of dyspnea. Contents, interobserver agreement and physiologic correlates of two new clinical indexes. Chest. 1984;85:751–8.
19. Tashkin DP, Roth MD, Clements PJ, et al., for the Scleroderma Lung Study II Investigators. Mycophenolate mofetil versus oral cyclophosphamide in scleroderma-related interstitial lung disease: Scleroderma lung study II (SLS-II), a double-blind, parallel group, mmunomodu controlled trial. Lancet Resp Med. 2016. [Epub ahead of print]
20. Kim HJ, Li G, Gjertson D, et al. Classification of parenchymal abnormality in scleroderma lung using a novel approach to denoise images collected via a multicenter study. Acad Radiol. 2008;15:1004–16.
21. Zaldivar MM, Pauels K, von Hundelshausen P, et al. CXC chemokine ligand 4 (Cxcl4) is a platelet-derived mediator of experimental liver fibrosis. Hepatology. 2010;51:1345–53.
22. Patsouras MD, Skiara MP, Grikak EP, et al. Elevated expression of platelet-derived chemokines in patients with antiphospholipid syndrome. J Autoimmun. 2015;65:30–7.
23. van Bon L, Cossu M, Scharstuhl A, et al. Low heme oxygenase-1 levels in patients with systemic sclerosis are associated with an altered Toll-like receptor response: another role for CXCL4? Rheumatol (Oxford). 2016 [Epub ahead of print].
24. Gourh P, Arnett FC, Assassi S, et al. Plasma cytokine profiles in systemic sclerosis: associations with autoantibody subsets and clinical manifestations. Arthritis Res Ther. 2009;11:R147.
25. R&D Systems: Quantikine ELISA Human CXCL4/PF4 Immunoassay. https://resources.rndsystems.com/pdfs/datasheets/dpf40.pdf (2016). Accessed 13 Sep 2016.

11

Effects of selexipag and its active metabolite in contrasting the profibrotic myofibroblast activity in cultured scleroderma skin fibroblasts

Maurizio Cutolo[1*], Barbara Ruaro[1], Paola Montagna[1], Renata Brizzolara[1], Emanuela Stratta[2], Amelia Chiara Trombetta[1], Stefano Scabini[2], Pier Paolo Tavilla[3], Aurora Parodi[3], Claudio Corallo[4], Nicola Giordano[4], Sabrina Paolino[1], Carmen Pizzorni[1], Alberto Sulli[1], Vanessa Smith[5] and Stefano Soldano[1]

Abstract

Background: Myofibroblasts contribute to fibrosis through the overproduction of extracellular matrix (ECM) proteins, primarily type I collagen (COL-1) and fibronectin (FN), a process which is mediated in systemic sclerosis (SSc) by the activation of fibrogenic intracellular signaling transduction molecules, including extracellular signal-regulated kinases 1 and 2 (Erk1/2) and protein kinase B (Akt). Selexipag is a prostacyclin receptor agonist synthesized for the treatment of pulmonary arterial hypertension. The study investigated the possibility for selexipag and its active metabolite (ACT-333679) to downregulate the profibrotic activity in primary cultures of SSc fibroblasts/myofibroblasts and the fibrogenic signaling molecules involved.

Methods: Fibroblasts from skin biopsies obtained with Ethics Committee (EC) approval from patients with SSc, after giving signed informed consent, were cultured until the 3rd culture passage and then either maintained in normal growth medium (untreated cells) or independently treated with different concentrations of selexipag (from 30 μM to 0.3 μM) or ACT-333679 (from 10 μM to 0.1 μM) for 48 h. Protein and gene expressions of α-smooth muscle actin (α-SMA), fibroblast specific protein-1 (S100A4), COL-1, and FN were investigated by western blotting and quantitative real-time PCR. Erk1/2 and Akt phosphorylation was investigated in untreated and ACT-333679-treated cells by western botting.

Results: Selexipag and ACT-333679 significantly reduced protein synthesis and gene expression of α-SMA, S100A4, and COL-1 in cultured SSc fibroblasts/myofibroblasts compared to untreated cells, whereas FN was significantly downregulated at the protein level. Interestingly, ACT-333679 significantly reduced the phosphorylation of Erk1/2 and Akt in cultured SSc fibroblasts/myofibroblasts.

Conclusions: Selexipag and mainly its active metabolite ACT-333679 were found for the first time to potentially interfere with the profibrotic activity of cultured SSc fibroblasts/myofibroblasts at least in vitro, possibly through the downregulation of fibrogenic Erk1/2 and Akt signaling molecules.

Keywords: Prostacyclin receptor agonists, Skin fibroblasts, Fibrosis, Systemic sclerosis, Connective tissue diseases

* Correspondence: mcutolo@unige.it
[1]Research Laboratory and Academic Division of Clinical Rheumatology, Department of Internal Medicine, University of Genova, Polyclinic San Martino Hospital, Genoa, Italy
Full list of author information is available at the end of the article

Background

Fibrosis is a common feature in diseases characterized by chronic tissue inflammation and damage, including systemic sclerosis (SSc) [1]. In SSc, fibrosis follows the microvascular/endothelial damage with activation of fibroblasts and their transition into profibrotic myofibroblasts [1–3]. After their phenotype transition, myofibroblasts acquire an increased persistent capability to synthesize and accumulate extracellular matrix (ECM) proteins, such as type I collagen (COL-1), and fibronectin (FN), beginning an aberrant "wound healing" process that contributes to fibrogenesis and finally to the systemic SSc fibrosis [4–6].

Myofibroblast transition and ECM overproduction are known to be induced by several profibrotic mediators, including transforming growth factor-β (TGFβ), endothelin-1 (ET-1), cytokines and chemokines (such as IL-6 and CCL18), whose circulating levels are increased in patients with SSc. These mediators have been shown to regulate the progression of fibrosis through the activation of intracellular signaling transduction pathways, such as those involving the activation of mitogen-activated protein kinase (MAPK), phosphatidylinositol 3-kinase (PI3K)/Akt and Wnt/β-catenin signaling [7–10]. Based on this knowledge, the blockage of fibroblast-to-myofibroblast transition and the attenuation of the profibrotic myofibroblast activity and related ECM overproduction might represent important steps in reducing the fibrotic process at least in SSc [11, 12].

Prostacyclin is an endothelium-derived eicosanoid that contributes to the maintenance of cardiovascular homeostasis, promotes both the proliferation and the differentiation of vascular smooth muscle cells, and acts as an inflammatory modulator [13]. The prostacyclin effects are mainly mediated by the activation of the prostacyclin I_2 receptor (IP receptor) and the subsequent accumulation of intracellular cyclic adenosine monophosphate (cAMP) [14]. The IP receptor is a member of the G protein coupled receptor superfamily highly expressed in several cell types, including vascular smooth muscle cells, leukocytes, monocytes, and fibroblasts [14–18].

Selexipag is an IP receptor agonist characterized by a non-prostanoid structure and it has been synthesized for the treatment of pulmonary arterial hypertension (PAH) [19]. Selexipag has one major active metabolite, ACT-333679, which is also a selective IP receptor agonist, and both compounds are characterized by specific binding and high affinity to this receptor [20].

This study investigated the effects of selexipag and ACT-333679 in reducing the activity of cultured skin SSc fibroblasts and their ECM protein overproduction, through the ability to interfere with the activation of those intracellular signaling transduction molecules involved in the regulation and progression of fibrosis, primarily MAPK family members (i.e. extracellular signal-regulated kinases 1 and 2 (Erk1/2)) and protein kinase B (PKB or Akt).

Methods

Patients with SSc and HSs

Six female patients with SSc (mean age 63 ± 10 years), who fulfilled the new European League Against Rheumatism (EULAR)/American College of Rheumatology (ACR) criteria for SSc, and five sex-matched healthy volunteer subjects (HSs) (mean age 57 ± 8 years) were recruited from the Divisions of Rheumatology and Dermatology at the University of Genova in accordance with the Declaration of Helsinki, after providing signed informed consent and following the local Ethical Board Committee approval (protocol ID: 237REG2015) [21]. Patients with SSc had an "active" nailfold videocapillaroscopic (NVC) pattern and their demographic and clinical characteristics are summarized in Table 1.

Cell cultures and treatments

Skin fibroblasts were isolated from fullthickness biopsies of the clinically involved skin of one third of the distal forearm of patients with SSc and of HSs, in accordance with the EULAR scleroderma trials and research (EUSTAR) protocol and our recent studies [5, 22, 23].

For the in vitro experiments, human SSc and HS skin fibroblasts were grown in Roswell Park Memorial Institute (RPMI) 1640 medium supplemented with 10% fetal bovine serum (FBS), 1% penicillin-streptomycin, and L-glutamine (Lonza Clonetic, Switzerland) and used at the 3rd culture passage.

The fibroblasts isolated from the biopsy sample from each patient with SSc were independently cultured up to 80% of confluence and then maintained in serum-free medium for 4 h. After starvation, a portion of these cells was maintained in growth medium at 5% of FBS without treatment (untreated cells) and another portion was treated for 48 h with three different concentrations of selexipag (30 μM, 3 μM, or 0.3 μM); a further portion of cells was treated for 48 h with three different concentrations of ACT-333679 (10 μM, 1 μM or 0.1 μM) (Actelion Pharmaceutics, Switzerland), in accordance with recent studies [15, 24–26].

The fibroblasts isolated from the biopsy sample from each HS were cultured up to 80% of confluence and maintained in growth medium at 5% FBS for 48 h, after starvation in serum-free medium for 4 h.

To assess the activation of intracellular signaling transduction molecules involved in the regulation of fibrosis, human SSc skin fibroblasts were cultured up to 80% of confluence and after starvation in serum-free medium for 4 h, the cells were maintained in growth medium at 5% FBS without any treatment (untreated cells) or treated with three different concentrations of ACT-333679 (10 μM,

Table 1 Demographic and clinical characteristics of patients with systemic sclerosis (SSc)

	Sample ID					
Parameters	SSc1	SSc2	SSc3	SSc4	SSc5	SSc6
Age	51	58	56	78	65	72
Sex	F	F	F	F	F	F
RP duration (months)	108	168	36	720	180	288
Disease duration (months)	108	168	24	48	36	288
Skin involvement	lcSSc	lcSSc	lcSSc	lcSSc	lcSSc	lcSSc
mRSS score	17	4	14	14	5	17
VCP pattern	Active	Active	Active	Active	Active	Active
ANA	Positive	Positive	Positive	Positive	Positive	Positive
Autoantibody	Scl70	CENP	Fibrillarin	CENP	CENP	CENP
Organ involvement	Yes (lung, esophagus)	No	No	No	No	No
Therapy	Ca_{2+} antagonists, ACE inhibitors, immunosuppressors, ERAs, aspirin, vitamin D	Aspirin, aminaphtone, angiotensin receptor blockers	Aminaphtone, vitamin D	Aspirin, steroids, ACE inhibitors, aminaphtone, MTX	Aspirin	Aminaphtone, vitamin D

Demographic and clinical parameters of patients with SSc enrolled into the study
F female, *RP* Raynaud's phenomenon, *lcSSc* "limited" cutaneous systemic sclerosis skin involvement, *mRSS* modified Rodnan skin score, *VCP* nailfold videocapillaroscopy, *ANA* anti-nuclear antibody, *Scl70* anti-topoisomerase antibody, *CENP* anti-centromere antibody, *ACE* angiotensin converting enzyme, *ERA* endothelin receptor antagonist, *MTX* methotrexate

1 μM, or 0.1 μM, Actelion Pharmaceutics) for 15 min, 30 min, and 48 h.

Immunocytochemistry analysis

SSc and HS skin fibroblasts were cultured in Flexi PERM chamber slides (5×10^3 cells/spot) (Millipore, Billerica, MA, USA) and treated as described in "Cell cultures and treatments". At the end of treatment, the cells were fixed in 2% paraformaldehyde and incubated with primary antibodies (dilution 1:100) to human α-smooth muscle actin (α-SMA) (Dako Cytomation, Denmark), COL-1 (Enzo Life Science, UK), and FN (Sigma-Aldrich, Milan, Italy). Linked antibodies were detected by biotinylated universal secondary antibody and then with the HRP-streptavidine complex (Vector Laboratories, CA, USA). The analysis of α-SMA expression and ECM protein synthesis was performed in each experimental condition evaluating the same number of cells by light microscopy (magnification × 20) (Leica, Cambridge, UK).

Western blotting

For the evaluation of myofibroblast phenotype markers and ECM proteins, cultured human SSc skin fibroblasts were lysed with NucleoSpin RNA/protein (Macherey-Nagel, Duren, Germany), whereas to assess the Erk1/2 and Akt activation, cultured cells were lysed in ice using Radio-Immunoprecipitation Assay (RIPA) buffer (HEPES 20 mM, NaCl 0.15 M, Glycerol 10%, EDTA 1 mM, aprotinin 10 μg/ml, leupeptin 10 μg/ml, pepstatin 1 μg/ml, PMSF 1 mM, Na_3Vo_4 1 mM, Sigma-Aldrich). The protein quantification was performed by the Bradford method. For every condition, 15 μg of protein was separated by electrophoresis on 8% and 4–16% gradient trisglycine gels (GenScript, New York, NY, USA) and transferred onto Hybond-C-nitrocellulose membrane (Life Technologies Ltd., Paisley, UK). After 1 h in a phosphate buffer solution (PBS)1x containing tritonX 0.1% and nonfat powdered milk 5% (Sigma-Aldrich), the membranes were incubated overnight at 4 °C with primary antibodies anti-human α-SMA (dilution 1:1000; Cell Signaling, MA, USA), fibroblast specific protein-1 (FSP1 or S100A4, dilution 1:500; Santa Cruz Biotechnology, CA, USA), COL-1 (dilution 1:600; Enzo Life Science), and FN (dilution 1:1000; Sigma-Aldrich).

Primary antibodies anti-human phospho-Erk1/2 (dilution 1:2000), Erk1/2 (dilution 1:600), phospho-Akt (dilution 1:300), and Akt (dilution 1:500) (Santa Cruz Biotechnology) were used to investigate the activation of intracellular signaling transduction pathways. The membranes were subsequently incubated with secondary antibodies (dilution 1:2000; Cell Signaling) and also incubated with primary HRP-conjugated antibody to human glyceraldehyde 3-phosphate dehydrogenase (GAPDH) (dilution 1:5000; Cell Signaling) to confirm similar loading of protein samples into the gels and the efficiency in the electrophoretic transfer.

Protein synthesis was detected using the enhanced chemiluminescence system (Luminata Crescendo, Millipore) and the densitometric analysis was performed by the UVITEC Image Analysis System (UVITEC, Cambridge, UK). Western blotting was performed in six independent experiments on cultured human SSc skin fibroblasts.

Quantitative real-time polymerase chain reaction (qRT-PCR)

Total RNA was obtained from cultured human SSc skin fibroblasts using NucleoSpin RNA/protein (Macherey-Nagel) and quantified by nanodrop, which was also used to evaluate the RNA integrity, in accordance with the manufacturer's protocol (Thermo Scientific, Wilmington, USA). For each experimental condition, firststrand complementary DNA (cDNA) was synthesized from 1 μg of total RNA using QuantiTect Reverse Transcription Kit (Qiagen, Milan, Italy).

The qRT-PCR was performed on an Eppendorf Realplex 4 Mastercycler using Real MasterMix SYBR Green detection system (Eppendorf, Milan, Italy) in a total volume of 10 μL loaded in triplicate. Primers for *α-SMA* (NM_001613), *S100A4* (NM_002961), *COL-1* (NM_000088), *FN* (NM_002026), and *βactin* (NM_001101, housekeeping gene) were supplied by Primerdesign (Primerdesign, UK).

The gene expression values were calculated using the comparative ΔΔ cycle threshold (ΔΔCT) method and corresponded to the expression level (fold increase) of the target gene compared to untreated cells, taken as the unit value [27]. In all qRT-PCR assays, the melting curve was performed to confirm the specificity of the SYBR green assay, and the qRT-PCR was performed on six independent experiments on cultured human SSc skin fibroblasts.

Statistical analysis

The statistical analysis was carried out by the nonparametric Mann-Whitney test to compare unpaired treatments. Any p value lower than 0.05 was considered as statistically significant. Results of western blotting and qRT-PCR were analyzed as mean ± standard deviation (SD).

Results

Selexipag and ACT-333679 reduced α-SMA and S100A4 protein synthesis and gene expression in cultured human SSc skin fibroblasts

Cultured SSc skin fibroblasts maintained in growth medium for 48 h without treatment (untreated cells) had increased expression of α-SMA compared to cultured HS fibroblasts, indicating their ongoing differentiation and transition into activated myofibroblasts (Fig. 1a). In cultured SSc fibroblasts, selexipag and ACT-333679 reduced the protein expression of α-SMA compared to untreated cells at all tested concentrations, as observed by immunocytochemistry analysis (Fig. 1b).

In these cells, the effects of selexipag and ACT-333679 on both the protein synthesis and the gene expression of α-SMA and S100A4 (specific myofibroblast markers) were evaluated by western blotting and qRT-PCR.

Selexipag significantly reduced the protein synthesis of α-SMA at all tested concentrations compared to untreated cells ($p < 0.05$ for all) and that of S100A4 at the concentration of 3 μM and 0.3 μM ($p < 0.05$ compared to untreated cells) (Fig. 2).

Similarly to selexipag, all tested concentrations of ACT-333679 significantly reduced the protein synthesis of α-SMA and S100A4 compared to untreated cells (α-SMA, $p < 0.05$ for all concentrations; S100A4, $p < 0.05$ for ACT-333679 10 μM and 1 μM, $p < 0.01$ for ACT-333679 0.1 μM) (Fig. 2).

At the gene expression level, selexipag 30 μM, 3 μM, and 0.3 μM significantly downregulated *α-SMA* ($p < 0.05$ for all), whereas only the concentrations of 3 μM and 0.3 μM induced significant downregulation in the gene expression of *S100A4* compared to untreated cells ($p < 0.05$) (Fig. 3).

At the same time, ACT-333679 downregulated the gene expression of these myofibroblast phenotype markers. ACT-333679 1 μM and 0.1 μM significantly reduced the gene expression of *α-SMA* compared to untreated cells ($p < 0.05$, for both concentrations), whereas the downregulation induced by ACT-333679 10 μM was not statistically significant (Fig. 3). However, all three tested concentrations of ACT-333679 significantly downregulated the gene expression of *S100A4* compared to untreated cells ($p < 0.05$ for ACT-333679 10 μM and 1 μM; $p < 0.01$ for ACT-333679 0.1 μM) (Fig. 3).

Selexipag and ACT-333679 decreased the ECM protein synthesis and gene expression in cultured human SSc skin fibroblasts

As observed on immunocytochemistry analysis, cultured SSc skin fibroblasts maintained in growth medium for 48 h without treatment (untreated cells) had increased production of both COL-1 and FN compared to HS skin fibroblasts, confirming their ongoing activated profibrotic phenotype (Fig. 1a).

In cultured SSc fibroblasts, selexipag and ACT-333679 reduced the synthesis of both COL-1 and FN compared to untreated cells (Fig. 2). Selexipag 3 μM and 0.3 μM and ACT-333679 10 μM, 1 μM, and 0.1 μM induced significant reduction of COL-1 synthesis ($p < 0.05$ vs. untreated cells), whereas FN production was significantly decreased by all tested concentrations of selexipag and ACT-333679 ($p < 0.05$ vs. untreated cells, for all concentrations of both compounds) (Fig. 2). All these data were obtained by western blotting.

At the gene expression level, selexipag 3 μM and 0.3 μM significantly downregulated *COL-1* compared to untreated cells ($p < 0.05$ for both) (Fig. 3). ACT-333679 10 μM, 1 μM, and 0.1 μM significantly downregulated the gene expression of *COL-1* compared to untreated

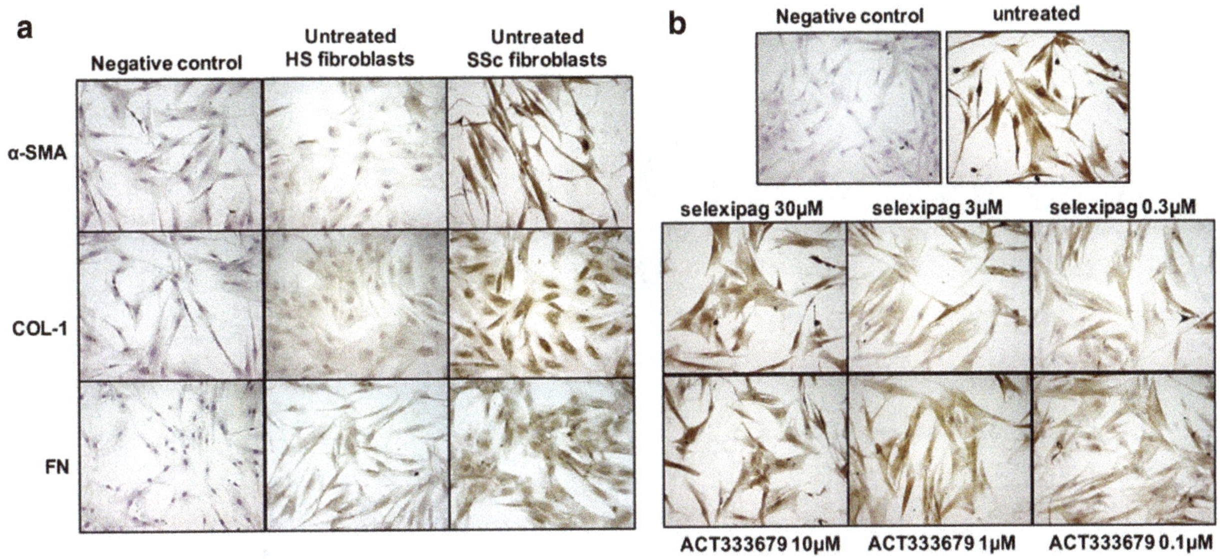

Fig. 1 Evaluation of α-smooth muscle actin (α-SMA), type I collagen (COL-1), and fibronectin (FN) in cultured human skin fibroblasts isolated from patients with systemic sclerosis (SSc) and healthy subjects (HSs). **a** Immunocytochemistry analysis of α-SMA, COL-1 and FN in cultured human SSc and HS skin fibroblasts maintained in normal growth medium without treatment for 48 h. **b** Immunocytochemistry analysis of α-SMA in cultured human SSc skin fibroblasts maintained in normal growth medium (untreated), treated with selexipag at the concentration of 30 μM, 3 μM, and 0.3 μM, and treated with ACT-333679 at the concentration of 10 μM, 1 μM, and 0.1 μM for 48 h

cells ($p < 0.05$ for all) (Fig. 3). No significant modulatory effects of selexipag and ACT-333679 were observed on *FN* gene expression (Fig. 3).

ACT-333679 reduced both Erk1/2 and Akt phosphorylation in cultured human SSc skin fibroblasts

Since ACT-333679 is the major active metabolite of selexipag, its possible modulatory effect on Erk1/2 and Akt activation was directly investigated in cultured SSc skin fibroblasts.

Cultured untreated SSc fibroblasts showed the activation of both Erk1/2 and Akt at 48 h, as observed through their increased phosphorylation state (Fig. 4a). Interestingly, ACT-333679 significantly reduced the phosphorylation of both Erk1/2 and Akt compared to untreated cells ($p < 0.05$ for all concentrations) (Fig. 4a). Moreover, cultured SSc fibroblasts were treated for 15 min and 30 min in the presence or absence of ACT-333679, in order to understand whether these mediators were activated early.

It was interesting to note that cultured untreated SSc fibroblasts showed a significant increase in Erk1/2 phosphorylation after 15 min and 30 min ($p < 0.01$ vs. time zero (T0) for all time points), whereas ACT-333679 treatment was shown to significantly reduce Erk1/2 phosphorylation after 30 min of treatment ($p < 0.05$ vs. untreated cells for all tested concentrations) (Fig. 4b).

At the same time, cultured untreated SSc fibroblasts had a rapid and significant increase in Akt phosphorylation after 15 min and 30 min ($p < 0.01$ vs. T0 for both time points), and ACT-333679 already contrasted this increased Akt phosphorylation after 15 min, and significantly after 30 min of treatment ($p < 0.01$ vs. untreated cells, for all tested concentrations) (Fig. 4b).

Discussion

The results of the study show for the first time that selexipag and mainly its active metabolite ACT-333679 can potentially downregulate the profibrotic activity of cultured SSc fibroblasts/myofibroblasts through the reduction of Erk1/2 and Akt phosphorylation/activation at least in vitro.

The effect was characterized after treatment by the reduced synthesis of specific myofibroblast markers, such as α-SMA and S100A4, and then of ECM proteins, COL-1 and FN.

Of note, cultured SSc skin fibroblasts, maintained for 48 h in growth medium, expressed high levels of α-SMA compared to cultured HS skin fibroblasts, confirming their ongoing transition into activated myofibroblasts.

Therefore, the ability of selexipag and ACT-333679 to downregulate the gene expression and the protein synthesis of α-SMA and S100A4, seems to suggest a possible role for this IP receptor agonist to interfere with the fibroblast-to-myofibroblast transition.

It is recognized that in wound healing and in fibrotic diseases, including SSc, the transition of fibroblasts into profibrotic α-SMA^{+}myofibroblasts is a fundamental event, making these cells the key mediators of fibrogenesis [28, 29]. The profibrotic capability of myofibroblasts is

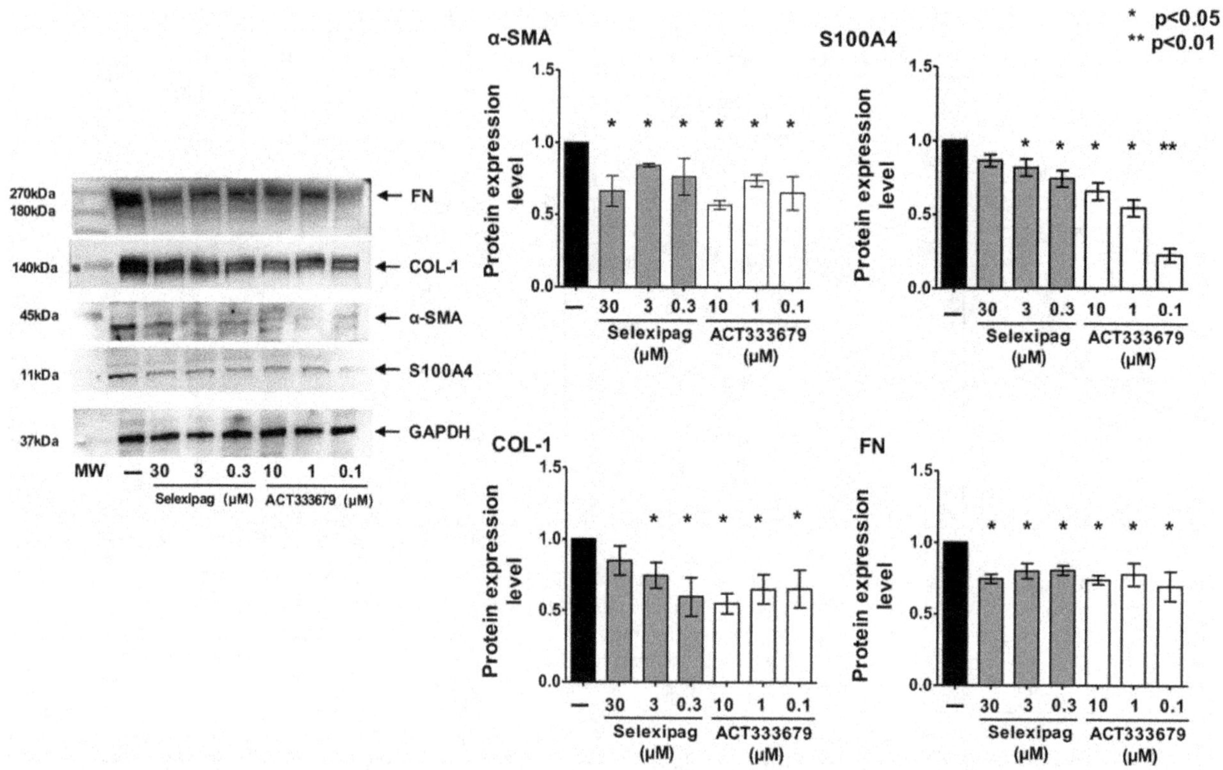

Fig. 2 Evaluation of the protein synthesis of myofibroblast phenotype markers and extracellular matrix macromolecules in cultured human systemic sclerosis (SSc) skin fibroblasts. Western blotting and related densitometric analysis of the protein synthesis of α-smooth muscle actin (α-SMA), S100A4, type I collagen (COL-1) and fibronectin (FN) in cultured human SSc skin fibroblasts maintained in normal growth medium (untreated), treated with selexipag at the concentration of 30 μM, 3 μM, and 0.3 μM, and treated with ACT-333679 at the concentration of 10 μM, 1 μM, and 0.1 μM, for 48 h. For each experimental condition, the value of the synthesis of α-SMA, S100A4, COL-1, and FN was normalized to that of the corresponding glyceraldehyde 3-phosphate dehydrogenase (GAPDH). The resulting value with each treatment was compared to that of the untreated cells (taken as a unit value), in order to obtain the level of protein synthesis. A molecular weight (MW) lane was also included. The final results represent the mean ± standard deviation (SD) of the values obtained from six independent experiments on cultured human SSc skin fibroblasts: $*p < 0.05$ and $**p < 0.01$ vs. untreated cells. kDa, kiloDalton

linked to their overproduction and deposition of ECM macromolecules, primarily COL-1 and FN, in the affected tissues [30, 31]. The present in vitro study confirmed that cultured SSc α-SMA$^+$fibroblasts are characterized by greater ECM protein synthesis compared to cultured HS fibroblasts.

Therefore, the ability of selexipag and ACT-333679 to significantly reduce the protein synthesis of COL-1 and FN in cultured SSc skin fibroblasts/myofibroblasts might suggest a possible antifibrotic action of the IP receptor agonist.

Selexipag and ACT-333679 bind selectively and with higher affinity to the IP receptor compared to other prostacyclin analogs (such as beraprost or treprostinil), targeting the pathway of prostacyclin activation and leading to vasodilatory and anti-proliferative effects, as observed in several mouse models of PAH [20, 30, 31]. In addition, ACT-333679 is present at 3-fold to 4-fold higher levels and is approximately 37-fold more potent in inducing in vitro activation of human IP receptor than the parent compound, suggesting that the metabolite is the major one responsible for the selexipag effects in humans [32, 33]. In accordance with these observations, the results of the present in vitro study showed that in cultured SSc skin fibroblasts/myofibroblasts, ACT-333679 induced the same effects as selexipag, but at a concentration three times lower than that of the parent compound (selexipag 3 μM and 0.3 μM, ACT-333679 1 μM and 0.1 μM). The concentrations of selexipag and especially ACT-333679 were in accordance with several in vitro studies [15, 24–26]. Moreover, the lowest ACT-333679 concentration (0.1 μM) is in range with the values of its bioavailability which were well-tolerated by the HSs and were indicated by the area under the curve during a dose interval of administration (AUC_t), as reported in several studies [25, 26].

It is interesting to note that selexipag and ACT-333679 did not have a dose-dependent effect in reducing the profibrotic activity of cultured SSc skin fibroblasts/myofibroblasts. A possible explanation of this might be related to the intrinsic variability in the cellular response to treatments with selexipag and ACT-333679 in cultured skin fibroblasts isolated from each

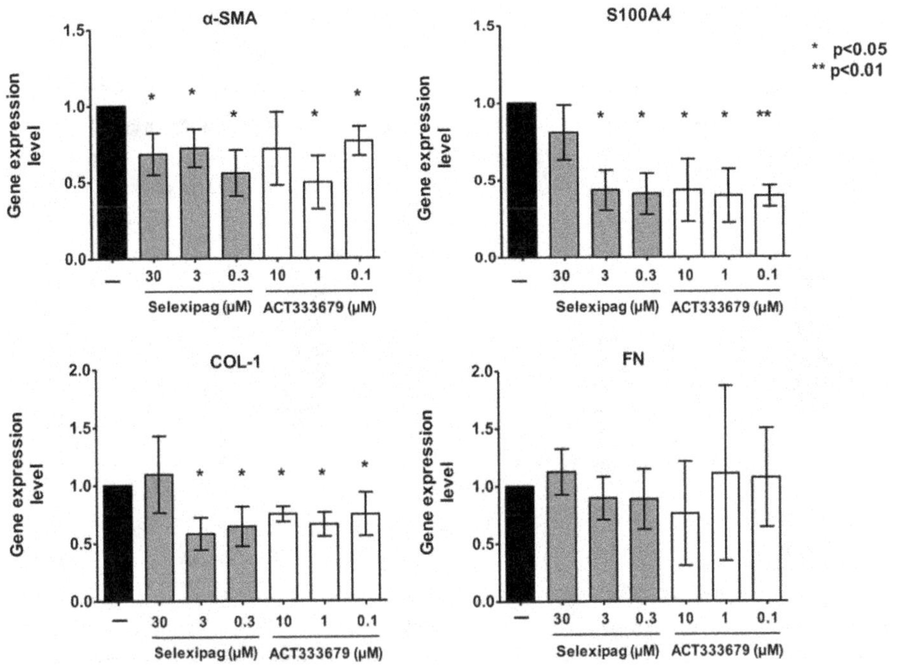

Fig. 3 Evaluation of the gene expression of myofibroblast phenotype markers and extracellular matrix macromolecules in cultured human systemic sclerosis (SSc) skin fibroblasts. Quantitative real-time polymerase chain reaction (qRT-PCR) and related analysis of the gene expression of α-smooth muscle actin (*α-SMA*), *S100A4*, type I collagen (*COL-1*) and fibronectin (*FN*) in cultured human SSc skin fibroblasts maintained in normal growth medium (untreated), treated with selexipag at the concentration of 30 μM, 3 μM, and 0.3 μM, and treated with ACT-333679 at the concentration of 10 μM, 1 μM, and 0.1 μM, for 48 h. The final results represent the mean ± standard deviation (SD) of the values obtained from six independent experiments on cultured human SSc skin fibroblasts: $*p < 0.05$ and $**p < 0.01$ vs. untreated cells

enrolled patient with SSc. Therefore, the variability might be reduced by increasing the number of patients with SSc and the related experiments.

Another possible explanation for the absence of a dose-response effect might depend on the expression level and activity of the IP receptor on the cell surface of cultured SSc skin fibroblasts/myofibroblasts. In a recent study it has been observed that several cell types, including pulmonary arterial smooth muscle cells (PASMCs), displayed a moderate degree of constitutive IP receptor internalization and treatment with prostacyclin analogs (such as beraprost, treprostinil) induced strong depletion of this receptor from the cell surface, whereas the non-prostanoid agonists selexipag and ACT-333679 did not induce these effects [15]. Moreover, ACT-333679 1 μM and 10 μM induced the same increase in the expression of the IP receptor on the cell surface, which was higher than that induced by ACT-333679 0.1 μM [15]. Based on this observation, it might be possible to hypothesize that the concentrations of selexipag 0.3 μM and 3 μM and ACT-333679 0.1 μM and 1 μM might be sufficient to bind to all the IP receptors on the cell surface, inducing the activation of an intracellular signaling cascade that involves increase in cAMP production. On the other hand, ACT-333679 at the concentration of 0.1 μM, 1 μM, and 10 μM induced overlapping effects in terms of cAMP production and efficacy to contrast proliferation and fibrosis-related readouts in human PASMCs in a saturable manner, determining an efficacy plateau [15].

Another important result of our in vitro study is that selexipag and ACT-333679 exerted their effects efficiently targeting the profibrotic activity of fibroblasts/myofibroblasts of the skin, which represents one of the tissues affected by the fibrotic process. These observations suggest that prostacyclin pathways may play an important role in fibrotic diseases, including pulmonary fibrosis, as already observed for the prostacyclin analog iloprost, which reduces COL-1 synthesis through the increase in cAMP production in SSc skin fibroblasts [34].

FN is a multifunctional macromolecule produced by fibroblasts that can modulate fibroblast-mediated collagen gel contraction. According to this process, the activation of the IP receptor was recently shown to inhibit FN release and fibroblast-mediated collagen gel contraction, suggesting its possible contribution in tissue remodeling through the action on fibroblasts [35]. The effects of selexipag and ACT-333679, as observed at 48 h and limited to the reduction in protein synthesis, might suggest that their downregulatory effects on FN gene expression should be a very early event, as already observed in the in vitro study by Kamio et al. [35]. In this study the authors demonstrated how the prostacyclin analog beraprost induced

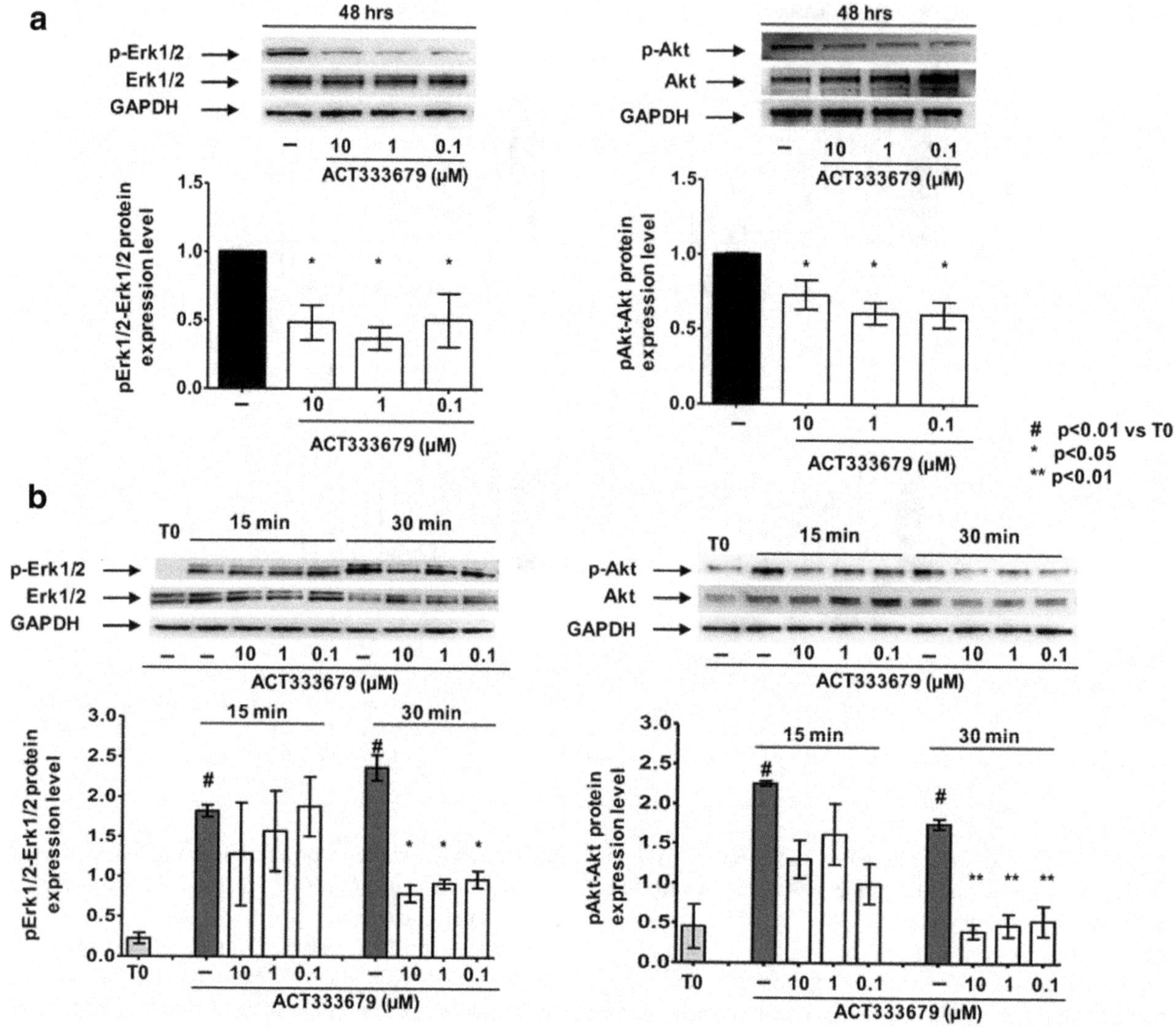

Fig. 4 Evaluation of the extracellular signal-regulated kinases 1 and 2 (Erk1/2) and protein kinase B (Akt) activation in cultured human systemic sclerosis (SSc) skin fibroblasts. **a** Western blotting and related densitometric analysis of phospho-Erk1/2 (p-Erk1/2), Erk1/2, phospho-Akt (p-Akt) and Akt in cultured human SSc skin fibroblasts maintained in normal growth medium (untreated) or treated with ACT-333679 at the concentration of 10 μM, 1 μM, and 0.1 μM for 48 h. The expression of phosphorylated proteins (p-Erk1/2 and p-Akt) was first normalized to that of the naïve proteins (Erk1/2 and Akt) and then normalized to that of the related expression of glyceraldehyde 3-phosphate dehydrogenase (GAPDH). The resulting value of each treatment was compared to that of the untreated cells (taken as the unit value): $*p < 0.05$ vs. untreated cells. **b** Western blotting and related densitometric analysis of phospho-Erk1/2 (p-Erk1/2), Erk1/2, phospho-Akt (p-Akt) and Akt, in cultured human SSc skin fibroblasts maintained in normal growth medium (untreated) or treated with ACT-333679 at the concentration of 10 μM, 1 μM, and 0.1 μM for 15 min and 30 min. The expression of phosphorylated proteins (p-Erk1/2 and p-Akt) was normalized to that of the naïve proteins (Erk1/2 and Akt). The resulting value was then normalized to that of the related expression of GAPDH: $^{\#}p < 0.01$ vs. time zero (T0); $*p < 0.05$ and $**p < 0.01$ vs. untreated cells. The final results represent the mean ± standard deviation (SD) of the values obtained from six independent experiments on cultured human SSc skin fibroblasts

downregulation of FN messenger RNA (mRNA) expression after 5 h of treatment, whereas the reduction in FN release was observed after 48 h of treatment [35]. This result might be due to the activation of post-transcriptional mechanisms induced by prostacyclin analogs and IP receptor agonists, which may be interesting to investigate. Based on this observation, even shorter in vitro experiments should be performed (at 4 h and 12 h).

Several molecules and growth factors contribute to the induction of the profibrotic phenotype of fibroblasts, including TGFβ1, ET-1 and cytokines (such as IL-6), through the activation of fibrogenic intracellular signaling pathways [7]. Among the molecules involved in these intracellular signaling pathways, Erk1/2 and Akt play an important role in mediating the effects of TGFβ1 and ET-1, which are considered key inducers of the fibrotic process and the levels of which are increased in SSc [7, 36]. As recently demonstrated, cultured SSc fibroblasts are characterized by increased phosphorylation of Erk1/2 and Akt when compared to HS fibroblasts suggesting the involvement of these molecules in mediating the activated profibrotic phenotype of SSc myofibroblasts [36].

The results of our in vitro study showed that cultured SSc fibroblasts/myofibroblasts are characterized by early phosphorylation and related activation of both Erk1/2 and Akt (15 min and 30 min) that was still present at a later time point (48 h).

Erk1/2 are members of the MAPK family implicated in several profibrotic signaling pathways [7, 37]. Previous investigations suggested that the activation of Erk1/2, induced by TGFβ1, is responsible for the overexpression of α-SMA and COL-1 in cultured fibroblasts, promoting the transition of these cells into profibrotic myofibroblasts [38]. In addition, several studies have reported that Erk1/2 can mediate the ET-1-induced expression of collagen isoforms and contractile proteins involved in the myofibroblast contraction and migration through the activation of the activator protein-1 (AP-1) transcription factor, contributing to the profibrotic effects of ET-1 [39–41].

Akt is a serine-threonine kinase that can engage multiple downstream signaling substrates and pathways, including the PI3K pathway, a Smad-independent intracellular signaling pathway that mediates TGFβ-induced fibrosis [7]. Very recent studies showed that the phosphorylation and the related activation of Akt are primarily implicated in fibroblast/myofibroblast differentiation, migration and proliferation of pulmonary and cardiac fibroblasts stimulated with TGFβ and ET-1 [42, 43].

Moreover, in previous investigations, the inhibition of PI3K/Akt phosphorylation was found to interfere with the expression of α-SMA in SSc lung fibroblasts and the ability of these cells to contract the collagen gel matrix mediated by ET-1 [44, 45].

Accordingly, the ability of ACT-333679 to significantly reduce the phosphorylation of both Erk1/2 and Akt in cultured SSc fibroblasts/myofibroblasts found in our study, seems to further suggest that the effects of this IP receptor agonist on these cells might involve downregulation in the profibrotic signaling pathways.

One limitation of the study is that the antifibrotic effects of selexipag and ACT-333679 were investigated in in vitro cultures of human skin fibroblasts, so they should also be replicated on lung fibroblasts, since this IP receptor agonist was synthesized mainly for the treatment of PAH.

If confirmed on lung fibroblasts, the vasodilator activity exerted by selexipag in SSc patients with PAH should be integrated by important antifibrotic lung effects, possibly exerting disease-modifying effects over the long term. Moreover, to give an overview of selexipag and its vasodilator effect, it is necessary to cite a recent randomized, placebo-controlled phase II study that showed how selexipag did not reduce the number of Raynaud's phenomenon (RP) attacks compared to placebo in adults with RP secondary to SSc, probably due to the differences between vascular effects in the systemic circulation compared to the pulmonary vasculature [46]. It is interesting to note that other therapies targeting the prostacyclin pathways can have positive or negative effects on RP based on the route of administration; in accordance with this observation, different studies highlighted that intravenous iloprost administration showed efficacy in reducing the number, severity, and duration of RP attacks whereas oral administration did not have any of these effects [47, 48]. Therefore, the route of administration of selexipag and other molecules targeting prostacyclin pathway may have an impact on the efficacy as indicated by the treatment response.

In addition, since Erk1/2 and Akt have been demonstrated to contribute to the intracellular signaling pathways responsible for the profibrotic effects exerted by TGFβ1 and ET-1, it might be interesting to investigate whether selexipag and ACT-333679 may contrast this action in cultured fibroblasts, both alone and in combination with selective TGFβ1 signaling blocking agents or ET-1 receptor antagonists, such as macitentan.

Moreover, based on present results, a new study is currently in progress to investigate the functional relevance of selexipag and its active metabolite, evaluating their ability to reduce the enhanced contractile fibrotic phenotype of SSc skin fibroblasts/myofibroblasts.

Conclusions

In conclusion, the in vitro study showed, for the first time, the potential antifibrotic effects of selexipag and its active metabolite in cultured SSc skin fibroblasts/myofibroblasts that might be determined through interference in the activation of the Erk1/2 and Akt signaling pathways. The action was characterized by the reduction in specific markers of activated myofibroblast phenotype and the ECM protein production.

Abbreviations

ACR: American College of Rheumatology; Akt: Protein kinase B; cAMP: Cyclic adenosine monophosphate; CCL18: Chemokine (C-C motif) ligand-18; cDNA: Complementary deoxyribonucleic acid; COL-1: Type I collagen; ECM: Extracellular matrix; Erk1/2: Extracellular signal-regulated kinases 1 and 2; ET-1: Endothelin-1; EULAR: European League Against Rheumatism; EUSTAR: European League Against Rheumatism scleroderma trials and research; FBS: Fetal bovine serum; FN: Fibronectin; GAPDH: Glyceraldehyde 3-phosphate dehydrogenase; HEPES: 4-(2-Hydroxyethyl)-1-piperazineethanesulfonic acid; HRP: Horseradish peroxidase; HS: Healthy subject; IL6: Interleukine-6; IP: Prostacyclin receptor; MAPK: Mitogen-activated protein kinase; NaCl2: Sodium chlorine; PAH: Pulmonary arterial hypertension; p-Akt: Phosphorylated protein kinase B; PBS: Phosphate buffer solution;

p-Erk1/2: Phosphorylated extracellular signal-regulated kinases 1 and 2; qRT-PCR: Quantitative real-time polymerase chain reaction; S100A4: Fibroblast specific protein-1; SSc: Systemic sclerosis; SYBR: Syber; TGF: Transforming growth factor; α-SMA: Alpha smooth muscle actin; μM: Micromolar

Acknowledgements
Selexipag and ACT-333679 powders for in vitro research have been kindly provided by Actelion Pharmaceuticals Ltd.
Dr. Sara De Gregorio was involved in the production of the figures and graphics in the manuscript.

Funding
MC received funds for the study from Actelion Pharmaceuticals Lds.

Authors' contributions
MC planned the study design, analyzed the results, and wrote the manuscript; BR contributed to the enrolment of patients with SSc and harvested information about clinical and demographic parameters; PM performed the qRT-PCR; RB performed the immunocytochemistry analysis and fibroblast isolation; ES and SSca performed skin biopsies in patients with SSc; PPT and AP performed skin biopsies in healthy subjects; ACT performed the statistical analysis; CC, NC, and VS revised the manuscript for critical and important intellectual content; SP, CP, and AS contributed to the enrollment of patients with SSc and revised the manuscript; SSol planned the study design, performed cell cultures and treatments and western blotting, contributed to the data analysis, and wrote the manuscript. All authors read and approved the final manuscript.

Authors' information
MC: full professor in Rheumatology, Director of the Research Laboratory and Academic Division of Clinical Rheumatology, Department of Internal Medicine, University of Genova, Polyclinic San Martino Hospital; BR: PhD student in Immunology, Division of Clinical Rheumatology, Department of Internal Medicine, University of Genova, Polyclinic San Martino Hospital; MP: PhD in Internal Medicine and Autoimmunity, Division of Clinical Rheumatology, Department of Internal Medicine, University of Genova, Polyclinic San Martino Hospital; RB: PhD in Internal Medicine and Autoimmunity, Division of Clinical Rheumatology, Department of Internal Medicine, University of Genova, Polyclinic San Martino Hospital; ES: trainee in Oncologic Surgery, Department of Surgery, Polyclinic San Martino Hospital; ACT: PhD student in Immunology, Division of Clinical Rheumatology, Department of Internal Medicine, University of Genova, Polyclinic San Martino Hospital; SSca: Hospital doctor and medical executive in Oncologic Surgery, Department of Surgery, Polyclinic San Martino Hospital; PPT: medical surgeon in Dermatology, Unit of Dermatology, University of Genova, Polyclinic San Martino Hospital AP: full professor of Dermatology, Unit of Dermatology, University of Genova, Polyclinic San Martino Hospital; CC: PhD in Rheumatology, Department of Medicine, Surgery and Neurosciences, Scleroderma Unit, University of Siena; NG: associate professor in Medical Science, Surgery and Neurosciences, Department of Medicine, Surgery and Neurosciences, Scleroderma Unit, University of Siena; SP: assistant professor in Rheumatology, Division of Clinical Rheumatology, Department of Internal Medicine, University of Genova, Polyclinic San Martino Hospital; CP: assistant professor in Rheumatology, Division of Clinical Rheumatology, Department of Internal Medicine, University of Genova, Polyclinic San Martino Hospital; AS: associate professor in Rheumatology, Division of Clinical Rheumatology, Department of Internal Medicine, University of Genova, Polyclinic San Martino Hospital; VS: associate professor in Rheumatology, Department of Rheumatology, Ghent University Hospital; SSol: PhD in Internal Medicine, Autoimmunity and Digestive System Diseases, Division of Clinical Rheumatology, Department of Internal Medicine, University of Genova, Polyclinic San Martino Hospital.

Competing interests
MC obtained funds for research from BMS, Actelion, Celgene, and Boehringer. BR, PM, RB, ES, ACT, SSca, PPT, AP CC, NG, SP, CP, AS, VS, and SSol have no competitive interests.

Author details
[1]Research Laboratory and Academic Division of Clinical Rheumatology, Department of Internal Medicine, University of Genova, Polyclinic San Martino Hospital, Genoa, Italy. [2]Oncologic Surgery, Department of Surgery, Polyclinic San Martino Hospital, Genoa, Italy. [3]Department of Health Science, Unit of Dermatology, University of Genova, Polyclinic San Martino Hospital, Genoa, Italy. [4]Department of Medicine, Surgery and Neurosciences, Scleroderma Unit, University of Siena, Siena, Italy. [5]Department of Rheumatology, Ghent University Hospital, Ghent, Belgium.

References
1. Ho YY, Lagares D, Tager AM, Kapoor M. Fibrosis—a lethal component of systemic sclerosis. Nature. 2014;10:390–402.
2. Distler JHW, Feghali-Bostwick C, Soare A, Asano Y, Distler O, Abraham DJ. Frontiers of antifibrotic therapy in systemic sclerosis. Arthritis Rheumatol. 2017;69:257–67.
3. Cutolo M, Ruaro B, Smith V. Macrocirculation versus microcirculation and digital ulcers in systemic sclerosis patients: macro-microcirculation and scleroderma. Rheumatology (Oxford). 2017;23 https://doi.org/10.1093/rheumatology/kex165. [Epub ahead of print]
4. Stempien-Otero A, Kim DH, Davis J. Molecular networks underlying myofibroblast fate and fibrosis. J Mol Cell Cardiol. 2016;97:153–61.
5. Cutolo M, Montagna P, Brizzolara R, Smith V, Alessandri E, Villaggio B, et al. Effects of macitentan and its active metabolite on cultured human systemic sclerosis and control skin fibroblasts. J Rheumatol. 2015;42:456–63.
6. Yang L, Serada S, Fujimoto M, Terao M, Kotobuki Y, Kitaba S, et al. Periostin facilitates skin sclerosis via PI3K/Akt dependent mechanism in a mouse model of scleroderma. PLoS One. 2012;7:e41994.
7. He W, Dai C. Key fibrogenic signalling. Curr Pathobil Rep. 2015;3:183–92.
8. Beyer C, Zenzmaier C, Palumbo-Zerr K, Mancuso R, Distler A, Dees C, et al. Stimulation of the soluble guanylate cyclase (sGC) inhibits fibrosis by blocking non-canonical TGFβ signalling. Ann Rheum Dis. 2015;74:1408–16.
9. Cipriani P, Di Benedetto P, Ruscitti P, Verzella D, Fischietti M, Zazzeroni F, et al. Macitentan inhibits the transforming growth factor-β profibrotic action, blocking the signaling mediated by the ETR/TβRI complex in systemic sclerosis dermal fibroblasts. Arthritis Res Ther. 2015;17:247. https://doi.org/10.1186/s13075-015-0754-7.
10. Edeling M, Ragi G, Huang S, Pavenstädt H, Susztak K. Developmental signalling pathways in renal fibrosis: the roles of Notch, Wnt and Hedgehog. Nat Rev Nephrol. 2016;12:426–39.
11. Denton CP. Systemic sclerosis: from pathogenesis to targeted therapy. Clin Exp Rheumatol. 2015;33(Suppl. 92):S3–7.
12. Soldano S, Paolino S, Pizzorni C, Trombetta AC, Montagna P, Brizzolara R, et al. Dual endothelin receptor antagonists contrast the effects induced by endothelin-1 on cultured human microvascular endothelial cells. Clin Exp Rheumatol. 2017;35:484–93.
13. Narumiya S. Physiology and pathophysiology of prostanoid receptors. Proc Jpn Acad Ser B Phys Biol Sci. 2007;83:296–319.
14. Wise H. Multiple signalling options for prostacyclin. Acta Pharmacol Sin. 2003;24:625–30.
15. Gatfield J, Menyhart K, Wanner D, Gnerre C, Monnier L, Morrison K, et al. Selexipag active metabolite ACT-333679 displays strong anticontractile and antiremodeling effects but low β-arrestin recruitment and desensitization potential. J Pharmacol Exp Ther. 2017;362:186–99.
16. Li R, Cindrova-Davies T, Skepper JN, Sellers LA. Prostacyclin induces apoptosis of vascular smooth cells by cAMP-mediated inhibition of extracellular signal-regulated kinase activity and can counteract the mitogen activity of endothelin-1 or basic growth factor. Circul Res. 2004;94:759–67.
17. Niina Y, Ito T, Oono T, Nakamura T, Fijimori N, Igarashi H, et al. A sustained prostacyclin analog, ONO-1301, attenuates pancreatic fibrosis in experimental chronic pancreatitis induced by dibutyltin dichloride in rats. Pancreatology. 2014;14:201–10.
18. Chen Y, Yang S, Yao W, Zhu H, Xu X, Meng G, Zhang W. Prostacyclin analogue beraprost inhibits cardiac fibroblast proliferation depending on prostacyclin receptor activation through a TGF β-Smad signal pathway. PLoS One. 2014;9:e98483.
19. Simonneau G, Torbicki A, Hoeper MM, Delcroix M, Karlócai K, Galiè N, Degano B, et al. Selexipag, an oral, selective IP receptor agonist for the treatment of pulmonary arterial hypertension. Eur Respir J. 2012;40:874–80.

20. Provencher S, Granton JT. Current treatment approaches to pulmonary arterial hypertension. Can J Cardiol. 2015;31:460–77.
21. van den Hoogen F, Khanna D, Fransen J, Johnson SR, Baron M, Tyndall A, et al. 2013 Classification criteria for systemic sclerosis: an American College of Rheumatology/European League Against Rheumatism collaborative initiative. Arthritis Rheum. 2013;65:2737–47.
22. Beyer C, Distler JH, Allanore Y, Aringer M, Avouac J, Czirijak L, et al. EUSTAR biobanking: recommendations for the collection, storage and distribution of biospecimens in scleroderma research. Ann Rheum Dis. 2011;70:1178–82.
23. Soldano S, Montagna P, Villaggio B, Parodi A, Gianotti G, Sulli A, et al. Endothelin and sex hormones modulate the fibronectin synthesis by cultured human skin scleroderma fibroblasts. Ann Rheum Dis. 2009;68:599–602.
24. Morrison K, Studer R, Emst R, Haag F, Kauser K, Clozel M. Different effects of selexipag and prostacyclin analogs in rat pulmonary artery. J Pharmacol Exp Ther. 2012;343:547–55.
25. Bruderer S, Hurst N, Kaufmann P, Dingemanse J. Multiple-dose up-titration study to evaluate the safety, tolerability, pharmacokinetics, and pharmacodynamics of selexipag, an orally available selective prostacyclin receptor agonist, in healthy subjects. Pharmacology. 2014;94:148–56.
26. Boehler M, Bruderer S, Ulč I, Dingemanse J. Biocomparison study of adult and paediatric dose strengths of the prostacyclin receptor agonist selexipag. Eur J Drug Metab Pharmacokinet. 2018;43:115–20.
27. Livak KJ, Schmittgen TD. Analysis of relative gene expression data using real-time quantitative PCR and the 2-ΔΔCT method. Method. 2001;25:402–8.
28. Kuwano K, Hashino A, Noda K, Kosugi K, Kuwabara K. A long-acting and highly selective prostacyclin receptor agonist prodrug, 2-{4-[(5, 6-diphenylpyrazin-2-yl)(isopropyl) amino] butoxy}-N-(methylsulfonyl) acetamide (NS-304), ameliorates rat pulmonary hypertension with unique relaxant responses of its active form,{4-[(5, 6-diphenylpyrazin- 2-yl)(isopropyl) amino] butoxy} acetic acid (MRE-269), on rat pulmonary artery. J Pharmacol Exp Ther. 2008;326:691–9.
29. Stitham J, Arehart E, Gleim SR, Li N, Douville K, Hwa J. New insights into human prostacyclin receptor structure and function through natural and synthetic mutations of transmembrane charged residues. Br J Pharmacol. 2007;152:513–22.
30. O'Connell C, Amar D, Boucly A, Savale L, Jaïs X, Chaumais MC, et al. Comparative safety and tolerability of prostacyclins in pulmonary hypertension. Drug Saf. 2016;39:287–94.
31. Morrison K, Haag F, Ernst R, Iglarz M, Clozel M. Selective prostacyclin receptor agonist selexipag, in contrast to prostacyclin analogs, does not evoke paradoxical vasoconstriction of rat femoral artery. J Pharmacol Exp Ther. 2018. https://doi.org/10.1124/jpet.117.246058. [Epub ahead of print].
32. Darby I, Zakuan N, Billet F, Desmoulière A. The myofibroblasts, a key cell in normal and pathological tissue repair. Cell Mol Life Sci. 2016;73:1145–57.
33. Kendall RT, Feghali-Bostwick CA. Fibroblasts in fibrosis: novel roles and mediators. Front Pharmacol. 2014;5:123. https://doi.org/10.3389/fphar.2014.00123.
34. Stratton R, Shiwen X, Martini G, Holmes A, Leask A, Haberberger T, et al. Iloprost suppresses connective tissue growth factor production in fibroblasts and in the skin of scleroderma patients. J Clin Invest. 2001; 108:241–50.
35. Kamio K, Liu X, Sugiura H, Togo S, Kobayashi T, Kawasaki S, et al. Prostacyclin analogs inhibit fibroblast contraction of collagen gels through the cAMP-PKA pathway. Am J Respir Cell Mol Biol. 2007;37:113–20.
36. Jing J, Dou TT, Yang JQ, Chen XB, Cao HL, Min M, et al. Role of endothelin-1 in skin fibrosis of systemic sclerosis. Eur Cyt Netw. 2015;26:10–4.
37. Zeisberg M, Kalluri R. Cellular mechanisms of fibrosis. Common and organ-specific mechanisms associated with tissue fibrosis. Am J Physiol Cell Physiol. 2013;304:C216–25.
38. Lafyatis R. Transforming growth factor β—at the centre of systemic sclerosis. Nat Rev Rheumatol. 2014;10:706–19.
39. Rodriguez-Pascual F, Busnadiego O, Gonzalez-Santamaria J. The profibrotic role of endothelin-1: is the door still open for the treatment of fibrotic diseases? Life Sci. 2014;118:156–64.
40. Ahmedat AS, Warnken M, Seemann WK, Mohr K, Kostenis E, Juergens UR, et al. Pro-fibrotic processes in human lung fibroblasts are driven by an autocrine/paracrine endothelinergic system. Br J Pharmacol. 2013; 168:471–87.
41. Lagares D, Busnadiego O, Garcia-Fernandez RA, Lamas S, Rodriguez-Pascual F. Adenoviral gene transfer of endothelin-1 in the lung induces pulmonary fibrosis through the activation of focal adhesion kinase. Am J Respir Cell Mol Biol. 2012;47:834–42.
42. Tsoyi K, Chu SG, Patino-Jaramillo NG, Wilder J, Villalba J, Doyle-Eisele M, et al. Syndecan-2 attenuates radiation-induced pulmonary fibrosis and inhibits fibroblast activation by regulating PI3K/Akt/ROCK pathway via CD148. Am J Respir Cell Mol Biol. 2017; https://doi.org/10.1165/rcmb.2017-0088OC.
43. Phosri S, Arieyawong A, Bunrukchai K, Parichatikanond W, Nishimura A, Nishida M, Mangmool S. Stimulation of adenosine A_{2B} receptor inhibits endothelin-1-induced cardiac fibroblast proliferation and α-smooth muscle actin synthesis through the cAMP/Epac/PI3K/Akt-signaling pathway. Front Pharmacol. 2017;8:428. https://doi.org/10.3389/fphar.2017.00428.
44. Horowitz JC, Ajayi IO, Kulasekaran P, Rogers DS, White JB, Townsend SK, et al. Survivin expression induced by endothelin-1 promotes myofibroblast resistance to apoptosis. Int J Biochem Cell Biol. 2012;44:158–69.
45. Shi-Wen X, Chen Y, Denton CP, Eastwood M, Renzoni EA, Bou-Gharios G, et al. Endothelin-1 promotes myofibroblast induction through the ETA receptor via a rac/phosphoinositide 3-kinase/Akt-dependent pathway and is essential for the enhanced contractile phenotype of fibrotic fibroblasts. Mol Biol Cell. 2004;15:2707–19.
46. Denton CP, Hachulla É, Riemekasten G, Schwarting A, Frenoux JM, Frey A, et al. Efficacy and safety of selexipag in adults with Raynaud's phenomenon secondary to systemic sclerosis: a randomized, placebo-controlled, phase II study. Arthritis Rheumatol. 2017;69:2370–9.
47. Black CM, Halkier-Sørensen L, Belch JJ, Ullman S, Madhok R, Smit AJ, et al. Oral iloprost in Raynaud's phenomenon secondary to systemic sclerosis: a multicentre, placebo-controlled, dose-comparison study. Br J Rheumatol. 1998;37:952–60.
48. Wigley FM, Korn JH, Csuka ME, Medsger TA Jr, Rothfield NF, Ellman M, et al. Oral iloprost treatment in patients with Raynaud's phenomenon secondary to systemic sclerosis: a multicenter, placebo-controlled, double-blind study. Arthritis Rheum. 1998;41:670–7.

12

High-frequency ultrasound of the skin in systemic sclerosis: an exploratory study to examine correlation with disease activity and to define the minimally detectable difference

Hongyan Li[1,3†], Daniel E. Furst[2†], Hongtao Jin[1†], Chao Sun[1], Xiaoping Wang[1], Lin Yang[1], Jingjing He[1], Yanru Wang[1] and Aijing Liu[1*]

Abstract

Background: Thickened skin is a major clinical feature in patients with systemic sclerosis (SSc). We investigated changes of skin thickness in patients with SSc using both high frequency ultrasound (HFU) and the modified Rodnan skin score (mRSS) to evaluate the feasibility of application of HFU in skin involvement and the relationship between HFU and clinical profiles.

Methods: We recruited 31 consecutive patients with SSc and 31 age-matched and sex-matched healthy controls in this prospective, cross-sectional study. Skin thickness was measured by an 18-MHz ultrasonic probe at five different skin sites. Total skin thickness (TST) and skin thickness using categorical mRSS scores were recorded and compared to HFU. The European Scleroderma Trial and Research (EUSTAR) group Disease Activity Index (EUSTAR-DAI) and other clinical manifestations were assessed and analyzed.

Results: TST in patients with SSc was thicker than in healthy controls ($P < 0.001$), and correlated positively with total mRSS and the EUSTAR-DAI and correlated negatively with disease duration ($P < 0.05$). Patients with higher TST had higher EUSTAR-DAI, mRSS, C-reactive protein (CRP) and lower diffusing capacity of the lung for carbon monoxide (DLCO) ($P < 0.05$). Even in patients who on clinical assessment were assigned an mRSS that suggested the skin thickness was normal. This was also true to mRSS locally of 1 and 2 ($P < 0.01$). The area under the receiver operator characteristic (ROC) curve was 0.831 and yielded sensitivity of 77.4% and specificity of 87.1% at the predicted probability of 7.4 mm as the optimal cutoff point to access skin thickness.

Conclusions: In the study, HFU was able to measure skin thickness, it correlated quantitatively with a valid measure of SSc activity, and a minimal detectable difference was identified.

Keywords: Systemic sclerosis, High frequency ultrasound, Disease activity, Skin thickness, Minimal detectable difference

* Correspondence: laj111@126.com
†Hongyan Li, Daniel E. Furst and Hongtao Jin contributed equally to this work.
[1]Department of Immunology and Rheumatology, the Second Hospital of Hebei Medical University, Shijiazhuang, Hebei, China
Full list of author information is available at the end of the article

Background

Systemic sclerosis (SSc) is an autoimmune disorder of unknown etiology, characterized by thickening and hardening of the skin and variable involvement of internal organs, with fibrosis and vasculopathy being the major pathological changes [1]. Skin tightening is the basic clinical hallmark for the diagnosis of SSc and is used to classify subtypes of the disease as well [2, 3].

Skin involvement in early diffuse SSc predicts the extent of visceral involvement, prognosis and mortality [4]. Improvement in the skin score (the semi-quantitative method used to assess skin thickening by palpation) indicates a favorable disease course and vice versa [5].

The modified Rodnan skin score (mRSS) was established by Rodnan in 1979 and is a validated method to evaluate skin thickening in SSc worldwide [6–8]. The mRSS is a popular parameter for reflecting changes in cutaneous involvement in patients with SSc because it is intuitive, comprehensive and repeatable in studies [8–10]. Improvement in the mRSS is associated with prolonged lifespan and with a good prognosis [5]. Nevertheless, the mRSS has some disadvantages such as lack of objectivity, bias among different examiners and failure to detect small degrees of skin change. Other techniques that are more sensitive, objective and reliable for assessment and evaluation are in development [11].

In recent years, high-frequency ultrasound (HFU) has frequently been applied beyond the musculoskeletal system. For example, HFU is used to detect skin thickness in patients with SSc because it can separate epidermis, dermis and subcutaneous layers [12, 13]. Moreover, it may allow early diagnosis of SSc skin involvement, because increasing skin thickness identified ultrasonically implies increasing disease severity [14–16]. However, HFU is subject to sampling artifacts and incompleteness, so its validity is disputed [17].

Using the validated European Scleroderma Trial and Research (EUSTAR) group Disease Activity Index (EUSTAR-DAI) in a cross-sectional analysis, with a large range of disease duration, we wished to compare HFU with the mRSS to further investigate skin thickness as a reflection of disease activity or severity, and to define a minimally detectable difference (MDD) by HFU.

Methods

Patients

We prospectively recruited 31 Chinese patients with SSc and 31 healthy controls matched by age, gender, and body mass index (BMI) from the Second Hospital of Hebei Medical University, between October 2015 and November 2016. Patients met the American College of Rheumatology (ACR)/European League Against Rheumatism (EULAR) 2013 criteria for SSc [18]. Patients were assessed using the mRSS, skin HFU, clinical profiling and serum assessment at enrollment (see below). Disease duration was calculated from onset of the first non-Raynaud's sign or symptom typical of SSc. Exclusion criteria included (1) overlap with other connective tissue disease as defined by validated criteria; (2) skin thickening due to morphea, eosinophilic fasciitis, scleromyxedema, diabetes mellitus, etc.; (3) infection or ulceration of local skin and widespread edema due to nephrotic syndrome or chronic heart failure; (4) non-provision of voluntary informed consent; and (5) use of corticosteroids or immunosuppressive drugs in the 3 months before admission to the study. Ethics approval was obtained from the ethics committee of the Second Hospital of Hebei Medical University and all participants voluntarily signed a written informed consent conform.

mRSS

Skin involvement in each patient was semi-quantitatively assessed using the mRSS, by one of the three experienced rheumatologists who were well-trained to be concordant in skin scoring skill and blinded to the HFU results. The mRSS was applied by palpation of 17 skin regions (face, anterior chest, abdomen and bilateral upper arms, forearms, hand dorsa, fingers, thighs, legs and dorsum of the foot) and was scored on a 0–3 categorical scale (maximum = 51) [8, 19, 20].

Skin HFU

Skin thickness including the epidermis and dermis was assessed in both patients and controls by two experienced rheumatologists, who had been engaged in musculoskeletal ultrasound for more than 4 years and were blinded to the clinical data of the subjects. The ultrasound system (ESaote, Italy) was equipped with an 18-MHz probe and all subjects were examined at five anatomical sites—the dorsal skin of the right forearm 3 cm proximal to the wrist, the area between metacarpophalangeal joints II and III of the right hand, the dorsal skin of the proximal phalanx of the right second finger, the skin of the right leg 12 cm proximal to the ankle joint and the sternum 2 cm distal to the upper part of the manubrium [19, 21, 22] (see ultrasound images in Fig. 1). Average values of regional skin thickness and total skin thickness (TST) were measured at three assessments performed horizontally and vertically and were recorded in millimeters, respectively.

Clinical profiles

Demographic, clinical and laboratory data on patients were systematically collected and the EUSTAR-DAI was calculated according to the EUSTAR 2016 revised standard for disease activity of patients with SSc [23]. The EUSTAR-DAI sums to a maximum weighted 10 points, including six aspects of disease: difference in (Δ) skin mRSS ≥ 18 given a score of 1.5, digital ulcers (DU) given

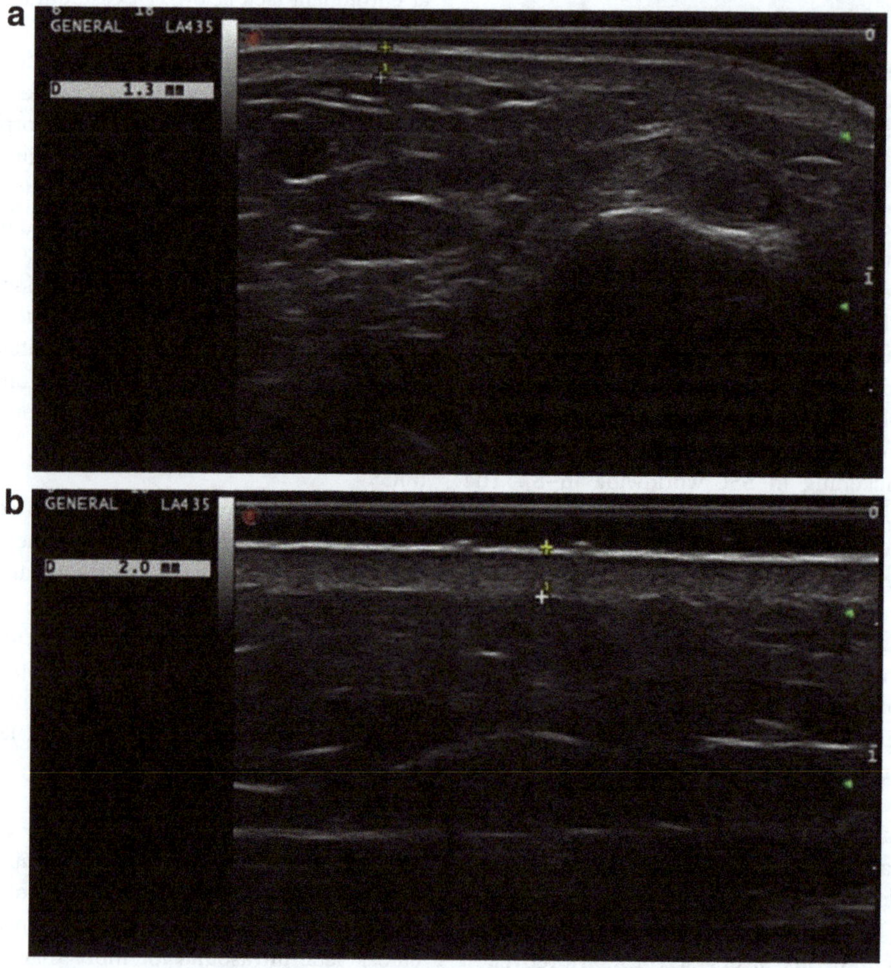

Fig. 1 High-frequency ultrasound, 18-MHz echograms (vertical images) highlight the epidermis and dermis at the forearm in a healthy control and a patient with systemic sclerosis. The skin thickness was 1.3 mm (between the plus sign) in the control (**a**), and 2.0 mm (between the plus sign) in the patient (**b**)

a score of 1.5, tendon friction rubs (TFR) given a score of 2.25, C-reactive protein (CRP) > 1 mg/dL given a score of 2.25 and percentage diffusing capacity of the lung for carbon monoxide (DLCO) < 70% predicted value given a score of 1.0. A EUSTAR-DAI score ≥ 2.5 was defined as active disease [23].

Statistical analysis

Statistical analyses were conducted using PRISM 5 software. Data were expressed as mean +/− standard deviation or median (interquartile range). Student's *t* test or the Mann-Whitney U test was performed to compare two groups. Nonparametric testing among three groups was performed using one-way analysis of variance (ANOVA). The Pearson or Spearman methods were used to test correlation. Sensitivity and specificity of skin thickness detection by HFU were evaluated by using receiver operating characteristic (ROC) curve analysis. P values <0.05 were considered statistically significant. No correction was made for repeated analyses.

Results

Demographics

The mean age of the patients with SSc was 47.23 ± 14.36 years and the average disease duration was 24.0 (32.4) months. Among the 31 patients, 27 were female and 4 were male.

Skin thickness assessed by HFU

We compared total skin thickness (TST) assessed by HFU in the patients with SSc with the total mRSS and found that both demonstrated that the skin was significantly thicker than in healthy controls ($P < 0.001$). However, when measuring localized skin thickness (e.g. on the arm, leg or chest), the skin thickness on the leg was not statistically significant compared to controls (Figs. 2 and 3, Table 1).

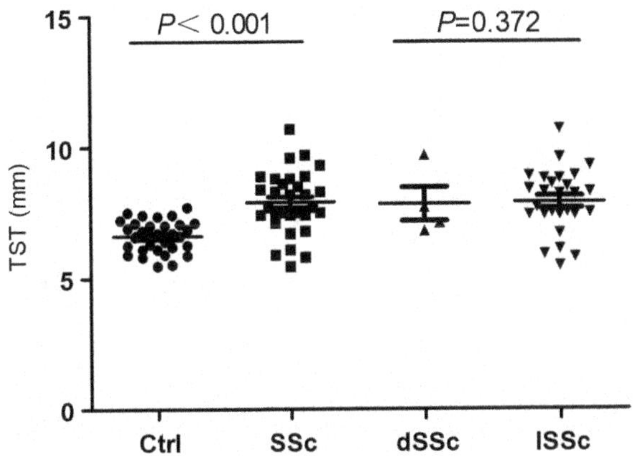

Fig. 2 Total skin thickness (TST) evaluated by high-frequency ultrasound in patients with systemic sclerosis (SSc) and healthy controls (Ctrl) (SSc vs Ctrl, $P < 0.001$), and patients with diffuse SSc (dSSc) and patients with limited SSc (lSSc) (dSSc vs lSSc, $P > 0.05$)

Of note, there were also significant differences between patients with limited cutaneous SSc (lSSc) and controls when we divided patients into those with diffuse cutaneous SSc (dSSc, $n = 4$) and those with lSSc ($n = 27$) according to skin involvement. There was no difference in the TST between patients with dSSc and those with lSSc (Fig. 2).

To address skin profiles in patients with different disease duration, the association between ultrasound (US)-defined thickness and disease duration was analyzed. As expected, the TST was negatively correlated with disease duration, with the correlation coefficient indicating moderate to good correlation ($r = -0.605$, $P < 0.001$) (Additional file 1: Figure S4).

TST in patients with different mRSS

To detect whether the skin in patients with a clinically normal skin score (mRSS = 0) was thicker than in the healthy controls, we examined the mRSS at five skin sites and local skin thickness assessed by HFU in patients with SSc dichotomously. Of interest, patients with skin thickness score on the mRSS as mRSS = 0, mRSS = 1 and mRSS = 2, all definitely had thicker skin than the controls ($P < 0.05$) (Fig. 4). Although localized skin thickness in the group scored as mRSS = 3 was thicker compared with controls, it was not statistically significant ($P = 0.057$), probably because there were only three skin sites (mRSS = 3) among the total 155 sites.

Comparing HFU-TST and mRSS in lcSSc

We also compared skin thickness using the full semi-quantitative range of mRSS (0–3+) and HFU in lSSc. Compared with the healthy controls, a skin thickness of mRSS = 0 in patients with SSc assessed by HFU was still thicker than in the normal controls ($P = 0.001$), suggesting skin involvement happened prior to being able to detect it clinically.

Receiver operating characteristic (ROC) curve analysis for HFU to detect the minimally detectable difference (MDD)

To address the efficiency of TST in SSc, we calculated the sensitivity and specificity for the TST in patients with SSc and the controls using ROC curve analysis. The area under the curve (AUC) was 0.831, standard error was 0.057 ($P < 0.001$), and the 95% confidence intervals (CI) were 0.719 and 0.942 (see Additional file 2: Figure S1). The positive predictive value and negative predictive value were 85.71% and 79.41%, and sensitivity and specificity were 77.40% and 87.10%, respectively. The cutoff value (MDD) for evaluation of thickened skin was 7.4 mm.

The clinical features of the patients with SSc with TST greater than the cutoff from the ROC analysis compared to patients with SSc with TST below the cutoff are shown in Table 2. Patients with greater TST had a higher EUSTAR-DAI, a higher mRSS, higher CRP and lower DLCO ($P < 0.05$) (see also Table 2).

Correlation between TST and clinical parameters

There was low-to-moderate, statistically significant, positive correlation between the TST and mRSS ($r = 0.416$, $P =$

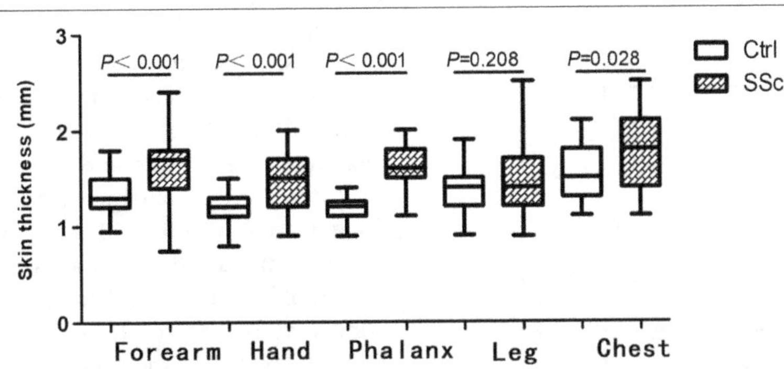

Fig. 3 Local skin thickness evaluated by high-frequency ultrasound in patients with systemic sclerosis (SSc) and healthy controls (Ctrl) (SSc vs Ctrl, $P < 0.05$ for all, with the exclusion of the leg). Data are presented for different skin areas, showing the 25th and 75th percentiles of measures as boxes, the median (line within the box) and the minimum and maximum values (whiskers)

Table 1 Skin thickness assessed by HFU in patients with SSc and healthy controls

	SSc (skin thickness, mm, $n = 31$)	Ctrl (skin thickness, mm, n = 31)	*P*	Range	
Forearm	1.70(0.40)	1.36 ± 0.19	< 0.001*	0.74–2.40	0.95–1.80
Hand	1.50(0.50)	1.20(0.20)	< 0.001*	0.90–2.00	0.79–1.50
Phalanx	1.60(0.30)	1.20(0.15)	< 0.001*	1.10–2.00	0.90–1.40
Leg	1.40(0.50)	1.40(0.30)	0.208	0.89–2.50	0.90–1.40
Chest	1.80(0.70)	1.50(0.50)	0.028*	1.10–2.50	1.10–1.60
TST	7.89 ± 1.20	6.61 ± 0.61	< 0.001*	5.47–10.70	5.47–7.70

HFU high-frequency ultrasound, *SSc* systemic sclerosis, *Ctrl* controls *TST* total skin thickness
*Compared with the healthy controls, $P < 0.05$

0.020) and between the TST and EUSTAR-DAI ($r = 0.436$, $P = 0.014$). The results indicated that to some extent, skin thickness assessed by ultrasound could reflect disease activity. The TST was significantly negatively correlated with disease duration, as we have described before: see Additional file 3: Figure S2, Additional file 4: Figure S3 and Additional file 1: Figure S4.

Discussion

Skin thickening evaluated by the mRSS is a measurement used often in the clinic to assess patients with either lSSc or dSSc [7, 8, 24]. Unfortunately, relatively large intra-observer or inter-observer variability decreases its applicability for individual patients in the clinic. The coefficient of variation is about 20%, indicating that a change needs to be greater than 20% to be greater than the variability of the measure (similar to the joint counts in rheumatoid arthritis) and is further confounding by edema and the need for a 6–9-month trial [25].

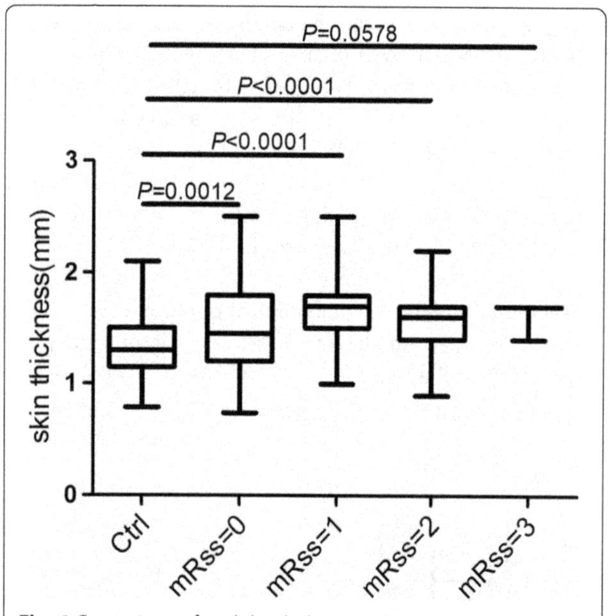

Fig. 4 Comparisons of total skin thickness (TST) evaluated by high-frequency ultrasound in healthy control and patients with systemic sclerosis (SSc) with scales of the modified Rodnan skin score (mRSS). Boxes represent the 25th and 75th percentile of measures, and the median (line within the box) and the minimum and maximum values (whiskers) are shown. TST with mRSS = 0, mRSS = 1 and mRSS = 2 in the patients were all significantly higher than in the controls ($P = 0.0012$, $P < 0.0001$ and $P < 0.0001$, respectively). No significant difference was found between patients with mRSS = 3 and the controls ($P = 0.0578$)

In our study, using an 18-MHz ultrasonic probe, we calculated inter-observer and intra-observer correlation coefficients of 0.88 and 0.93. This corresponds to an intra-observer coefficient of variation of 2.2%, significantly better than that for the mRSS.

Scheja et al. demonstrated in a study of 41 patients with SSc that inter-observer variability when using ultrasound to assess skin thickness in the phalanx, hand and forearm was only 1%, 4.2% and 0.0016%, respectively when using a 20 MHz probe [26]. In addition, Moore et al., who established a 17-point skin HFU scoring system calculated correlation coefficients of 0.93 and 0.95 for inter-observer and intra-observer dermal measurements [14]. These findings support our study results.

ROC analysis defined a minimum detectable difference (MDD) for HFU assessment of skin thickness in SSc in this data set. The AUC was 0.831 ($P < 0.001$) with the best deflection-point at 7.4 mm. Sensitivity was 77.4% and specificity was 87.1% to separate active from inactive disease using the EUSTAR-DAI at a cut point of 2.5. Thus, we identified a skin thickness of 7.4 mm as the MDD that best separated normal skin from skin affected by SSc when we used phalanx/hand/forearm/leg/chest as a composite measure, which were previously defined as the five sites of ultrasound assessment [21, 22].

In view of the facts that more patients with lSSc were recruited into the study, we utilized the composite phalanx/hand/forearm site and local phalanx site separately for extensive ROC analyses (see Additional file 5: Figure S5 and Additional file 6: Figure S6). For skin thickness at the phalanx/hand/forearm sites, the AUC was 0.869 and the cutoff value was 4.3 mm, with the same sensitivity compared as the five sites (77.4%) but with higher specificity (93.5%). For the local phalanx site, the AUC was 0.946 and the cutoff value was 1.3 mm, with 87.1% sensitivity and much more higher specificity (96.8%) to discriminate thickened skin from normal skin. These

Table 2 Clinical profiles of patients with SSc with TST higher and lower than the cutoff in ROC analysis

Feature	Elevated TST ($n = 24$)	Normal TST ($n = 7$)	P
Male/female	4/20	0/7	0.247
Age (years)	50.21 ± 14.01	37.00 ± 11.02	0.187
Duration	24.00 (26.40)	56.06 ± 30.17	0.002*
DAI	5.24 ± 2.36	1.84 (1.92)	0.048*
mRSS	10.00 (6.00)	4.00 (5.00)	0.031*
RP	21	7	0.325
ILD	16	1	0.014*
PAH	5	3	0.214
DU	4	2	0.483
Muscular involvement	5	3	0.214
Synovitis	10	2	0.531
Scl-70(+)	10	3	0.955
CRP (mg/L)	8.60 (10.48)	3.52 (4.93)	0.038*
ESR (mm/h)	23.00 (16.25)	48.71 ± 43.19	0.723

SSc systemic sclerosis, *TST* total skin thickness, *DAI* European Scleroderma Trial and Research group Disease Activity Index, *RP* Raynaud's phenomenon, *ILD* interstitial lung disease, *PAH* pulmonary artery hypertension, *DU* digital ulcers, *CRP* C-reactive protein, *ESR* erythrocyte sedimentation rate
*$P < 0.05$

figures suggest that a better distinction can be shown using fewer ultrasound sites in patients with lSSc, especially if the sites assessed are tailored to the type of patient and to the sites of clinical disease.

In the present study, we demonstrated that TST in patients with SSc is significantly greater than in healthy controls ($P < 0.001$), similar to other research [15, 16]. There were also statistically significantly differences locally, at the forearm, hand, phalanx and chest. There was no difference in skin thickness on the legs in patients with SSc and normal controls. This may have been because in the study there were small numbers of patients recruited with lower extremity involvement, but further research will be needed to examine this finding.

The TST correlated positively with the mRSS and correlated negatively with disease duration, similar to data reported by others [22]. Skin thickness reduced as skin went from interstitial edema through thickening to atrophy [21]. This point could be illustrated by the correlation between the mRSS and TST. The coefficient for correlation between the mRSS and HFU decreased from 0.63 (in patients with disease duration less than 1 year) to 0.40 (in patients with disease duration of 1–3 years) over time in a longitudinal study by Hesselstrant et al. [22]. We found that patients with a normal clinical skin score (mRSS = 0) still had some increased thickening identified by HFU ($P < 0.01$), as have others [27]. This finding may help explain the weaker correlation between the mRSS and HFU over time.

The mRSS is considered by many to be one of the most important aspects in the classification of different SSc subtypes [28]. Sedky et al. showed that ultrasound TST in patients with dSSc was thicker than in those with lSSc ($P = 0.002$), especially in the chest wall [16]. We did not find differences between dSSC and lSSc using HFU-TST. However, the number of patients with dSSc was small ($N = 4$), so the power to identify differences between dSSc and lSSc was very low.

The skin thickness measured by HFU in the chest wall of patients with SSc was greater than in normal controls ($P < 0.05$), despite the fact that 87.1% of our patients had lSSc and thus, by definition, these patients did not have clinical skin thickening on the chest (See Table 2). The meaning of this relative skin thickening at the chest in patients with lSSc as assessed by HFU will require further research in longitudinal studies, although it is congruent with the finding that even when mRSS = 0 in dSSc, the skin is measured as thicker when assessed by HFU.

There was low-to-moderate, positive correlation between HFU-TST and the EUSTAR-DAI ($r = 0.436$, $P = 0.014$) in patients with SSc; this suggests that thickened skin could predict more active disease, although this degree of correlation indicates either the need for many more patients or that active disease is predicted by more than only skin thickness. HFU-TST was also only moderately positively correlated with the mRSS ($r = 0.416$, $P = 0.020$) and the correlation remained in the multivariate regression model ($t = 0.335$, $P = 0.044$). This supports the possibility that the mRSS might reflect the increased skin thickness primarily in the early disease phase and that skin thickness and the mRSS could become disconnected over time [17, 22, 29].

It may be important to recognize and treat SSc in its edematous phase during which patients are more responsive to medication compared with the sclerotic or atrophic phase [29]. Hesselstrand et al. reported that patients in the edematous phase of their disease (usually short duration) had increased skin thickness assessed by HFU, but with low echogenicity (which represents high water content, i.e. more interstitial fluid). It is intriguing in this study that skin thickness negatively correlated with skin echogenicity measured by ultrasound ($P = 0.001$). That relationship implies that the edema results in increased skin thickness and decreased skin echogenicity. Over time, echogenicity increased, correlating with increasing fibrosis [29]. Although our patients had early disease, the finding that TST negatively correlated with disease duration in our data set indicates that these patients had a range of degrees of edema and fibrosis, going from the edematous to the fibrotic/atropic phase as disease duration increased. Overall, the this suggests that objective HFU techniques may be able to differentiate early edematous disease from early fibrosis and may even be able to detect thickening that is not clinically evident. These findings will need corroboration and significant research to ascertain their meaning.

Overall, the mRSS is simple to perform for the assessment of skin changes, it can estimate skin thickness and it samples large areas of the skin, but observer bias and low sensitivity detracts from its accuracy [30]. HFU may be able to examine both skin thickness and interstitial edema, which may mean this modality is able to better examine prognosis and determine drug response [31]. However, standardized imaging, decreasing operator variability, definition of appropriate skin sites and examination of a large range of patients need significant further research [21].

This study has some limitations. First, it is cross-sectional and a longitudinal study would be beneficial, which is being planned. Second, it involves relatively few patients from a single center. However, it is an exploratory effort and has given insights into the MDD and has identified some degree of correlation with a measure of disease activity. A study of more patients is needed, involving a broader set of clinical measures such as the Clinical Response Index for SSc (CRISS) or including gastrointestinal, specific myocardial and lung involvement. Third, we needed to use total skin measurement using HFU because our data precluded separation of the epidermis and dermis. An analysis in a group of patients with earlier more diffuse disease may help address this issue. Further we found no difference between limited and diffuse disease using HFU and the mRSS and did not find differences when assessing skin on the legs and thus, inclusion of more patients with diffuse disease and lower extremity involvement would have been helpful.

Conclusions

HFU was able to measure skin thickness quantitatively and it correlates with a valid measure of SSc activity, and a minimal detectable difference has been identified. With further research, HFU may be used to effectively and more objectively evaluate skin changes and could be used to predict visceral involvement.

Additional files

Additional file 1: Figure S4. Correlation between the TST and disease duration in patients with SSc. There was negative correlation between the TST and disease duration ($r = -0.605$, $P < 0.001$). (TIF 3162 kb)

Additional file 2: Figure S1. ROC analysis of TST in patients with SSc at the phalanx/hand/forearm/leg/chest sites. The area under the curve (AUC) was 0.831, the cutoff value was 7.4 mm, with sensitivity and specificity of 77.40% and 87.10%, respectively. (TIF 40 kb)

Additional file 3: Figure S2. Correlation between TST and DAI in patients with SSc. There was positive correlation between the TST and EUSTAR-DAI ($r = 0.436$, $P = 0.014$). (TIF 3195 kb)

Additional file 4: Figure S3. Correlation between the TST and mRSS in patients with SSc. There was positive correlation between the TST and mRSS ($r = 0.416$, $P = 0.020$). (TIF 3144 kb)

Additional file 5: Figure S5. ROC analysis of the TST in patients with SSc at the phalanx/hand/forearm sites. The AUC was 0.869 and the cutoff value was 4.3 mm, with 77.4% sensitivity and 93.5% specificity. (TIF 40 kb)

Abbreviations

ACR: American College of Rheumatology; ANOVA: One-way analysis of variance; AUC: Area under the curve; BMI: Body mass index; CRISS: Clinical Response Index for SSc; CRP: C-reactive protein; DLCO: Diffusing capacity of the lung for carbon monoxide; dSSc: Diffuse cutaneous systemic sclerosis; DU: Digital ulcers; EULAR: European League Against Rheumatism; EUSTAR-DAI: European Scleroderma Trial and Research-Disease Activity Index; HFU: High-frequency ultrasound; lSSc: Limited cutaneous SSc; MDD: Minimally detectable difference; mRSS: Modified Rodnan skin score; ROC: Receiver operating characteristic; SSc: Systemic sclerosis; TFR: Tendon friction rubs; TFR: Tendon friction rubs; TST: Total skin thickness

Acknowledgements

We thank the health professional staff and the patients from the Department of Immunology and Rheumatology, the Second Hospital of Hebei Medical University for their participation.

Funding

This work was supported by the New Technology Foundation of the Second Hospital of Hebei Medical University (820), China.

Authors' contributions

H-YL, D-EF and H-TJ contributed equally to the manuscript. A-JL conceptualized, designed, and supervised the project. CS and H-YL performed the ultrasound and A-JL applied the modified Rodnan skin score. D-EF gave teaching and training on applying the mRSS. H-YL, D-EF and H-TJ wrote the manuscript, with contributions from all authors. X-PW, LY, J-JH, Y-RW and H-TJ participated in the sample collection and clinical analysis. All authors read and approved the manuscript.

Competing interests

The authors declare that they have no competing interests.

Author details

[1]Department of Immunology and Rheumatology, the Second Hospital of Hebei Medical University, Shijiazhuang, Hebei, China. [2]Department of Rheumatology, Geffen School of Medicine, University of California, Los Angeles, CA, USA. [3]The Affiliated Jiangning Hospital of Nanjing Medical University, Nanjing, Jiangsu, China.

References

1. Varga J, Trajonowski M. Pathogenesis of systemic sclerosis: recent insights. J Scleroderma Relat Disord. 2017;2:137–52.
2. van den Hoogen F, Khanna D, Fransen J, et al. 2013 Classification criteria for systemic sclerosis: an American College of Rheumatology/European League against Rheumatism collaborative initiative. Arthritis Rheum. 2013;65:2737–47.
3. Hudson M, Fritzler MJ. Diagnostic criteria of systemic sclerosis. J Autoimmun. 2014;48–49:38–41.
4. Ionescu R, Rednic S, Damjanov N, et al. Repeated teaching courses of the modified Rodnan skin score in systemic sclerosis. Clin Exp Rheumatol. 2010; 28(2 Suppl 58):S37–41.
5. Steen VD, Medsger TA Jr. Improvement in skin thickening in systemic sclerosis associated with improved survival. Arthritis Rheum. 2001;44:2828–35.
6. Amjadi S, Maranian P, Furst D, et al. Course of the modified Rodnan skin thickness score in systemic sclerosis clinical trials: analysis of three large multicenter, double-blind, randomized controlled trials. Arthritis Rheum. 2009;60:2490–8.
7. Khanna D, Furst DE, Clements PJ, et al. Standardization of the modified Rodnan skin score for use in clinical trials of systemic sclerosis. J Scleroderma Relat Disord. 2017;2:11–8.

8. Kaldas M, Khanna PP, Furst DE, et al. Sensitivity to change of the modified Rodnan skin score in diffuse systemic sclerosis–assessment of individual body sites in two large randomized controlled trials. Rheumatology (Oxford). 2009;48:1143–6.
9. Jordan S, Distler JH, Maurer B, et al. Effects and safety of rituximab in systemic sclerosis: an analysis from the European scleroderma trial and research (EUSTAR) group. Ann Rheum Dis. 2015;74:1188–94.
10. Jung M, Bonner A, Hudson M, et al. Myopathy is a poor prognostic feature in systemic sclerosis: results from the Canadian Scleroderma Research Group (CSRG) cohort. Scand J Rheumatol. 2014;43:217–20.
11. Porta F, Gargani L, Kaloudi O, et al. The new frontiers of ultrasound in the complex world of vasculitides and scleroderma. Rheumatology (Oxford). 2012;51(Suppl 7):vii26–30.
12. Kaloudi O, Bandinelli F, Filippucci E, et al. High frequency ultrasound measurement of digital dermal thickness in systemic sclerosis. Ann Rheum Dis. 2010;69:1140–3.
13. Elhai M, Guerini H, Bazeli R, et al. Ultrasonographic hand features in systemic sclerosis and correlates with clinical, biologic, and radiographic findings. Arthritis Care Res (Hoboken). 2012;64:1244–9.
14. Moore TL, Lunt M, Mc Manus B, et al. Seventeen-point dermal ultrasound scoring system–a reliable measure of skin thickness in patients with systemic sclerosis. Rheumatology (Oxford). 2003;42:1559–63.
15. Sulli A, Ruaro B, Alessandri E, et al. Correlation between nailfold microangiopathy severity, finger dermal thickness and fingertip blood perfusion in systemic sclerosis patients. Ann Rheum Dis. 2014;73:247–51.
16. Sedky MM, Fawzy SM, El Baki NA, et al. Systemic sclerosis: an ultrasonographic study of skin and subcutaneous tissue in relation to clinical findings. Skin Res Technol. 2013;19:e78–84.
17. Ch'ng SS, Roddy J, Keen HI. A systematic review of ultrasonography as an outcome measure of skin involvement in systemic sclerosis. Int J Rheum Dis. 2013;16:264–72.
18. van den Hoogen F, Khanna D, Fransen J, et al. 2013 Cassification criteria for systemic sclerosis: an American college of rheumatology/European league against rheumatism collaborative initiative. Ann Rheum Dis. 2013;72:1747–55.
19. Vinet É, Bernatsky S, Hudson M, et al. Effect of menopause on the modified Rodnan skin score in systemic sclerosis. Arthritis Res Ther. 2014;16:R130.
20. Liu H, Hou Y, Zhu QL, et al. A preliminary study of skin ultrasound in diffuse cutaneous systemic sclerosis: does skin echogenicity matter? PLoS One. 2017;12:e0174481.
21. Akesson A, Hesselstrand R, Scheja A, et al. Longitudinal development of skin involvement and reliability of high frequency ultrasound in systemic sclerosis. Ann Rheum Dis. 2004;63:791–6.
22. Hesselstrand R, Carlestam J, Wildt M, et al. High frequency ultrasound of skin involvement in systemic sclerosis – a follow-up study. Arthritis Res Ther. 2015;17:329.
23. Valentini G, Iudici M, Walker UA, et al. The European scleroderma trials and research group (EUSTAR) task force for the development of revised activity criteria for systemic sclerosis: derivation and validation of a preliminarily revised EUSTAR activity index. Ann Rheum Dis. 2017;76:270–6.
24. Dobrota R, Maurer B, Graf N, et al. Prediction of improvement in skin fibrosis in diffuse cutaneous systemic sclerosis: a EUSTAR analysis. Ann Rheum Dis. 2016;75:1743–8.
25. Czirják L, Nagy Z, Aringer M, et al. The EUSTAR model for teaching and implementing the modified Rodnan skin score in systemic sclerosis. Ann Rheum Dis. 2007;66:966–9.
26. Scheja A, Akesson A. Comparison of high frequency (20 MHz) ultrasound and palpation for the assessment of skin involvement in systemic sclerosis (scleroderma). Clin Exp Rheumatol. 1997;15:283–8.
27. Sulli A, Ruaro B, Smith V, et al. Subclinical dermal involvement is detectable by high frequency ultrasound even in patients with limited cutaneous systemic sclerosis. Arthritis Res Ther. 2017;19:61.
28. Cutolo M, Sulli A, Smith V. Assessing microvascular changes in systemic sclerosis diagnosis and management. Nat Rev Rheumatol. 2010;6:578–87.
29. Hesselstrand R, Scheja A, Wildt M, et al. High frequency ultrasound of skin involvement in systemic sclerosis reflects oedema, extension and severity in early disease. Rheumatology (Oxford). 2008;47:84–7.
30. Hou Y, Zhu QL, Liu H, et al. A preliminary study of acoustic radiation force impulse quantification for the assessment of skin in diffuse cutaneous systemic sclerosis. J Rheumatol. 2015;42:449–55.
31. Furst DE, Clements PJ, Steen VD, et al. The modified Rodnan skin score is an accurate reflection of skin biopsy thickness in systemic sclerosis. J Rheumatol. 1998;25:84–8.

Safety and tolerability of an anti-CD19 monoclonal antibody, MEDI-551, in subjects with systemic sclerosis: a phase I, randomized, placebo-controlled, escalating single-dose study

Elena Schiopu[1*], Soumya Chatterjee[2], Vivien Hsu[3], Armando Flor[4], Daniel Cimbora[4], Kaushik Patra[4], Wenliang Yao[4], Jing Li[5], Katie Streicher[4], Kathleen McKeever[4,6], Barbara White[4,7], Eliezer Katz[4], Jorn Drappa[4], Sarah Sweeny[4] and Ronald Herbst[4]

Abstract

Background: Systemic sclerosis (SSc) is a clinically heterogeneous, life-threatening disease characterized by fibrosis, microvasculopathy, and autoimmunity. Extensive nonclinical and clinical data implicate B cells in the pathogenesis of SSc. MEDI-551 is an investigational humanized monoclonal antibody that targets the B cell surface antigen CD19 and mediates antibody-dependent, cell-mediated cytotoxicity of B cells. This clinical study evaluated the safety and tolerability, pharmacokinetics, and pharmacodynamics of MEDI-551 in subjects with SSc.

Methods: This phase I multicenter, randomized, double-blind, placebo-controlled, single escalating dose study enrolled adult subjects with either limited or diffuse cutaneous SSc. A single intravenous dose of MEDI-551 was administered, and safety and tolerability were evaluated. MEDI-551 pharmacokinetics (PK), pharmacodynamics, and immunogenicity were also assessed. Safety assessments included the incidence of adverse events and changes in clinical and laboratory results. MEDI-551 serum concentrations, effects on circulating and tissue B cells and plasma cells (PCs), and antidrug antibodies were analyzed. Modified Rodnan skin score (MRSS) and pulmonary function tests were used to explore the clinical effect of MEDI-551.

Results: The study enrolled 28 subjects with SSc (mean age, 47.3 years; 67.9 % female). Twenty-four received a single dose of MEDI-551 (0.1–10.0 mg/kg) and four received placebo. Treatment-emergent adverse events (TEAEs) occurred in 95.8 % of subjects in the MEDI-551 group and in 75.0 % of subjects in the placebo group; the majority of TEAEs were mild or moderate in severity. Two serious adverse events were considered possibly related to the study drug. One death, deemed not related to the study drug, occurred in a MEDI-551-treated subject. MEDI-551 exhibited linear PK in the dose range of 1.0 to 10.0 mg/kg, and more rapid clearance at lower doses. Dose-dependent depletion of circulating B cells and plasma cells was observed. MRSS assessments suggest a possible clinical effect of MEDI-551 on affected skin.

Conclusions: A single escalating dose of MEDI-551 was tolerable and safe in this subject population. B cell depletion was achieved and was dose dependent. A signal of clinical effect was observed. Based on these results, further investigation of MEDI-551 as a disease-modifying treatment for SSc is warranted.

Keywords: B cells, CD19, Pharmacokinetics, Pharmacodynamics, Scleroderma, Systemic sclerosis

* Correspondence: eschiopu@yahoo.com
[1]Department of Internal Medicine, University of Michigan, 1500 E Medical Center Dr, SPC 5370, Ann Arbor, MI 48109, USA
Full list of author information is available at the end of the article

Background

Systemic sclerosis (SSc), a connective tissue disorder, is characterized by autoimmune processes, obliterative microvasculopathy, and fibrosis that affects the skin and internal organs [1, 2]. Disease manifestations are highly heterogeneous and include digital vasculopathy, variable degrees of skin and musculoskeletal involvement, interstitial and vascular lung disease, scleroderma renal crisis, and gastrointestinal disease. Patients with SSc experience a substantial increase in mortality, and there is a lack of effective therapeutic options for these patients [3–5].

Clinical and animal study data suggest a pathogenic role of B cell activation and autoantibody production in SSc, identifying B cells as a promising target for therapeutic intervention [6–10]. B cell and plasma cell (PC) infiltrates have been reported in affected skin and lung tissue obtained from patients with SSc [11–15]. B cells found in SSc patients are highly active, as evidenced by hypergammaglobulinemia, polyclonal B cell hyperactivity, and the presence of autoantibodies [16, 17]. Enhanced B cell signaling in SSc patients is associated with increased production of profibrotic cytokines, such as interleukin (IL)-6 and transforming growth factor (TGF)-β [18, 19]. A wide variety of SSc-associated autoantibodies produced by plasma cells have been identified in patients; several are associated with particular clinical pictures and prognoses, and there is evidence for the involvement of certain autoantibodies in the pathogenic processes of fibrosis and vasculopathy underlying SSc [8, 20].

Several clinical studies examined the effects of the B cell-depleting agent rituximab, an anti-CD20 antibody, in patients with SSc. Positive effects on skin thickness and pulmonary function were reported and, in some studies, a significant effect ($p \leq 0.01$) was achieved [11, 12, 21–23]. Clearly, more data, particularly from well-designed, randomized, double-blind, placebo-controlled clinical studies, are needed to understand the potential for B cell depletion as a therapeutic avenue in SSc.

The B cell surface antigen CD19 is expressed throughout B cell development, from pre-B cells through plasmablasts and in some plasma cells. CD19, a key positive regulator of B cell signaling, is overexpressed in SSc patients, and even modest overexpression of CD19 in transgenic mice induced production of SSc-associated autoantibodies [24]. A novel B cell-depleting agent, MEDI-551 (MedImmune; Gaithersburg, MD, USA) targets CD19 and is a humanized, afucosylated immunoglobulin (Ig)G1k monoclonal antibody with enhanced affinity for the human FcγRIIIA and murine FcγRIV receptors. MEDI-551 mediates antibody-dependent cellular cytotoxicity (ADCC) targeting B cells in vitro and in transgenic mice that express human CD19 [25, 26]. In a murine model of experimental SSc, wherein production of pathogenic autoantibodies requires CD19+ B cells, MEDI-551 was effective in reducing circulating and target tissue-infiltrating B cells, total serum immunoglobulin, autoantibodies, and deposition of complement proteins in target tissues. Furthermore, the benefit to organs affected by SSc was evident in those mice with kidney pathology, wherein treatment with MEDI-551 induced sustained reversion of proteinuria and reduction of Ig deposition in glomeruli (Tracy Delaney, written communication, May 2009).

This phase I clinical study of MEDI-551 in subjects with SSc was designed to assess the safety and tolerability, pharmacokinetics (PK), pharmacodynamics (PD), and immunogenicity of MEDI-551, and to explore potential activity of MEDI-551 on SSc disease measures.

Methods

Study design

This phase I, multicenter, randomized, double-blind, placebo-controlled dose escalation study of a single intravenous (IV) dose of MEDI-551 enrolled adult subjects with SSc. The primary objective was to evaluate the safety and tolerability of MEDI-551 in adults with SSc. Secondary objectives included evaluation of the PK, PD, and immunogenicity of MEDI-551. Assessing possible effects of MEDI-551 on measures of disease activity and disease-relevant biomarkers were exploratory end points.

The study was conducted in accordance with the Declaration of Helsinki, International Council for Harmonisation Guidance for Good Clinical Practice, and all local laws (www.clinicaltrials.gov identifier: NCT00946699). The ethics committee from each participating hospital approved the study protocol and all amendments (IRB numbers: HUM00040791 and HUM00031527; see Appendix). All subjects provided written informed consent before study participation.

Following a screening period of up to 21 days, the investigator or designee entered eligible subjects' names and relevant information into an interactive voice-response system (IVRS). The IVRS then assigned subjects in a 6:1 ratio (except for groups 1 [n = 1] and 2 [4:1]) to one of five ascending-dose groups. Subjects received a single IV dose of MEDI-551 or placebo on day 1 (Fig. 1). Study site personnel and subjects were blinded to treatment; the study sponsor's staff members were not blinded. MEDI-551 was administered over ≥60 minutes for doses up to 1 mg/kg, and over ≥120 minutes for doses >1 mg/kg. Assessments for safety, PK, and PD took place at scheduled visits over the 12-week posttreatment period (days 1, 3, 15, 29, 57, and 85). Dose-escalation decisions were made no earlier than day 29 and were based on the incidence of treatment-emergent adverse events (TEAEs), serious adverse events (SAEs), and safety laboratory data.

Subjects with reduced B cell counts at day 85 were eligible to enter a long-term follow-up (LTFU) period,

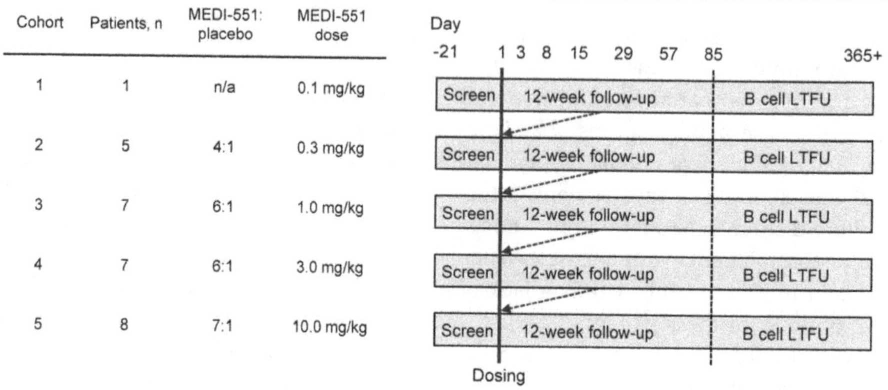

Fig. 1 Study design. Number of subjects in each group includes those who received MEDI-551 and those who received placebo. *LTFU* long-term follow-up

returning once monthly during the first 3 months and every 3 months thereafter for safety evaluations and B cell assessment. Early versions of the protocol specified that subjects in whom B cell counts had not returned to ≥25 % of the baseline value or ≥50 % of the lower limit of normal (LLN) at day 85 were eligible to participate in the LTFU period. During the study, the protocol was amended to include in the LTFU any subject whose B cell count on day 85 was lower than on day 1, in response to feedback from the US Food and Drug Administration to more fully characterize B cell repletion. Subjects who completed the study under earlier versions of the protocol were asked to re-enter the study and consent to blood sampling. This included two subjects who had received placebo. Subjects were followed over the LTFU period until B cell counts were at least equal to baseline values. The investigator and medical monitor were permitted to conjointly decide to discontinue LTFU if baseline B cell counts were reached in a subject after 18 months.

Subjects in the first three dose groups did not receive prophylactic premedication for the prevention of infusion-related reactions (IRRs). Following the occurrence of a grade 3 IRR in the first subject in the MEDI-551 3.0-mg/kg group, the remaining subjects received oral acetaminophen 500 to 600 mg, oral diphenhydramine 25 to 50 mg, and IV methylprednisolone 100 mg or equivalent glucocorticoid 30 to 60 minutes before study drug administration.

Subjects

Eligible subjects were aged at least 18 years, fulfilled the College of Rheumatology/European League Against Rheumatism classification criteria for SSc [2], had at least moderate skin thickening (modified Rodnan skin score [MRSS] [27] ≥2) in at least one area suitable for a repeat skin biopsy, had B cell counts in peripheral blood of ≥50 % LLN at screening, had forced vital capacity (FVC) of ≥55 % predicted and diffusing capacity for carbon monoxide (DL_{co}) of ≥40 % predicted. Subjects were not eligible if they had pulmonary hypertension requiring treatment, scleroderma renal crisis within the previous year, significant malabsorption, Herpes zoster infection in the previous 3 months, a history of severe viral infection, active hepatitis or human immunodeficiency virus (HIV) infection, or evidence of active or latent tuberculosis without appropriate treatment.

Safety evaluations

Adverse events (AEs) and serious AEs (SAEs) were recorded through study exit. Investigators determined the severity of AEs (according to the National Cancer Institute Common Terminology Criteria for Adverse Events version 4.0 criteria) and their causal relationship to the study drug. Vital signs were measured at each visit from day 1 to day 85. Physical examinations were performed on days 1 and 85. Samples for clinical laboratory tests (serum chemistry, hematology, and urinalysis) were collected at each visit through day 85, except for day 3. Electrocardiograms (ECGs) were obtained on days 3 and 85. Samples for IgM, IgG, IgA, and IgE levels were obtained on days 29 and 85, and during the LTFU period. Clinical laboratory safety tests, including those used in screening, were conducted by a central laboratory. Throughout the study, a Safety Monitoring Committee comprising physicians, some employed by MedImmune, met monthly and ad hoc to independently review cumulative safety surveillance data and the medical monitor's decisions on dose escalation, and to make recommendations regarding study progression.

Immunogenicity evaluations

The presence of antidrug antibodies (ADAs) was evaluated in blood samples collected prior to dosing on day 1, on days 29, 57, and 85, and during the B cell LTFU period. An electrochemiluminescent, solution-phase, bridging immunoassay that employed technology by Meso Scale Diagnostics (Rockville, MD, USA) was developed and validated by MedImmune for the detection, confirmation, and titration of ADAs to MEDI-551 in human serum. Study samples that tested positive for ADAs and were confirmed in a screening assay were then analyzed in a titration assay, wherein samples were serially diluted with negative control serum and the highest dilution with detectable ADAs was determined. Subjects were considered to be positive for ADAs if ADAs were detected in the titration assay at sample dilutions ≥1:50.

Pharmacokinetic evaluations

Blood samples for PK analysis were collected before infusion and 30 minutes after the end of infusion on day 1, and on days 3, 8, 15, 29, 57, and 85. MEDI-551 concentration was measured in human serum samples using a colorimetric sandwich enzyme-linked immunosorbent assay (ELISA) developed and validated by MedImmune. The upper and lower limits of quantification were determined to be 4105 ng/mL and 100 ng/mL, respectively. Method validation met the acceptance criteria for accuracy, precision, selectivity (evaluated in serum from normal individuals and in serum samples from subjects with scleroderma), specificity, dilutional linearity, robustness, and stability of MEDI-551 in human serum.

Pharmacodynamic evaluations

Peripheral blood samples for B cell analysis were collected prior to dosing on day 1, and on days 3, 8, 15, 29, 57, and 85. For subjects who entered the LTFU period, blood samples for B cell analysis were collected once monthly for 3 months then every 3 months thereafter, until counts returned to baseline (day 1) values. The presence of MEDI-551 in samples interferes with CD19-based detection of B cells by flow cytometry. Therefore, immunodetection of the B cell surface marker CD20, which is co-expressed with CD19 on B cells throughout most of their development, was used to monitor B cells by flow cytometry following MEDI-551 treatment. The absolute number of CD20+ B cells per microliter was derived from the percentage of CD20+ cells and the absolute number of lymphocytes. The absolute number of lymphocytes was calculated using white blood cell counts and total number of CD45+ cells. Flow cytometry was performed at two central laboratory facilities (LabCorp; Cranford, NY, USA and Mechelen, Belgium).

The plasma cell (PC) gene signature was previously described as a robust, sensitive, and accurate measure of PCs in clinical samples [28]. The PC gene signature is based on expression analysis of five genes (IGHA1, IGJ, IGKC, IGKV4-1, and TNFRSF17) expressed predominantly in PCs. The PC gene signature was evaluated by whole-genome microarray in blood samples obtained on days 1, 3, 29, and 85, and during the LTFU period. For each subject at each time point after day 1, the PC gene signature was calculated as the median of the percentage change from baseline of the genes in each panel, and is interpreted as a change in PC abundance.

Disease assessments

The MRSS, a validated measure of SSc disease activity in skin [29], is a clinician-rated assessment of skin thickness at 17 body sites, including the fingers, hands, forearms, arms, face, chest, abdomen, thighs, legs, and feet, with each site scored from 0 to 3 (0 = normal skin, 1 = mild thickness, 2 = moderate thickness, and 3 = severe thickness). The MRSS is the sum of scores at all 17 sites, for a maximum score of 51. The MRSS is responsive to therapeutic intervention, and a change of 3 to 5 points was found to be the minimum clinically significant difference [30].

Pulmonary function tests to measure FVC and DL_{CO} [31, 32] were performed according to the guidelines of the American Thoracic Society and European Respiratory Society [33] at screening and on days 29 and 85, and the percentage of predicted normal values was calculated.

Statistical analyses

Sample size determination was based on typical design of a phase I study. A minimum of 27 subjects were planned for enrollment, with a maximum of 35 subjects if additional eligible subjects were available by closure of enrollment. Results were presented descriptively (no formal statistical hypothesis testing) for the as-treated population (i.e., subjects who received ≥1 dose of study drug) by actual treatment received. Treatment-emergent AEs were defined as those with onset immediately following study drug administration through end of study, and were coded using the Medical Dictionary for Regulatory Activities, version 17.0.

Noncompartmental PK data analyses were performed, with time 0 defined as the beginning of the infusion. Postdose maximum observed concentration (C_{max}), area under the concentration-time curve from dosing to the last measurable time point (AUC_{last}), postdose AUC extrapolated to infinity (AUC_{inf}), systemic clearance (CL), elimination half-life ($t_{½}$), and steady-state volume of distribution (V_{ss}) were determined. The incidence of detectable ADAs was summarized by treatment group.

For analysis of the PD effect of MEDI-551 on peripheral B cells, B cell depletion was defined as a reduction in B cell counts by ≥90 % from day 1 values. Time to depletion was defined as the time to the first observation of ≥90 % reduction from baseline in B cell counts in a subject, and duration of depletion was defined as the interval between first and last observations of ≥90 % reduction from day 1 values in B cell counts in a subject.

Results

Subjects

The study enrolled 28 subjects at 13 sites in the US, UK, and Canada and was conducted from 19 March 2010 to 19 March 2014 (Fig. 2). Group 1 consisted of a single subject who received MEDI-551 0.1 mg/kg. Groups 2 through 5 each comprised four to seven subjects, randomized to receive increasing doses of MEDI-551 or placebo. In total, 24 subjects received MEDI-551 and four subjects received placebo. All subjects received a single dose of study drug according to their assigned treatment. All 28 subjects remained on study through day 85, and 24 subjects entered the LTFU period for B cell monitoring. Reasons for discontinuation included lost to follow-up (one subject in the placebo group), withdrawal of consent (one subject in the 1-mg/kg group, one subject in the 3-mg/kg group), and death (one subject in the 3-mg/kg group).

Demographics and baseline characteristics were summarized for the entire study population and by treatment group (Table 1). Overall, the clinical and other baseline characteristics, including B cell counts, were similar between treatment groups. The overall study population was predominantly female (67.9 %) and white (85.7 %), with a mean age of 47.3 years. Most subjects (85.7 %) were diagnosed with diffuse cutaneous (as opposed to limited cutaneous) SSc, and mean disease duration was 5.4 years from onset of non-Raynaud's symptoms. Most subjects (75.0 %) were positive for antinuclear autoantibodies. The study subjects had skin thickening (mean MRSS, 23.0) and mildly reduced lung function (mean 82.5 % predicted FVC; mean 72.0 % predicted DL_{co}) at baseline.

Safety

The majority of subjects in the combined MEDI-551 group (n = 23 [95.8 %]) and in the placebo group (n = 3 [75.0 %]) experienced ≥1 TEAE during the study (Table 2). The majority of TEAEs (111/127 events [87.4 %]) reported by MEDI-551-treated subjects were mild or moderate (grade 1 or 2) in severity. In the MEDI-551 group, seven subjects (29.2 %) experienced a grade 3 TEAE (14 events) and one subject (4.2 %) experienced a grade 4 TEAE (one event). No subject in the placebo group experienced a TEAE worse than grade 2 (14 events total).

The most frequent TEAEs (regardless of relationship to the study drug) were nausea (n = 4 [16.7 %], MEDI-551; n = 0, placebo), fatigue (n = 4 [16.7 %], MEDI-551; n = 1 [25.0 %], placebo), IRRs (n = 4 [16.7 %], MEDI-551; n = 0, placebo), arthralgia (n = 4 [16.7 %], MEDI-551; n = 1 [25.0 %], placebo), and pain in extremity (n = 4 [16.7 %], MEDI-551; n = 1 [25.0 %], placebo). In the MEDI-551 group, 14 subjects (58 %) experienced a total of 20 TEAEs that were considered by investigators to be related to the study drug (Table 2). Most were single events, with the exception of IRRs in four subjects and cough in two subjects. No subjects in the placebo group experienced a treatment-related TEAE.

In the MEDI-551 group, six subjects (25 %) experienced a total of 15 SAEs. Of these, 13 events (atrial fibrillation, colitis, ischemic colitis, diarrhea, gastric antral vascular ectasia, noncardiac chest pain, prostate cancer, cervical myelopathy, acute renal failure, scleroderma renal crisis, respiratory failure, and two occurrences of skin ulcer) were considered to be not related to the study drug. The two SAEs deemed possibly related to the study drug were supraventricular tachycardia (grade 2, onset day 2, duration 1 day, occurring in a subject in the MEDI-551 0.3-mg/kg group) and subclavian vein thrombosis (grade 3, onset day 2, duration 27 days, occurring in a subject in the MEDI-551 1.0-mg/kg group);

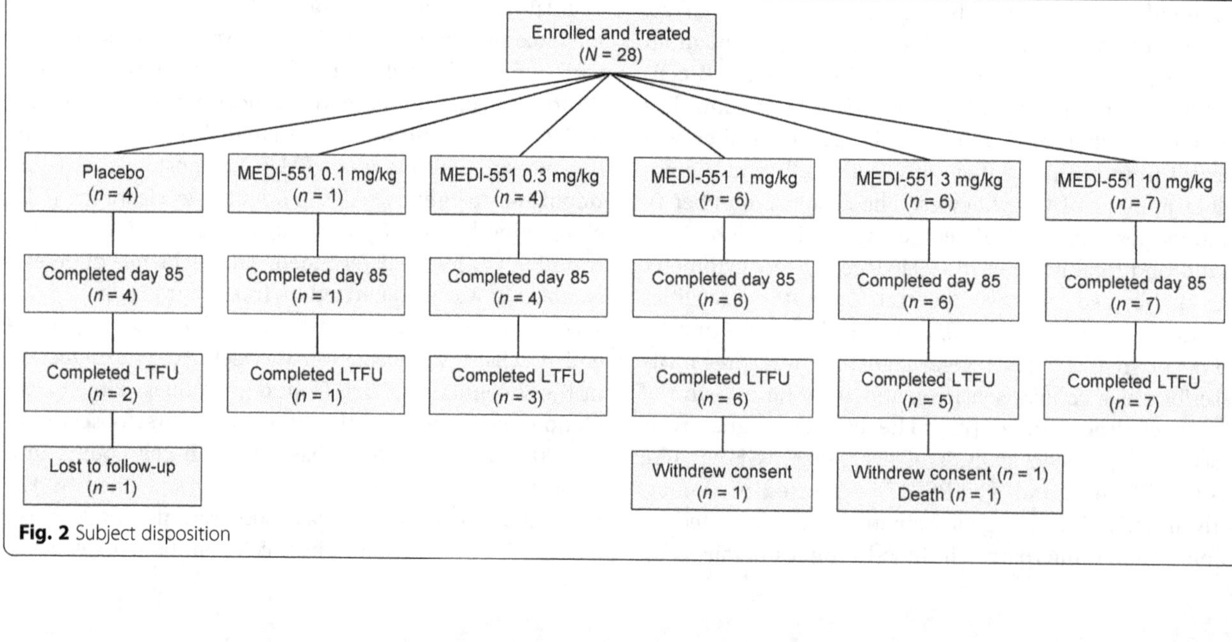

Fig. 2 Subject disposition

Table 1 Baseline characteristics of study subjects

Characteristic	Placebo	MEDI-551 ($n = 24$)					Total
		0.1 mg/kg	0.3 mg/kg	1.0 mg/kg	3.0 mg/kg	10 mg/kg	
	($n = 4$)	($n = 1$)	($n = 4$)	($n = 6$)	($n = 6$)	($n = 7$)	($N = 28$)
Age, years, mean (SD)	42.3 (14.4)	52.0 (NA)	47.3 (11.6)	48.8 (9.8)	49.8 (9.3)	46.0 (8.6)	47.3 (9.7)
Female, n (%)	2 (50.0)	0 (0.0)	3 (75.0)	3 (50.0)	5 (83.3)	6 (85.7)	19 (67.9)
White, n (%)	4 (100.0)	1 (100.0)	2 (50.0)	6 (100.0)	5 (83.3)	6 (85.7)	24 (85.7)
Weight, kg, mean (SD)	84.7 (7.9)	114.2 (NA)	75.3 (4.4)	68.2 (18.7)	73.4 (14.6)	71.7 (20.5)	75.2 (17.1)
Diffuse cutaneous SSc, n (%)	3 (75.0)	1 (100.0)	3 (75.0)	5 (83.3)	6 (100.0)	6 (85.7)	24 (85.7)
Disease duration, years, mean (SD)	5.6 (6.2)	5.3 (NA)	5.7 (3.35)	6.7 (4.7)	3.7 (3.0)	5.4 (5.1)	5.4 (4.3)
Positive antinuclear antibody, n (%)	2 (50.0)	0 (0.0)	4 (100.0)	4 (66.7)	4 (66.7)	7 (100.0)	21 (75.0)
Positive anti-Scl70 antibody, n (%)	3 (75.0)	0 (0.0)	1 (25.0)	2 (33.3)	4 (66.7)	2 (28.6)	12 (42.9)
Elevated acute phase reactants (ESR, CRP), n (%)	2 (50.0)	1 (100.0)	1 (25.0)	4 (66.7)	3 (50.0)	3 (42.9)	14 (50.0)
MRSS, mean (SD)	22.8 (7.5)	31.0 (NA)	23.5 (7.6)	20.0 (9.8)	23.3 (12.8)	24.0 (5.1)	23.0 (8.5)
FVC, % predicted, mean (SD)	87.9 (10.9)	83.0 (NA)	87.0 (10.9)	75.0 (19.0)	83.8 (21.9)	82.1 (22.8)	82.5 (17.8)
DL_{CO}, % predicted, mean (SD)	69.8 (30.2)	98.0 (NA)	79.5 (20.9)	54.5 (10.0)	74.8 (29.2)	77.9 (20.7)	72.0 (23.1)
CD19 B cell count, cells/uL, mean (SD)	223.8 (209.5)	182.0 (NA)	187.3 (149.9)	119.2 (115.7)	175.8 (116.1)	175.3 (211.8)	172.3 (152.9)
CD20 B cell count, cells/uL, mean (SD)	221.0 (210.7)	174.0 (NA)	180.0 (135.3)	115.8 (113.9)	177.0 (116.5)	173.3 (211.4)	169.6 (151.3)

CRP C-reactive protein, DL_{CO} diffusing capacity for carbon monoxide, *ESR* erythrocyte sedimentation rate, *FVC* forced vital capacity, *MRSS* modified Rodnan skin score, *NA* not available, *SSc* systemic scleroderma

in both cases, an alternate etiology was provided. No SAEs occurred in the placebo group.

One subject died on study. This subject, who had received MEDI-551 3.0 mg/kg, experienced an SAE of scleroderma renal crisis (onset day 62) that led to death 47 days later. This subject also experienced SAEs of gastric antral vascular ectasia (grade 3, onset day 62) and respiratory failure (grade 4, onset day 67). Both the investigator and the study sponsor assessed these events as not related to MEDI-551, with an alternative etiology of underlying disease.

No subject experienced hypersensitivity (including anaphylaxis), immune complex disease, cytopenia (neutropenia, thrombocytopenia), or progressive multifocal leukoencephalopathy. The TEAEs categorized as "infections and infestations" occurred at similar frequency in the MEDI-551 (n = 11 [45.8 %]) and placebo (n = 2 [50.0 %]) groups; all were grade 1 or 2. Four out of 12 subjects (33.3 %) in the MEDI-551 group who were not premedicated experienced an IRR. Three of these subjects (two in the 1.0-mg/kg group and one in the 3.0-mg/kg group) received reduced doses of MEDI-551 because of the IRR. All IRRs but one were grade 1 or grade 2 in severity, none were serious, all were treated with antihistamine, anxiolytic, and/or analgesic medications, and all resolved within 2 days. The one grade 3 IRR occurred in a subject in the MEDI-551 3.0-mg/kg group, which prompted the protocol amendment requiring premedication to mitigate IRRs. After this protocol amendment was implemented, none of the subsequent 12 subjects who received MEDI-551 experienced an IRR. No subjects in the placebo group experienced an IRR.

Analysis of IgG, IgA, IgM, and IgE levels revealed that, in the total MEDI-551 group, seven subjects with normal baseline values had low posttreatment values. These included two subjects with IgG values less than the normal range at day 85 and one subject with IgG values less than the normal range at B cell recovery; one subject with an IgA value less than the normal range at day 85 and one subject with an IgA value less than the normal range at B cell recovery; and two subjects with IgM values less than the normal range at days 29 and 85. No subject in the placebo group with a normal baseline value had a low posttreatment value.

Of the four subjects in the MEDI-551 group who experienced IRRs, vital sign abnormalities, including elevated blood pressure, respiratory rate, or heart rate, were reported on the day of infusion for three subjects; vital signs were not collected on the day of infusion for the fourth subject. One subject in the MEDI-551 0.3-mg/kg group had an elevated heart rate on day 3 that was reported as an SAE (supraventricular tachycardia) and was assessed as possibly related to MEDI-551, although an alternate etiology of preexisting supraventricular tachycardia was provided.

Two subjects (8.3 %) in the MEDI-551 group had a clinically significant abnormal ECG finding on day 3 that was reported as a TEAE. A subject in the MEDI-551 0.3-mg/kg group with a history of supraventricular tachycardia, hypertension, and palpitations experienced an SAE of supraventricular tachycardia (onset day 2) that persisted on day 3 and resolved after treatment with metoprolol. A subject in the MEDI-551 10.0-mg/kg

Table 2 Treatment-emergent and treatment-related adverse events

Adverse event, n (%)	Placebo	MEDI-551					
		0.1 mg/kg	0.3 mg/kg	1.0 mg/kg	3.0 mg/kg	10 mg/kg	Total
	(*n* = 4)	(*n* = 1)	(*n* = 4)	(*n* = 6)	(*n* = 6)	(*n* = 7)	(*N* = 24)
≥1 TEAE	3 (75.0)	1 (100.0)	4 (100.0)	6 (100.0)	5 (83.3)	7 (100.0)	23 (95.8)
≥1 grade 3 TEAE	0	1 (100.0)	0	2 (33.3)	2 (33.3)	2 (28.6)	7 (29.2)
≥1 grade 4 TEAE	0	0	0	0	1 (16.7)	0	1 (4.2)
Death	0	0	0	0	1 (16.7)	0	0
≥1 SAE	0	1 (100.0)	1 (25.0)	1 (16.7)	2 (33.3)	1 (14.3)	6 (25.0)
≥1 study drug-related TEAE	0	0	2 (50.0)	4 (66.7)	4 (66.7)	4 (57.1)	14 (58.3)
≥1 study drug-related SAE	0	0	1 (25.0)	1 (16.7)	0	0	2 (8.3)
Treatment-related TEAEs and SAEs, by MedDRA preferred term							
Infusion-related reaction	0	0	1 (25.0)	2 (33.3)	1 (16.7)	0	4 (16.7)
Cough	0	0	0	0	0	2 (28.6)	2 (8.3)
Diarrhea	0	0	0	0	1 (16.7)	0	1 (4.2)
Fatigue	0	0	0	0	0	1 (14.3)	1 (4.2)
Flushing	0	0	0	1 (16.7)	0	0	1 (4.2)
Headache	0	0	0	0	0	1 (14.3)	1 (4.2)
Hot flush	0	0	0	1 (16.7)	0	0	1 (4.2)
Hyperglycemia	0	0	0	0	1 (16.7)	0	1 (4.2)
Lip swelling	0	0	0	0	1 (16.7)	0	1 (4.2)
Night sweats	0	0	0	0	0	1 (14.3)	1 (4.2)
Rash	0	0	0	0	1 (16.7)	0	1 (4.2)
Subclavian vein thrombosis	0	0	0	1 (16.7)	0	0	1 (4.2)
Supraventricular extrasystoles	0	0	0	0	0	1 (14.3)	1 (4.2)
Supraventricular tachycardia	0	0	1 (25.0)	0	0	0	1 (4.2)
Tongue ulceration	0	0	0	0	0	1 (14.3)	1 (4.2)
Upper respiratory tract infection	0	0	0	0	1 (16.7)	0	1 (4.2)

MedDRA Medical Dictionary for Regulatory Activities, *SAE* serious adverse event, *TEAE* treatment-emergent adverse event,

group with a history of tachycardia and exercise-induced pulmonary hypertension experienced a TEAE of supraventricular extrasystoles (onset day 2) and had an abnormal, clinically significant ECG finding of premature supraventricular complexes on day 3. No subject in the placebo group had a clinically significant abnormal ECG finding before or after dosing.

Immunogenicity

No subjects were positive for anti-MEDI-551 ADAs prior to dosing, nor were any subjects in the placebo group positive at any time after dosing. Among subjects who received MEDI-551, four (16.7 %) were found to be positive at one or more time points after dosing, with no apparent relationship to dose level (one subject in the 0.3-mg/kg group, one in the 1-mg/kg group, one in the 3-mg/kg group, and one in the 10-mg/kg group). The subjects in the MEDI-551 0.3- and 1.0-mg/kg groups were positive for ADAs on days 29, 57, and 85, and were negative thereafter. The subject in the MEDI-551 3.0-mg/kg group was positive on days 29 and 57; no further data were available. The subject in the MEDI-551 10.0-mg/kg group was positive on day 29, negative on days 57 and 85, and became positive again on day 365, with no further data available.

Of the four ADA-positive subjects, two (one in the 0.3-mg/kg group and one in the 10.0-mg/kg group) received the full dose of MEDI-551, and two (one in the 1.0-mg/kg group and one in the 3.0-mg/kg group) received a reduced dose (90.0 % and 39.7 % of the intended doses, respectively) owing to the occurrence of an IRR. In the two subjects who received full doses, MEDI-551 serum concentration-time profiles were similar to those of other members of the respective dose group. In the two subjects who received a reduced dose, serum concentration-time profiles were less than other members of the dose group. The ADA-positive subjects in the MEDI-551 0.3-mg/kg and 10.0-mg/kg groups who received full MEDI-551 doses and the subject in the MEDI-551 1.0-mg/kg group who received 90 % of the intended dose displayed B cell depletion patterns similar to those of other members of their respective groups. The ADA-positive subject in the MEDI-551 3.0-mg/kg group who received 39.7 % of the intended dose showed evidence of reduced B cell depletion relative to other members of the group.

Pharmacokinetics

MEDI-551 serum concentration-time profiles following a single IV administration of MEDI-551 are shown in Fig. 3, and PK parameters are summarized in Table 3. MEDI-551 exhibited nonlinear PK for all dose levels, ranging from 0.1 to 10.0 mg/kg. A dose-proportional increase in C_{max} values was observed, but both the $AUC_{0\text{-last}}$ and $AUC_{0\text{-inf}}$ values demonstrated more than dose-proportional increases for all dose levels. Mean CL decreased from 6.2 to 3.5 mL/kg/day when the dose of MEDI-551 was increased from 0.1 to 10.0 mg/kg. For MEDI-551 doses of 1.0 mg/kg or greater, parallel terminal elimination phases and similar half-lives (11.3–13.5 days) were observed, whereas the terminal elimination half-life of MEDI-551 was shorter at lower doses (6.8 and 7.1 days for the 0.1- and 0.3-mg/kg groups, respectively). The mean V_{ss} ranged between 53.7 and 71.6 mL/kg across the dose groups.

Pharmacodynamics

A single IV administration of MEDI-551 at all dose levels resulted in rapid and sustained decreases in the number of circulating B cells in all subjects (Fig. 4; Table 4). Higher doses of MEDI-551 were associated with a greater proportion of subjects achieving B cell depletion: two of four (50 %) subjects in the 0.3-mg/kg dose group, five of six (83.3 %) in the 1- and 3-mg/kg dose groups, and seven of seven (100 %) in the 10-mg/kg dose group achieved dose depletion. In the 0.3-mg/kg, 1.0-mg/kg, 3.0-mg/kg, and 10.0-mg/kg dose groups, respectively, the median times to B cell depletion were 43.5, 57, 29, and 28 days, with median durations of B cell depletion of 14, 29, 119, and 231 days. The mean values for the maximum observed B cell reduction from baseline were 89.7 %, 93.0 %, 93.4 %, and 98.3 % for the 0.3-mg/kg, 1.0-mg/kg, 3.0-mg/kg, and 10.0-mg/kg dose groups, respectively. The single subject who received MEDI-551 0.1 mg/kg displayed B cell depletion kinetics similar to that of subjects in the 0.3-mg/kg group. As expected, B cell counts in the placebo group were variable, and no trend over time was apparent (data not shown).

Day 85 CD20+ B cell counts were available for 23 MEDI-551-treated subjects and for three placebo subjects. Day 85 CD20+ B cell counts in the MEDI-551 group ranged from 0 to 104.5 % of day 1 values, while those in the placebo group ranged from 63.5 to 137.8 % of day 1 values. Twenty-two subjects in the MEDI-551 group and two subjects in the placebo group participated in the LTFU period (Fig. 2). During the LTFU period, 16 (72.7 %) MEDI-551-treated subjects exhibited recovery of B cell counts to baseline levels. Among the six MEDI-551-treated subjects for whom full B cell recovery was not observed, four (18.2 %) were released from the LTFU period prior to full B cell recovery by mutual agreement of the investigator and sponsor after at least 18 months of follow-up, based on observed trends in B cell recovery and clinical judgement; two (9.1 %) withdrew consent (Fig. 2) and could not be fully assessed for B cell recovery. The two placebo subjects

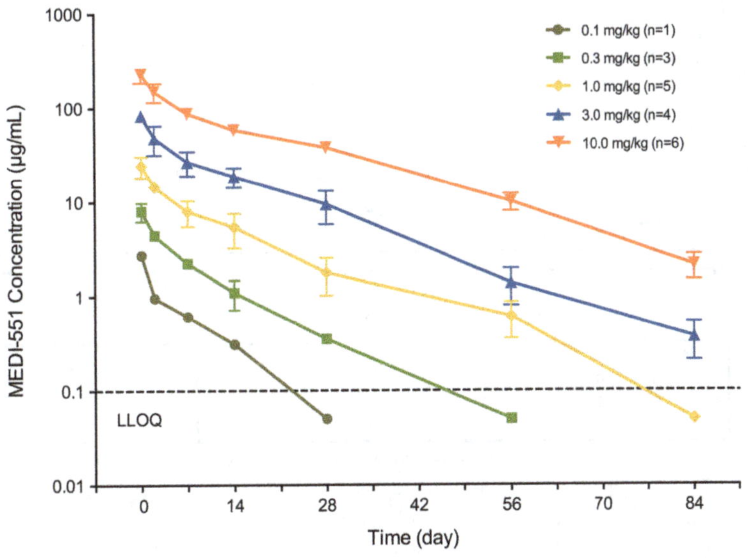

Fig. 3 Pharmacokinetics of MEDI-551. Serum concentration-time profile of MEDI-551 following a single IV administration

Table 3 Pharmacokinetic parameters for MEDI-551

MEDI-551 dose, mean (SD)	*n*	C_{max}, µg/mL	$AUC_{0\text{-last}}$, µg•d/mL	$AUC_{0\text{-inf}}$, µg•d/mL	CL, mL/kg/d	$T_{½}$, day	V_{ss}, mL/kg
0.1 mg/kg	1	2.7	13.0	16.1	6.2	6.8	53.7
0.3 mg/kg	3[a]	8.0 (1.8)	45.7 (12.9)	50.6 (13.2)	6.2 (1.5)	7.1 (1.8)	58.9 (24.5)
1.0 mg/kg	5[b]	22.5 (7.1)	202.0 (79.2)	211.0 (77.0)	5.3 (2.2)	11.3 (3.7)	69.3 (11.4)
3.0 mg/kg	4[c]	83.6 (10.6)	781.0 (230.0)	789.0 (230.0)	4.1 (1.3)	11.3 (1.0)	63.4 (22.4)
10.0 mg/kg	6[d]	227.0 (43.0)	2840.0 (260.0)	2890.0 (267.0)	3.5 (0.4)	13.5 (1.1)	71.6 (8.2)

$AUC_{0\text{-inf}}$ area under the concentration-time curve extrapolated to infinity after dosing, $AUC_{0\text{-last}}$ area under the concentration-time curve from dosing to last measurable time point, *CL* systemic clearance, C_{max} maximum observed concentration, $t_{½}$ terminal elimination half-life, V_{ss} steady-state volume of distribution

[a] $n = 4$ for C_{max}

[b] $n = 6$ for C_{max}

[c] $n = 5$ for $t_{½}$

[d] $n = 7$ for C_{max}

who participated in the LTFU period exhibited B cell counts that equaled or exceeded baseline counts at day 85 or at the first LTFU assessment. Subjects exited the study after B cell repletion was achieved; as a result, the number of subjects with available B cell data declined during LTFU (Fig. 4). The prolongation of B cell depletion in the 1.0-mg/kg group is likely related to the reduced number of subjects with data available at later time points.

Circulating plasma cells, as measured by the PC gene signature in whole blood, were reduced following MEDI-551 administration (Fig. 5). Plasma cell gene signatures were reduced to 25 to 50 % of baseline on day 3 and 8 to 20 % of baseline on day 29, with a greater degree of reduction observed with higher MEDI-551 doses. At day 85, the PC gene signature had partially recovered in the 0.1-, 0.3-, and 1.0-mg/kg groups, but had declined further in the higher-dose groups. After day 85, PC gene signatures recovered to near baseline levels. A reduction in the PC gene signature was not observed for the placebo group (Fig. 5).

Disease assessments

Potential effects of MEDI-551 on skin thickness, as measured by the MRSS, were assessed as an exploratory end point. The mean MRSS change from baseline to day 85 was -5.4 points (SD 4.2) in the combined MEDI-551 group and 2.3 points (SD 6.1) in the placebo group. In the MEDI-551 dose groups, mean changes from baseline ranged from -14.0 to -3.6, with no clear relationship to dose level (Table 5).

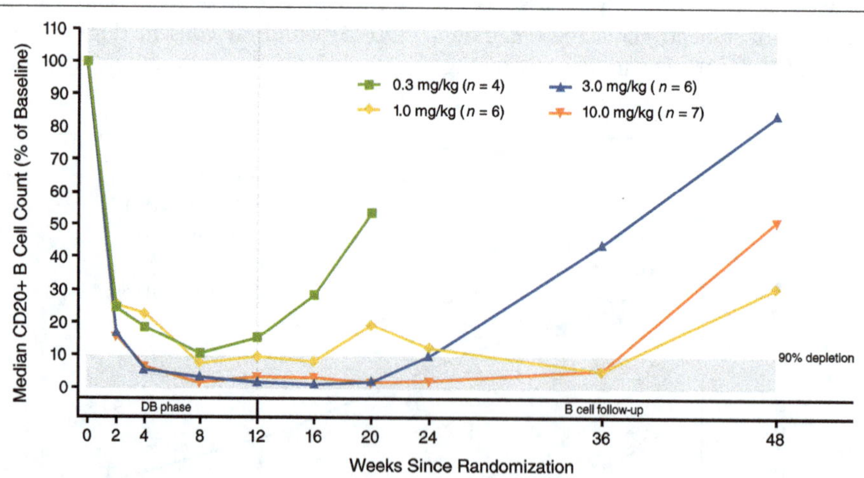

	0	2	4	8	12	16	20	24	36	48
0.3 mg/kg	4	4	4	4	4	2	2	-	-	-
1.0 mg/kg	6	5	6	6	6	2	3	3	1	1
3.0 mg/kg	6	5	6	6	5	5	2	3	4	2
10.0 mg/kg	7	7	7	7	7	6	6	7	7	7

Subjects (*n*) with CD20+ B Cell Count

Fig. 4 Effect of MEDI-551 on peripheral B cells. Median B cell counts over time, by MEDI-551 dose. B cell counts are presented as % of day 1 values. The data plotted represent only those subjects for which B cell counts are available at each time point. The number of subjects in the analysis in each group at each time point is tabulated below the graph. This number declines over time as subjects exit the study following B cell repletion

Table 4 Summary of B cell depletion activity of MEDI-551

MEDI-551 Dose	Subjects, *n*	Subjects achieving depletion,[a] n (%)	Time to depletion,[b,c] median (range), days	Duration of depletion,[b,d] median (range), days	Maximum B cell reduction,[e] mean % (SD)
0.3 mg/kg	4	2 (50.0)	43.5 (30–57)	13.5 (0–27)	89.7 (3.9)
1.0 mg/kg	6	5 (83.3)	57.0 (29–67)	29.0 (0–209)	93.0 (10.2)
3.0 mg/kg	6	5 (83.3)	29.0 (7–85)	119 (0–154)	93.4 (10.9)
10.0 mg/kg	7	7 (100.0)	28.0 (3–86)	231 (30–264)	98.3 (3.2)

[a]Defined as ≥ 90 % reduction in B cell counts from the day 1 value
[b]Among subjects who achieved B cell depletion
[c]Defined as the time to the first observation of ≥90 % reduction from the day 1 value
[d]Defined as the interval between the first and last observation of ≥90 % reduction in B cell count from the day 1 value. Subjects with B cell depletion at only a single assessment had a duration of depletion of zero
[e]Values represent mean of the maximum degree of B cell reduction for subjects in the group, at any time after dosing, expressed as % reduction of day 1 values

Potential effects of MEDI-551 on pulmonary function were also examined. Mean percent predicted FVC values (standard deviation [SD]) in subjects who received MEDI-551 were 81.6 % (18.8) at baseline (n = 24) and 81.2 % (18.9) at day 85 (n = 21) versus 87.9 % (10.9) at baseline (n = 4) and 89.3 % (12.3) at day 85 (n = 4) in the placebo group. Mean percent predicted DL_{CO} (SD) in subjects who received MEDI-551 was 72.4 % (22.5) at baseline and 65.8 % (23.6) at day 85 versus 69.8 % (30.2) at baseline and 66.2 % (25.9) at day 85 in the placebo group.

Discussion

In this phase I study of MEDI-551 in subjects with SSc, single MEDI-551 doses from 0.1 to 10 mg/kg were safe and well tolerated. Most subjects in both the MEDI-551 and placebo groups experienced TEAEs following treatment, and most of the events were mild or moderate in severity. Two SAEs, supraventricular tachycardia in a subject on MEDI-551 0.3 mg/kg and subclavian vein thrombosis in a subject on MEDI-551 1.0 mg/kg, were deemed possibly related to MEDI-551 because of close temporal association with dosing. However, both subjects had relevant medical histories that may have contributed to the events: the subject with supraventricular tachycardia had a history of this condition, and the subject who experienced subclavian vein thrombosis had a prothrombin 20210A mutation, which has been associated with increased risk of thrombosis [34]. The single death reported in this study, which followed the occurrence of scleroderma renal crisis in a subject in the 3.0-mg/kg dose group, was deemed unrelated to MEDI-551 treatment and was attributed to underlying disease. Clinically significant abnormal ECG findings were observed

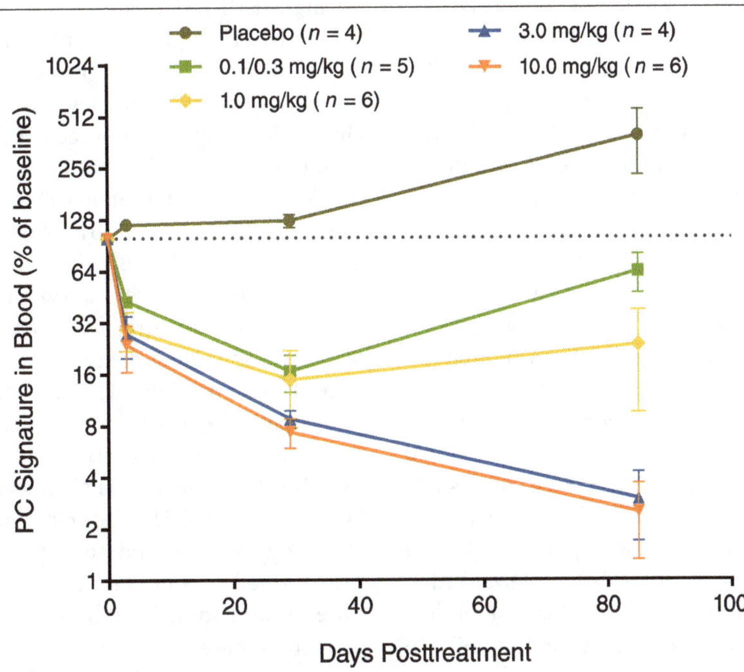

Fig. 5 Effect of MEDI-551 on plasma cell signature in blood. Mean values are plotted. *Bars* represent standard error of the mean. *PC* plasma cells

Table 5 Summary of MRSS values by treatment

Treatment group	*n*	MRSS, mean (SD)		
		Day 1	Day 85	Change from day 1 to day 85
Placebo	4	22.8 (7.5)	25.0 (7.2)	2.3 (6.1)
MEDI-551 0.1 mg/kg	1	31.0 (NA)	17.0 (NA)	-14.0 (NA)
MEDI-551 0.3 mg/	4	23.5 (7.6)	17.3 (5.1)	-6.3 (3.5)
MEDI-551 1.0 mg/kg	6	20.0 (9.8)	15.5 (8.7)	-4.5 (1.5)
MEDI-551 3.0 mg/kg	6[a]	23.3 (12.8)	17.8 (13.1)	-6.6 (3.0)
MEDI-551 10.0 mg/kg	7	24.0 (5.1)	20.4 (7.7)	-3.6 (5.7)
Combined MEDI-551	24[b]	23.0 (8.7)	17.9 (8.5)	-5.4 (4.2)

MRSS modified Rodnan skin score
[a]At day 85, $n = 5$
[b]At day 85, $n = 23$

in two MEDI-551-treated subjects; however, both had relevant cardiac history as well as abnormal baseline ECG findings.

Infusion-related reactions are a significant risk with biologic agents. Rituximab and alemtuzumab, for example, are associated with particularly high rates of IRRs, with a 77 % incidence in oncology subjects and a 92 % incidence in multiple sclerosis subjects, respectively [35, 36]. In the present study, IRRs were the most frequently reported TEAE associated with MEDI-551, with an incidence of 16.7 %. Premedication with antihistamines, acetaminophen, and glucocorticoids is often used to reduce the risk of IRRs to therapeutic antibodies [37]. In fact, no subjects in this study who received such premedication experienced an IRR. Type I (immediate) hypersensitivity reactions (i.e., anaphylaxis) are especially concerning, as they can be fatal if not diagnosed and treated promptly. Rituximab is associated with a relatively high frequency of these reactions (5–10 %) [38], which may be related to its chimeric nature [39]. Such reactions were not observed with MEDI-551 in this study, with the caveat that the sample size was small.

B cell depletion therapy is associated with a reduction of immunoglobulin levels and an increased risk of infection. Analysis of the long-term use of rituximab in a large cohort of rheumatoid arthritis (RA) patients determined an event rate for serious infections of approximately four per 100 patient-years [40]. Although no serious infections occurred during the present study, given the small size and relatively short duration of the study, an event rate similar to that of rituximab would not be expected to result in a serious infection in study participants. Rituximab has been linked to reduced immunoglobulin levels: in the large RA group, 22.4 % of rituximab-treated patients developed low IgM and a smaller proportion developed low IgG (3.5 %) or low IgA (1.1 %) that persisted for at least 4 months [40]. In the present study, seven patients with normal baseline levels exhibited low IgG, IgA, and/or IgM levels following MEDI-551 treatment, and the duration of the immunoglobulin reductions ranged from a single visit to longer than 6 months. However, as other immunosuppressive medications were permitted during this study, the effects on immunoglobulin levels may not be completely attributable to MEDI-551.

A low risk of progressive multifocal leukoencephalopathy (PML) has been associated with rituximab use in patients with autoimmune disease [41, 42]. Similarly, late-onset neutropenia has been reported following rituximab therapy, although the risk appears to be somewhat less in patients with autoimmune disease (4 %) [43] than in oncology (8–27 % incidence rate from six studies) [44]. The present study, a small, single-dose phase I study, was not designed to assess these rare SAEs. However, no cases of PML or neutropenia were observed following MEDI-551 treatment.

MEDI-551 displayed nonlinear PK characterized by slower clearance at higher doses (≥1.0 mg/kg), suggesting saturation of a clearance mechanism. The terminal elimination half-life approached 2 weeks at the highest dose tested (10 mg/kg), similar to numerous other therapeutic monoclonal antibodies [45].

In this study, MEDI-551 exhibited durable PD effects in which circulating B cells (as measured by immunocytochemistry/flow cytometry) and PCs (as measured by the PC gene signature) [28] were depleted. The time to onset, duration, and degree of depletion with MEDI-551 were dose dependent. The hypothesized roles of B cells in SSc pathogenesis have been discussed in the literature [6–9], and the implications for B cell depletion by MEDI-551 are clear. The significance of the depletion of PCs with MEDI-551 is not clear in relation to the pathophysiology of SSc and to a potential treatment effect. Autoantibodies produced by PCs are found in most SSc patients, and some have been shown to have profibrotic, pro-inflammatory, or other effects suggestive of a pathogenic role in the disease [8]. The effect of CD20-targeting agents such as rituximab on autoantibody production is not fully understood. Rituximab treatment is associated with reduction in pathogenic autoantibody titers in autoimmune disease [46], suggesting that rituximab does affect some antibody-producing cells. Additionally, studies in transgenic mice identified a subset of short-lived PCs that reside in the spleen and lymph nodes (as opposed to bone marrow), express CD20, produce autoantibodies, and are sensitive to rituximab [47]. On the other hand, CD20-targeted B cell depletion has also been reported to spare PCs in patients with autoimmune disease treated with rituximab [48, 49] and in mice [50], and response to rituximab is reduced in patients with RA with higher levels of a plasmablast-specific marker, *IgJ* [51]. Relative to CD20, CD19 is expressed on a broader range of B cell subsets, including earlier-stage precursor cells and later-stage differentiated cells, such as plasmablasts and some PCs [52, 53]. Further research is needed to understand the contributions of PCs to disease processes and to establish the difference, if one exists, in the therapeutic effect of CD20-depleting versus CD19-depleting agents.

We previously reported analyses of B cell and PC gene signatures in serial skin biopsy samples obtained before and after treatment from subjects in this study, which showed a PD effect of MEDI-551 on both cell types in affected skin [28]. It is not yet clear whether the B cell or PC tissue infiltrates observed in the skin and lungs of SSc patients [11–15] contribute to the pathophysiology of SSc. Potential mechanisms for the contribution of tissue-localized B cells to disease pathology have been proposed, including antigen-presenting cell function and cytokine secretion [54, 55]. Interestingly, a recent study showed that co-culture of B cells with dermal fibroblasts from patients with SSc induces collagen production and secretion of the profibrotic cytokines IL-6 and TGF-β1; furthermore, this effect is dependent on direct contact between B cells and fibroblasts [56, 57]. The demonstration of a PD effect of MEDI-551 on B cells in affected skin raises the possibility of both systemic and local effects on disease processes.

The results of this study should be interpreted with regard to certain study limitations. Although we observed a potential trend of improvement in skin thickness in subjects treated with MEDI-551 (and not in subjects who received placebo), it is important to acknowledge the small sample size and relatively short study duration. Additionally, differences in baseline characteristics between the treatment groups and the potential effect of concomitant immunosuppressive therapy received by subjects during the study are potentially confounding factors.

Conclusions

The safety and tolerability of a single escalating dose of MEDI-551 in this population of subjects with SSc are encouraging and should be further studied in a larger patient population. The PD effect on B cells, implicated in the pathogenesis of this disease, provides rationale for further study of MEDI-551 as a potentially disease-modifying treatment for SSc.

Appendix

List of Institutional Review Boards/Ethics Committees

Bannatyne Campus Research Ethics Boards; Winnipeg, Manitoba, Canada

BRANY Institutional Review Board; Lake Success, NY, USA

Cleveland Clinic Institutional Review Board; Cleveland, OH, USA

Duke Medicine Institutional Review Board for Clinical Investigations; Durham, NC, USA

Institutional Review Board for Human Research Subject, Louisiana State University Health Sciences Center; Shreveport, LO, USA

Office of Sponsored Research Institutional Review Board; Loma Linda, CA, USA

Stanford University Panel on Medical Human Subjects; Stanford, CA, USA

UCL/UCLH/Royal Free Joint Biomedical Research Unit; London, United Kingdom

University of Connecticut Human Subjects Protection Office Institutional Review Board; Farmington, CT, USA

University of Michigan IRBMED; Ann Arbor, MI, USA

Western Institutional Review Board; Olympia, WA, USA

Abbreviations

ADA, antidrug antibody; ADCC, antibody-dependent cellular cytotoxicity; AE, adverse event; AUC_{inf}, postdose AUC extrapolated to infinity; AUC_{last}, area under the concentration-time curve from dosing to last measurable time point; CL, systemic clearance; C_{max}, maximum observed concentration; DL_{CO}, diffusing capacity for carbon monoxide; ECG, electrocardiogram; FVC, forced vital capacity; HIV, human immunodeficiency virus; Ig, immunoglobulin; IL, interleukin; IRR, infusion-related reaction; IV, intravenous; LLN, lower limit of normal; LTFU, long-term follow-up; MRSS, modified Rodnan Skin Score; PC, plasma cell; PD, pharmacodynamic; PK, pharmacokinetic; PML, progressive multifocal leukoencephalopathy; RA, rheumatoid arthritis; SAE, serious adverse event; SD, standard deviation; SSc, systemic sclerosis; $t_{1/2}$, elimination half-life; TEAE, treatment-emergent adverse event; TGF, transforming growth factor; V_{ss}, steady-state volume of distribution

Acknowledgments

The authors thank James R. Seibold, MD, for his early participation in this study at the University of Michigan. The authors also thank Amy Zannikos, PharmD, of Peloton Advantage for medical writing and editorial support, which was funded by MedImmune. The authors acknowledge the deceased Dr. Dominique Ethgen for his significant contributions to the design and implementation of this study. The authors also acknowledge the following investigators, who participated in this study: Lorinda Chung (Stanford University School of Medicine, Palo Alto, CA, USA); Christopher Denton (Royal Free Hospital NHS Trust, London, UK); Samina Hayat (Louisiana State University, Shreveport, LA, USA); Thomas Geppert (Metroplex Clinical Research Center, Dallas, TX, USA); Avram Goldberg (NYU Langone Ambulatory Care, New Hyde Park, NY, USA); Emmanuel Katsaros (Loma Linda University Medical Center, Loma Linda, CA, USA); Alan Kivitz (Altoona Center for Clinical Research, Duncansville, PA, USA); David Robinson (Winnipeg Regional Health Authority-Health Sciences Centre, Winnipeg, Manitoba,

Canada); Naomi Rothfield (University of Connecticut Health Center, Farmington, CT, USA); and William St. Clair (Duke University Medical Center, Durham, NC, USA).

Source of funding
This study was sponsored by MedImmune. Elena Schiopu, Soumya Chatterjee, and Vivien Hsu received no honoraria or other form of financial support related to the development of this manuscript.

Authors' contributions
AF, BW, KM, and RH designed the study. ES was the principal investigator. ES, SC, and VH were study investigators and enrolled subjects. ES and SS collected and assembled the data. ES, AF, DC, KP, WY, JL, KS, EK, JD, SS, RH, KM, BW, SC, and VH participated in data analysis and interpretation. ES, AF, DC, KP, WY, JL, KS, EK, JD, SS, RH, KM, BW, SC, and VH contributed to the preparation, critical review, and revision of the manuscript. All authors granted final approval for submission of the manuscript.

Competing interests
ES, SC, and VH received research funding from MedImmune for this study and have no nonfinancial conflicts to declare in relation to this manuscript. AF, DC, KP, WY, JL, KS, EK, JD, SS, and RH are employees of MedImmune and may own stock or stock options in that company. KM and BW were employees of MedImmune at the time of this study.

Author details
[1]Department of Internal Medicine, University of Michigan, 1500 E Medical Center Dr, SPC 5370, Ann Arbor, MI 48109, USA. [2]Department of Rheumatologic and Immunologic Diseases, Cleveland Clinic, 9500 Euclid Ave, Cleveland, OH 44195, USA. [3]Clinical Research Center, Rutgers-Robert Wood Johnson Medical School, 125 Paterson St, New Brunswick, NJ 08901, USA. [4]Departments of Research and Clinical Biologics, MedImmune, 1 MedImmune Way, Gaithersburg, MD 20878, USA. [5]Department of Clinical Pharmacology and Drug Metabolism and Pharmacokinetics, MedImmune, 319 North Bernardo Ave, Mountain View, CA 94043, USA. [6]Present address: Ultragenyx Pharmaceutical, 60 Leveroni Ct, Novato, CA 94949, USA. [7]Present address: Corbus Pharmaceuticals, 100 River Ridge Dr, Norwood, MA 02062, USA.

References

1. Desbois AC, Cacoub P. Systemic sclerosis: an update in 2016. Autoimmun Rev. 2016;15(5):417–26.
2. van den Hoogen F, Khanna D, Fransen J, Johnson SR, Baron M, Tyndall A, et al. 2013 classification criteria for systemic sclerosis: an American College of Rheumatology/European League against Rheumatism collaborative initiative. Arthritis Rheum. 2013;65:2737–47.
3. Cappelli S, Bellando-Randone S, Guiducci S, Matucci-Cerinic M. Is immunosuppressive therapy the anchor treatment to achieve remission in systemic sclerosis? Rheumatology (Oxford). 2014;53:975–87.
4. Kowal-Bielecka O, Landewe R, Avouac J, Chwiesko S, Miniati I, Czirjak L, et al. EULAR recommendations for the treatment of systemic sclerosis: a report from the EULAR Scleroderma Trials and Research group (EUSTAR). Ann Rheum Dis. 2009;68:620–8.
5. Mayes MD, Lacey Jr JV, Beebe-Dimmer J, Gillespie BW, Cooper B, Laing TJ, et al. Prevalence, incidence, survival, and disease characteristics of systemic sclerosis in a large US population. Arthritis Rheum. 2003;48:2246–55.
6. Bosello S, De LG, Tolusso B, Lama G, Angelucci C, Sica G, et al. B cells in systemic sclerosis: a possible target for therapy. Autoimmun Rev. 2011;10: 624–30.
7. Hasegawa M. B lymphocytes: shedding new light on the pathogenesis of systemic sclerosis. J Dermatol. 2010;37:3–10.
8. Sakkas LI, Bogdanos DP. Systemic sclerosis: new evidence re-enforces the role of B cells. Autoimmun Rev. 2016;15:155–61.
9. Zuber JP, Spertini F. Immunological basis of systemic sclerosis. Rheumatology (Oxford). 2006;45 Suppl 3:iii23–5.
10. Sato S, Fujimoto M, Hasegawa M, Takehara K. Altered blood B lymphocyte homeostasis in systemic sclerosis: expanded naive B cells and diminished but activated memory B cells. Arthritis Rheum. 2004;50:1918–27.
11. Bosello S, De SM, Lama G, Spano C, Angelucci C, Tolusso B, et al. B cell depletion in diffuse progressive systemic sclerosis: safety, skin score modification and IL-6 modulation in an up to thirty-six months follow-up open-label trial. Arthritis Res Ther. 2010;12:R54.
12. Daoussis D, Liossis SN, Tsamandas AC, Kalogeropoulou C, Kazantzi A, Sirinian C, et al. Experience with rituximab in scleroderma: results from a 1-year, proof-of-principle study. Rheumatology (Oxford). 2010;49:271–80.
13. Fleischmajer R, Perlish JS, Reeves JR. Cellular infiltrates in scleroderma skin. Arthritis Rheum. 1977;20:975–84.
14. Lafyatis R, Kissin E, York M, Farina G, Viger K, Fritzler MJ, et al. B cell depletion with rituximab in patients with diffuse cutaneous systemic sclerosis. Arthritis Rheum. 2009;60:578–83.
15. Whitfield ML, Finlay DR, Murray JI, Troyanskaya OG, Chi JT, Pergamenschikov A, et al. Systemic and cell type-specific gene expression patterns in scleroderma skin. Proc Natl Acad Sci U S A. 2003;100:12319–24.
16. Lanteri A, Sobanski V, Langlois C, Lefevre G, Hauspie C, Sanges S, et al. Serum free light chains of immunoglobulins as biomarkers for systemic sclerosis characteristics, activity and severity. Autoimmun Rev. 2014;13:974–80.
17. Sato S, Fujimoto M, Hasegawa M, Takehara K, Tedder TF. Altered B lymphocyte function induces systemic autoimmunity in systemic sclerosis. Mol Immunol. 2004;41:1123–33.
18. Hasegawa M, Sato S, Takehara K. Augmented production of transforming growth factor-beta by cultured peripheral blood mononuclear cells from patients with systemic sclerosis. Arch Dermatol Res. 2004;296:89–93.
19. Matsushita T, Hasegawa M, Yanaba K, Kodera M, Takehara K, Sato S. Elevated serum BAFF levels in patients with systemic sclerosis: enhanced BAFF signaling in systemic sclerosis B lymphocytes. Arthritis Rheum. 2006;54:192–201.
20. Denton CP. Systemic sclerosis: from pathogenesis to targeted therapy. Clin Exp Rheumatol. 2015;33:S3–7.
21. Daoussis D, Liossis SN, Tsamandas AC, Kalogeropoulou C, Paliogianni F, Sirinian C, et al. Effect of long-term treatment with rituximab on pulmonary function and skin fibrosis in patients with diffuse systemic sclerosis. Clin Exp Rheumatol. 2012;30:S17–22.
22. Jordan S, Distler JH, Maurer B, Huscher D, van Laar JM, Allanore Y, et al. Effects and safety of rituximab in systemic sclerosis: an analysis from the European Scleroderma Trial and Research (EUSTAR) group. Ann Rheum Dis. 2015;74:1188–94.
23. Smith V, Van Praet JT, Vandooren B, Van der Cruyssen B, Naeyaert JM, Decuman S, et al. Rituximab in diffuse cutaneous systemic sclerosis: an open-label clinical and histopathological study. Ann Rheum Dis. 2010;69:193–7.
24. Sato S, Hasegawa M, Fujimoto M, Tedder TF, Takehara K. Quantitative genetic variation in CD19 expression correlates with autoimmunity. J Immunol. 2000;165:6635–43.
25. Herbst R, Wang Y, Gallagher S, Mittereder N, Kuta E, Damschroder M, et al. B-cell depletion in vitro and in vivo with an afucosylated anti-CD19 antibody. J Pharmacol Exp Ther. 2010;335:213–22.
26. Ward E, Mittereder N, Kuta E, Sims GP, Bowen MA, Dall'Acqua W, et al. A glycoengineered anti-CD19 antibody with potent antibody-dependent cellular cytotoxicity activity in vitro and lymphoma growth inhibition in vivo. Br J Haematol. 2011;155:426–37.
27. Clements PJ, Lachenbruch PA, Seibold JR, Zee B, Steen VD, Brennan P, et al. Skin thickness score in systemic sclerosis: an assessment of interobserver variability in 3 independent studies. J Rheumatol. 1993;20:1892–6.
28. Streicher K, Morehouse CA, Groves CJ, Rajan B, Pilataxi F, Lehmann KP, et al. The plasma cell signature in autoimmune disease. Arthritis Rheumatol. 2014; 66:173–84.
29. Clements P, Lachenbruch P, Siebold J, White B, Weiner S, Martin R, et al. Inter and intraobserver variability of total skin thickness score (modified Rodnan TSS) in systemic sclerosis. J Rheumatol. 1995;22:1281–5.
30. Khanna D, Furst DE, Hays RD, Park GS, Wong WK, Seibold JR, et al. Minimally important difference in diffuse systemic sclerosis: results from the D-penicillamine study. Ann Rheum Dis. 2006;65:1325–9.
31. Hankinson JL, Odencrantz JR, Fedan KB. Spirometric reference values from a sample of the general U.S. population. Am J Respir Crit Care Med. 1999;159: 179–87.
32. Hankinson JL, Crapo RO, Jensen RL. Spirometric reference values for the 6-s FVC maneuver. Chest. 2003;124:1805–11.
33. Miller MR, Hankinson J, Brusasco V, Burgos F, Casaburi R, Coates A, et al. Standardisation of spirometry. Eur Respir J. 2005;26:319–38.
34. Bertina RM. The prothrombin 20210 G to A variation and thrombosis. Curr Opin Hematol. 1998;5:339–42.

35. Rituxan [package insert]. South San Francisco, CA: Genentech, Inc., 2014.
36. Lemtrada [package insert]. Cambridge, MA: Genzyme Corporation, 2014.
37. Chung CH. Managing premedications and the risk for reactions to infusional monoclonal antibody therapy. Oncologist. 2008;13:725–32.
38. Brennan PJ, Rodriguez BT, Hsu FI, Sloane DE, Castells MC. Hypersensitivity reactions to mAbs: 105 desensitizations in 23 patients, from evaluation to treatment. J Allergy Clin Immunol. 2009;124:1259–66.
39. Baldo BA. Adverse events to monoclonal antibodies used for cancer therapy: Focus on hypersensitivity responses. Oncoimmunology. 2013;2:e26333.
40. van Vollenhoven RF, Emery P, Bingham III CO, Keystone EC, Fleischmann RM, Furst DE, et al. Long-term safety of rituximab in rheumatoid arthritis: 9.5-year follow-up of the global clinical trial programme with a focus on adverse events of interest in RA patients. Ann Rheum Dis. 2013;72:1496–502.
41. Clifford DB, Ances B, Costello C, Rosen-Schmidt S, Andersson M, Parks D, et al. Rituximab-associated progressive multifocal leukoencephalopathy in rheumatoid arthritis. Arch Neurol. 2011;68:1156–64.
42. Harris HE. Progressive multifocal leucoencephalopathy in a patient with systemic lupus erythematosus treated with rituximab. Rheumatology (Oxford). 2008;47:224–5.
43. Rios-Fernandez R, Gutierrez-Salmeron MT, Callejas-Rubio JL, Fernandez-Pugnaire M, Ortego-Centeno N. Late-onset neutropenia following rituximab treatment in patients with autoimmune diseases. Br J Dermatol. 2007;157: 1271–3.
44. Dunleavy K, Tay K, Wilson WH. Rituximab-associated neutropenia. Semin Hematol. 2010;47:180–6.
45. Keizer RJ, Huitema AD, Schellens JH, Beijnen JH. Clinical pharmacokinetics of therapeutic monoclonal antibodies. Clin Pharmacokinet. 2010;49:493–507.
46. Sfikakis PP, Boletis JN, Tsokos GC. Rituximab anti-B-cell therapy in systemic lupus erythematosus: pointing to the future. Curr Opin Rheumatol. 2005;17:550–7.
47. Huang H, Benoist C, Mathis D. Rituximab specifically depletes short-lived autoreactive plasma cells in a mouse model of inflammatory arthritis. Proc Natl Acad Sci U S A. 2010;107:4658–63.
48. Engel P, Gomez-Puerta JA, Ramos-Casals M, Lozano F, Bosch X. Therapeutic targeting of B cells for rheumatic autoimmune diseases. Pharmacol Rev. 2011;63:127–56.
49. Mahevas M, Michel M, Weill JC, Reynaud CA. Long-lived plasma cells in autoimmunity: lessons from B-cell depleting therapy. Front Immunol. 2013;4:494.
50. DiLillo DJ, Hamaguchi Y, Ueda Y, Yang K, Uchida J, Haas KM, et al. Maintenance of long-lived plasma cells and serological memory despite mature and memory B cell depletion during CD20 immunotherapy in mice. J Immunol. 2008;180:361–71.
51. Owczarczyk K, Lal P, Abbas AR, Wolslegel K, Holweg CT, Dummer W, et al. A plasmablast biomarker for nonresponse to antibody therapy to CD20 in rheumatoid arthritis. Sci Transl Med. 2011;3:101ra92.
52. Dalakas MC. B cells as therapeutic targets in autoimmune neurological disorders. Nat Clin Pract Neurol. 2008;4:557–67.
53. Tedder TF. CD19: a promising B cell target for rheumatoid arthritis. Nat Rev Rheumatol. 2009;5:572–7.
54. Eisenberg R, Looney RJ. The therapeutic potential of anti-CD20: What do B-cells do? Clin Immunol. 2005;117:207–13.
55. Sabahi R, Anolik JH. B-cell-targeted therapy for systemic lupus erythematosus. Drugs. 2006;66:1933–48.
56. Daoussis D, Liossis SN. B cells tell scleroderma fibroblasts to produce collagen. Arthritis Res Ther. 2013;15:125.
57. Francois A, Chatelus E, Wachsmann D, Sibilia J, Bahram S, Alsaleh G, et al. B lymphocytes and B-cell activating factor promote collagen and profibrotic markers expression by dermal fibroblasts in systemic sclerosis. Arthritis Res Ther. 2013;15:R168.

TIM-1 defines a human regulatory B cell population that is altered in frequency and function in systemic sclerosis patients

Octavio Aravena[1], Ashley Ferrier[1], Madhvi Menon[2], Claudia Mauri[2], Juan Carlos Aguillón[1], Lilian Soto[1,3] and Diego Catalán[1*]

Abstract

Background: Systemic sclerosis (SSc) is a systemic autoimmune disease characterized by excessive production of extracellular matrix by fibroblasts on skin and internal organs. Although Th2 cells have been involved in fibroblast stimulation, hyperactivated B cells may also play an important role. Regulatory B cells (Bregs) are cells capable of inhibiting inflammatory responses and controlling autoimmune diseases. Although many Breg populations have in common the ability to produce high amounts of IL-10, a unique surface marker defining most human Bregs is lacking. It has been described in mice that T cell Ig and mucin domain protein 1 (TIM-1) is an inclusive marker for Bregs, and that TIM-1+ B cells are able to prevent the development of autoimmunity. The aim of this work was to evaluate TIM-1 as a marker for human IL-10$^+$ Bregs, and to determine whether TIM-1+ B cells are defective in SSc patients.

Methods: SSc patients (n = 39) and 53 healthy subjects were recruited. TIM-1 and IL-10 expression was assessed in resting or activated peripheral blood CD19$^+$ B cells by flow cytometry. The regulatory function of TIM-1$^+$ or activated B cells from SSc patients and healthy subjects was assessed in autologous and allogenic co-cultures with CD4$^+$ T cells, where T cell proliferation and IFN-γ, IL-17, TNF-α and IL-4 production by T cells was measured by flow cytometry.

Results: TIM-1 and IL-10 were preferentially expressed in transitional B cells, but were upregulated in naïve and memory B cells upon stimulation. The frequency of transitional TIM-1$^+$ IL-10$^+$ B cells was significantly decreased in SSc patients compared to healthy controls. In addition, activated B cells from SSc patients induced stronger allogenic Th1 and Th2 responses than activated B cells from healthy controls. Finally, TIM-1$^+$ B cells, including transitional and non-transitional cells, exhibited a higher CD4$^+$ T cell suppressive ability than TIM-1$^-$ B cells in healthy controls, but not in SSc patients.

Conclusions: TIM-1 is a unique marker for the identification of a human IL-10$^+$ Breg subpopulation which is partially superimposed with transitional B cells. Alterations in TIM-1$^+$ B cells could contribute to the development of autoimmune diseases such as SSc.

Keywords: Regulatory B cells, TIM-1, Systemic sclerosis, IL-10

Background

B cells play a central role in immune homeostasis, not only as precursors of antibody-secreting plasma cells, but also by presenting antigens and activating T cells, secreting a multiplicity of cytokines, and performing immune regulatory functions [1, 2]. The maintenance of immune tolerance and prevention of autoimmunity is exerted by different subpopulations of regulatory B cells (Bregs), which include type 2 marginal zone precursors [3], CD1d^{high}CD5$^+$ B10 cells [4], plasmablasts [5], and plasma cells [6] in mice; and CD24^{high}CD38^{high} transitional B cells [7], CD24^{high}CD27$^+$ B10 cells [8], and CD25^{high}CD86^{high} B cells [9] in humans. Nearly all of them have been functionally classified as regulatory based on their ability to secrete interleukin (IL)-10, suppress the differentiation or activation of pro-inflammatory immune cells, such as monocytes, dendritic cells, CD4$^+$ T cells, and cytotoxic

* Correspondence: dfcatalan@med.uchile.cl
[1]Programa Disciplinario de Inmunología, Instituto de Ciencias Biomédicas (ICBM), Facultad de Medicina, Universidad de Chile, and Millennium Institute in Immunology and Immunotherapy, Santiago, Chile
Full list of author information is available at the end of the article

$CD8^+$ T cells and/or induce the differentiation or activation of regulatory T cells and invariant natural killer T (iNKT) [10]. However, a unique marker common to most human Breg populations has not been found so far.

Studies in mice have postulated T cell Ig and mucin domain protein 1 (TIM-1) as an inclusive marker for IL-10^+ Bregs [11–13]. TIM-1 binds to phosphatidylserine, which is flipped to the outer leaflet of apoptotic cell membranes, conveying phagocytosis by macrophages and IL-10 expression by B cells [11, 14]. Adoptive transfer of TIM-1^+ B cells prevents allograft rejection and attenuates the development of experimental autoimmune encephalomyelitis (EAE) [12], while susceptible mice with a mutated TIM-1 molecule develop accelerated lupus [13]. Although TIM-1 $^+$ cells have been found to be enriched in IL-10-expressing human B cells [15–17], their regulatory function and their association with systemic autoimmune diseases have been insufficiently characterized.

Systemic Sclerosis (SSc) is a systemic autoimmune disease with pathophysiological features based on three phenomena: autoimmunity, fibrosis and vasculopathy, which in conjunction lead to a complex pattern of manifestations that include an excessive deposition of extracellular matrix on skin and internal organs, transient vasoconstriction events, and the production of a wide spectrum of autoantibodies [18]. This disease is classified in limited cutaneous (lcSSc) and diffuse cutaneous (dcSSc), according to the degree of skin sclerosis, internal organ involvement, and autoantibody profile [18].

Patients with SSc have a high frequency of circulating and skin-infiltrating type 2 $CD4^+$ T helper cells (Th2) producing profibrotic cytokines such as IL-4 [19, 20]. More recently, IL-17 and IL-22-producing $CD4^+$ T cells (Th17 and Th22, respectively) were also found to be expanded in blood from patients with SSc and have been related to SSc pathogenesis [21, 22]. Furthermore, regulatory cells, such as $CD4^+$ regulatory T cells (Tregs), that keep those pathogenic populations in check, are defective in patients with SSc [23].

B cells exhibit a hyperactivated phenotype in patients with SSc, with high expression of activation molecules and inflammatory cytokines [24, 25], but low expression of IL-10 [26–28]. Moreover, several reports have confirmed the benefits of B cell depletion therapies on skin fibrosis and lung function in patients with SSc [29]. However, it is not known whether Bregs from patients with SSc are able to restrain the activation of pro-inflammatory $CD4^+$ T cell responses.

Transitional B cells have been previously ascribed with regulatory functions; however, only around 15% of them produce IL-10 [7]. Therefore, we set out to investigate whether TIM-1 could better identify the IL-10-producing population amongst transitional B cells. In addition, we investigated the presence of functional alterations in TIM-1-expressing B cells in Th2-driven systemic autoimmune disease with hyperactivated B cells such as SSc. Results herein show that TIM-1 identifies most IL-10^+ B cells amongst transitional B cells. We also show that the frequency of TIM-1^+ transitional B cells, but not of other B cell subsets, was reduced in patients with SSc compared to healthy controls. In addition, we observed that activated B cells from patients with SSc potentiate Th1 and Th2 responses, instead of suppressing $CD4^+$ T cell responses as in healthy donors. Finally, while transitional and non-transitional TIM-1^+ B cells from healthy subjects suppressed $CD4^+$ T cell activation, TIM-1^+ B cells from patients with SSc did not, suggesting a functional defect of Bregs in this disease.

Methods

Patients and controls

Peripheral blood samples from 39 patients with SSc meeting the American College of Rheumatology/European League Against Rheumatism Classification Criteria for SSc [30], and 53 healthy controls, were obtained for B cell characterization, and purification of B and T cells. Characteristics of SSc and healthy controls can be found in Table 1. This study was approved by the Ethical Committees of the Hospital Clínico and Facultad de Medicina, Universidad de Chile, and UCLH-National Health Service Trust, London, UK. All subjects gave written informed consent in accordance with the Declaration of Helsinki.

Flow cytometry and cell sorting

Dead cells were excluded from flow cytometry analysis and cell sorting using the LIVE/DEAD® staining kit (Thermo Fisher Scientific, Waltham, MA, USA). The following anti-human antibodies were used for flow cytometry or cell sorting: anti-CD19 FITC (clone HIB19), anti-CD24 PECy7 (clone ML5), anti-CD38 APC (clone HB-7), anti-IL-10 PE (clone JES3-9D7), anti-TIM-1 PE (clone 1D12), anti-CD3 APC (clone SK7), anti-interferon (IFN)-γ (clone 4S.B3), anti-IL-4 PE (clone MP4-25D2), and anti-IL-17 PerCP (clone BL168) (BioLegend, San Diego, CA, USA). To assess co-expression of IL-10 and TIM-1 on B cells, an anti-TIM-1 Alexa Fluor 488 antibody (clone 219211; R&D Systems Inc, MN, USA) was used. Intracellular cytokines were stained using Permeabilization and IC Fixation Buffers (eBioscience, San Diego, CA, USA). Samples were acquired and sorted with a FACSAria III cell sorter (Becton Dickinson, NJ, USA), and data was analyzed with the FloJo X Software (OR, USA).

B and T cell isolation

Untouched $CD19^+$ B cells and $CD4^+$ T cells were isolated from fresh heparinized whole blood or buffy coats with the RosetteSep Human B cell or $CD4^+$ T Cell Enrichment Cocktail kits, respectively (Stemcell Technologies, Vancouver, Canada).

Table 1 Main demographic and clinical characteristics of the patients with systemic sclerosis and healthy controls

Characteristics	Patients (n = 39)	Controls (n = 53)
Female/male, *n*	30/9	28/25
Age, mean ± SD	48.4 ± 11.3	40.0 ± 13.7
Disease duration, months, mean ± SD	95.4 ± 100.7	
lcSSc/dcSSc, *n*	26/13	
Rodnan score, mean ± SD	13.8 ± 6.8	
Corrected DLCO[a], mean ± SD	19.7 ± 6.7	
ANA pattern[b], *n* (%)		
Speckled	10/34 (29.4)	
Nucleolar	9/34 (26.5)	
Homogeneous	9/34 (26.5)	
Centromere	16/34 (47.1)	
Anti-Scl-70 positivity	6/33 (18.2)	
Organ involvement, *n* (%)		
Peripheral vascular	16 (41.6)	
Gastrointestinal tract	27 (69.2)	
Lung	21 (53.8)	
Heart	16 (41.0)	
Kidney	4 (10.2)	
Therapy, *n*/total number		
Prednisone	3/39	
Azathioprine + prednisone	2/39	
Methotrexate	4/39	
D-penicillamine	1/39	
Methotrexate + D-penicillamine	1/39	
Methotrexate + D-penicillamine + prednisone	1/39	
Hydroxychloroquine	4/39	
Methotrexate + hydroxychloroquine	1/39	
Only symptomatic treatment	22/39	

[a]Measured in 25 patients. [b]Some patients have more than one pattern. *SD* standard deviation, *lcSSc* limited cutaneous systemic sclerosis, *dcSSc* diffuse cutaneous systemic sclerosis, *Corrected DLCO* Diffusing capacity for carbon monoxide correction of predicted value for hemoglobin, *ANA* antinuclear antibody

B cell activation

Isolated B cells were cultured for 48 hours in RPMI 1640 medium supplemented with 10% fetal bovine serum (HyClone, GE Healthcare, USA) at a 1×10^6 cells/ml density, 37 °C and 5% CO_2, in presence or absence of 5 μg/ml polyclonal anti-human IgG + IgM goat antibodies (Jackson Immunoresearch, West Grove, PA, USA) to activate the B cell receptor (BCR) and 3 μg/ml ODN 2006 Class B CpG oligonucleotide to activate Toll-like receptor 9 (TLR9) (Invivogen, San Diego, CA, USA). To evaluate IL-10 secretion by ELISA (Biolegend), cells were stimulated with 50 ng/ml phorbol 12-myristate 13-acetate (PMA) and 1 μg/ml ionomycin (Sigma-Aldrich, Saint Louis, MO, USA) for the last 5 hours of culture, and for intracellular detection of cytokines by flow cytometry, 1 μg/ml brefeldin A (eBioscience) was simultaneously added.

$CD4^+$ T cell and B cell co-cultures

For autologous co-cultures, total B cells and $CD4^+$ T cells from healthy donors were isolated. B cells were cultured for 48 hours in absence of stimulus or were stimulated with anti-BCR antibodies plus CpG, as indicated above. Next, B cells were harvested, washed thoroughly and plated at a 1:1 ratio with 5,6-carboxylfluorescein diacetate succinimidyl ester (CFSE)-labeled autologous $CD4^+$ T cells (1×10^6 total cells/ml) and anti-CD3/anti-CD28 antibody-conjugated beads (Life Technologies, Paisley, UK) for 5 days. To assess the regulatory ability of activated B cells from patients with SSc, an allogenic assay was performed. B cells from patients with SSc or sex-matched and age-matched healthy donors, either unstimulated or stimulated for 48 hours, were co-cultured for 4 days at a 1:1 ratio with CFSE-labeled $CD4^+$ T cells from a single healthy donor, in order to exclude the intrinsic cytokine profile of $CD4^+$ T cells from patients with SSc [21]. In some cases, TIM-1^+ and TIM-1^- $CD19^+$ B cells from patients with SSc or healthy donors were sorted by fluorescence-activated cell sorting, and immediately plated with autologous CFSE-labelled $CD4^+$ T cells at a 1:1 ratio and anti-CD3/anti-CD28 beads for 5 days. In another experiment, TIM-1^+ $CD24^{high}$ $CD38^{high}$ transitional B cells, TIM-1^- $CD24^{high}$ $CD38^{high}$ transitional B cells and TIM-1^+ $CD24^{med/low}$ $CD38^{med/low}$ non-transitional B cells from healthy donors were isolated by cell sorting and were cultured with autologous $CD4^+$ $CD25^-$ T cells stimulated with 0.5 ug/ml plate-bound anti-CD3 antibody, at a 1:2 ratio for 3 days. For all co-cultures, 50 ng/ml PMA, 1 μg/ml ionomycin and 1 μg/ml brefeldin A was added for the last 5 hours, and intracellular IFN-γ, IL-4, IL-17 or TNF-α expression in $CD4^+$ T cells was determined by flow cytometry. An inhibition index was calculated according to the following formula:

Inhibition index = 1 - (Percentage of cytokine-producing CD4+ T cells in presence of B cells/Percentage of cytokine-producing CD4+ T cells activated with anti-CD3/anti-CD28 alone).

Statistical analyses

The two-tailed unpaired or paired Student *t* test was used when appropriate to make comparisons between two conditions or between patients with SSc and healthy controls. Analysis of variance (ANOVA) for repeated measures with Bonferroni post-test correction was used for comparisons between B cell subpopulations. The Spearman test was used to test for correlation between continuous variables. A P value $<0.05$was considered significant. All analyses were performed with GraphPad Prism 6 (La Jolla, CA, USA).

Results

Patients with SSc exhibit reduced peripheral blood TIM-1 + transitional B cells

First, the expression of TIM-1 was evaluated on different human circulating B cell subpopulations. For this purpose, peripheral blood mononuclear cells were isolated and $CD19^+$ B cell subpopulations were defined by flow cytometry according to the expression of CD24 and CD38 in: $CD19^+$ $CD24^{high}$ $CD38^{high}$ transitional B cells, $CD19^+$ $CD24^{med}$ $CD38^{med}$ naïve B cells, $CD19^+$ $CD24^{high}$ $CD38^{med}$ memory B cells, and $CD19^+$ $CD24^-$ $CD38^{high}$ plasmablasts, as described elsewhere [31] (Fig. 1a). As shown in Fig. 1a, TIM-1 was expressed in all subpopulations except plasmablasts. Transitional B cells exhibited a markedly higher frequency of TIM-1-expressing cells (around 35%), compared to naïve and memory cells (Fig. 1a).

Defects in different subsets of Bregs have been described in several autoimmune diseases [7, 32]. Our group has previously reported that compared to healthy controls, patients with SSc, have an increased frequency of transitional B cells, but a decreased proportion of IL-10-producing transitional B cells after short stimulation with PMA and ionomycin, and also a decreased frequency of $CD25^{high}$ $CD27^{high}$ $CD86^{high}$ $CD1d^{high}$ B cells, which are regarded as regulatory [9, 28]. To assess whether defects in the expression of TIM-1 in B cells are associated with the development of SSc, frequencies of TIM-1^+ B cells in peripheral blood of patients with SSc and healthy controls were compared. Reduced frequency of B cells expressing TIM-1 was observed exclusively in the transitional subpopulation in patients with SSc (Fig. 1b).

The hyperactivated phenotype of B cells in SSc has been attributed to exacerbated activity of the activating molecule CD19, and CD19 expression levels have been found to be increased in naïve and memory B cell subpopulations in patients with SSc [24, 33, 34]. Recently, we have demonstrated that CD19, together with activation markers CD86 and CD40, are upregulated in transitional B cells from patients with SSc [28]. Correlation analysis was performed to find out if there is a relationship between reduced expression of TIM-1 and the hyperactivated phenotype of SSc B cells. Although there was no significant correlation between the expression of TIM-1 and CD86 or CD40 (data not shown), there was direct correlation between the expression of TIM-1 and CD19 in transitional B cells (Fig. 1c).

BCR and TLR9 activation induces an increase in TIM-1 expression that is impaired in B cells from patients with SSc

Combined stimulation of the BCR and TLR9 in human B cells induces robust IL-10 secretion and equips them with the ability to suppress T cell activation [35]. Therefore, the possibility that TIM-1, as a marker of Bregs, could change its expression after B cell activation was explored. A significant increase in TIM-1 expression upon activation of BCR and TLR9 was observed in all studied B cell subpopulations except plasmablasts (Fig. 2a). Similar to constitutive TIM-1 expression on transitional B cells, the percentage of transitional B cells expressing TIM-1 after activation of BCR and TLR9 was lower in patients with SSc than in healthy controls (Fig. 2b).

Activation of B cells has been involved with lung and skin fibrosis in a murine model of SSc [36]. Accordingly, lungs from SSc-associated interstitial lung disease and skin samples from patients with SSc exhibit B cell infiltration [37, 38]. Moreover, B cell depletion therapy has shown a beneficial effect on lung function and skin fibrosis in patients with SSc [39]. Therefore, we assessed a possible association between TIM-1 expression and parameters related to lung and skin fibrosis. Interestingly, TIM-1 expression levels on transitional B cells, either unstimulated or stimulated, were higher in patients with SSc who presented with the diffuse cutaneous form of the disease (Fig. 2c). Moreover, there was correlation between worse respiratory function, measured as a lower DLCO, and higher TIM-1 expression levels on stimulated transitional B cells (Fig. 2d). Likewise, there was direct correlation between TIM-1 levels on unstimulated or stimulated transitional B cells and the Rodnan score, which mirrors the degree of skin fibrosis (Fig. 2e). There was no significant association between TIM-1 expression on B cells and the presence of autoantibodies or involvement of internal organs.

A subpopulation of human transitional B cells co-express TIM-1 and IL-10, an ability that is compromised in B cells from patients with SSc

So far, the main common trait for all human regulatory B cell populations is the expression of IL-10. In order to verify whether human TIM-1 is preferentially expressed on IL-10-producing B cells, as previously shown in mice [14], B cells were isolated and stimulated with PMA and ionomycin, and co-expression of surface TIM-1 and intracellular IL-10 was assessed by flow cytometry. As previously described [7], transitional B cells were the subpopulation most enriched in IL-10^+ cells (Fig. 3a, upper panel). More importantly, TIM-1 was expressed in the majority of transitional IL-10^+ B cells, while naïve, memor, and plasmablast TIM-1^+ B cells did not show major IL-10 expression (Fig. 3a, upper panel). Furthermore, about 60% of transitional B cells, but also around 30% of memory B cells, co-expressed IL-10 and TIM-1 after activation with CpG and anti-BCR (Additional file 1: Figure S1). In contrast, patients with SSc had significantly decreased TIM-1^+ IL-10^+ transitional B cell frequencies after 5 hours of incubation with PMA and ionomycin (Fig. 3a, lower panel and graph). Thus, similar to murine B cells, TIM-1 was preferentially expressed in IL-10-producing B cells from healthy donors, but not from patients with SSc.

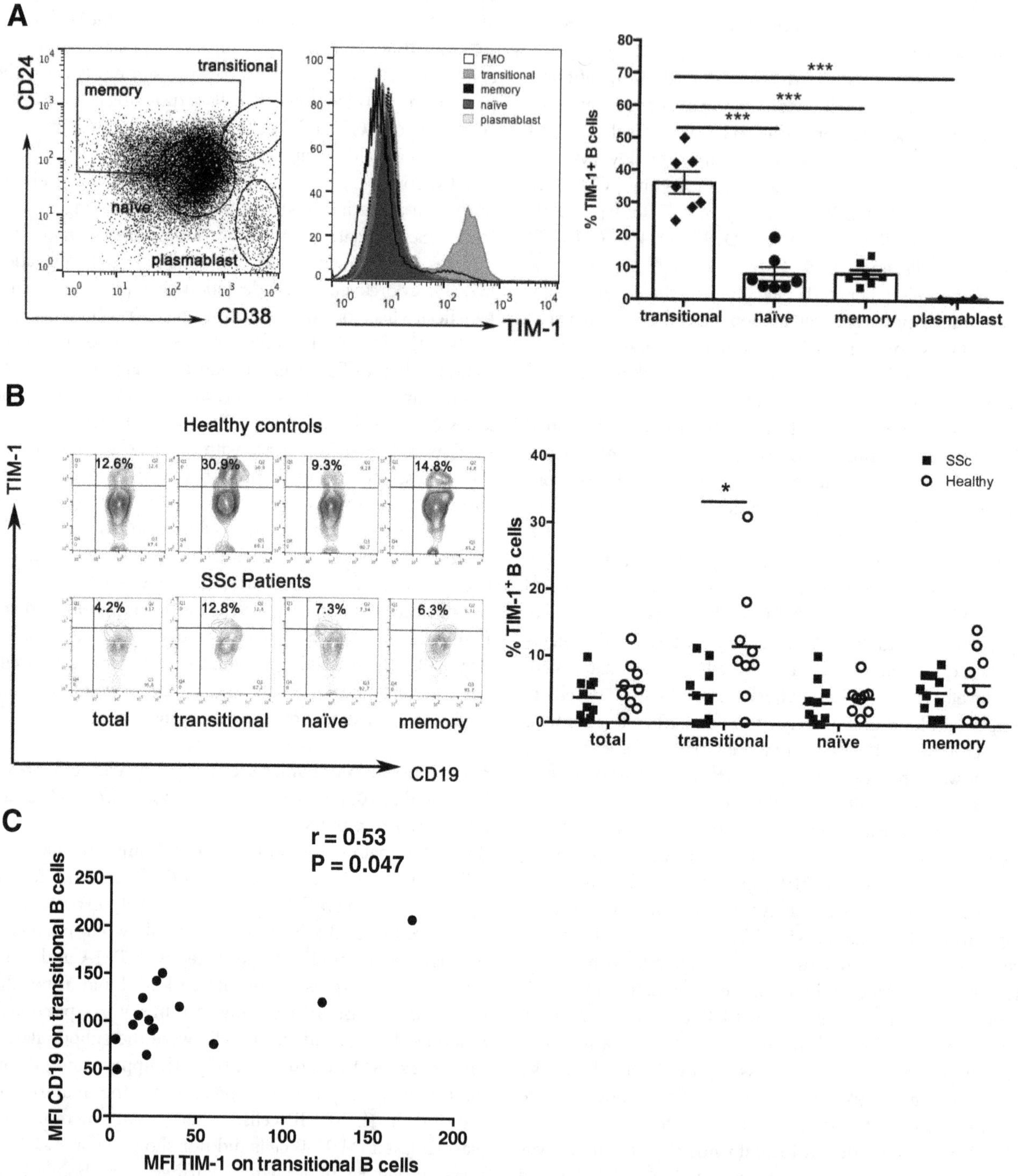

Fig. 1 T cell Ig and mucin domain protein 1 (*TIM-1*) expression by healthy and systemic sclerosis (*SSc*) B cell subpopulations. **a** *Left* representative dot-plot indicating the gating strategy to identify transitional, naïve, memory, and plasmablast B cell subpopulations according to the expression of CD24 and CD38. *Middle* representative histograms show the expression of TIM-1 in different B cell subpopulations. *Right* percentage of TIM-1-expressing B cells from healthy donors in each indicated subpopulation, n = 7. **b**. Representative dot-plots (*left*) and graph (*right*) show the frequency of TIM-1$^+$ cells on different B cell subpopulations from healthy subjects and patients with SSc. **c** Correlation between the expression levels of TIM-1 and CD19 in transitional B cells from patients with SSc. *FMO* fluorescence minus one staining control, *MFI* mean fluorescence intensity. *$P < 0.05$, ***$P < 0.001$

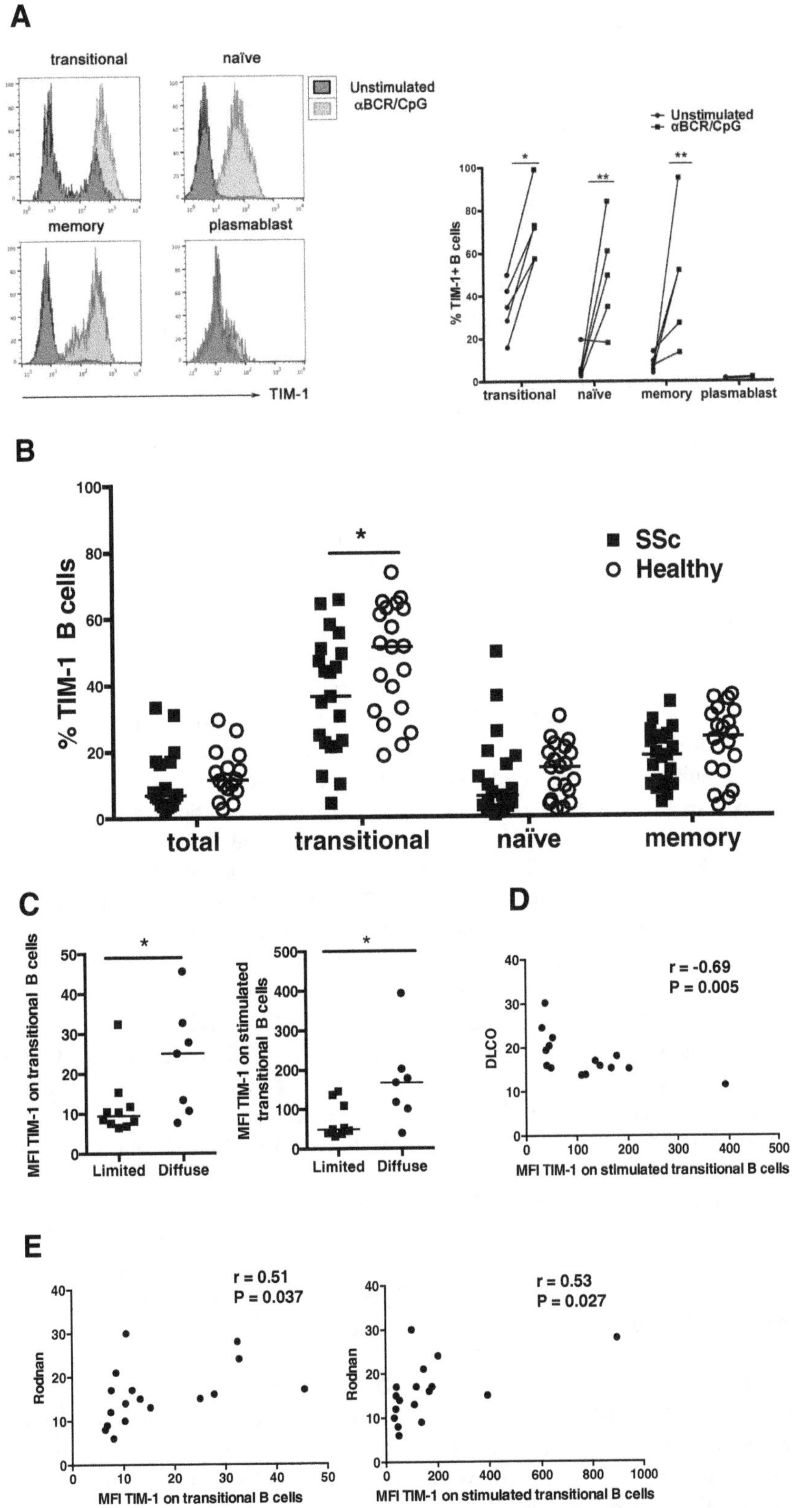

Fig. 2 (See legend on next page.)

(See figure on previous page.)
Fig. 2 T cell Ig and mucin domain protein 1 (*TIM-1*) expression upon B cell receptor (BCR) and Toll-like receptor-9 (TLR9) activation in healthy subjects and patients with systemic sclerosis (*SSc*). **a. a** Representative histograms (*left*) and summarizing graph (*right*) show the percentage of TIM-1-expressing B cells from healthy subjects in different subpopulations, left unstimulated or activated with an anti-BCR antibody (*αBCR*) and CpG for 48 hours. **b** Percentage of TIM-1$^+$ total, transitional, naïve and memory B cells from healthy controls and patients with SSc after stimulation with αBCR and CpG for 48 hours. **c** Expression levels of TIM-1 on unstimulated (*left*) or stimulated (*right*) transitional B cells from patients with SSc with the diffuse or limited form of the disease. **d** Correlation between the expression levels of TIM-1 in stimulated transitional B cells from patients with SSc and the diffusing capacity for carbon monoxide (DLCO). **e.** Correlation between the expression levels of TIM-1 in unstimulated (*left*) or stimulated (*right*) transitional B cells from patients with SSc and the Rodnan score of skin involvement. *MFI* mean fluorescence intensity. $^*P < 0.05$, $^{**}P < 0.01$

These differences are in line with decreased IL-10 secretion by B cells stimulated with PMA/ionomycin, and a reduced frequency of IL-10-producing transitional B cells, either stimulated with PMA/ionomycin alone or pre-activated with an anti-BCR antibody and CpG, observed in patients with SSc (Fig. 3b-c).

B cells from patients with SSc activated via BCR and TLR9 are unable to inhibit allogenic CD4$^+$ T cell responses

B cells activated either with CpG plus anti-BCR, or with anti-BCR alone, have been demonstrated to suppress CD4 + T cell proliferation [40, 41]. Thus, the effect of activated B cells expressing high levels of TIM-1 and IL-10 after stimulation with anti-BCR plus CpG, over polyclonally activated autologous CD4$^+$ T cells was evaluated. Significantly lower T cell proliferation and IFN-γ and IL-4 expression was observed in co-cultures with activated B cells compared to unstimulated B cells, while no differences were detected in IL-17 expression (Fig. 4a).

Thereafter, the regulatory ability of activated B cells was compared between patients with SSc and healthy controls. B cells from patients with SSc or healthy donors, either unstimulated or stimulated for 48 hours with anti-BCR plus CpG, were co-cultured with CD4$^+$ T cells from a single third-party healthy donor. As shown in Fig. 4b, stimulated B cells from patients with SSc induced greater proliferation and production of IFN-γ and IL-4 by allogenic CD4+ T cells, compared to healthy controls (Fig. 4b). These results indicate that stimulatory conditions that induce B cells to upregulate TIM-1 and IL-10, and endow them with regulatory functions, generate a Th1 and Th2 activation profile in B cells from patients with SSc.

TIM-1$^+$ B cells from healthy subjects, but not from patients with SSc, inhibit autologous CD4$^+$ T cell responses

As TIM-1 defines an important population of IL-10-producing B cells, the regulatory properties of TIM-1$^+$ B cells were evaluated. First, total TIM-1$^+$ or TIM-1$^-$ B cells from healthy subjects or patients with SSc were isolated by cell sorting. TIM-1$^+$ or TIM-1$^-$ B cells were co-cultured at a 1:1 ratio with autologous CD4$^+$ T cells, which were stimulated with anti-CD3/anti-CD28 beads. No differences were observed in the proliferative response of CD4$^+$ T cells co-cultured with TIM-1$^+$ or TIM-1$^-$ B cells from healthy controls; however, TIM-1$^+$ B cells strongly suppressed the expression of pro-inflammatory cytokines by CD4$^+$ T cells, such as IFN-γ, TNF-α, and IL-17, compared to TIM-1$^-$ B cells (Fig. 5a). There was only modest inhibition of IL-4 production by CD4$^+$ T cells with both TIM-1$^+$ and TIM-1$^-$ B cells (Fig. 5a). Conversely, TIM-1$^+$ and TIM-1$^-$ B cells from patients with SSc did not suppress CD4$^+$ T cell proliferation or production of any of the cytokines assessed (Fig. 5b).

Human TIM-1$^+$ B cells and transitional B cells exhibit a different suppressive profile

As transitional B cells have been demonstrated to suppress T cell activation [7], and TIM-1 is mainly expressed on this subpopulation along with IL-10, an assay was performed to address whether TIM-1$^+$ or transitional B cells, or both subpopulations, are responsible for the regulatory effect previously described for transitional B cells. Three B cell subpopulations were sorted: TIM-1$^+$ CD24^{high} CD38^{high} (TIM-1$^+$ transitional), TIM-1$^-$ CD24^{high} CD38^{high} (TIM-1$^-$ transitional), and TIM-1$^+$ CD24$^{med/low}$ CD38$^{med/low}$ (TIM-1$^+$ non-transitional). The sorted cells were co-cultured with autologous anti-CD3-activated CD4$^+$ CD25$^-$ T cells for 3 days, and the expression of IFN-γ and TNF-α was assessed by flow cytometry. As shown in Fig. 5c, although the three subpopulations suppressed the expression of IFN-γ, both TIM-1$^+$ subpopulations tended to achieve it in a stronger way (Fig. 5c). In contrast, on evaluation of TNF-α suppression, even though the inhibition was modest and there was wide inter-individual variation, TIM-1$^+$ non-transitional cells appeared to be more potent (Fig. 5c). These results suggest that TIM-1 identifies a population of human Bregs different from transitional B cells.

Discussion

TIM-1 is an inclusive marker for IL-10$^+$ Bregs and an important receptor for Breg induction and function in mice, probably by sensing of apoptotic cells and induction of IL-10 expression on B cells, in order to preserve tolerance to self-antigens and prevent autoimmunity [11, 12]. In humans, few studies have evaluated TIM-1 expression in B cells. Liu et al. report that TIM-1 is

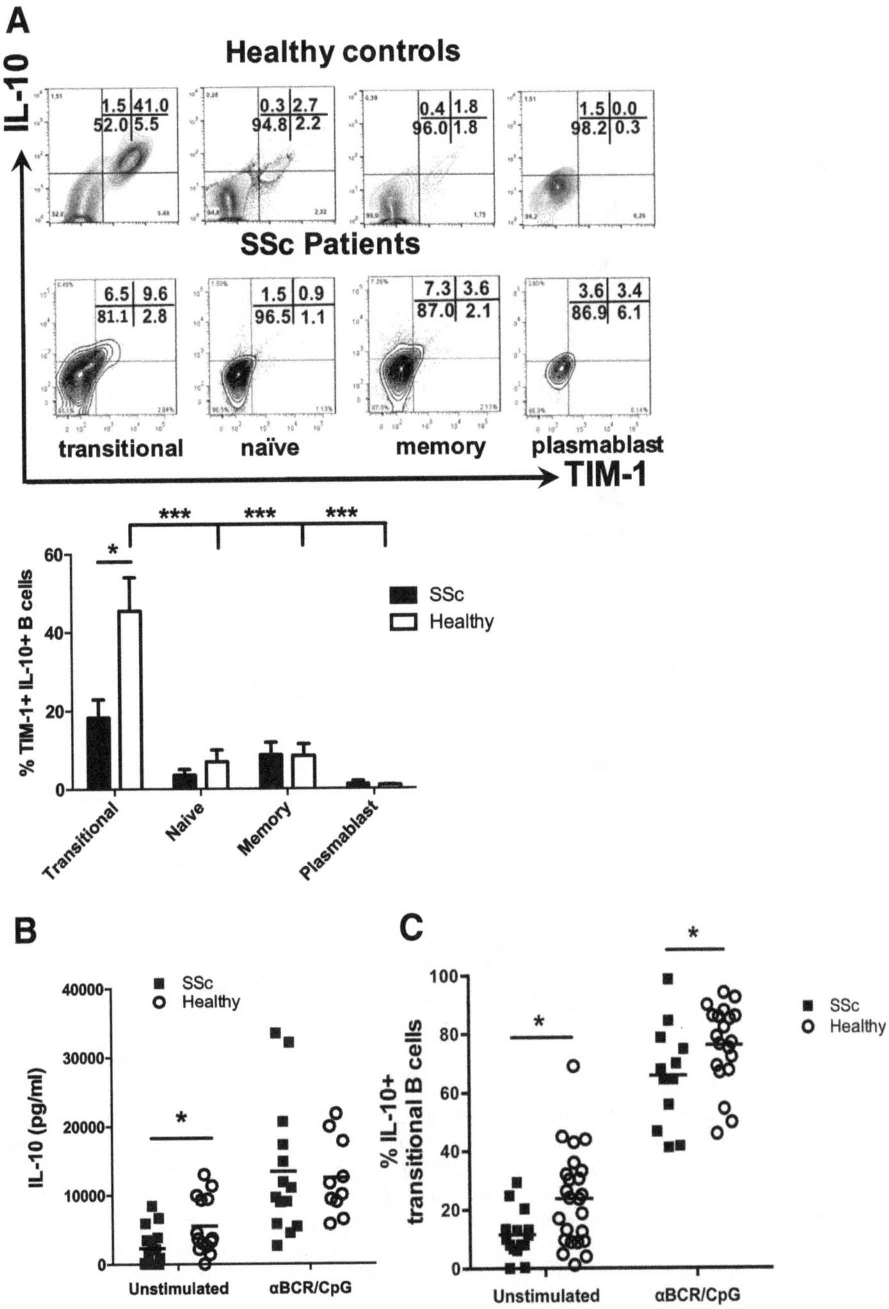

Fig. 3 Co-expression of IL-10 and T cell Ig and mucin domain protein 1 (*TIM-1*) in B cell subpopulations from healthy subjects and patients with systemic sclerosis (*SSc*). **a** Representative dot-plots (*above*) and column graph (*below*) show the percentage of TIM-1 and IL-10 expression on different B cell subpopulations from healthy controls and patients with SSc stimulated with phorbol 12-myristate 13-acetate (PMA) and ionomycin for 5 hours (n = 3 patients with SSc, n = 5 healthy controls). **b** Levels of IL-10 secreted by total B cells from healthy controls and patients with SSc stimulated with PMA and ionomycin alone or after incubation with an anti-B-cell receptor antibody (*αBCR*) and CpG for 48 hours. **c**. Percentage of IL-10$^+$ transitional B cells from healthy controls and patients with SSc stimulated under the same conditions as in **b**. *$P < 0.05$, ***$P < 0.001$

expressed in over 75% of peripheral IL-10$^+$ B cells and less than 25% of IL-10$^-$ B cells from healthy subjects [15]. In contrast, Kristensen et al. found that up to 40% of IL-10$^+$ B cells express TIM-1, which is almost absent from IL-10$^-$ B cells [16]. Similar to this observation, we show that among total B cells, around 50% of PMA/ionomycin-activated IL-10$^+$ B cells are TIM-1$^+$, whereas TIM-1 is expressed in only 10% of IL-10$^-$ B cells. The different antibody clone used to stain TIM-1 in the earlier work could explain this divergence.

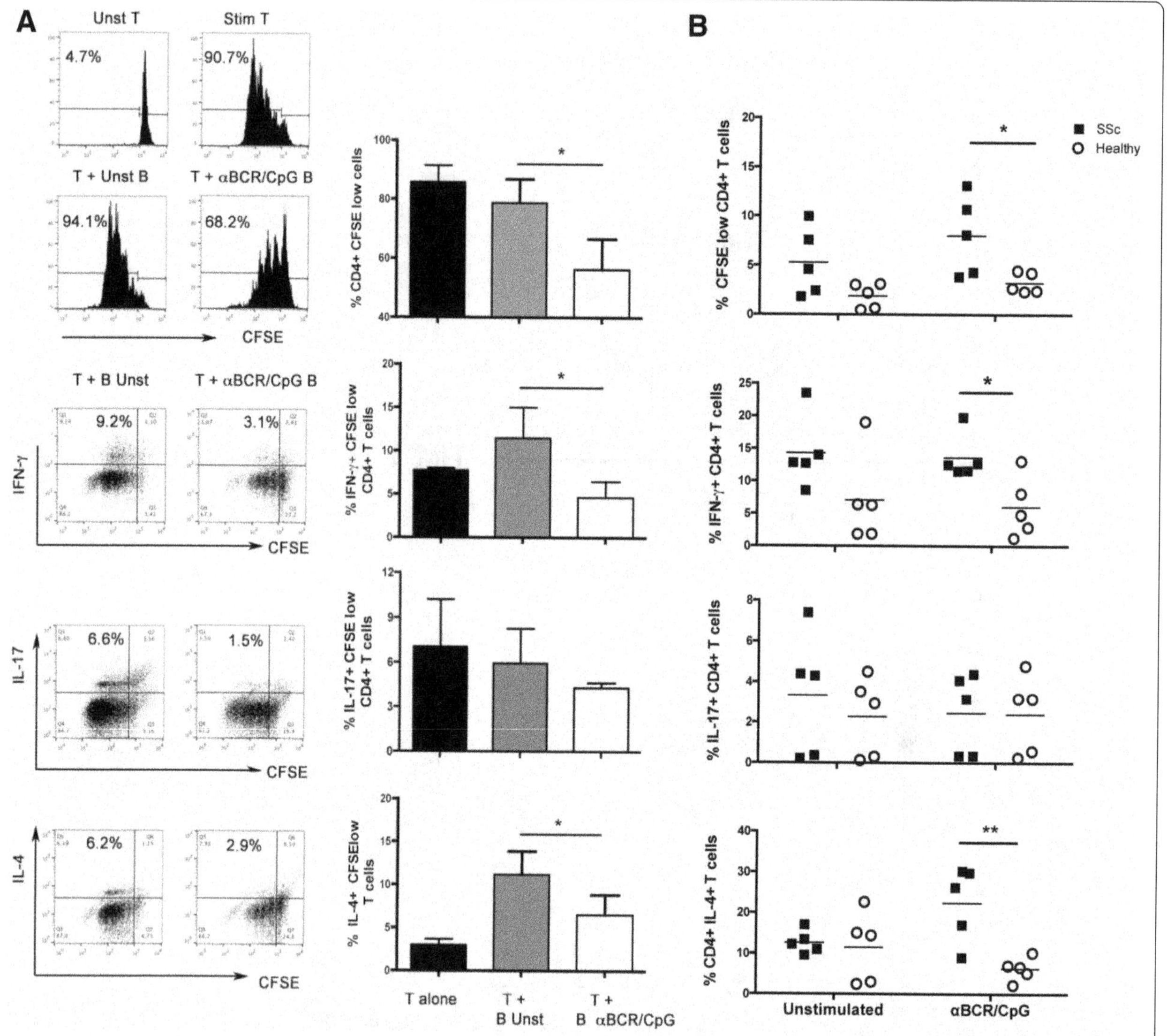

Fig. 4 Modulation of CD4$^+$ T cells by stimulated B cells from healthy controls and patients systemic sclerosis (*SSc*). **a** Representative histogram and dot-plots (*left*), and graphs (*right*) showing the effect of B cells from a healthy control stimulated with an anti-B-cell receptor antibody (*αBCR*) and CpG for 48 hours, in the proliferation (measured as percentage of 5, 6-carboxylfluorescein diacetate succinimidyl ester (*CFSE*)^{low} cells) (n = 5) and in the production of interferon (*IFN*)-γ (n = 7), IL-17 (n = 4) and IL-4 (n = 6) by autologous CD4$^+$ T cells stimulated with anti-CD3 and anti-CD28 antibodies for 5 days. CD4$^+$ T cells cultured alone (*unst T*) or only with stimulating antibodies (*stim T*) were used as negative and positive controls, respectively. **b** Graphs represent the percentage of allogenic CD4$^+$ T cells proliferating and producing IFN-γ, IL-17, and IL-4 after 4-day co-culture with B cells from patients with SSc and healthy controls, stimulated with αBCR and CpG, or left unstimulated for 48 hours. *$P < 0.05$, **$P < 0.01$

It has been shown that murine TIM-1$^+$ B cells are able to suppress Th1 responses in vivo and promote Th2 and Treg responses in an allograft transplantation setting [12]. Also, TIM-1$^+$ B cells inhibit Th1 and Th17 responses in vivo in the EAE model [13]. In humans, TIM-1 has been used as a surface marker to isolate Bregs and explore their in vitro suppressive function in HIV-infected patients, demonstrating an inhibition of antigen-specific IFN-γ and TNF-α production by CD8$^+$ and CD4$^+$ T cells [15]. Similarly, TIM-1$^+$ B cells from patients with HBV-induced hepatocellular carcinoma do not suppress granzyme and perforin production by CD4$^+$ T cells [17]. To determine whether TIM-1 identifies previously described regulatory B cell subpopulations, we evaluated TIM-1 expression in plasmablasts, transitional, naïve and memory B cells. Of interest, the transitional subpopulation, one of the better characterized human Breg subsets, was by far the most enriched in TIM-1$^+$ cells, and the majority of TIM-1$^+$ transitional B cells also co-expressed IL-10.

In addition, we found that TIM-1$^+$ B cells from healthy donors have a potent suppressive capacity compared to their TIM-1$^-$ counterparts, inhibiting the production of

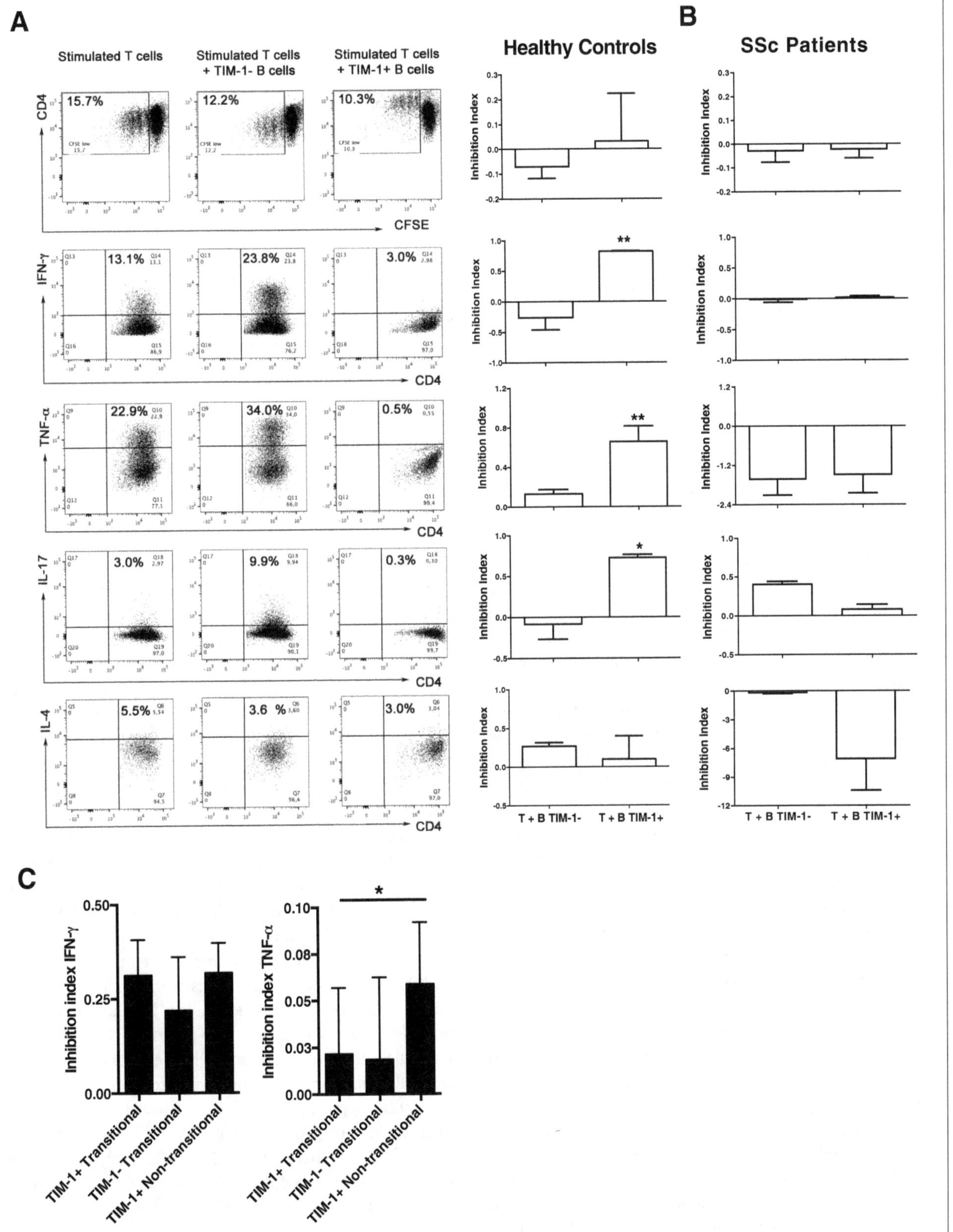

Fig. 5 (See legend on next page.)

(See figure on previous page.)
Fig. 5 Suppressive function of T cell Ig and mucin domain protein 1 (*TIM-1*)$^+$ B cells from healthy controls and patients with systemic sclerosis (*SSc*) over T cells. **a** *Left* representative dot-plots show the effect of TIM-1$^+$ and TIM-1$^-$ purified B cells from healthy controls in the proliferation (measured as percentage of 5, 6-carboxylfluorescein diacetate succinimidyl ester (*CFSE*)^{low} cells) and in the production of interferon (*IFN*)-γ, TNF-α, IL-17, and IL-4 by autologous CD4+ T cells stimulated with anti-CD3 and anti-CD28 antibodies for 5 days. *Right* suppressive effect of TIM-1$^+$ and TIM-1$^-$ B cells from healthy donors in the proliferation and the production of IFN-γ, TNF-α, IL-17, and IL-4 by autologous stimulated CD4$^+$ T, calculated as the inhibition index (1 – (percentage of activated CD4$^+$ T cells in presence of B cells/percentage of activated CD4$^+$ T cells with anti-CD3 plus anti-CD28 alone)) (n = 3). **b** Suppressive effect of TIM-1$^+$ and TIM-1$^-$ B cells from patients with SSc in the proliferation, and the production of IFN-γ, TNF-α, IL-17, and IL-4 by autologous stimulated CD4$^+$ T, calculated as inhibition index (n = 3). **c** Inhibition of the expression of IFN-γ and TNF-α by autologous activated CD4$^+$ T cells by the indicated B cell subpopulations from healthy donors (n = 3). **P* < 0.05, ***P* < 0.01

IFN-γ, TNF-α and IL-17 by activated CD4$^+$ T cells. It is noteworthy that TIM-1$^-$ transitional B cells are also able to suppress IFN-γ production by autologous CD4$^+$ T cells, although not equivalently to TIM-1$^+$ transitional B cells, and that non-transitional TIM-1$^+$ B cells also suppress IFN-γ and TNF-α production, revealing that transitional B cells and TIM-1$^+$ B cells probably correspond to two different, but partially superimposed, regulatory subpopulations. According to previous studies, IL-10 appears to be crucial in the inhibitory functions of TIM-1$^+$ and transitional B cells [7, 15, 17]; however, the involvement of other mechanisms cannot be excluded.

After stimulation of BCR and TLR9 receptors, naïve and memory B cells acquired TIM-1 expression, together with upregulation of IL-10 production. Even upon stimulation, transitional B cells comprise the highest frequency of TIM-1$^+$ and IL-10$^+$ cells. Such TIM-1 induction upon BCR activation was previously demonstrated in murine germinal center B cells [42], and could be a possible explanation for the positive correlation we observed in transitional B cells from patients with SSc, between the expression levels of TIM-1 and CD19, a B cell activating co-receptor that has been previously reported to be upregulated in SSc B cells [28, 33]. These results could imply a general mechanism to favor IL-10 production by B cells in the context of an ongoing inflammatory response, where an accumulation of apoptotic cells carrying potential autoantigens and TLR ligands, bears the inherent risk of developing autoimmunity [43].

Until now, there have been only two studies published in which the frequency of TIM-1$^+$ B cells has been evaluated in autoimmune disease [16, 44]. In the first, peripheral blood TIM-1$^+$ IL-10$^+$ B cells from patients with Graves' disease and Hashimoto's thyroiditis were found to be elevated compared to healthy donors [16]. In contrast, in patients with myasthenia gravis, the frequency of peripheral blood TIM-1$^+$ B cells was lower than in healthy controls, and was negatively correlated with disease severity [44]. SSc is a systemic autoimmune disease with hyperactivated B cells having a prominent role in its pathogenicity [24, 25], and in consequence, it is a good model for the study of Breg frequency and function. According to our results, patients with SSc have reduced frequencies of TIM-1$^+$ IL-10$^+$ B cells, but only within the transitional subpopulation, both in resting cells and after stimulation of the BCR and TLR9 receptor. Differences between our study and the one in autoimmune thyroid disease may be due to the completely disparate pathogenic mechanisms behind organ-specific autoimmune diseases such as Graves' disease and Hashimoto's thyroiditis, and a systemic disease such as SSc. Additionally, this could also be due to the fact that no characterization of B cell subpopulations expressing TIM-1 was performed in that study.

We also found that TIM-1 expression levels on transitional B cells are higher in the diffuse form of the disease, and that they are directly correlated with parameters related to the degree of skin and lung fibrosis and inflammation, such as the Rodnan score and DLCO, respectively. These results are in line with our results showing upregulation of TIM-1 after TLR9 and BCR activation, and with evidence from mouse models showing increased frequency of Bregs in response to inflammation [10, 45].

Our results show that TIM-1$^+$ B cells from patients with SSc are unable to suppress CD4$^+$ T cell activation, and that stimulated B cells from patients with SSc induced stronger activation of Th1 and Th2 allogenic responses than those from healthy controls. Two studies have described reduced frequencies of IL-10-producing Bregs in patients with SSc, upon stimulation with CD40L and CpG [26], or CpG alone [27]. In the latter work, the authors described altered activation of STAT-3 and p38 MAPK, two signaling molecules involved in IL-10 production, after stimulation of the BCR and TLR9 receptor [27]. This evidence, together with our results, points to defective regulatory functions in Bregs from patients with SSc, which could be partially explained by their inability to increase TIM-1 and IL-10, and probably other inhibitory molecules, upon stimulation, while expressing activation molecules and pro-inflammatory cytokines, such as IL-6 [25, 28], tipping the balance toward a more pro-inflammatory or pro-fibrotic profile. Although it has been proposed that hyperactivated B cells directly or indirectly help CD4$^+$ T cells to differentiate into a Th2 profile in SSc [29], this assumption had not been tested until now.

Conclusions

Overall, we have demonstrated that TIM-1 is a viable marker for IL-10$^+$ Bregs in humans and that TIM-1$^+$ B cells are decreased in frequency and have an impaired regulatory function in patients with SSc. The results presented herein do not only contribute to the characterization of a novel marker for a subpopulation of B cells with regulatory properties, but also open new routes to explore cell-based therapies, given that the surface expression of TIM-1 allows the isolation of Bregs, which could be expanded ex vivo and re-infused to patients with autoimmune disorders such as SSc, with the aim of replacing defective tolerance mechanisms.

Abbreviations

BCR: B-cell receptor; Bregs: regulatory B cells; CFSE: 5, 6-carboxylfluorescein diacetate succinimidyl ester; dcSSc: diffuse cutaneous systemic sclerosis; DLCO: Diffusing capacity for carbon monoxide; EAE: experimental autoimmune encephalomyelitis; ELISA: enzyme-linked immunosorbent assay; FMO: fluorescence minus one; IFN: interferon; IL: interleukin; lcSSc: limited cutaneous systemic sclerosis; PMA: phorbol 12-myristate 13-acetate; SSc: systemic sclerosis; Th: helper T cells; TIM-1: T cell Ig and mucin domain protein 1; TLR9: Toll-like receptor 9, Tregs, regulatory T cells

Acknowledgements

We gratefully acknowledge Dr. Katina Schinnerling for critically reviewing the manuscript, Mr. Claudio Pérez for helping to obtain the blood samples, Dr. Bárbara Pesce and Jamie Evans for their help in cell sorting and flow cytometry data acquisition and analysis, and Mrs. Nancy Fabres and Mrs. Juana Orellana for their excellent technical assistance.

Funding

This study was supported by FONDECYT-CHILE Grant N°11121497 and Millennium Institute in Immunology and Immunotherapy P09-016-F.

Authors' contributions

OA performed the majority of the experiments and characterizations, analyzed the data, and contributed to drafting the manuscript. AF helped in the execution of co-culture and ELISA assays and in data analysis and interpretation. MM performed the experiments with transitional or non-transitional TIM-1$^{+/-}$ subpopulations and contributed to drafting the manuscript. CM and JCA participated in the conception and design of the study and in writing the manuscript. LS participated in the study design and in the recruitment and characterization of patients. DC participated in the conception and design of the study, interpretation of data, and in writing the manuscript. All authors read and approved the final manuscript.

Competing interests

The authors declare that they have no competing interests.

Author details

[1]Programa Disciplinario de Inmunología, Instituto de Ciencias Biomédicas (ICBM), Facultad de Medicina, Universidad de Chile, and Millennium Institute in Immunology and Immunotherapy, Santiago, Chile. [2]Centre for Rheumatology Research, Department of Medicine, University College London, London, UK. [3]Departamento de Medicina, Hospital Clínico, Universidad de Chile, Santiago, Chile.

References

1. Mauri C, Bosma A. Immune regulatory function of B cells. Annu Rev Immunol. 2012;30:221–41.
2. Mauri C, Menon M. The expanding family of regulatory B cells. Int Immunol. 2015;27(10):479–86.
3. Evans JG, Chavez-Rueda KA, Eddaoudi A, Meyer-Bahlburg A, Rawlings DJ, Ehrenstein MR, Mauri C. Novel suppressive function of transitional 2 B cells in experimental arthritis. J Immunol. 2007;178(12):7868–78.
4. Yanaba K, Bouaziz JD, Haas KM, Poe JC, Fujimoto M, Tedder TF. A regulatory B cell subset with a unique CD1dhiCD5+ phenotype controls T cell-dependent inflammatory responses. Immunity. 2008;28(5):639–50.
5. Matsumoto M, Baba A, Yokota T, Nishikawa H, Ohkawa Y, Kayama H, Kallies A, Nutt SL, Sakaguchi S, Takeda K, et al. Interleukin-10-producing plasmablasts exert regulatory function in autoimmune inflammation. Immunity. 2014;41(6):1040–51.
6. Shen P, Roch T, Lampropoulou V, O'Connor RA, Stervbo U, Hilgenberg E, Ries S, Dang VD, Jaimes Y, Daridon C, et al. IL-35-producing B cells are critical regulators of immunity during autoimmune and infectious diseases. Nature. 2014;507(7492):366–70.
7. Blair PA, Norena LY, Flores-Borja F, Rawlings DJ, Isenberg DA, Ehrenstein MR, Mauri C. CD19(+)CD24(hi)CD38(hi) B cells exhibit regulatory capacity in healthy individuals but are functionally impaired in systemic lupus erythematosus patients. Immunity. 2010;32(1):129–40.
8. Iwata Y, Matsushita T, Horikawa M, Dilillo DJ, Yanaba K, Venturi GM, Szabolcs PM, Bernstein SH, Magro CM, Williams AD, et al. Characterization of a rare IL-10-competent B-cell subset in humans that parallels mouse regulatory B10 cells. Blood. 2011;117(2):530–41.
9. Kessel A, Haj T, Peri R, Snir A, Melamed D, Sabo E, Toubi E. Human CD19(+)CD25(high) B regulatory cells suppress proliferation of CD4(+) T cells and enhance Foxp3 and CTLA-4 expression in T-regulatory cells. Autoimmun Rev. 2012;11(9):670–7.
10. Rosser EC, Mauri C. Regulatory B cells: origin, phenotype, and function. Immunity. 2015;42(4):607–12.
11. Xiao S, Brooks CR, Sobel RA, Kuchroo VK. Tim-1 is essential for induction and maintenance of IL-10 in regulatory B cells and their regulation of tissue inflammation. J Immunol. 2015;194(4):1602–8.
12. Ding Q, Yeung M, Camirand G, Zeng Q, Akiba H, Yagita H, Chalasani G, Sayegh MH, Najafian N, Rothstein DM. Regulatory B cells are identified by expression of TIM-1 and can be induced through TIM-1 ligation to promote tolerance in mice. J Clin Invest. 2011;121(9):3645–56.
13. Xiao S, Brooks CR, Zhu C, Wu C, Sweere JM, Petecka S, Yeste A, Quintana FJ, Ichimura T, Sobel RA, et al. Defect in regulatory B-cell function and development of systemic autoimmunity in T-cell Ig mucin 1 (Tim-1) mucin domain-mutant mice. Proc Natl Acad Sci U S A. 2012;109(30):12105–10.
14. Yeung MY, Ding Q, Brooks CR, Xiao S, Workman CJ, Vignali DA, Ueno T, Padera RF, Kuchroo VK, Najafian N, et al. TIM-1 signaling is required for maintenance and induction of regulatory B cells. Am J Transplant. 2015; 15(4):942–53.
15. Liu J, Zhan W, Kim CJ, Clayton K, Zhao H, Lee E, Cao JC, Ziegler B, Gregor A, Yue FY, et al. IL-10-producing B cells are induced early in HIV-1 infection and suppress HIV-1-specific T cell responses. PLoS One. 2014;9(2):e89236.
16. Kristensen B, Hegedus L, Lundy SK, Brimnes MK, Smith TJ, Nielsen CH. Characterization of regulatory B cells in Graves' disease and Hashimoto's thyroiditis. PLoS One. 2015;10(5):e0127949.
17. Xue H, Lin F, Tan H, Zhu ZQ, Zhang ZY, Zhao L. Overrepresentation of IL-10-expressing B cells suppresses cytotoxic CD4+ T cell activity in HBV-induced hepatocellular carcinoma. PLoS One. 2016;11(5):e0154815.
18. Gabrielli A, Avvedimento EV, Krieg T. Scleroderma. N Engl J Med. 2009; 360(19):1989–2003.
19. Parel Y, Aurrand-Lions M, Scheja A, Dayer JM, Roosnek E, Chizzolini C. Presence of CD4 + CD8+ double-positive T cells with very high interleukin-4 production potential in lesional skin of patients with systemic sclerosis. Arthritis Rheum. 2007;56(10):3459–67.
20. Chizzolini C, Parel Y, De Luca C, Tyndall A, Akesson A, Scheja A, Dayer JM. Systemic sclerosis Th2 cells inhibit collagen production by dermal fibroblasts via membrane-associated tumor necrosis factor alpha. Arthritis Rheum. 2003;48(9):2593–604.
21. Truchetet ME, Brembilla NC, Montanari E, Allanore Y, Chizzolini C. Increased frequency of circulating Th22 in addition to Th17 and Th2 lymphocytes in systemic sclerosis: association with interstitial lung disease. Arthritis Res Ther. 2011;13(5):R166.

22. Liu M, Yang J, Xing X, Cui X, Li M. Interleukin-17A promotes functional activation of systemic sclerosis patient-derived dermal vascular smooth muscle cells by extracellular-regulated protein kinases signalling pathway. Arthritis Res Ther. 2014;16(6):4223.
23. Radstake TR, van Bon L, Broen J, Wenink M, Santegoets K, Deng Y, Hussaini A, Simms R, Cruikshank WW, Lafyatis R. Increased frequency and compromised function of T regulatory cells in systemic sclerosis (SSc) is related to a diminished CD69 and TGFbeta expression. PLoS One. 2009;4(6):e5981.
24. Sato S, Fujimoto M, Hasegawa M, Takehara K. Altered blood B lymphocyte homeostasis in systemic sclerosis: expanded naive B cells and diminished but activated memory B cells. Arthritis Rheum. 2004;50(6):1918–27.
25. Matsushita T, Hasegawa M, Yanaba K, Kodera M, Takehara K, Sato S. Elevated serum BAFF levels in patients with systemic sclerosis: enhanced BAFF signaling in systemic sclerosis B lymphocytes. Arthritis Rheum. 2006;54(1):192–201.
26. Matsushita T, Hamaguchi Y, Hasegawa M, Takehara K, Fujimoto M. Decreased levels of regulatory B cells in patients with systemic sclerosis: association with autoantibody production and disease activity. Rheumatology (Oxford). 2015;55(2):263–7.
27. Mavropoulos A, Simopoulou T, Varna A, Liaskos C, Katsiari CG, Bogdanos DP, Sakkas LI. Breg cells are numerically decreased and functionally impaired in patients with systemic sclerosis. Arthritis Rheumatol. 2016;68(2):494–504.
28. Soto L, Ferrier A, Aravena O, Fonseca E, Berendsen J, Biere A, Bueno D, Ramos V, Aguillon JC, Catalan D. Systemic sclerosis patients present alterations in the expression of molecules involved in B-cell regulation. Front Immunol. 2015;6:496.
29. Sakkas LI, Bogdanos DP. Systemic sclerosis: New evidence re-enforces the role of B cells. Autoimmun Rev. 2016;15(2):155–61.
30. van den Hoogen F, Khanna D, Fransen J, Johnson SR, Baron M, Tyndall A, Matucci-Cerinic M, Naden RP, Medsger Jr TA, Carreira PE, et al. 2013 classification criteria for systemic sclerosis: an American College of Rheumatology/European League against Rheumatism collaborative initiative. Arthritis Rheum. 2013;65(11):2737–47.
31. Sims GP, Ettinger R, Shirota Y, Yarboro CH, Illei GG, Lipsky PE. Identification and characterization of circulating human transitional B cells. Blood. 2005; 105(11):4390–8.
32. Flores-Borja F, Bosma A, Ng D, Reddy V, Ehrenstein MR, Isenberg DA, Mauri C. CD19 + CD24hiCD38hi B cells maintain regulatory T cells while limiting TH1 and TH17 differentiation. Sci Transl Med. 2013;5(173):173ra123.
33. Sato S, Hasegawa M, Fujimoto M, Tedder TF, Takehara K. Quantitative genetic variation in CD19 expression correlates with autoimmunity. J Immunol. 2000;165(11):6635–43.
34. Saito E, Fujimoto M, Hasegawa M, Komura K, Hamaguchi Y, Kaburagi Y, Nagaoka T, Takehara K, Tedder TF, Sato S. CD19-dependent B lymphocyte signaling thresholds influence skin fibrosis and autoimmunity in the tight-skin mouse. J Clin Invest. 2002;109(11):1453–62.
35. Liu BS, Cao Y, Huizinga TW, Hafler DA, Toes RE. TLR-mediated STAT3 and ERK activation controls IL-10 secretion by human B cells. Eur J Immunol. 2014;44(7):2121–9.
36. Yoshizaki A, Iwata Y, Komura K, Ogawa F, Hara T, Muroi E, Takenaka M, Shimizu K, Hasegawa M, Fujimoto M, et al. CD19 regulates skin and lung fibrosis via Toll-like receptor signaling in a model of bleomycin-induced scleroderma. Am J Pathol. 2008;172(6):1650–63.
37. Lafyatis R, O'Hara C, Feghali-Bostwick CA, Matteson E. B cell infiltration in systemic sclerosis-associated interstitial lung disease. Arthritis Rheum. 2007;56(9):3167–8.
38. Whitfield ML, Finlay DR, Murray JI, Troyanskaya OG, Chi JT, Pergamenschikov A, McCalmont TH, Brown PO, Botstein D, Connolly MK. Systemic and cell type-specific gene expression patterns in scleroderma skin. Proc Natl Acad Sci U S A. 2003;100(21):12319–24.
39. Daoussis D, Melissaropoulos K, Sakellaropoulos G, Antonopoulos I, Markatseli TE, Simopoulou T, Georgiou P, Andonopoulos AP, Drosos AA, Sakkas L, et al. A multicenter, open-label, comparative study of B-cell depletion therapy with Rituximab for systemic sclerosis-associated interstitial lung disease. Semin Arthritis Rheum. 2016. doi:10.1016/j.semarthrit.2016.10.003 [Epub ahead of print].
40. Bouaziz JD, Calbo S, Maho-Vaillant M, Saussine A, Bagot M, Bensussan A, Musette P. IL-10 produced by activated human B cells regulates CD4(+) T-cell activation in vitro. Eur J Immunol. 2010;40(10):2686–91.
41. Tretter T, Venigalla RK, Eckstein V, Saffrich R, Sertel S, Ho AD, Lorenz HM. Induction of CD4+ T-cell anergy and apoptosis by activated human B cells. Blood. 2008;112(12):4555–64.
42. Wong SH, Barlow JL, Nabarro S, Fallon PG, McKenzie AN. Tim-1 is induced on germinal centre B cells through B-cell receptor signalling but is not essential for the germinal centre response. Immunology. 2010;131(1):77–88.
43. Munoz LE, Lauber K, Schiller M, Manfredi AA, Herrmann M. The role of defective clearance of apoptotic cells in systemic autoimmunity. Nat Rev Rheumatol. 2010;6(5):280–9.
44. Zhang Y, Zhang X, Xia Y, Jia X, Li H, Zhang Y, Shao Z, Xin N, Guo M, Chen J, et al. CD19+ Tim-1+ B cells are decreased and negatively correlated with disease severity in Myasthenia Gravis patients. Immunol Res. 2016.
45. Rosser EC, Oleinika K, Tonon S, Doyle R, Bosma A, Carter NA, Harris KA, Jones SA, Klein N, Mauri C. Regulatory B cells are induced by gut microbiota-driven interleukin-1beta and interleukin-6 production. Nat Med. 2014;20(11):1334–9.

15

α2AP regulates vascular alteration by inhibiting VEGF signaling in systemic sclerosis: the roles of α2AP in vascular dysfunction in systemic sclerosis

Yosuke Kanno[1*], En Shu[2], Hiroyuki Kanoh[2], Ayaka Matsuda[1] and Mariko Seishima[2]

Abstract

Background: Systemic sclerosis (SSc) is a connective tissues disease of unknown origin characterized by vascular damage and extensive fibrosis. Recently, we demonstrated that α2-antiplasmin (α2AP) is associated with the development of fibrosis in SSc. We herein investigate the roles of α2AP in vascular dysfunction in SSc.

Methods: Vascular damage in mice was determined by the levels of blood vessels and blood flow. Vascular functions in vascular endothelial cells (ECs) were determined by the levels of tube formation, cell proliferation, and endothelial junction-associated protein (VE-cadherin and PECAM1) production.

Results: The administration of α2AP induced vascular damage in mice. Conversely, the α2AP neutralization improved vascular damage in a bleomycin-induced mouse model of SSc. Additionally, we showed that the SSc fibroblast-conditioned media induced the reduction of tube formation, cell proliferation, and endothelial junction-associated protein production in ECs, and that α2AP neutralization improved them. We also examined the mechanisms underlying the effects of α2AP on vascular alteration in SSc and found that α2AP attenuated vascular endothelial growth factor-induced tube formation, cell proliferation, and endothelial junction-associated protein production through the adipose triglyceride lipase/tyrosine phosphatase SHP2 axis in ECs.

Conclusion: Our findings demonstrate that α2AP is associated with vascular alteration, and that the blocking of α2AP improves vascular dysfunction in SSc.

Keywords: Alpha2-antiplasmin, Systemic sclerosis, Vascular dysfunction, VEGF

Background

Systemic sclerosis (SSc) is a connective tissue disease characterized by vascular damage and fibrosis of skin and visceral organs [1]. Vascular damage, such as the reduction of blood vessels and blood flow, occurs in the early stages of the disease, and leads to extensive fibrosis [2]. However, the detailed mechanisms of SSc pathogenesis is unclear. Vascular endothelial growth factor (VEGF) is known to regulate the growth and activation of vascular endothelial cells (ECs), and plays a critical role in maintaining the vascular function. The expression of VEGF is elevated in various cells, such as fibroblasts, ECs, and immune cells, but vascular insufficiency manifests in SSc [2, 3]. The impairment of VEGF responses may cause vascular dysfunction in SSc. However, the detailed mechanisms are still not precisely understood.

Alpha2-antiplasmin (α2AP) functions as the main inhibitor of plasmin, resulting in the formation of a stable inactive complex, plasmin-α2AP and inhibits fibrinolysis [4]. α2AP is known to be synthesized in various tissues [5]. Recently, we found that α2AP induces TGF-β production through adipose triglyceride lipase (ATGL), which has been described as a member of the calcium-independent phospholipase A_2/adiponutrin/patatin-like

* Correspondence: ykanno@dwc.doshisha.ac.jp
[1]Department of Clinical Pathological Biochemistry, Faculty of Pharmaceutical Science, Doshisha Women's Collage of Liberal Arts, 97-1 Kodo, Kyo-tanabe, Kyoto 610-0395, Japan
Full list of author information is available at the end of the article

phospholipase domain-containing 2 (PNPLA2) family, and has a pro-fibrotic effects other than regulation of plasmin activity [6–10]. We also found that the expression of α2AP was elevated in the dermal fibroblasts obtained from SSc patients and the fibrotic tissue in SSc mouse models, and α2AP is associated with the development of fibrosis in SSc [7, 10]. Additionally, α2AP is known to play a critical role on angiogenesis, tissue repair, and vascular remodeling [11, 12], and may be also associated with vascular alteration in SSc. We herein investigated that the roles of α2AP in vascular dysfunction in SSc.

Methods

Mice experiments

We performed mice experiments as previously described [10]. The saline, bleomycin (5 mg/kg) plus control IgG (100 μg/kg) or bleomycin (5 mg/kg) plus anti-α2AP antibodies (100 μg/kg) (R&D Systems, MN, USA) were administered subcutaneously into the shaved backs of mice (male, 8-week-old C57BL/6 J mice) in the same site daily for up to 3 weeks. In parallel experiments, the saline or α2AP (15 μg/kg) (Calbiochem, CA, USA) were administered subcutaneously into the shaved backs of mice (male, 8-week-old C57BL/6 J mice) in the same site daily for up to 3 weeks. The samples of skin were placed immediately in liquid nitrogen, and stored at −80 °C until further use.

Immunohistochemical staining of PECAM1

We performed immunohistochemical staining as previously described [10, 11]. Paraffin sections were labeled with anti-PECAM1 antibody, then secondarily labeled with FITC-conjugated anti-rabbit IgG (Thermo Scientific, CA, USA). We used Rabbit (DA1E) mAb IgG XP Isotype control (Cell Signaling Technology, MA, USA) as isotype control (Additional file 1: Figure S1). The signals in the skin section were detected using a laser-scanning microscope. Then, the signals obtained from the same rectangular area for the dermis in the skin section were analyzed using ImageJ.

Blood flow in the skin

Blood flow in the skin was measured for 10 seconds using a laser Doppler flowmeter (BRL-100; Bio Research Center, Tokyo, Japan), and determined by calculating the average of two-time measurements in each skin sample.

Cell culture

Human normal and SSc dermal fibroblasts were obtained from patients with SSc (S4) and healthy control (N3) as previously described [10, 11]. Dermal fibroblasts were seeded onto the 10-cm diameter dishes and maintained in 10 mL Dulbecco's modified Eagle medium (DMEM) containing 10% FCS at 37 °C in a humidified atmosphere with 5% CO_2/95% air. After 5 days, the media were collected. In other studies, vascular ECs (UV♀2) were seeded onto 35-mm diameter dishes and maintained in 2 mL DMEM containing 10% FCS at 37 ° C in a humidified atmosphere with 5% CO_2/95% air. After 5 days, the media were replaced with serum-free DMEM. Then, the cells were used for experiments.

Tube formation assay

Matrigel (Becton, Dickinson and Company, NJ, USA) was added to each well of a 96-well plate. ECs were seeded on Matrigel coated plates, and were treated with the conditioned media (CM) of dermal fibroblasts, VEGF, or α2AP at the indicated concentration for 24 hours. The length of capillary like structure was analyzed by using ImageJ.

Cell proliferation assays

ECs were seeded on a 96-well plate, and the ECs were treated with the CM of dermal fibroblasts, VEGF, or α2AP at the indicated concentration for 24 hours. Cell proliferation was determined by counting cells number.

Western blot analysis

Cells were washed twice with cold PBS, harvested, and then sonicated in lysis buffer containing 10 mM Tris–HCl buffer (pH 7.5), 1% SDS, 1% Triton X-100, and a protease inhibitor cocktail (Roche, Mannheim, Germany). The skin samples from mice were homogenized and sonicated in the lysis buffer. The protein concentration in each lysate was measured using a BCA protein assay kit (Pierce, IL, USA). Proteins in the supernatant were separated by electrophoresis on 10% SDS-polyacrylamide gels and transferred to a PVDF membrane. We detected PECAM1, vascular endothelial cadherin, GAPDH, phospho-VEGFR2, VEGFR2, phospho-Akt, Akt, phospho-ERK1/2, ERK1/2, phospho-p38, p38, phospho-SHP2, SHP2, and ATGL by incubation with the respective antibodies followed by incubation with horseradish peroxidase-conjugated antibodies to rabbit IgG (Amersham Pharmacia Biotech, Uppsala, Sweden).

ATGL siRNAs study

SSc dermal fibroblasts were transfected with ATGL siRNA (Santa Cruz Biotechnology, CA, USA) using Lipofectamine 2000 (Invitrogen, CA, USA) according to the manufacturer's instructions. A non-specific siRNA was employed as the control. At 24 hours after transfection, the cells were used for experiments.

Statistical analysis

All data were expressed as mean ± SEM. The significance of the effect of each treatment ($P < 0.05$) was determined by analysis of variance (ANOVA) followed by the least significant difference test.

Results

Effect of α2AP on vascular damage in mice

To clarify the effects of α2AP on vascular damage, such as the reduction of blood vessels and blood flow, we examined the expression of the vascular EC marker, platelet-endothelial cell adhesion molecule 1 (PECAM1, CD31) and blood flow following the administration of α2AP in mice. The administration of α2AP induced the reduction of PECAM1 expression within the dermis (Fig. 1a, b) and blood flow in the skin (Fig. 1c).

Effect of blocking α2AP on vascular damage in a bleomycin-induced mouse model of SSc

We examined the effects of α2AP neutralization on vascular damage in a bleomycin-induced mouse model of SSc. The administration of bleomycin induced the reduction of PECAM1 expression (Fig. 2a, b) and blood flow (Fig. 2c) in the skin of SSc model mice, and the blocking of α2AP by α2AP-neutralizing antibodies improved the bleomycin-induced reduction of PECAM1 expression within the dermis (Fig. 2a, b) and blood flow (Fig. 2c) in the skin of SSc model mice.

Effect of blocking α2AP on the SSc dermal fibroblast-induced vascular dysfunction in ECs

We examined whether or not the CM from SSc dermal fibroblasts induces vascular dysfunction, including the reduction of tube formation, cell proliferation, and endothelial junction-associated protein (PECAM1 and vascular endothelial cadherin) production. The tube formation (Fig. 3a, b), cell proliferation (Fig. 3c), and endothelial junction-associated protein production (Fig. 3d) in SSc dermal fibroblast CM-stimulated ECs were lower than those in normal dermal fibroblast CM-stimulated ECs. These data suggest the SSc dermal fibroblasts induced vascular dysfunction. Next, we examined the effects of α2AP neutralization on the SSc dermal fibroblast CM-induced reduction of tube formation, cell proliferation, and endothelial junction-associated protein production. The α2AP neutralization improved the SSc dermal fibroblast CM-induced reduction of tube formation (Fig. 3e, f), cell proliferation (Fig. 3g), and endothelial junction-associated protein production (Fig. 3h).

Effect of α2AP on the VEGF-induced pro-angiogenic effects in ECs

We examined the effects of α2AP on the VEGF-regulated tube formation, cell proliferation, and endothelial junction-associated protein production in ECs. We confirmed that VEGF induced tube formation (Fig. 4a, b), cell proliferation (Fig. 4c), and endothelial junction-associated protein production (Fig. 4d) in ECs, and found that α2AP attenuated VEGF-induced tube formation (Fig. 4a, b), cell proliferation (Fig. 4c), and endothelial junction-associated protein production (Fig. 4d) in ECs.

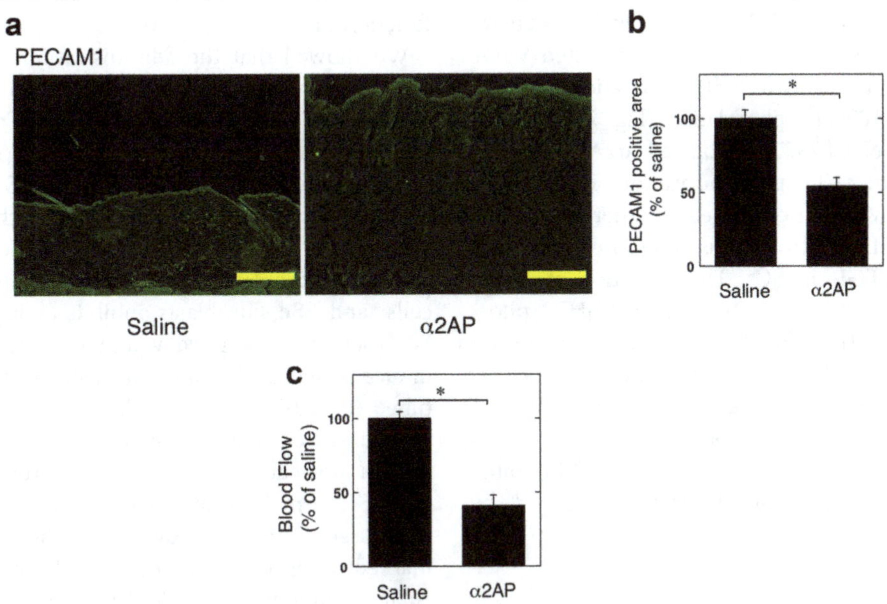

Fig. 1 Effect of α2AP on vascular damage in mice. **a** The skin sections from saline or α2AP-administered mice were stained with antibodies to PECAM1. **b** The histogram shows quantitative representations of PECAM1 (n = 6). **c** Blood flow in the skin of saline or α2AP-administered mice (n = 4). The data represent the mean ± SEM. * $P < 0.01$. Scale bar, 200 μm

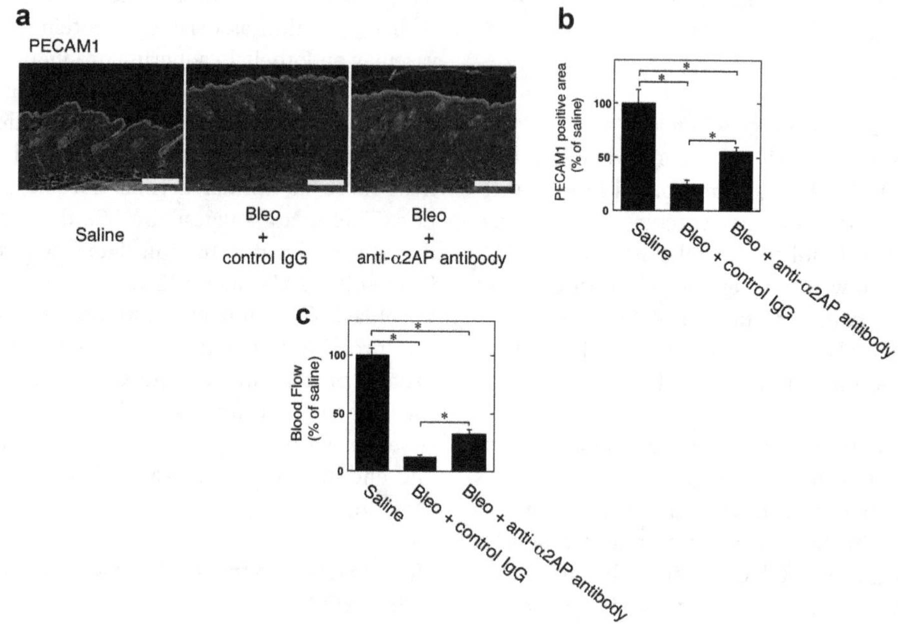

Fig. 2 Effect of blocking α2AP on vascular damage in a bleomycin-induced mouse model of systemic sclerosis. **a** The skin sections from mice treated with saline, bleomycin plus control IgG, or bleomycin plus α2AP-neutralizing antibodies were stained with antibodies to PECAM1. **b** The histogram shows quantitative representations of PECAM1 (n = 6). **c** Blood flow in the skin of mice treated with saline (n = 5), bleomycin plus control IgG (n = 4), or bleomycin plus α2AP-neutralizing antibodies (n = 4). The data represent the mean ± SEM. * $P < 0.01$. Scale bar, 200 μm

Effect of α2AP on VEGF signaling through ATGL/SHP2 axis in ECs

We also examined the effects of α2AP on VEGF signaling in ECs, and found that α2AP inhibited VEGF-induced VEGFR2, Akt, ERK1/2, and p38 phosphorylation in ECs (Fig. 5a). It has been reported that src-homology domain-2 containing tyrosine phosphatase 2 (SHP2) activation inhibits VEGF signaling [13]. Therefore, we examined whether or not α2AP-inhibited VEGF signaling is associated with SHP2 activation in ECs. α2AP induced SHP2 phosphorylation (Fig. 5b) and the SHP2 inhibitor, NSC87877, abrogated α2AP-inhibited Akt, ERK1/2, and p38 phosphorylation induced by VEGF (Fig. 5c). We then examined whether or not the α2AP-induced SHP2 activation is associated with the α2AP receptor, ATGL, in ECs. The reduction of ATGL using siRNA attenuated the α2AP-induced SHP2 phosphorylation in ECs (Fig. 5d). We also examined the effects of the irreversible ATGL inhibitor, bromoenol lactone (BEL), on α2AP-activated SHP2 in ECs. BEL attenuated α2AP-induced SHP2 phosphorylation in ECs (Fig. 5e). Additionally, BEL abrogated α2AP-inhibited Akt, ERK1/2, and p38 phosphorylation induced by VEGF in ECs (Fig. 5f).

Discussion

SSc is a chronic immune disorder characterized by vascular dysfunction and fibrosis of the skin and internal organs [1]. Recently, we showed that α2AP is associated with the development of fibrosis in SSc [6–8, 10]. α2AP is also associated with angiogenesis [11], vascular remodeling [12], the production of IgG, IgM, and IgE [14, 15], and the recruitment of lymphocytes and neutrophils [15–17]. These observations suggest that α2AP may be a critical regulator in the pathogenesis of SSc. We herein demonstrated that α2AP is associated with vascular dysfunction in SSc.

We showed that the administration of α2AP induced vascular damage such as the reduction of blood vessels and blood flow in mice (Fig. 1). Conversely, α2AP neutralization improved vascular damage in a bleomycin-induced mouse model of SSc (Fig. 2). These data suggest that α2AP may be one of the factors initiating vascular damage in SSc.

In SSc, fibroblasts are likely to be important effector cells, and SSc fibroblasts inhibit angiogenesis [18, 19]. We therefore examined whether or not SSc fibroblasts induce vascular dysfunction, such as the reduction of tube formation, cell proliferation, and endothelial junction-associated protein production, using CM from human normal and SSc dermal fibroblasts. We found that SSc dermal fibroblasts induced vascular dysfunction (Fig. 3a–d). We also showed that the blocking of α2AP markedly improved SSc dermal fibroblast-induced vascular dysfunction (Fig. 3e–h). In a previous study, we showed that the expression of α2AP was elevated in SSc dermal fibroblasts [10]. The SSc fibroblast-derived α2AP may cause vascular dysfunction in the disease.

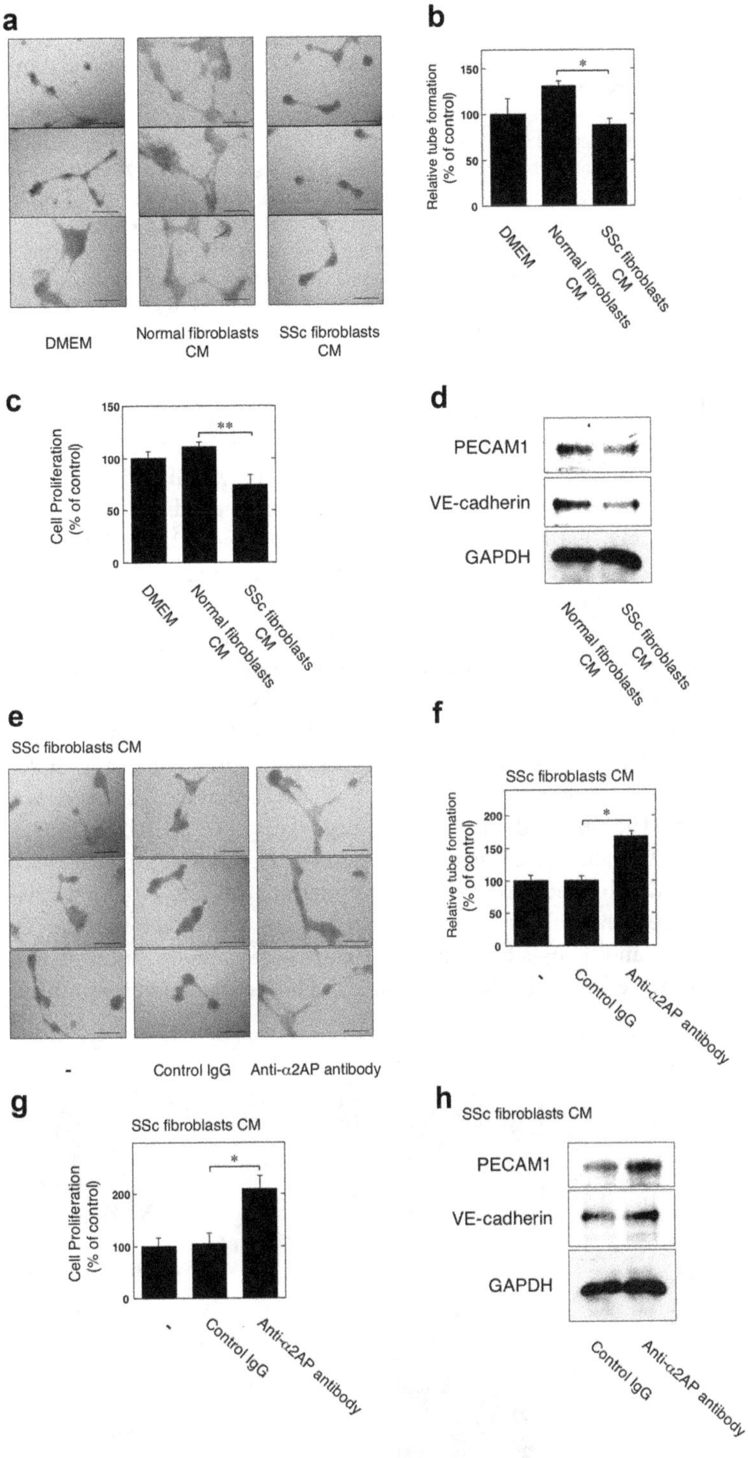

Fig. 3 (See legend on next page.)

(See figure on previous page.)
Fig. 3 Effect of blocking α2AP on the systemic sclerosis (SSc) dermal fibroblast-induced vascular dysfunction in endothelial cells (ECs). **a** ECs were seeded on 96-well Matrigel coated plates. ECs were cultured with the condition media (CM) of human normal dermal fibroblasts or human SSc dermal fibroblasts for 24 hours. **b** Tube formation in ECs was measured as described in Materials and Methods (n = 6). **c** ECs were cultured with the CM of the human normal dermal fibroblasts or the human SSc dermal fibroblasts for 24 hours. The cell proliferation was assessed as described in Materials and Methods (n = 3). **d** ECs were cultured with the CM of human normal dermal fibroblasts or human SSc dermal fibroblasts for 24 hours. The expression of each protein was examined by western blot analysis. **e** ECs were seeded on 96-well Matrigel-coated plates. ECs were cultured with the CM of human SSc dermal fibroblasts, and were stimulated by control IgG (1 μg/mL) or α2AP-neutralizing antibodies (1 μg/mL) for 24 hours. **f** Tube formation in ECs was measured as described in Materials and Methods (n = 6). **g** ECs were cultured with the CM of the human SSc dermal fibroblasts, and were stimulated by control IgG (1 μg/mL) or α2AP-neutralizing antibodies (1 μg/mL) for 24 hours. Cell proliferation was assessed as described in Materials and Methods (n = 8). **h** ECs were cultured with the CM of human SSc dermal fibroblasts and were stimulated by control IgG (1 μg/mL) or α2AP-neutralizing antibodies (1 μg/mL) for 24 hours. The expression of each protein was examined by western blot analysis. Data represent the mean ± SEM. * $P < 0.01$, ** $P < 0.05$. Scale bar, 50 μm

It has been reported that the expression of VEGF, which is a main regulator of angiogenesis, is elevated in SSc patients [2, 3]. However, angiogenesis is disturbed in SSc, and the mechanism of dysregulated angiogenesis in the presence of elevated VEGF remains poorly understood. We showed that α2AP attenuated VEGF-induced pro-angiogenic effects such as tube formation, cell proliferation, and endothelial junction-associated protein production in ECs (Fig. 4). Additionally, we showed that α2AP inhibited VEGF signaling (VEGFR2, Akt, ERK1/2, and p38 activation) (Fig. 5a). It has been reported that the activation of SHP2 inhibits VEGF signaling and regulates vascular endothelial functions [13]. In this study, we found that α2AP induced SHP2 activation (Fig. 5b), and the inhibition of SHP2 recovered α2AP-attenuated VEGF signaling (Fig. 5c). We also found that α2AP inhibited VEGF signaling through SHP2 activation. We previously showed that α2AP induces cell differentiation and TGF-β production through ATGL [8]. Therefore, we examined whether or not ATGL is associated with α2AP-induced SHP2 activation using siRNA and its inhibitor. Both reduction and inhibition of ATGL attenuated the α2AP-induced SHP2 activation (Fig. 5d, e). Additionally, the inhibition of ATGL recovered the α2AP-inhibited VEGF signaling (Fig. 5f). These data suggest that α2AP induced SHP2 activation through ATGL, and the α2AP-activated SHP2 inhibited VEGF signaling (Fig. 5g). The increase of α2AP expression in SSc may cause impairment of the VEGF response, and lead to vascular dysfunction.

Additionally, plasmin is known to regulate vascular endothelial functions, and influence the progression of various cardiovascular diseases through fibrinolysis, the degradation of matrix proteins, and the activation of growth factors [20]. The levels of plasmin-α2AP and D-dimer are elevated in patients with SSc [21, 22], and plasmin may also affect vascular dysfunction in SSc. α2AP may cause vascular disorder not only through inhibition of VEGF responses but also through plasmin inhibition.

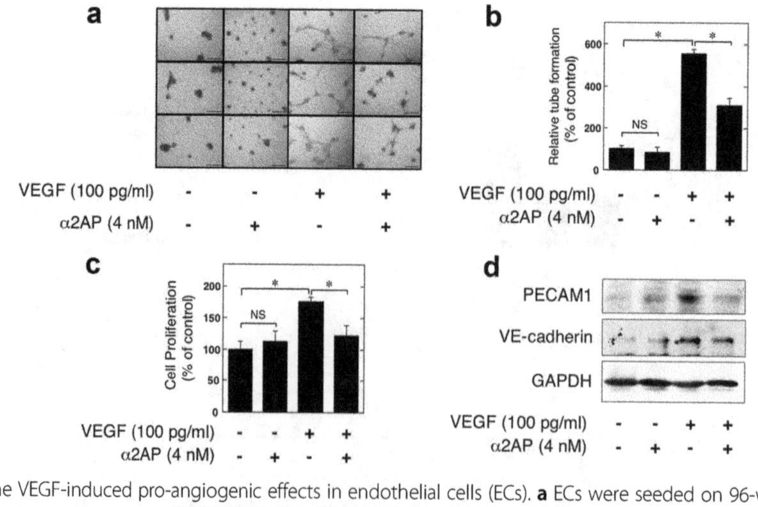

Fig. 4 Effect of α2AP on the VEGF-induced pro-angiogenic effects in endothelial cells (ECs). **a** ECs were seeded on 96-well Matrigel-coated plates. ECs were cultured in the absence or presence of VEGF (100 pg/mL) or α2AP (4 nM) as indicated for 24 hours. **b** Tube formation in ECs was measured as described in Materials and Methods (n = 6). **c** ECs were cultured for 24 hours in the absence or presence of VEGF (100 pg/mL) or α2AP (4 nM). Cell proliferation was assessed as described in Materials and Methods (n = 3). **d** ECs were cultured for 24 hours in the absence or presence of VEGF (100 pg/mL) or α2AP (4 nM). The expression of each protein was examined by western blot analysis. The data represent the mean ± SEM. * $P < 0.01$. NS, not significant. Scale bar, 50 μm

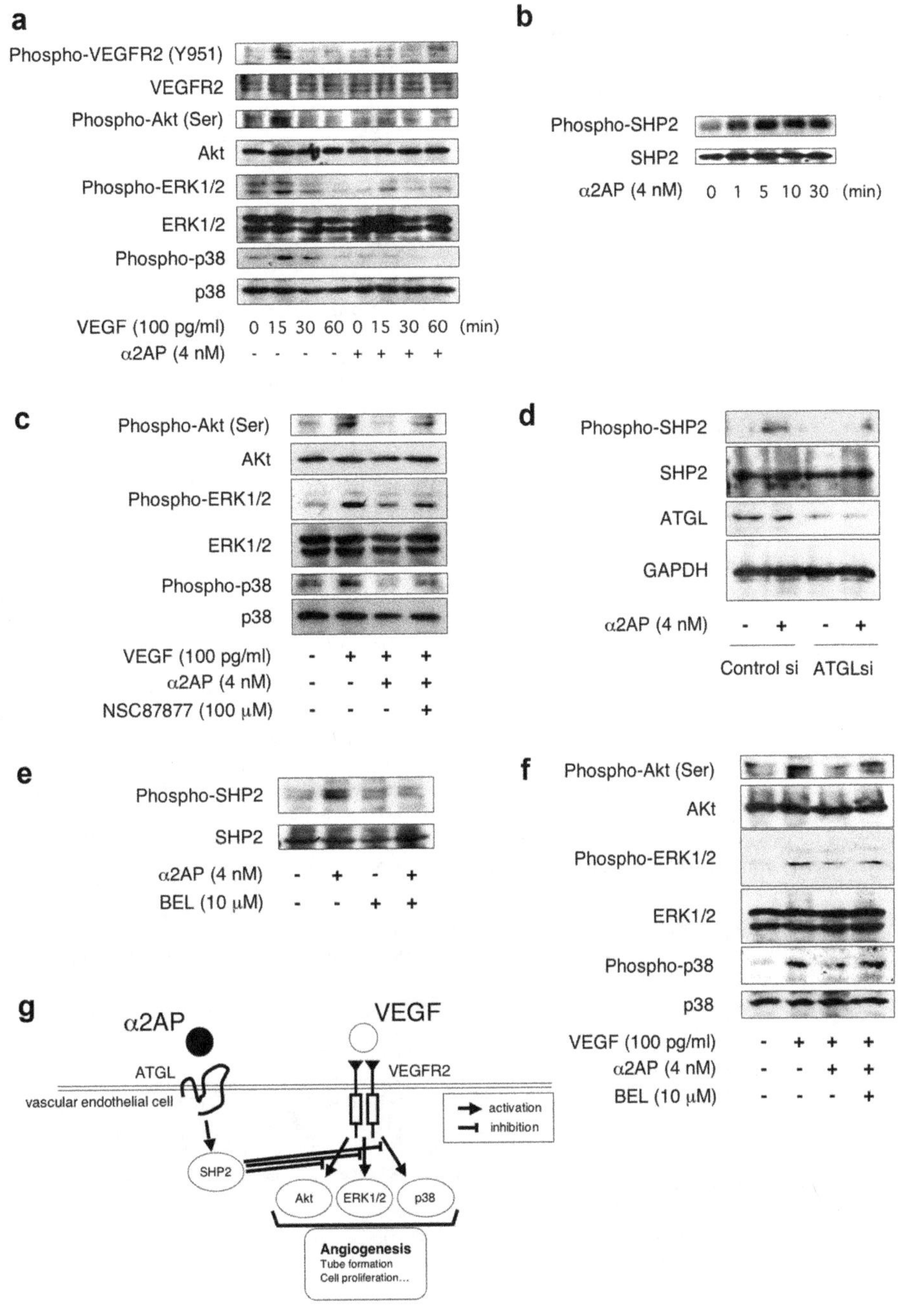

Fig. 5 Effect of α2AP on the VEGF signaling through ATGL/SHP2 axis in endothelial cells (ECs). **a** ECs were pretreated with 4 nM α2AP for 30 minutes and then stimulated with 100 pg/mL VEGF for the indicated periods. Phosphorylation of each protein was examined by western blot analysis. **b** ECs were stimulated with 4 nM α2AP for the indicated periods. Phosphorylation of SHP2 was examined by western blot analysis. **c** ECs were cultured for 30 minutes in the absence or presence of 4 nM α2AP or 100 μM NSC87877, and then stimulated with 100 pg/mL VEGF for 15 minutes. Phosphorylation of each protein was examined by western blot analysis. **d** ECs were transfected with control or ATGL siRNA. At 24 hours after transfection, the cells were stimulated with 4 nM α2AP for 5 minutes. The expression of each protein was examined by western blot analysis. **e** ECs were pretreated with 10 μM BEL for 30 minutes and then stimulated with 4 nM α2AP for 5 minutes. Phosphorylation of SHP2 was examined by western blot analysis. **f** ECs were pretreated with 4 nM α2AP or 10 μM BEL for 30 minutes and then stimulated with 100 pg/mL VEGF for 15 minutes. Phosphorylation of each protein was examined by western blot analysis. **g** The proposed mechanism of α2AP-attenuated vascular endothelial functions. VEGF induced Akt, ERK1/2, and p38 activation and led to pro-angiogenic effects, such as tube formation, cell proliferation, and endothelial junction-associated protein production in ECs. On the other hand, α2AP activated SHP2 through ATGL, and then α2AP-induced SHP2 activation inhibited VEGF signaling in ECs. α2AP inhibited VEGF signaling through the ATGL/SHP2 axis, and may cause impairment of vascular functions

Conclusion

α2AP functions as an inducer of vascular damage in mice. Blocking of α2AP improved vascular damage in an SSc mice model and SSc dermal fibroblast-induced vascular dysfunction. Additionally, α2AP regulated vascular alteration by inhibiting VEGF signaling through the ATGL/SHP2 axis. Our findings may eventually provide new insights into the development of clinical therapies for SSc.

Abbreviations

ATGL: adipose triglyceride lipase; BEL: bromoenol lactone; CM: conditioned media; EC: endothelial cell; PECAM1: platelet-endothelial cell adhesion molecule 1; PNPLA2: patatin-like phospholipase domain-contain 2; SHP2: src-homology domain-2 containing tyrosine phosphatase 2; SSc: systemic sclerosis; VEGF: vascular endothelial growth factor; α2AP: α2-antiplasmin

Acknowledgements

We thank the support of the Takeda Science Foundation.

Funding

This work was supported by the Takeda Science Foundation.

Authors' contributions

YK conceived and designed the experiment, and was involved in human and mice experiments, analyzed the data, data interpretation, and writing of the manuscript. ES was involved in human experiments, data interpretation, and writing of the manuscript. HK was involved in human experiments, data interpretation, and writing of the manuscript. AM was involved in mice experiments and analyzed the data. MS was involved in human experiments, data interpretation, and writing of the manuscript. All authors read and approved the final manuscript.

Competing interests

The authors declare that they have no competing interests.

Author details

[1]Department of Clinical Pathological Biochemistry, Faculty of Pharmaceutical Science, Doshisha Women's Collage of Liberal Arts, 97-1 Kodo, Kyo-tanabe, Kyoto 610-0395, Japan. [2]Department of Dermatology, Gifu University Graduate School of Medicine, 1-1 Yanagido, Gifu 501-1194, Japan.

References

1. Desbois AC, Cacoub P. Systemic sclerosis: an update in 2016. Autoimmun Rev. 2016;15:417–26.
2. Liakouli V, Cipriani P, Marrelli A, Alvaro S, Ruscitti P, Giacomelli R. Angiogenic cytokines and growth factors in systemic sclerosis. Autoimmun Rev. 2011;10: 590–4.
3. Trojanowska M. Cellular and molecular aspects of vascular dysfunction in systemic sclerosis. Nat Rev Rheumatol. 2010;6:453–60.
4. Collen D. Identification and some properties of a new fast-reacting plasmin inhibitor in human plasma. Eur J Biochem. 1976;69:209–16.
5. Menoud PA, Sappino N, Boudal-Khoshbeen M, Vassalli JD, Sappino AP. The kidney is a major site of alpha(2)-antiplasmin production. J Clin Invest. 1996; 97:2478–84.
6. Kanno Y, Kuroki A, Okada K, Tomogane K, Ueshima S, Matsuo O, et al. alpha2-Antiplasmin is involved in the production of transforming growth factor beta1 and fibrosis. J Thromb Haemost. 2007;5:2266–73.
7. Kanno Y, Kawashita E, Minamida M, Kaneiwa A, Okada K, Ueshima S, et al. alpha2-antiplasmin is associated with the progression of fibrosis. Am J Pathol. 2010;176:238–45.
8. Kanno Y, Kawashita E, Kokado A, Okada K, Ueshima S, Matsuo O, et al. Alpha2-antiplasmin regulates the development of dermal fibrosis in mice by prostaglandin F(2α) synthesis through adipose triglyceride lipase/calcium-independent phospholipase A(2). Arthritis Rheum. 2013;65:492–502.
9. Kanno Y, Kawashita E, Kokado A, Kuretake H, Ikeda K, Okada K, et al. α2AP mediated myofibroblast formation and the development of renal fibrosis in unilateral ureteral obstruction. Sci Rep. 2014;4:5967.
10. Kanno Y, Shu E, Kanoh H, Seishima M. The antifibrotic effect of α2AP neutralization in systemic sclerosis dermal fibroblasts and mouse models of systemic sclerosis. J Invest Dermatol. 2016;136:762–9.
11. Kanno Y, Hirade K, Ishisaki A, Nakajima K, Suga H, Into T, et al. Lack of alpha2-antiplasmin improves cutaneous wound healing via over-released vascular endothelial growth factor-induced angiogenesis in wound lesions. J Thromb Haemost. 2006;4:1602–10.
12. Hou Y, Okada K, Okamoto C, Ueshima S, Matsuo O. Alpha2-antiplasmin is a critical regulator of angiotensin II-mediated vascular remodeling. Arterioscler Thromb Vasc Biol. 2008;28:1257–62.
13. Fraineau S, Monvoisin A, Clarhaut J, Talbot J, Simonneau C, Kanthou C, et al. The vitamin K-dependent anticoagulant factor, protein S, inhibits multiple VEGF-A-induced angiogenesis events in a Mer- and SHP2-dependent manner. Blood. 2012;120:5073–83.
14. Zhabin SG, Gorin VS. The effects of alpha 2-antiplasmin complex and alpha 2-antiplasmin on the secretion of IgG and IgM by cultured human mononuclear cells. J Clin Lab Immunol. 1997;49:77–82.
15. Okada K, Ueshima S, Kawao N, Yano M, Tamura Y, Tanaka M, et al. Lack of both α2-antiplasmin and plasminogen activator inhibitor type-1 induces high IgE production. Life Sci. 2013;93:89–95.
16. Kager LM, Weehuizen TA, Wiersinga WJ, Roelofs JJ, Meijers JC, Dondorp AM, et al. Endogenous α2-antiplasmin is protective during severe gram-negative sepsis (melioidosis). Am J Respir Crit Care Med. 2013;188:967–75.
17. Eddy JL, Schroeder JA, Zimbler DL, Bellows LE, Lathem WW. Impact of the Pla protease substrate α2-antiplasmin on the progression of primary pneumonic plague. Infect Immun. 2015;83:4837–47.
18. Gilbane AJ, Denton CP, Holmes AM. Scleroderma pathogenesis: a pivotal role for fibroblasts as effector cells. Arthritis Res Ther. 2013;15:215.
19. Serratì S, Cinelli M, Margheri F, Guiducci S, Del Rosso A, Pucci M, et al. Systemic sclerosis fibroblasts inhibit in vitro angiogenesis by MMP-12-dependent cleavage of the endothelial cell urokinase receptor. J Pathol. 2006;210:240–8.
20. Plow EF, Hoover-Plow J. The functions of plasminogen in cardiovascular disease. Trends Cardiovasc Med. 2004;14:180–6.
21. Jinnin M, Ihn H, Yamane K, Asano Y, Yazawa N, Tamaki K. Plasma plasmin-alpha2-plasmin inhibitor complex levels are increased in systemic sclerosis patients with pulmonary hypertension. Rheumatology (Oxford). 2003;42: 240–3.
22. Marie I, Borg JY, Hellot MF, Levesque H. Plasma D-dimer concentration in patients with systemic sclerosis. Br J Dermatol. 2008;158:392–5.

16

Proangiogenic effects of soluble α-Klotho on systemic sclerosis dermal microvascular endothelial cells

Celestina Mazzotta[1*], Mirko Manetti[2], Irene Rosa[1,2], Eloisa Romano[1], Jelena Blagojevic[1], Silvia Bellando-Randone[1], Cosimo Bruni[1], Gemma Lepri[1], Serena Guiducci[1], Lidia Ibba-Manneschi[2] and Marco Matucci-Cerinic[1]

Abstract

Background: Systemic sclerosis (SSc) is characterized by endothelial cell (EC) apoptosis, impaired angiogenesis and peripheral microvasculopathy. Soluble α-Klotho (sKl) is a pleiotropic molecule with multiple effects on ECs, including antioxidant and vasculoprotective activities. On the EC surface, sKl interacts with vascular endothelial growth factor (VEGF) receptor-2 (VEGFR-2) and transient receptor potential canonical-1 (TRPC-1) cation channel to control EC homeostasis. Here, we investigated whether sKl might act as a protective factor to improve angiogenesis in dermal microvascular endothelial cells (MVECs) from SSc patients (SSc-MVECs).

Methods: Wound healing assay was performed on healthy dermal MVECs (H-MVECs) challenged with sera from healthy controls or SSc patients with or without the addition of sKl. Capillary morphogenesis on Matrigel was assessed in H-MVECs and SSc-MVECs at basal conditions and treated with sKl, as well as in H-MVECs challenged with healthy or SSc sera in presence or absence of sKl. The expression of α-Klotho, $VEGF_{165}b$, VEGFR-2, TRPC-1, Ki67 and active caspase-3 in H-MVECs and SSc-MVECs was investigated by western blotting. Immunostaining for α-Klotho was performed in H-MVECs and SSc-MVECs, and in healthy and SSc skin sections.

Results: Treatment with sKl effectively counteracted the inihibitory effects of SSc sera on wound healing ability and angiogenic performance of H-MVECs. The addition of sKl significantly improved angiogenesis and maintained over time capillary-like tube formation in vitro by SSc-MVECs. Stimulation of SSc-MVECs with sKl resulted in the upregulation of the proliferation marker Ki67 in parallel with the downregulation of proapoptotic active caspase-3. The expression of α-Klotho was significantly lower in SSc-MVECs than in H-MVECs. The expression of TRPC-1 was also significantly decreased, while that of VEGFR-2 and $VEGF_{165}b$ was significantly increased, in SSc-MVECs compared with H-MVECs. Challenge with sKl either significantly increased TRPC-1 or decreased $VEGF_{165}b$ in SSc-MVECs. Ex vivo analyses revealed that α-Klotho immunostaining was almost absent in the dermal microvascular network of SSc skin compared with control skin.

Conclusions: Our findings provide the first evidence that α-Klotho is significantly decreased in the microvasculature in SSc skin and that sKl administration may effectively improve SSc-MVEC functions in vitro by acting as a powerful proangiogenic factor.

Keywords: α-Klotho, Endothelial cells, Angiogenesis, Systemic sclerosis

* Correspondence: mazzottacelestina@gmail.com
[1]Department of Experimental and Clinical Medicine, Division of Rheumatology, University of Florence, AOUC, Largo Brambilla 3, 50134 Florence, Italy
Full list of author information is available at the end of the article

Background

Systemic sclerosis (SSc) is an autoimmune connective tissue disease characterized by alterations in the microcirculation, deregulation of immune response and fibrosis of the skin and internal organs [1]. According to the degree of skin involvement, SSc is categorized into limited and diffuse cutaneous SSc subsets (lcSSc and dcSSc, respectively) [2, 3]. Vascular damage occurs early in the course of SSc, with chronic tissue ischemia and lack of compensatory angiogenesis, progressing until the loss of dermal capillaries and formation of non-healing digital ulcers [4].

Angiogenesis, a process controlled by a tight balance between proangiogenic and anti-angiogenic signals, is essential for wound healing [5]. Among proangiogenic molecules, vascular endothelial growth factor (VEGF) has a pivotal role in postnatal neovascularization, which comprises angiogenesis and vasculogenesis [6–8]. Indeed, angiogenesis is the formation of new blood vessels by sprouting of pre-existing mature endothelial cells (ECs), while vasculogenesis is a process involving the recruitment and differentiation of bone marrow (BM)-derived endothelial precursor cells (EPCs) [9, 10]. In this context, several studies have reported that VEGF levels are significantly elevated in serum in SSc despite the lack of adaptive angiogenesis [11–15]. Moreover, microvascular ECs (MVECs) isolated from skin in SSc display a defective angiogenic capacity in vitro, including impaired proliferation, migration and capillary-like tube formation, even in response to exogenous VEGF stimulation [4].

A recent study demonstrated that soluble α-Klotho (sKl) protein interacts directly both with VEGF receptor-2 (VEGFR-2) and transient receptor potential canonical-1 (TRPC-1) cation channel on the surface of ECs [16]. The resulting heterotrimeric molecular complex is incorporated into ECs in response to VEGF stimulation and is involved in stabilizing the entry of Ca^{2+} in order to maintain EC integrity [16] (Fig. 1).

The *α-Klotho* gene encodes a type I single-pass-transmembrane protein composed of a large extracellular domain (130 kDa), a transmembrane domain and a very short intracellular domain (10 amino acids) [17–19]. The extracellular domain has homologies with the family of 1-glycosidases and is subjected to ectodomain shedding. As a result, the entire extracellular domain is released into the extracellular space and is detectable in blood, urine and cerebrospinal fluid [20–22]. Therefore, α-Klotho protein has transmembrane (tKl) and soluble circulating (sKl) forms with different properties.

The full-length tKl functions as an obligatory co-receptor for fibroblast growth factor 23 (FGF23) forming a complex with FGF receptors and FGF23 that regulates phosphate homeostasis by inhibiting 1,25$(OH)_2$ vitamin D_3 synthesis and inducing phosphaturia [23–25]. sKl functions instead as a humoral factor with pleiotropic activities, such as the suppression of growth factor signaling and oxidative stress and the regulation of ion channels and transporters [26, 27]. Moreover, sKl increases endothelial nitric oxide (NO) production, improves endothelium-dependent vasodilatation, induces resistance to lipid peroxidation and exerts anti-inflammatory and anti-cancer effects [28]. In addition,

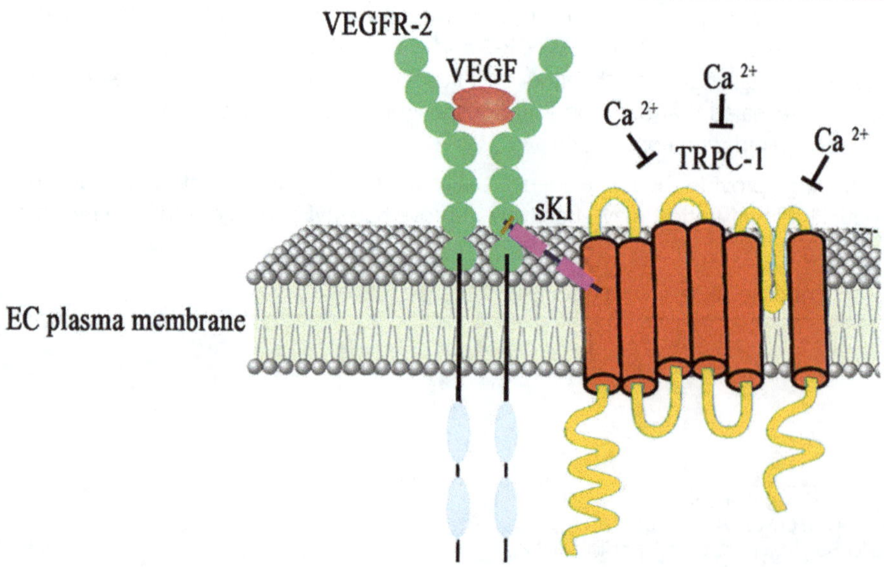

Fig. 1 Schematic representation of the molecular complex formed by vascular endothelial growth factor (*VEGF*)-bound VEGF receptor-2 (*VEGFR-2*), transient receptor potential canonical-1 (*TRPC-1*) and soluble α-Klotho (*sKl*) on the surface of endothelial cells (*ECs*). This molecular complex regulates the influx of Ca^{2+} and the permeability of the plasma membrane contributing to the maintenance of EC integrity

sKl negatively regulates insulin/insulin-like growth factor-1 signaling with consequent inhibition of cellular senescence through the inactivation of Akt and the induction of p53 and p21 expression [20].

Insulin, by stimulating the proteolytic activities of a disintegrin and metalloprotease (ADAM)-10 and ADAM-17, may enhance tKl shedding and the release of the extracellular domain of α-Klotho [29]. Circulating α-Klotho may derive also by alternative mRNA splicing of exon 3 with generation of a different transcript called secreted α-Klotho, which has a half-length of the full-length transcript [17, 18, 30] and is believed to act as a hormone regulating the functions of cells or tissues that do not express α-Klotho. On ECs sKl plays the role of antioxidant with the ability to downregulate generation of reactive oxygen species (ROS) and mediate vasculoprotective effects [31, 32].

Based on these facts, the aim of the present study was to examine whether sKl could exert positive effects on dermal MVECs from patients with SSc by promoting in vitro angiogenesis.

Methods

Patients and controls

Serum samples were obtained from five patients with lcSSc (n = 3) or dcSSc (n = 2) (median age 61 years, range 35–76 years) [2] and from five age-matched and sex-matched healthy individuals. The patients enrolled were not on corticosteroids, immunosuppressants or other disease-modifying drugs. Peripheral blood samples were collected without any additive, left to clot for 30 minutes before centrifugation at 1500 g for 15 minutes, and serum was collected and stored in aliquots at −80 °C until used.

Paraffin-embedded sections of lesional forearm skin biopsies were obtained from 15 patients with SSc (13 women and 2 men; n = 10 with lcSSc and n = 5 with dcSSc, median age 45.3 years, range 29–67 years, and median disease duration 5 years, range 1–14 years) and 13 age-matched and sex-matched healthy donors. The study was approved by the Ethical Committee of the Azienda Ospedaliero-Universitaria Careggi (AOUC), Florence, Italy, and all subjects provided written informed consent. The study was conducted in accordance with the Declaration of Helsinki.

Isolation of dermal MVECs and cell culture

Dermal MVECs were isolated from skin biopsies from five patients with dcSSc (SSc-MVECs) and from five healthy subjects (H-MVECs). Briefly, skin samples were mechanically cleaned to remove the adipose and epidermal layers, in order to obtain a pure specimen of vascularized dermis, and were treated as described elsewhere [33]. The samples were placed at 37 °C in a humidified atmosphere with 5% CO_2. After one day of culture in EC basal medium (EBM-2, catalog number LOCC3156; Euroclone, Milan, Italy) supplemented with 20% fetal bovine serum (FBS), 5 ng/ml H-epidermal growth factor (hEGF; Clonetics Corporation, San Diego, CA, USA), 1 µg/ml hydrocortisone acetate, 100 U/ml penicillin, 100 µg/ml streptomycin and 25 µg/ml amphotericin B without addition of further angiogenic growth factors, small colonies of polygonal elements were detected. Non-adherent cells were removed and fresh EC complete medium was added. To maintain optimal culture conditions, the medium was changed every third day, and after 2 weeks of primary culture a monolayer of cells was obtained. MVECs from primary cultures were further identified using immunomagnetic beads recognizing CD31. Isolated cells were purified as MVECs by labeling with anti-factor VIII-related antigen and anti-CD105, followed by reprobing with anti-CD31 antibodies. Dermal MVECs were maintained in EC complete medium and were used between the third and seventh passages in culture.

In vitro wound healing assay

Wound healing assay was performed on confluent H-MVECs in basal condition and challenged with serum from healthy controls (n = 5) or patients with SSc (n = 5 (n = 3 with lcSSc and n = 2 with dcSSc)) with or without the addition of recombinant human sKl protein (5 ng/ml) (Active Human α-Klotho protein fragment, catalog number ab84072; Abcam, Cambridge, UK). H-MVECs were seeded onto 6-well tissue culture plates and cultured in EBM-2 medium with 10% FBS until 80–90% of confluence. The cells were then rinsed with phosphate-buffered saline (PBS) and starved in low serum medium (0.5% FBS) overnight. The day after, a wound was made on the cellular monolayer using a sterile 200-µl pipet tip followed by a wash with EBM-2 basal medium to remove detached cells. Wound healing capacity was assessed by capturing phase-contrast images of the wounded area at the beginning (T0) and at 24 hours (T24) under a Leica inverted microscope (Leica Microsystems, Mannheim, Germany), and comparing the images to quantify the migration rate of the cells after wounding. All experimental conditions were performed in triplicate.

In vitro capillary morphogenesis assay

In vitro capillary morphogenesis assay was performed in 96-well plates covered with Matrigel (BD Biosciences, San Jose, CA, USA). Matrigel (50 µl; 10–12 mg/ml) was pipetted into culture wells and polymerized for 30 minutes at 37 °C, as described elsewhere [13]. H-MVECs and SSc-MVECs (30×10^3 cells/well) were incubated in basal EBM-2 medium containing 10% FBS or serum from five patients with SSc or five healthy subjects, with or without the addition of recombinant human sKl protein (5 ng/ml). Stimulation with recombinant human $VEGF_{165}$ (10 ng/ml) (R&D Systems, Minneapolis, MN, USA) was used as positive control of angiogenesis. All conditions were performed in triplicate and the plates were photographed at 24 and 48 hours. Results were quantified at the same time by measuring the percent field occupancy of capillary projections, as determined by image analysis. Six to nine photographic fields from three plates were scanned for each point.

Western blotting

H-MVECs and SSc-MVECs were cultured until confluence, detached with trypsin-EDTA, washed with PBS, pelleted and subjected to total protein extraction. In some experimental conditions, H-MVECs and SSc-MVECs were stimulated with recombinant human sKl protein (5 ng/ml) (catalog number ab84072; Abcam) for 24 and 48 hours before protein extraction. Twenty-five micrograms of total proteins were electrophoresed on NuPAGE 4 to 12% Bis-Tris Gel (Invitrogen, Carlsbad, CA, USA) and blotted onto polyvinylidene difluoride membranes (Invitrogen). The membranes were blocked with blocking solution included in the Western Breeze Chromogenic Western Blot Immunodetection Kit (Invitrogen) for 40 minutes at room temperature on a rotary shaker and subsequently incubated for 1 hour at room temperature with rabbit monoclonal anti-human α-Klotho (1:500 dilution; catalog number ab181373; Abcam), mouse monoclonal anti-human $VEGF_{165}b$ (1:500 dilution; catalog number ab14994; Abcam), rabbit polyclonal anti-human VEGFR-2 (1:100 dilution; catalog number ab45010; Abcam), rabbit monoclonal anti-human TRPC-1 (1:1000 dilution; catalog number ab51255; Abcam), rabbit monoclonal anti-human Ki67 (1:1000 dilution; catalog number ab92742; Abcam), rabbit polyclonal anti-human caspase-3 (1:1000 dilution; catalog number 9662; Cell Signaling Technology, Danvers, MA, USA), and rabbit polyclonal anti-human α-tubulin (1:1000 dilution; catalog number ab18251; Abcam) antibodies, assuming α-tubulin as control invariant protein. Immunodetection was performed as described in the Western Breeze Chromogenic Immunodetection protocol (Invitrogen). ImageJ software was used for densitometric analysis of the bands and the values were normalized to α-tubulin.

Immunohistochemical analysis

After deparaffinization and rehydration, skin sections (5 μm thick) were boiled for 10 minutes in sodium citrate buffer (10 mM, pH 6.0) for antigen retrieval and treated with 3% H_2O_2 in methanol for 15 minutes at room temperature to block endogenous peroxidase activity. Sections were then washed and incubated with Ultra V block (UltraVision Large Volume Detection System Anti-Polyvalent, HRP, catalog number TP-125-HL; LabVision, Fremont, CA, USA) for 10 minutes at room temperature according to the manufacturer's protocol. After blocking non-specific site binding, slides were incubated overnight at 4 °C with rabbit monoclonal anti-human α-Klotho antibody (1:20 dilution; catalog number ab181373; Abcam) diluted in 1% bovine serum albumin (BSA) in PBS.

The day after, tissue sections were washed three times in PBS and incubated with biotinylated secondary antibodies (UltraVision Large Volume Detection System Anti-Polyvalent, HRP; LabVision) for 10 minutes at room temperature. Subsequently, the slides were washed three times in PBS and incubated with streptavidin peroxidase (UltraVision Large Volume Detection System Anti-Polyvalent, HRP; LabVision) for 10 minutes at room temperature. Immunoreactivity was developed using 3-amino-9-ethylcarbazole (AEC kit, catalog number TA-125-SA; LabVision) as chromogen. Skin sections were finally counterstained with Mayer's hematoxylin (Bio-Optica, Milan, Italy), washed, mounted in an aqueous mounting medium and observed under a Leica DM4000 B microscope (Leica Microsystems). Sections not exposed to primary antibodies or incubated with isotype-matched and concentration-matched non-immune rabbit IgG (Sigma-Aldrich, St. Louis, MO, USA) were included as negative controls for antibody specificity.

Light microscopy images were captured with a Leica DFC310 FX 1.4-megapixel digital color camera equipped with the Leica software application suite LAS V3.8 (Leica Microsystems). α-Klotho immunostaining was quantified in a semi-quantitative manner, where 0 indicates no staining, 1 indicates weak staining, 2 indicates moderate staining and 3 indicates strong staining in microvessels at eight randomly chosen high-power fields (×40 original magnification) per sample. Two different examiners performed blinded evaluation. When there was interobserver disagreement, the specimen was reviewed again by both observers and the disagreement resolved.

Immunocytochemical analysis

MVECs were seeded onto glass coverslips, grown to 70% confluence, fixed with 3.7% buffered paraformaldehyde and permeabilized with 0.1% Triton X-100 in PBS. Slides were then washed, treated with 3% H_2O_2 in PBS for 15 minutes at room temperature and subsequently blocked with Ultra V block (UltraVision Large Volume Detection System Anti-Polyvalent, HRP; LabVision) for 10 minutes. Cells were incubated overnight at 4 °C with rabbit monoclonal anti-human α-Klotho antibody (catalog number ab181373; Abcam) at 1:20 dilution in 1%

BSA in PBS, followed by incubation with biotinylated secondary antibodies and streptavidin peroxidase (UltraVision Large Volume Detection System Anti-Polyvalent, HRP; LabVision) at room temperature.

Immunoreactivity was developed with 3-amino-9-ethylcarbazole (AEC kit; LabVision). Irrelevant isotype-matched and concentration-matched rabbit IgG (Sigma-Aldrich) were used as negative controls. Nuclei were counterstained with Mayer's hematoxylin (Bio-Optica). Immunolabeled cells were examined with a Leica DM4000 B microscope (Leica Microsystems) and photomicrographs were captured with a Leica DFC310 FX 1.4-megapixel digital colour camera equipped with the Leica software application suite LAS V3.8 (Leica Microsystems).

Statistical analysis

Data are expressed as the mean ± standard deviation (SD) or the mean ± standard error of the mean (SEM). Student's t test and Tukey's multiple comparisons test were used where appropriate for statistical evaluation of the differences between independent groups. A p value less than 0.05 was considered statistically significant.

Results

Effects of sKl on wound healing capacity of MVECs

The in vitro wound healing assay was performed to evaluate the ability of H-MVECs to repair the injured area in standard conditions or under challenge with serum from healthy subjects or patients with SSc, in the presence or absence of sKl (Fig. 2a–l). After 24 hours, H-MVECs cultured in standard conditions and challenged with sKl had increased ability to repair the wounded area when compared to basal H-MVECs without sKl ($p = 0.039$) (Fig. 2b, d, m). Moreover, the addition of sKl to H-MVECs treated with healthy serum improved the wound healing process compared with H-MVECs treated with healthy serum alone ($p = 0.018$) (Fig. 2f, h, m). H-MVECs challenged with serum from

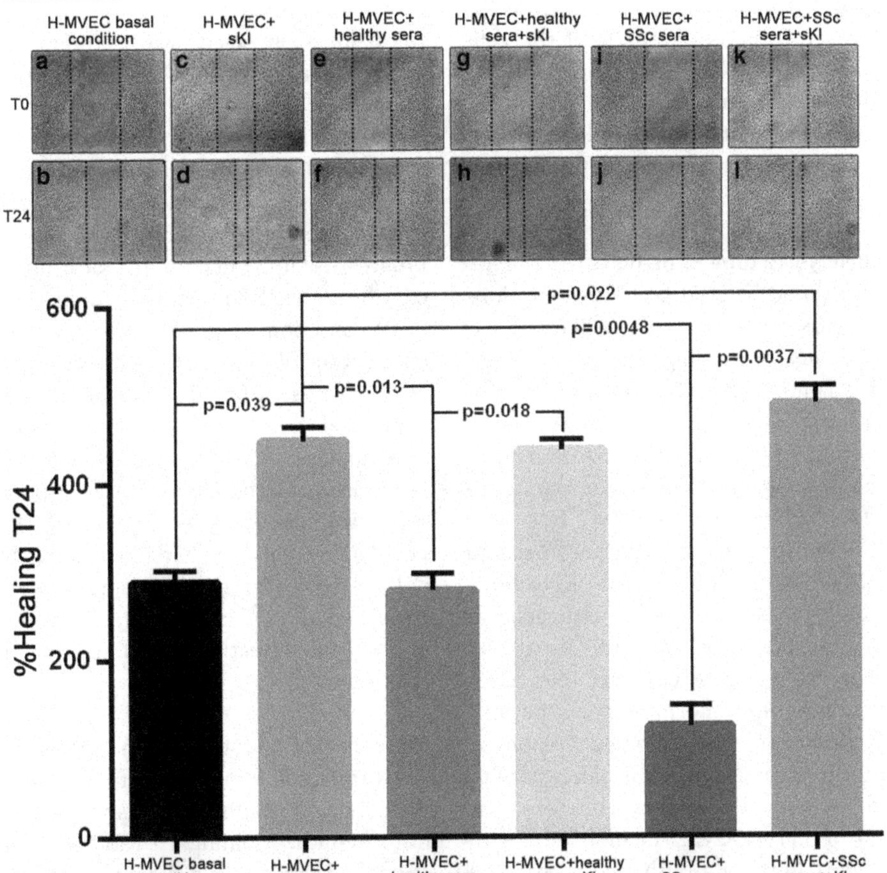

Fig. 2 Soluble α-Klotho (*sKl*) improves the wound healing capacity of healthy dermal microvascular endothelial cells (*H-MVECs*) and counteracts the inhibitory effects of serum from patients with systemic sclerosis (*SSc*). Wound healing capacity of H-MVECs was assayed at basal conditions and in the presence of serum from healthy controls (n = 5) and patients with SSc (n = 5), with or without the addition of sKl. **a–l** Representative images of the wounded area at 0 hours and 24 hours after scratching. **m** Quantitative analysis of the percentage of wound repair. Data are means ± SD of three independent experiments performed in triplicate with each one of the five H-MVEC lines. Tukey's multiple comparisons test was used for statistical analysis; p values are indicated

patients with SSc lost the ability to repair the wounded area (Fig. 2j) in respect to H-MVECs at basal condition and H-MVECs cultured with healthy serum ($p = 0.0048$ and $p = 0.0008$, respectively) (Fig. 2b, f, m). Interestingly, the administration of sKl to H-MVECs challenged with serum from patients with SSc significantly improved wound healing compared to H-MVECs treated with serum from patients with SSc alone ($p = 0.0037$) (Fig. 2j, l, m) and compared to H-MVECs with sKl or H-MVECs treated with healthy serum in the presence of sKl ($p = 0.022$ and $p = 0.031$, respectively) (Fig. 2d, h, m).

These results suggest that sKl acts as a powerful pro-reparative factor exhibiting the most significant effects in a pathological microenvironment such as in the presence of serum from patients with SSc, by improving cell migration and cell growth toward the center of the wound. We also observed that H-MVECs cultured in standard condition or with healthy serum in the presence of sKl had a high proliferation rate in the first 24 hours, and subsequently the cells detached from the culture plate, and after 48 hours only 30% of the cells were still adherent to the plate (data not shown), suggesting that sKl may contribute to regulate cell overgrowth over time in normal conditions, while in pathological conditions it may foster and sustain reparative processes.

Effects of sKl on capillary-like tube formation

As previously demonstrated [34, 35], at basal conditions the ability of H-MVECs to form capillary-like tubular structures after 24 hours of seeding on Matrigel was significantly greater compared with SSc-MVECs ($p < 0.0001$) (Fig. 3a, g). Furthermore, in the first 24 hours, the addition of sKl significantly increased the angiogenic ability of H-MVECs compared to basal conditions ($p = 0.008$) (Fig. 3a, b, l), but after 48 hours the tubular structures were degenerated (Fig. 3j). For SSc-MVECs, the addition of sKl significantly improved angiogenesis compared with cells at basal conditions ($p < 0.0001$), by over time restoring and maintaining the sprouting of capillary-like tubes organized into a honeycomb morphological pattern (Fig. 3g, h, k, l). Moreover, the angiogenic response of H-MVECs cultured with serum from patients with SSc was impaired in respect to either H-MVECs at basal conditions or H-MVECs challenged with healthy serum ($p = 0.04$ for both comparisons) (Fig. 3a, c, e). The negative effect of serum from patients with SSc on H-MVECs was reversed by the addition of sKl as demonstrated by the production of an endothelial network comparable to those observed in basal H-MVECs and H-MVECs cultured with healthy serum (Fig. 3f).

Consistent with the wound healing assay data, sKl had a different effect in normal or pathological conditions. In fact, in H-MVECs the addition of sKl induced angiogenesis up to 24 hours, while at 48 hours it had an inhibitory effect on cell proliferation by regulating cell overgrowth. Conversely, in SSc-MVECs sKl ameliorated the production of elongated processes and improved the organization of cellular branching cords by maintaining its positive effect over time.

Differential regulation of proliferative and apoptotic pathways by administration of sKl to H-MVECs and SSc-MVECs

In order to investigate the effects of sKl administration on H-MVEC and SSc-MVEC proliferation and apoptosis, we analyzed the protein expression levels of the proliferative marker Ki67 and proapoptotic active caspase-3 at basal condition and after stimulation with sKl for 24 and 48 hours. As displayed in Fig. 4a, compared with the basal condition, challenge with sKl for 24 hours increased Ki67 expression levels in H-MVECs ($p < 0.05$). Conversely, Ki67 protein levels were significantly decreased in H-MVECs treated with sKl for 48 hours in respect to basal H-MVECs ($p < 0.05$) (Fig. 4a).

Ki67 protein expression was strongly reduced in basal SSc-MVECs compared with basal H-MVECs (Fig. 4a). The addition of sKl to SSc-MVECs resulted in significant progressive upregulation of Ki67 up to 48 hours ($p < 0.05$ for either 24-hour or 48-hour treatment versus the basal condition) (Fig. 4a). As shown in Fig. 4b, 24-hour stimulation of H-MVECs with sKl significantly reduced active caspase-3 ($p < 0.05$ versus basal H-MVECs), while challenge with sKl for 48 hours resulted in significant upregulation of active caspase-3 ($p < 0.05$ versus basal H-MVECs). At baseline, active caspase-3 protein levels were significantly higher in SSc-MVECs compared with H-MVECs (Fig. 4b). Treatment of SSc-MVECs with sKl led to a significant progressive decrease in active caspase-3 up to 48 hours ($p < 0.05$ for either 24-hour or 48-hour treatment versus the basal condition) (Fig. 4b).

Expression of α-Klotho in skin biopsies

The expression of α-Klotho in skin biopsies from patients with SSc and healthy controls was evaluated by immunohistochemical staining. α-Klotho immunostaining was strongly decreased in different cellular components of the skin in SSc, including dermal fibroblasts, as compared with healthy skin (Fig. 5a). Moreover, α-Klotho immunostaining was almost absent in the dermal microvascular network of the skin in SSc compared with healthy controls (Fig. 5a). As displayed in Fig. 5b, semi-quantitative analysis of immunostaining revealed significantly lower expression

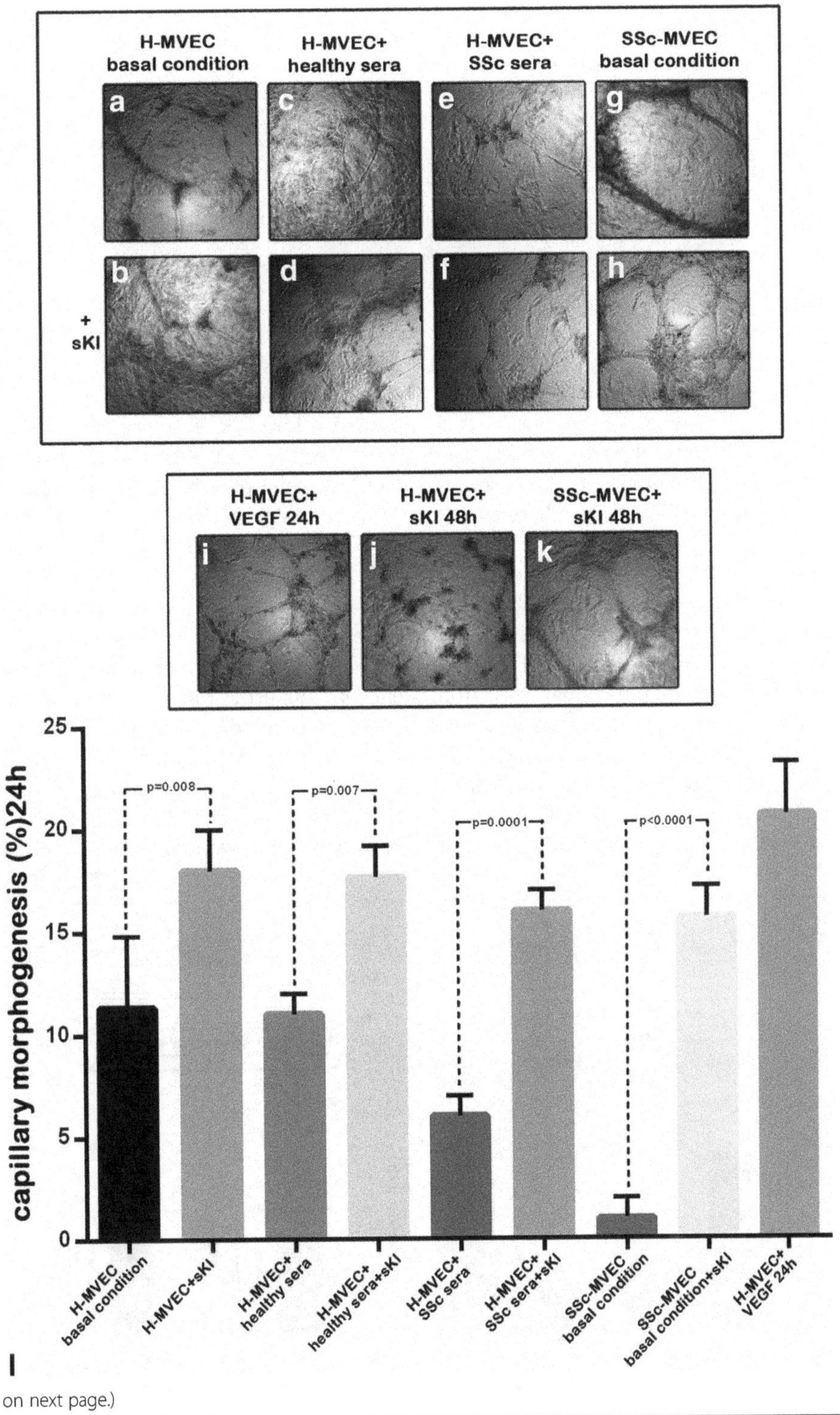

Fig. 3 (See legend on next page.)

(See figure on previous page.)

Fig. 3 Effects of soluble α-Klotho (*sKl*) on the ability of dermal microvascular endothelial cells from healthy controls (*H-MVECs*) and patients with systemic sclerosis (SSc) (*SSc-MVECs*) to form capillary-like tubes on Matrigel. In vitro capillary morphogenesis of H-MVECs was evaluated at basal conditions and after challenge with serum from healthy controls (n = 5) and patients with SSc (n = 5), with or without the addition of sKl. Stimulation with vascular endothelial growth factor (*VEGF*)$_{165}$ was included as a positive control for angiogenesis. In vitro capillary morphogenesis of SSc-MVECs was evaluated at basal conditions and after stimulation with sKl. **a–i** Representative images of the capillary network formed on Matrigel at 24 hours after plating are shown for each experimental point. **j, k** Representative images of H-MVECs (**j**) and SSc-MVECs (**k**) stimulated with sKl at 48 hours from plating on Matrigel. **l** Quantitative analysis of capillary morphogenesis on Matrigel as percent field occupancy of capillary projections at 24 hours after plating. Data are means ± SD of three independent experiments performed in triplicate with each one of the five H-MVEC and five SSc-MVEC lines. Tukey's multiple comparisons test was used for statistical analysis; *p* values are indicated

of α-Klotho in the dermal microvessels in patients with SSc compared with controls ($p = 0.002$).

Protein expression levels of α-Klotho, VEGF$_{165}$b, VEGFR-2 and TRPC-1 in MVECs

It has been demonstrated that sKl plays a pivotal role in the maintenance of EC integrity through direct interaction with VEGFR-2 and TRPC-1 cation channel and consequent formation of a heterotrimeric complex, which is incorporated into ECs in response to VEGF [16]. As the expression levels of the anti-angiogenic VEGF$_{165}$b isoform have been reported to be selectively increased in SSc-MVECs compared with H-MVECs [13], and considering that there are no anti-human α-Klotho antibodies suitable for a co-immunoprecipitation assay, we evaluated the expression of α-Klotho, VEGF$_{165}$b, VEGFR-2 and TRPC-1 proteins in H-MVECs and SSc-MVECs (Fig. 6a–f). In protein lysates from SSc-MVECs, the expression of α-Klotho was significantly decreased compared to H-MVECs ($p = 0.0003$) (Fig. 6c). Immunocytochemical analysis confirmed these results showing lower expression of α-Klotho at cytoplasmic subcellular level in SSc-MVECs compared with H-MVECs (Fig. 6a and b). Moreover, TRPC-1 protein expression was significantly lower in SSc-MVECs than in H-MVECs ($p = 0.0013$), while protein levels of VEGFR-2 and VEGF$_{165}$b were both significantly higher in SSc-MVECs compared to H-MVECs ($p = 0.026$ and $p = 0.0001$, respectively) (Fig. 6d, e, f).

As we have shown that stimulation with sKl may ameliorate in vitro angiogenesis in SSc-MVECs, we further investigated whether sKl could mediate these proangiogenic effects though the modulation of VEGF$_{165}$b and TRPC-1 expression. As displayed in Fig. 7a, challenge of SSc-MVECs with sKl resulted in a significant progressive decrease in VEGF$_{165}$b protein up to 48 hours ($p < 0.05$ for either 24-hour or 48-hour treatment versus the basal condition). Moreover, there was a significant progressive

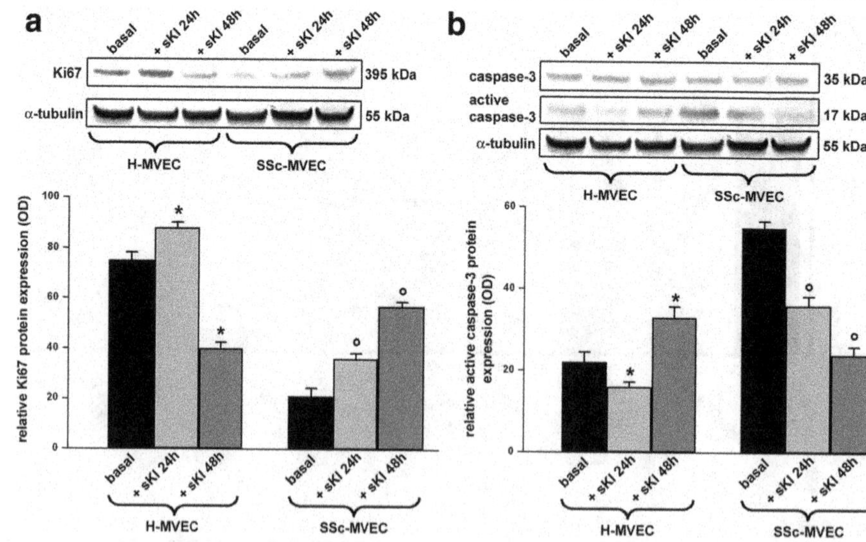

Fig. 4 Expression of the proliferative marker Ki67 and proapoptotic active caspase-3 in dermal microvascular endothelial cells from healthy controls (*H-MVECs*) and patients with systemic sclerosis (SSc) (*SSc-MVECs*). **a, b** Western blotting of total protein extracts from H-MVECs and SSc-MVECs at basal condition and treated with recombinant human soluble α-Klotho (*sKl*) protein for 24 and 48 hours assayed with anti-Ki67 (**a**) and anti-caspase 3 (**b**) antibodies. Representative immunoblots are shown. The active fragment of casapase-3 is identified at the expected molecular weight of 17 kDa. The densitometric analysis of the bands normalized to α-tubulin is reported in the histograms. Data are mean ± SD of optical density (*OD*) in arbitrary units. Student's *t* test was used for statistical analysis; *$p < 0.05$ versus basal H-MVECs, °$p < 0.05$ versus basal SSc-MVECs. Results are representative of three independent experiments performed with each one of the five H-MVEC and five SSc-MVEC lines

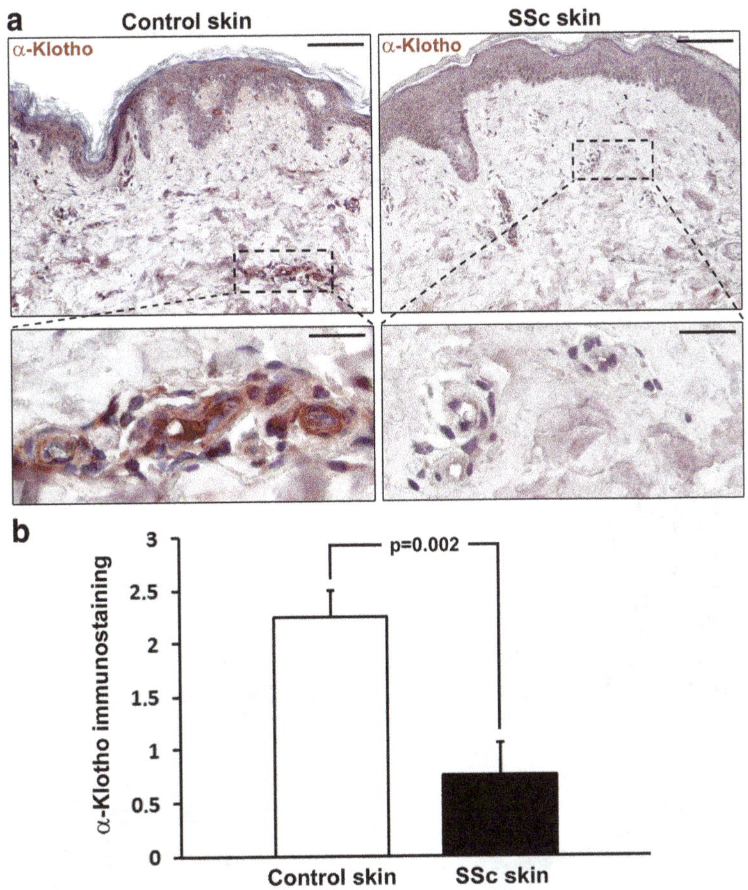

Fig. 5 Decreased expression of α-Klotho in the skin of patients with systemic sclerosis (*SSc*). **a** Representative microphotographs of skin sections from healthy controls and patients with SSc immunostained with rabbit monoclonal anti-human α-Klotho antibody and counterstained with hematoxylin. *Boxed area* (*upper panels*) is shown at higher magnification in the respective *lower panels*. α-Klotho immunostaining is decreased in dermal microvessels of the skin in SSc compared with healthy control skin. *Scale bar* 100 μm (*upper panels*) and 20 μm (*lower panels*). **b** Semi-quantitative analysis of α-Klotho immunostaining in dermal microvessels. Data are mean ± SEM of immunostaining score performed on skin sections from eight patients with SSc and eight healthy controls. Student's *t* test was used for statistical analysis; the *p* value is indicated

increase in TRPC-1 in SSc-MVECs challenged with sKl ($p < 0.05$ for either 24-hour or 48-hour treatment versus basal condition) (Fig. 7b). As far as H-MVECs are concerned, stimulation with sKl did not result in any significant changes in $VEGF_{165}b$ protein expression either at 24 or 48 hours, while TRPC-1 was significantly upregulated only after 24-hour treatment ($p < 0.05$ versus basal condition) (Fig. 7a, b).

These results suggest that either the downregulation of α-Klotho and TRPC-1 or the preferential binding of the upregulated anti-angiogenic $VEGF_{165}b$ isoform to VEGFR-2 may prevent the formation of the $VEGF_{165}$/VEGFR-2/TRPC-1/sKl molecular complex on the plasma membrane of SSc-MVECs, with consequent negative effects on cellular homeostasis and angiogenesis. According to our western blotting data, the proangiogenic effects exerted over time on SSc-MVECs by the addition of sKl might in part be explained by sKl-induced downregulation of $VEGF_{165}b$ and parallel upregulation of TRPC-1.

Discussion

This is the first report to investigate the possible protective and proangiogenic effects of sKl on vascular ECs from patients with SSc. Indeed, we have shown that sKl improves SSc-MVEC angiogenesis in vitro, with a robust positive effect persisting over time. In particular, by restoring vessel sprouting, treatment with sKl enhances the number and improves the morphology of capillary-like tubes formed by SSc-MVECs in vitro. On the contrary, we observed that in a physiological condition mirrored in vitro by H-MVECs, sKl stimulates angiogenesis only transiently, while inducing cell detachment with consequent vessel regression and dissociation over time.

This dualistic behavior of α-Klotho might depend on its ability to influence the activation of the normal cell

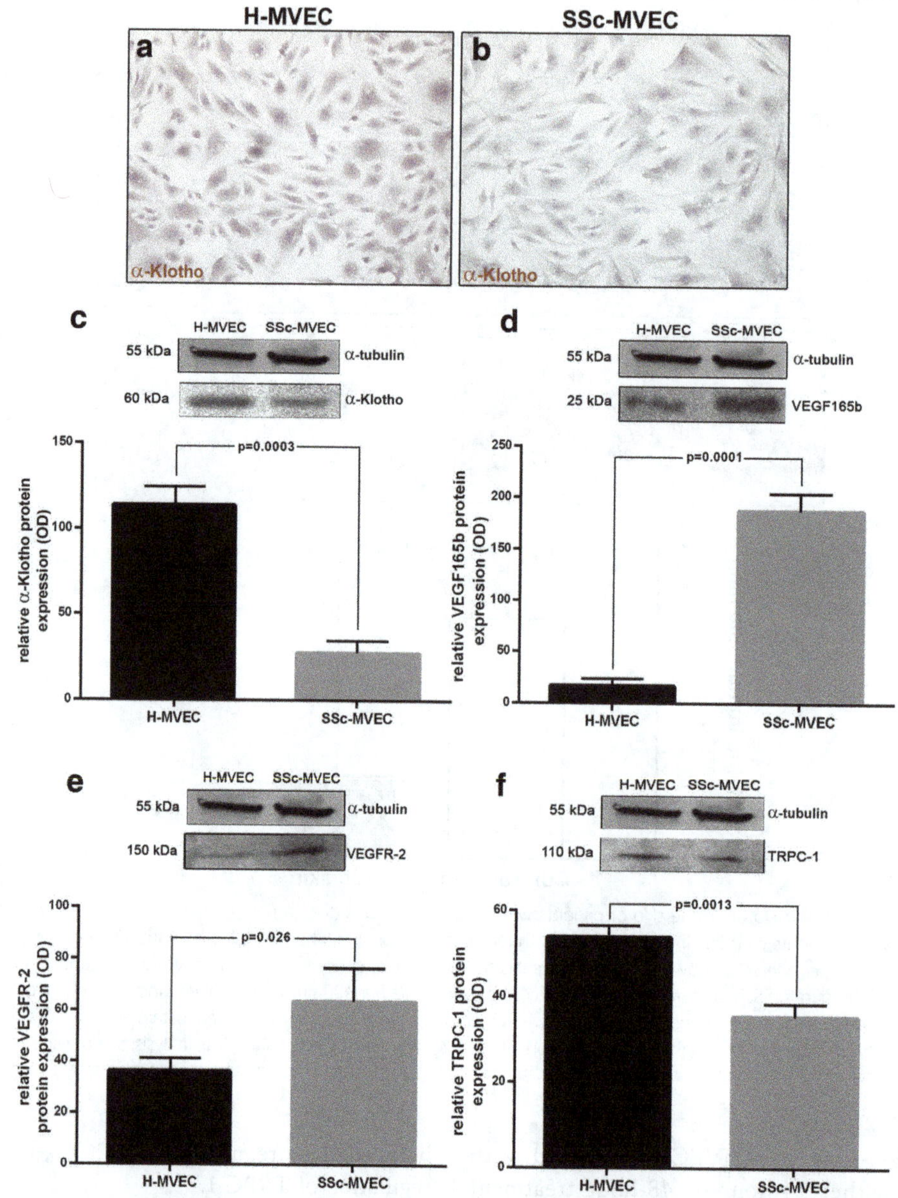

Fig. 6 Expression of α-Klotho, vascular endothelial growth factor (*VEGF*)$_{165}$b, VEGF receptor-2 (*VEGFR-2*) and transient receptor potential canonical-1 (*TRPC-1*) in dermal microvascular endothelial cells from healthy controls (*H-MVECs*) and patients with systemic sclerosis (SSc) (*SSc-MVECs*). **a**, **b** Representative microphotographs of immunocytochemical staining for α-Klotho in H-MVECs (**a**) and SSc-MVECs (**b**) detected with biotinylated secondary antibodies and streptavidin peroxidase. **c**-**f** Protein lysates from H-MVECs and SSc-MVECs were subjected to western blotting analysis using anti-α-Klotho (**c**), anti-VEGF$_{165}$b (**d**), anti-VEGFR-2 (**e**) and anti-TRPC-1 (**f**) antibodies. Representative immunoblots are shown. The densitometric analysis of the bands normalized to α-tubulin is reported in the histograms. Data are mean ± SD of optical density (*OD*) in arbitrary units. Student's *t* test was used for statistical analysis; *p* values are indicated in each panel. Results are representative of three independent experiments performed with each one of the five H-MVEC and five SSc-MVEC lines

cycle regulatory pathways, including p53/p21. Indeed, several reports have demonstrated that sKl attenuates cellular apoptosis and senescence in vascular cells via mitogen-activated kinase and extracellular signal-regulated kinase pathways [36, 37]. In fact, by regulating p53-mediated cell cycle arrest in the transition from G1 to S phase of cell replication [38], sKl may influence the p53/p21 pathway. In this context, our in vitro observations suggest that sKl may act preferentially as a protective and proangiogenic factor in pathological conditions, while exerting a regulatory role to maintain normal cell growth in physiological conditions. Indeed, a tight balance between survival and death signaling determines the cell fate [39], and continuous stimulation by growth factors to enhance proliferation is perceived by normal cells as a negative signal.

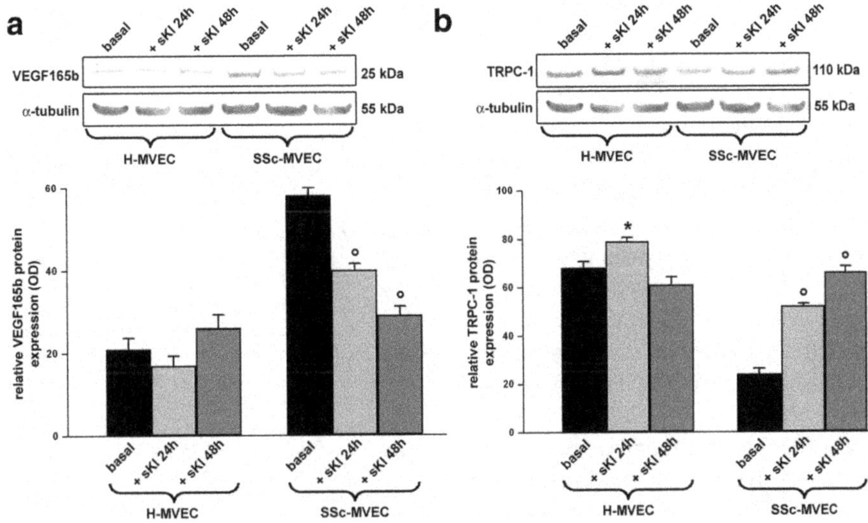

Fig. 7 Expression of vascular endothelial growth factor (*VEGF*)$_{165}$b and transient receptor potential canonical-1 (*TRPC-1*) in dermal microvascular endothelial cells from healthy controls (*H-MVECs*) and systemic sclerosis (SSc) patients (*SSc-MVECs*). **a**, **b** Western blotting of total protein extracts from H-MVECs and SSc-MVECs at basal condition and treated with recombinant human soluble α-Klotho (*sKl*) protein for 24 and 48 hours assayed with anti-VEGF$_{165}$b (**a**) and anti-TRPC-1 (**b**) antibodies. Representative immunoblots are shown. The densitometric analysis of the bands normalized to α-tubulin is reported in the histograms. Data are mean ± SD of optical density (*OD*) in arbitrary units. Student's *t* test was used for statistical analysis; *$p < 0.05$ versus basal H-MVECs, °$p < 0.05$ versus basal SSc-MVECs. Results are representative of three independent experiments performed with each one of the five H-MVEC and five SSc-MVEC lines

In all cell types the activation of apoptosis-regulatory genes is a physiological mechanism to control cell proliferation, and the deregulation of this complex mechanism is the primary cause of neoplastic transformation. Cultured non-transformed cells have a limited proliferative capacity, known as the Hayflick limit, which results in an irreversible proliferative arrest, called cellular senescence [40]. Indeed, according to this view, our Ki67 and active caspase-3 western blotting data show that while stimulation with sKl induces proliferation and inhibits apoptosis of SSc-MVECs over time, such pro-proliferative and anti-apoptotic effects are only transient in H-MVECs, being in fact rapidly followed by cell proliferation arrest and increased apoptosis.

Our ex vivo data demonstrated decreased expression of α-Klotho in skin biopsies from patients with SSc, in particular at microvascular level. In addition, in cultured SSc-MVECs α-Klotho was downregulated compared with H-MVECs, which instead exhibited strong expression of α-Klotho at cytoplasmic level. Interestingly, western blotting experiments on MVEC lysates confirmed the presence of a 60-kDa α-Klotho isoform that could derive from alternative splicing of exon 3; considering that, to the best of our knowledge, only the premature form of α-Klotho (130 kDa) was previously found in the endoplasmic reticulum and Golgi apparatus [22, 41].

In vascular ECs, α-Klotho upregulates the production of NO with protective effects against cell dysfunction [42, 43]. Of note, experimental models of parabiosis (i.e. the surgical connection of two animals to allow exchange of humoral factors) between α-*klotho* heterozygous and wild-type mice have shown complete recovery of endothelial function in α-*klotho* heterozygous mice, indicating the crucial role of α-Klotho as a humoral factor regulating EC homeostasis [44]. Moreover, in cultured ECs α-Klotho also regulates the homeostatic balance between ROS and antioxidant agents, and decreases hydrogen peroxide-induced apoptosis and cellular senescence [36]. In addition, α-Klotho has a protective effect against angiotensin II-induced ROS production and reduces the activation of superoxide anions [45, 46]. Thus, the downregulation of α-Klotho in the microvascular endothelium might substantially contribute to ROS generation, oxidative stress and tissue damage in the skin of patients with SSc.

In mouse models, α-Klotho also regulates the BM microenvironment, including macrophages, fibroblasts, ECs and extracellular matrix, with potential effects on hematopoiesis and EPC differentiation [47]. The differentiation and mobilization of EPCs from the BM is likely impaired in *kl-/kl-* mice, as shown by decreased numbers of EPC-like cells both in the BM compartment and in the peripheral blood [48]. Although conflicting data have been reported on the role of EPC dysfunction in SSc [49, 50], further evaluation of the possible role of sKl in EPCs from patients with SSc could be of interest.

sKl has been recently shown to maintain EC homeostasis in association with $VEGF_{165}$-bound VEGFR-2 and TRPC-1 by forming a heterotrimeric complex on the surface of ECs, which regulates Ca^{2+} influx, maintaining plasma membrane permeability and cell integrity [16]. As previously demonstrated [13], SSc-MVECs strongly express the anti-angiogenic $VEGF_{165}$b isoform that binds VEGFR-2 with the same affinity of $VEGF_{165}$ but does not activate proangiogenic downstream signaling cascades. Moreover, we showed here that TRPC-1 is downregulated in SSc-MVECs. Thus, either the downregulation of TRPC-1 or the preferential binding of the upregulated anti-angiogenic $VEGF_{165}$b isoform to VEGFR-2 may prevent the formation of the $VEGF_{165}$/VEGFR-2/TRPC-1/sKl molecular complex on the plasma membrane of SSc-MVECs, contributing to cell dysfunction and impairment of angiogenesis. Interestingly, here we also provide evidence that the exogenous addition of sKl to SSc-MVECs might improve the formation of the aforementioned complex through the downregulation of $VEGF_{165}$b and the parallel upregulation of TRPC-1 with a consequent boost of the angiogenic response.

Conclusions

In SSc, microvascular injury, chronic ischemia and tissue hypoxia lead to EC apoptosis and dysfunction, with several regulatory molecular pathways being involved in the pathogenic mechanisms underlying endothelial damage [51–55]. In this complex scenario, our study provides evidence that the administration of exogenous sKl may effectively improve SSc-MVEC functions in vitro by acting as a powerful proangiogenic factor fostering the formation of capillary-like tubes similar to those formed by H-MVECs. Further studies will be necessary to investigate how this pleiotropic protein may regulate the microvascular milieu in SSc and to clarify whether sKl administration might be useful to counteract SSc-related endothelial dysfunction. On the basis of our in vitro data, it will be of primary importance to test the potential utility of sKl peptide analogs as a novel therapeutic option to slow down the microvascular injury in patients with SSc.

Abbreviations

ADAM: A disintegrin and metalloprotease; BM: Bone marrow; BSA: Bovine serum albumin; dcSSc: Diffuse cutaneous systemic sclerosis; EBM: Endothelial cell basal medium; ECs: Endothelial cells; EPCs: Endothelial precursor cells; FBS: Fetal bovine serum; FGF23: Fibroblast growth factor 23; H-MVECs: Healthy microvascular endothelial cells; kDa: kiloDalton; lcSSc: Limited cutaneous systemic sclerosis; MVECs: Microvascular endothelial cells; NO: Nitric oxide; PBS: Phosphate-buffered saline; ROS: Reactive oxygen species; SD: Standard deviation; SEM: Standard error of the mean; sKl: Soluble α-Klotho; SSc: Systemic sclerosis; SSc-MVECs: Systemic sclerosis microvascular endothelial cells; tKl: Transmembrane α-Klotho; TRPC-1: Transient receptor potential canonical-1; VEGF: Vascular endothelial growth factor; VEGFR-2: Vascular endothelial growth factor receptor-2

Acknowledgements

Not applicable.

Funding

The authors received no specific funding for this work.

Authors' contributions

All authors meet the criteria for authorship. CM conceived the study, participated in study design and coordination, contributed to most of the experiments, analysis and interpretation of data, drafted and edited the manuscript and revised it critically for important intellectual content. MM contributed to dermal microvascular endothelial cell isolation, immunohistochemistry and immunocytochemistry, analysis and interpretation of data, drafted and edited the article and revised it critically for important intellectual content. IR contributed to western blotting experiments, immunohistochemistry and immunocytochemistry and helped to draft the manuscript. ER contributed to dermal microvascular endothelial cell isolation, western blotting experiments and analysis of data and helped to draft the manuscript. JB, SB-R, CB, GL and SG collected and supplied biological samples and clinical data, contributed to analysis of data and helped to draft the manuscript. LI-M contributed to immunohistochemistry, immunocytochemistry and interpretation of data and helped to draft the manuscript. MM-C participated in study design and coordination and interpretation of data, drafted the article and revised it critically for important intellectual content. All authors reviewed and approved the final manuscript and all authors agree to be accountable for all aspects of the study.

Authors' information

Qualifications: CM PhD; MM PhD; IR PhD; ER PhD; JB MD, PhD; SB-R MD, PhD; CB MD; GL MD; SG MD, PhD; LI-M MD; MM-C MD, PhD.

Competing interests

The authors declare that they have no competing interests.

Consent for publication

All authors approved the final version of the manuscript to be published.

Author details

[1]Department of Experimental and Clinical Medicine, Division of Rheumatology, University of Florence, AOUC, Largo Brambilla 3, 50134 Florence, Italy. [2]Department of Experimental and Clinical Medicine, Section of Anatomy and Histology, University of Florence, Largo Brambilla 3, 50134 Florence, Italy.

References

1. Balbir-Gurman A, Braun-Moscovici Y. Scleroderma - new aspects in pathogenesis and treatment. Best Pract Res Clin Rheumatol. 2012;26:13–24.
2. LeRoy EC, Black C, Fleischmajer R, Jablonska S, Krieg T, Medsger Jr TA, et al. Scleroderma (systemic sclerosis): classification, subsets and pathogenesis. J Rheumatol. 1988;15:202–5.
3. van den Hoogen F, Khanna D, Fransen J, Johnson SR, Baron M, Tyndall A, et al. 2013 Classification criteria for systemic sclerosis: an American College of Rheumatology/European League Against Rheumatism Collaborative initiative. Arthritis Rheum. 2013;65:2737–47.
4. Manetti M, Guiducci S, Ibba-Manneschi L, Matucci-Cerinic M. Impaired angiogenesis in systemic sclerosis: the emerging role of the antiangiogenic VEGF165b splice variant. Trends Cardiovasc Med. 2011;21:204–10.
5. Carmeliet P. Angiogenesis in life, disease and medicine. Nature. 2005; 438:932–6.

6. Folkman J. Angiogenesis in cancer, vascular, rheumatoid and other disease. Nat Med. 1995;1:27–31.
7. Rafii S. Circulating endothelial precursors: mystery, reality, and promise. J Clin Invest. 2000;105:17–9.
8. Isner JM, Asahara T. Angiogenesis and vasculogenesis as therapeutic strategies for postnatal neovascularization. J Clin Invest. 1999;103:1231–6.
9. Asahara T, Murohara T, Sullivan A, Silver M, van der Zee R, Li T, et al. Isolation of putative progenitor endothelial cells for angiogenesis. Science. 1997;275:965–7.
10. Cooper LT, Cooke JP, Dzau VJ. The vasculopathy of aging. J Gerontol. 1994; 49:B191–6.
11. De Santis M, Ceribelli A, Cavaciocchi F, Crotti C, Massarotti M, Belloli L, et al. Nailfold videocapillaroscopy and serum VEGF levels in scleroderma are associated with internal organ involvement. Auto Immun Highlights. 2016;7:5.
12. Bielecki M, Kowal K, Lapinska A, Chwiesko-Minarowska S, Chyczewski L, Kowal-Bielecka O. Peripheral blood mononuclear cells from patients with systemic sclerosis spontaneously secrete increased amounts of vascular endothelial growth factor (VEGF) already in the early stage of the disease. Adv Med Sci. 2011;56:255–63.
13. Manetti M, Guiducci S, Romano E, Ceccarelli C, Bellando-Randone S, Conforti ML, et al. Overexpression of VEGF165b, an inhibitory splice variant of vascular endothelial growth factor, leads to insufficient angiogenesis in patients with systemic sclerosis. Circ Res. 2011;109:e14–26.
14. Choi JJ, Min DJ, Cho ML, Min SY, Kim SJ, Lee SS, et al. Elevated vascular endothelial growth factor in systemic sclerosis. J Rheumatol. 2003;30:1529–33.
15. Distler O, Distler JH, Scheid A, Acker T, Hirth A, Rethage J, et al. Uncontrolled expression of vascular endothelial growth factor and its receptors leads to insufficient skin angiogenesis in patients with systemic sclerosis. Circ Res. 2004;95:109–16.
16. Kusaba T, Okigaki M, Matui A, Murakami M, Ishikawa K, Kimura T, et al. Klotho is associated with VEGF receptor-2 and the transient receptor potential canonical-1 Ca2+ channel to maintain endothelial integrity. Proc Natl Acad Sci U S A. 2010;107:19308–13.
17. Matsumura Y, Aizawa H, Shiraki-Iida T, Nagai R, Kuro-o M, Nabeshima Y. Identification of the human Klotho gene and its two transcripts encoding membrane and secreted Klotho protein. Biochem Biophys Res Commun. 1998;242:626–30.
18. Shiraki-Iida T, Aizawa H, Matsumura Y, Sekine S, Iida A, Anazawa H, et al. Structure of the mouse klotho gene and its two transcripts encoding membrane and secreted protein. FEBS Lett. 1998;424:6–10.
19. Kuro-o M, Matsumura Y, Aizawa H, Kawaguchi H, Suga T, Utsugi T, et al. Mutation of the mouse Klotho gene leads to a syndrome resembling ageing. Nature. 1997;390:45–51.
20. Kurosu H, Yamamoto M, Clark JD, Pastor JV, Nandi A, Gurnani P, et al. Suppression of aging in mice by the hormone Klotho. Science. 2005;309: 1829–33.
21. Imura A, Iwano A, Tohyama O, Tsuji Y, Nozaki K, Hashimoto N, et al. Secreted Klotho protein in sera and CSF: implication for post-translational cleavage in release of Klotho protein from cell membrane. FEBS Lett. 2004;565:143–7.
22. Li SA, Watanabe M, Yamada H, Nagai A, Kinuta M, Takei K. Immunohistochemical localization of Klotho protein in brain, kidney, and reproductive organs of mice. Cell Struct Funct. 2004;29:91–9.
23. Kurosu H, Ogawa Y, Miyoshi M, Yamamoto M, Nandi A, Rosenblatt KP, et al. Regulation of fibroblast growth factor-23 signaling by klotho. J Biol Chem. 2006;281:6120–3.
24. Kuro-o M. Klotho as a regulator of fibroblast growth factor signaling and phosphate/calcium metabolism. Curr Opin Nephrol Hypertens. 2006;15:437–41.
25. Hu MC, Kuro-o M, Moe OW. The emerging role of Klotho in clinical nephrology. Nephrol Dial Transplant. 2012;27:2650–7.
26. Yamamoto M, Clark JD, Pastor JV, Gurnani P, Nandi A, Kurosu H, et al. Regulation of oxidative stress by the anti-aging hormone klotho. J Biol Chem. 2005;280:38029–34.
27. Hsieh CC, Kuro-o M, Rosenblatt KP, Brobey R, Papaconstantinou J. The ASK1-Signalosome regulates p38 MAPK activity in response to levels of endogenous oxidative stress in the Klotho mouse models of aging. Aging (Albany NY). 2010;2:597–611.
28. Kuro-o M. Klotho in health and disease. Curr Opin Nephrol Hypertens. 2012; 21:362–8.
29. Chen CD, Podvin S, Gillespie E, Leeman SE, Abraham CR. Insulin stimulates the cleavage and release of the extracellular domain of Klotho by ADAM10 and ADAM17. Proc Natl Acad Sci U S A. 2007;104: 19796–801.
30. Ohyama Y, Kurabayashi M, Masuda H, Nakamura T, Aihara Y, Kaname T, et al. Molecular cloning of rat klotho cDNA: markedly decreased expression of klotho by acute inflammatory stress. Biochem Biophys Res Commun. 1998; 251:920–5.
31. Vervloet MG, Larsson TE. Fibroblast growth factor-23 and Klotho in chronic kidney disease. Kidney Int. 2011;1:130–5.
32. Wang Y, Kuro-o M, Sun Z. Klotho gene delivery suppresses Nox2 expression and attenuates oxidative stress in rat aortic smooth muscle cells via the cAMP-PKA pathway. Aging Cell. 2012;11:410–7.
33. Scott PA, Bicknell R. The isolation and culture of microvascular endothelium. J Cell Sci. 1993;105:269–73.
34. D'Alessio S, Fibbi G, Cinelli M, Guiducci S, Del Rosso A, Margheri F, et al. Matrix metalloproteinase 12-dependent cleavage of urokinase receptor in systemic sclerosis microvascular endothelial cells results in impaired angiogenesis. Arthritis Rheum. 2004;50:3275–85.
35. Margheri F, Manetti M, Serratì S, Nosi D, Pucci M, Matucci-Cerinic M, et al. Domain 1 of the urokinase-type plasminogen activator receptor is required for its morphologic and functional, beta2 integrin-mediated connection with actin cytoskeleton in human microvascular endothelial cells: failure of association in systemic sclerosis endothelial cells. Arthritis Rheum. 2006;54:3926–38.
36. Ikushima M, Rakugi H, Ishikawa K, Maekawa Y, Yamamoto K, Ohta J, et al. Anti-apoptotic and anti-senescence effects of klotho on vascular endothelial cells. Biochem Res Commun. 2006;339:827–32.
37. Maekawa Y, Ohishi M, Ikushima M, Yamamoto K, Yasuda O, Oguro R, et al. Klotho protein diminishes endothelial apoptosis and senescence via a mitogen-activated kinase pathway. Geriatric Gerontol Int. 2011;11:510–6.
38. de Oliveira RM. Klotho RNAi induces premature senescence of human cells via a p53/p21 dependent pathway. FEBS Lett. 2006;580:5753–8.
39. Safirstein R, DiMari J, Megyesi J, Price P. Mechanisms of renal repair and survival following acute injury. Semin Nephrol. 1998;18:519–22.
40. Rubin H. Cell aging in vivo and in vitro. Mech Ageing Dev. 1997;98:1–35.
41. Imura A, Tsuji Y, Murata M, Maeda R, Kubota K, Iwano A, et al. Alpha-Klotho as a regulator of calcium homeostasis. Science. 2007;316:1615–8.
42. Griffith TM, Edwards DH, Lewis MJ, Newby AC, Henderson AH. The nature of endothelium-derived vascular relaxant factor. Nature. 1984;308:645–7.
43. Palmer RM, Ferrige AG, Moncada S. Nitric oxide release accounts for the biological activity of endothelium-derived relaxing factor. Nature. 1987;327:524–6.
44. Saito Y, Nakamura T, Ohyama Y, Suzuki T, Iida A, Shiraki-Iida T, et al. In vivo klotho gene delivery protects against endothelial dysfunction in multiple risk factor syndrome. Biochem Biophys Res Commun. 2000;276:767–72.
45. Rakugi H, Matsukawa N, Ishikawa K, Yang J, Imai M, Ikushima M, et al. Anti-oxidative effect of Klotho on endothelial cells through cAMP activation. Endocrine. 2007;31:82–7.
46. Mukai Y, Shimokawa H, Higashi M, Morikawa K, Matoba T, Hiroki J, et al. Inhibition of renin-angiotensin system ameliorates endothelial dysfunction associated with aging in rats. Arterioscler Thromb Vasc Biol. 2002;22:1445–50.
47. Okada S, Yoshida T, Hong Z, Ishii G, Hatano M. Kuro-OM, et al. Impairment of B lymphopoiesis in precocious aging (klotho) mice. Int Immunol. 2000;12:861–71.
48. Shimada T, Takeshita Y, Murohara T, Sasaki K, Egami K, Shintani S, et al. Angiogenesis and vasculogenesis are impaired in the precocious-aging klotho mouse. Circulation. 2004;110:1148–55.
49. Kuwana M, Okazaki Y, Yasuoka H, Kawakami Y, Ikeda Y. Defective vasculogenesis in systemic sclerosis. Lancet. 2004;364:603–10.
50. Avouac J, Juin F, Wipff J, Couraud PO, Chiocchia G, Kahan A, et al. Circulating endothelial progenitor cells in systemic sclerosis: association with disease severity. Ann Rheum Dis. 2008;67:1455–60.
51. Manetti M, Guiducci S, Ibba-Manneschi L, Matucci-Cerinic M. Mechanisms in the loss of capillaries in systemic sclerosis: angiogenesis versus vasculogenesis. J Cell Mol Med. 2010;14:1241–54.
52. Cipriani P, Guiducci S, Miniati I, Cinelli M, Urbani S, Marrelli A, et al. Impairment of endothelial cell differentiation from bone marrow-derived mesenchymal stem cells: new insight into the pathogenesis of systemic sclerosis. Arthritis Rheum. 2007;56:1994–2004.

17

Epidemiology and disease characteristics of systemic sclerosis-related pulmonary arterial hypertension: results from a real-life screening programme

Kathleen Morrisroe[1,2], Wendy Stevens[2], Joanne Sahhar[3], Candice Rabusa[2], Mandana Nikpour[1,2*†], Susanna Proudman[4,5†] the Australian Scleroderma Interest Group (ASIG)

Abstract

Background: Pulmonary arterial hypertension (PAH) is the leading cause of death in systemic sclerosis (SSc). Annual screening with echocardiogram (ECHO) is recommended. We present the methodological aspects of a PAH screening programme in a large Australian SSc cohort, the epidemiology of SSc-PAH in this cohort, and an evaluation of factors influencing physician adherence to PAH screening guidelines.

Methods: Patient characteristics and results of PAH screening were determined in all patients enrolled in a SSc longitudinal cohort study. Adherence to PAH screening guidelines was assessed by a survey of Australian rheumatologists. Summary statistics, chi-square tests, univariate and multivariable logistic regression were used to determine the associations of risk factors with PAH.

Results: Among 1636 patients with SSc, 194 (11.9%) had PAH proven by right-heart catheter. Of these, 160 were detected by screening. The annual incidence of PAH was 1.4%. Patients with PAH diagnosed on subsequent screens, compared with patients in whom PAH was diagnosed on first screen, were more likely to have diffuse SSc ($p = 0.03$), be in a better World Health Organisation (WHO) Functional Class at PAH diagnosis ($p = 0.01$) and have less advanced PAH evidenced by higher mean six-minute walk distance ($p = 0.03$), lower mean pulmonary arterial pressure ($p = 0.009$), lower mean pulmonary vascular resistance ($p = 0.006$) and fewer non-trivial pericardial effusions ($p = 0.03$). Adherence to annual PAH screening using an ECHO-based algorithm was poor among Australian rheumatologists, with less than half screening their patients with SSc of more than ten years disease duration.

Conclusion: PAH is a common complication of SSc. Physician adherence to PAH screening recommendations remains poor. Identifying modifiable barriers to screening may improve adherence and ultimately patient outcomes.

Keywords: Systemic sclerosis, Scleroderma, Pulmonary arterial hypertension, Screening algorithm

* Correspondence: m.nikpour@unimelb.edu.au
[†]Equal contributors
[1]Department of Medicine, The University of Melbourne at St Vincent's Hospital (Melbourne), 41 Victoria Parade, Fitzroy 3065, Victoria, Australia
[2]Departments of Rheumatology and Medicine, The University of Melbourne at St Vincent's Hospital (Melbourne), 41 Victoria Parade, Fitzroy 3065, Victoria, Australia
Full list of author information is available at the end of the article

Background

Systemic sclerosis (SSc) is a multisystem connective tissue disease (CTD) characterised by vasculopathy and fibrosis [1]. There is no cure for SSc, leading to significant morbidity, mortality and poor health-related quality of life [2, 3].

Cardiopulmonary manifestations, namely interstitial lung disease (ILD) and pulmonary arterial hypertension (PAH), have replaced SSc renal crisis (SRC) as the leading cause of mortality in SSc [4, 5].

SSc-PAH occurs with a prevalence of 8–12% [6] and is the second most common cause of PAH after idiopathic PAH [7]. PAH is characterised by abnormal proliferation, vasoconstriction and thrombosis of the pulmonary vasculature, leading to elevated pulmonary vascular resistance (PVR), resulting in right-heart failure and death [8]. Despite new pulmonary vasodilator therapies that improve symptoms and survival [9–16], one-year and three-year survival remains poor (78% and 47%, respectively) [17, 18], less than that of idiopathic and other connective tissue disease (CTD)-associated PAH [18]. Risk factors for the development of SSc PAH include anti-centromere antibody, telangiectasia, calcinosis, oesphageal stricture, sicca symptoms, mild ILD and digital ulcers [19, 20], although none of these perform sufficiently well as indicators in the individual patient and are often inconsistent between studies.

Early recognition of SSc-PAH is difficult as early disease is clinically silent and the heterogeneous nature of SSc makes interpretation of fatigue and dyspnoea challenging [21]. Survival is improved even after adjustment for lead-time bias in SSc-PAH when diagnosed by screening compared with diagnosis during routine care [9–14]. Consequently, annual screening with transthoracic echocardiogram (TTE) and pulmonary function tests (PFTs) is recommended [22], regardless of the presence or absence of the aforementioned risk factors, to identify patients who should undergo right-heart catheterisation (RHC) to confirm the diagnosis.

Despite the documented benefit of PAH screening, physician adherence is suboptimal, with one study showing that only 34.7% of patients with SSc had a TTE and 53.1% had PFT in the twelve months prior to PAH diagnosis [23]. Adherence among Australian physicians is no better, with over 40% not adhering to annual screening and even fewer using RHC for PAH diagnosis [24]. Consequently, the Australian Scleroderma Cohort Study (ASCS), a longitudinal multi-centre study, was established in 2007 as a web-based screening platform for the cardiorespiratory manifestations of SSc.

In this paper, we present the methodological aspects of establishing the ASCS and the screening algorithm, the characteristics of patients with SSc with PAH in this cohort and an evaluation of the factors influencing Australian rheumatologists' adherence to screening guidelines.

Methods

Study centres

The ASCS is a nationwide project wherein patients with SSc are recruited from 13 participating centres across Australia. SSc experts were invited by a core group of rheumatologists to form the Australian Scleroderma Interest Group (ASIG) and to take part in the ASCS through recruitment of patients and collection of data at their centres. Physicians who are not at an ASIG centre and care for patients with SSc are invited to refer patients for the screening service, while ongoing care between screening visits remains their responsibility.

Patients

All patients with SSc, defined according to American College of Rheumatology (ACR)/European League Against Rheumatism (EULAR) criteria [25] or Leroy/Medsger criteria [26], and mixed connective tissue disease (MCTD), as originally described by Sharp et al. [27], are eligible for enrolment. Patients provide written informed consent for collection of de-identified data, chart review, and storage of serum and DNA for future studies. All human research ethics committees of the participating sites have approved ASCS.

Data collection and database

Comprehensive demographic and disease-related data are collected annually and entered into a custom-made database hosted by St. Vincent's Hospital Melbourne using a remote secure access token. A log is kept of all users and the database is backed up daily. Logic checks are used to detect errors in data entry and incomplete entries.

Screening algorithm for early detection of PAH

Participation in the ASCS mandates annual application of a PAH screening algorithm created by a panel of Australian rheumatologists, cardiologists and respiratory physicians (Fig. 1) based on the European Society of Cardiology (ESC)/European Respiratory Society (ERS) guidelines [28, 29]. According to Fig. 1, investigations are recommended for symptomatic patients with low probability of PAH, and irrespective of symptoms for patients with moderate or high probability of PAH [30].

Clinical decision support tool

If any value falls outside a predetermined range for systolic pulmonary arterial pressure (sPAP) on TTE, diffusing capacity of the lung for carbon monoxide (DLCO) corrected for haemoglobin, and/or forced vital capacity (FVC) according to the screening algorithm, an email to the treating physician is automatically generated, indicating why the alert has been triggered and recommending a course of action. If the physician chooses not to follow the algorithm he/she must justify this decision.

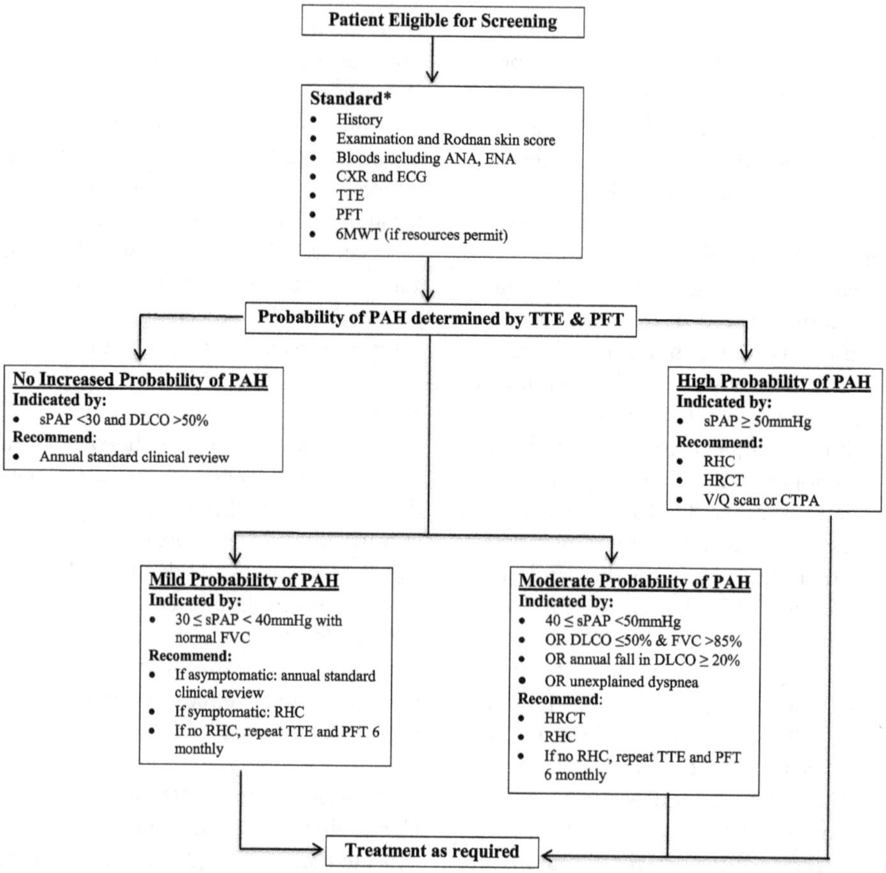

Fig. 1 Australian Scleroderma Cohort Study algorithm for screening for pulmonary hypertension. *ANA* antinuclear antibody, *ENA* extractable nuclear antibody, *CXR* chest radiograph, *ECG* electrocardiogram, *TTE* transthoracic echocardiogram, *PFT* pulmonary function test, *6MWT* six-minute walk test, *PAH* pulmonary arterial hypertension, *sPAP* systolic pulmonary arterial pressure, *DLCO* diffusing capacity of the lung for carbon monoxide corrected for haemoglobin, *RHC* right-heart catheterization, *HRCT* high-resolution chest computed tomography, *V/Q* ventilation perfusion, *CTPA* computed tomography pulmonary angiography

Adherence to published recommendations for annual PAH screening

Non-ASIG physicians' screening practices and adherence to published recommendations for PAH screening [24, 28, 29] were assessed by means of a cross-sectional survey (Additional file 1: Table S1 using survey monkey circulated through the Australian Rheumatology Association following the establishment of ASCS in 2007. The survey addressed existing screening practices based on SSc disease subtype and disease duration (early or late defined as <10 or ≥10 years from the first non-Raynaud's disease manifestation, respectively), barriers to screening encountered by physicians and suggestions for streamlining screening.

Statistics

For the purpose of statistical analysis, de-identified aggregated data are exported in.txt and.xml format. Characteristics of patients in the study are presented as mean (standard deviation (SD)) or number (percentage). We compared dichotomous variables using the chi-square test. Continuous variables were compared using the *t* test for normally distributed data and the Wilcoxon rank-sum (Mann-Whitney) test for non-parametric data. All-cause mortality was used for survival analyses. Kaplan-Meier (K-M) curves were used to estimate survival in patients with SSc-PAH diagnosed at first screen versus subsequent screen. The date of PAH diagnosis on RHC was considered the baseline from which survival was calculated. Log-rank and Wilcoxon tests were used to compare survival curves.

Results

Recruitment

A total of 1636 patients were recruited into ASCS from July 2007 to July 2016 (census date). Recruitment comprised new referrals from general practitioners for comprehensive specialist management, and from rheumatologists requesting the PAH screening service only. The number of patients recruited, relative to the predicted prevalence of SSc in Australia [31, 32] and population data from the Australian Bureau of Statistics [33] were estimated.

Patient characteristics and follow up

Of the 1636 patients, 1243 (75.9%) had been seen within the 18 months before the census date and were considered "current" (Table 1). The period of 18 months was selected to allow for delays in data entry. Patient characteristics and follow-up status are summarised in Table 1.

Patients with limited disease (lcSSc) were older at recruitment than patients with diffuse disease (dcSSc) (58.8 ± 12.2 vs 53.1 ± 13.1 years, $p < 0.001$) with longer disease duration from first non-Raynaud's clinical manifestation (12.2 ± 10.8 vs 8.1 ± 8.7 years, $p < 0.001$). ILD was more prevalent in the patients with dcSSc (40.9% vs 21.1%) but there was no significant difference in the prevalence of PAH (10.1% vs 12.7%, $p = 0.40$) (Table 2).

In total, 232 patients (14.2%) were diagnosed with pulmonary hypertension (PH). Of these, 194 patients (83.6%) had World Health Organisation (WHO) Group I PAH according to the criteria developed in Nice [34], 15 patients (6.5%) had exercise-induced PH, 18 patients (7.8%) had PH secondary to left ventricular dysfunction (WHO Group 2 PH) and 5 patients (2.2%) had PH secondary to ILD (WHO Group 3 PH). Only patients with WHO Group I PAH were analysed in this study.

At enrollment, 34 (2.1%) patients had previously been diagnosed with PAH and 122 (7.5%) were diagnosed at their first contact with ASCS. Among the latter, 89 (72.9%) had SSc disease duration of ≥4 years and the date of their last TTE was 1.6 ± 4.6 years before enrollment to ASCS, highlighting a lack of adherence to annual PAH screening in the community.

Outcomes of screening in the ASCS

A total of 4326 screening visits were analysed, to determine the success of, and adherence to the PAH screening algorithm (Table 3). Only patients not previously diagnosed with PAH were included. At the first screening visit, sufficient data to apply the screening algorithm were available for 1363 patients. Of these, 101 patients (7.4%) were at high risk of PAH, 121 patients (8.9%) at moderate risk, 358 patients (26.3%) at low risk and 470 patients (34.5%) at no increased risk based on TTE and PFT results. The number of patients with no tricuspid regurgitation (TR) on TTE, and hence inestimable sPAP, was high at 313 (22.9%).

At the first screening visit, 157 of the 580 (27.1%) patients at low (38/358), moderate (36/121), or high (83/101) risk of PAH underwent RHC. WHO Group 1 PAH was diagnosed in 122 patients (8.9% of the cohort), including 4 of 19 (21.0%) patients with a normal TTE and 10 of 24 patients (41.7%) with a missing sPAP on TTE due to lack of a TR jet. The patients in the latter two groups were referred for RHC due to reduced exercise capacity and/reduced DLCO. Only 4% of the patients with no TR were referred for RHC but 36.8% of these

Table 1 Characteristics of patients recruited up to July 2016 (n = 1636)

Characteristic	Number (%) or mean ± SD
Patient number	1636
Gender (female:male)	6.4:1 (86.1% vs 13.9%)
Race	
Caucasian	1390 (91.9%)
Asian	75 (4.9%)
Aboriginal-Islander	18 (1.2%)
Hispanic	11 (0.7%)
Other	19 (1.3%)
Age at recruitment, mean ± SD, years	57.2 ± 12.8
Disease duration at recruitment[a], years	10.9 ± 10.2
Recruited within 4 years of first non-Raynaud's feature	435
Age at diagnosis of PAH if present, years	62.9 ± 11.1
Number of study visits	
One	364 (22.3%)
Two	325 (19.9%)
Three	216 (13.2%)
Four	199 (12.2%)
Five	165 (10.1%)
Six	119 (7.3%)
Seven	71 (4.3%)
Eight	79 (4.8%)
Nine	84(5.2%)
Ten	14 (0.9%)
Duration of follow up, mean ± SD, years	3.7 ± 2.7
Patient status	
Current	1243 (76.5%)
Withdrawn	101 (6.2%)
Dead	220 (13.5%)
Lost to follow up	61 (3.8%)
Disease subtype	
Limited	1122 (68.6%)
Diffuse	377 (23.0%)
MCTD	83 (5.3%)
Autoantibody profile	
ANA positive (n = 1508)	1418 (94.0%)
Anti-centromere (n = 1497)	673 (44.9%)
Anti-Scl70 (n = 1483)	205 (13.8%)
Anti-RNAP (n = 794)	125 (13.1%)

[a]Disease duration from first non-Raynaud manifestation. Numbers of variables analysed (n =) are included in each section of the table to acknowledge any missing data. Patient status: current patients were defined as being seen in the last 2 years, withdrawn patients have withdrawn their consent from participating in the database and lost to follow up is defined as patients who, despite multiple attempts, we have been unable to contact for >18 months. *PAH* pulmonary arterial hypertension, *MCTD* mixed connective tissue disease, *ANA* antinuclear antibody, *Anti-RNAP* anti-RNA polymerase

Table 2 Characteristics of patients with SSc by disease subset

	Limited n = 1122 mean ± SD or %	Diffuse n = 377 mean ± SD or %	*P* value
Age at recruitment, years	58.8 ± 12.2	53.1 ± 13.1	<0.001
Female	89.5%	74.9%	<0.001
Disease duration[a] (non-Raynaud) at recruitment, years	12.2 ± 10.8	8.1 ± 8.7	<0.001
Anti-centromere pattern ANA	59.2%	9.6%	<0.001
Scl 70 positive	8.9%	31.1%	<0.001
RNA polymerase III positive	5.4%	39.6%	<0.001
ILD (HRCT scan)	236 (21.11%)	154 (40.9%)	<0.001
PAH (RHC)	142 (12.7%)	38 (10.1%)	0.40
Rodnan skin score (highest ever)	7.7 ± 5.4	22.7 ± 9.9	<0.001
Digital ulcers ever	39.6%	60.8%	<0.001
Joint contractures ever	28.5%	71.2%	<0.001
Renal crisis ever	0.9%	7.7%	<0.001
Gastro-oesophageal reflux	80.3%	82.7%	0.29
Anal incontinence	27.9%	25.6%	0.39

ANA antinuclear antibodies, *ILD* interstitial lung disease, *HRCT* high-resolution chest computed tomography, *PAH* pulmonary arterial hypertension, *RHC* right-heart catheterisation
[a]Disease duration defined as from first non-Raynaud's disease manifestation. Disease manifestations are defined as present if ever present from time of diagnosis of systemic sclerosis (SSc)

were diagnosed with WHO Group 1 PAH. At the physician's discretion and based on other indicators such as patient symptoms and TTE parameters, patients whose initial RHC was negative for PAH were considered for future RHC.

The screening algorithm correctly identified patients at increased risk of PAH and stratified them by level of risk. The higher the probability of PAH, the more likely PAH was to be identified on RHC (Table 3). A new diagnosis of WHO Group I PAH was made in 160 patients from 4326 (3.7%) screening visits (115/1122 with lcSSc, 32/377 with dcSSc and 10/83 with MCTD), giving a prevalence of PAH of 11.8% (10.3% in lcSSc, 8.5% in dcSSc and 12.0% in MCTD). The annual prevalence of PAH was 1.4% (1.2% in lcSSc, 0.9% in dcSSc, 0.4% in MCTD). All patients were treated with specific PAH therapy.

Characteristics of patients with PAH

Patients with PAH were significantly older than patients without PAH (63.1 vs 56.3 years, $p < 0.001$), had longer disease duration (13.6 vs 10.4 years, $p < 0.001$) and were in WHO Functional Class III/IV (85.0% vs 21.7%, $p < 0.001$) (Table 4). Clinical manifestations and autoantibody status are summarised in Table 4.

Characteristics of patients with PAH diagnosed on first screen compared with patients whose PAH was diagnosed on subsequent screens

To assess whether the ASCS screening programme succeeded in detecting PAH at an earlier stage, we divided our PAH cohort into those patients whose PAH was detected on first screening and those whose PAH was detected on the second or subsequent screen (Table 5).

We believe that PAH detected on first screen were likely to be a "delayed diagnosis" in patients who were referred to ASCS due to symptoms or clinical suspicion of PAH, whereas PAH detected on subsequent screens was more likely to be an "incident" PAH identified on earlier screening.

Patients diagnosed with PAH on subsequent screens compared with first screen were more likely to have dcSSc (35.1% vs 15.9%, $p = 0.03$), be in a better WHO functional class (54.1% vs 75.9% in Class III, 5.4% vs 16.2% in Class IV, $p = 0.01$) and have less advanced PAH at diagnosis evidenced by lower mPVR (3.8 vs 5.5, $p = 0.005$), higher mean 6MWD (340.6 vs 295.9, $p = 0.05$), lower mPAP (32.5 vs 38.2, $p = 0.005$), and fewer non-trivial pericardial effusions (2.7% vs 16.0%, $p = 0.03$).

PAH treatment with combination therapy and anticoagulation therapy was prescribed at a similar rate in those diagnosed at subsequent screens (36.8% and 28.9%, respectively) and those diagnosed at first screen (32.1% and 26.8%, respectively). Three-year survival from the time of PAH diagnosis was better in those diagnosed on subsequent screen compared with those diagnosed at first screen as outlined in Fig. 2 (94.7% vs 42.7%, $p < 0.001$) and mean time to death was longer in those diagnosed with PAH on subsequent screens compared with those diagnosed at first screen (4.7 ± 2.3 vs 2.3 ± 2.3, $p < 0.001$). PAH was the direct cause of death in 100% of patients diagnosed on subsequent screen and in 92.7% of those diagnosed on first screen ($p = 0.40$).

Adherence to the ASCS screening algorithm

ASIG physicians' adherence to PAH screening guidelines was high with 84.4% of patients undergoing annual screening over a ten-year period. Despite the screening algorithm (Fig. 1) mandating that patients at moderate or high risk of PAH should undergo RHC, only 29.7% (170/572) had RHC. Even among those in the high probability group, only 59.1% of patients underwent RHC. Physician justification for not performing RHC predominantly related to their WHO functional class. In 50.5% of cases, RHC was not performed as the patient was in WHO Functional Class I (31.6%), or Class II (14.7%) or was not dyspnoeic (4.2%). In 18.9% of cases, the physician referred the patient to another specialist for their opinion, most commonly a cardiologist or respiratory physician. In 16.8% of cases, the physician was deterred

Table 3 Diagnosis of WHO Group I PAH by risk stratification using the screening algorithm

		No increased probability[a]			Low probability of PAH[a]			Moderate probability of PAH[a]			High probability of PAH[a]			Missing sPAP			Total with PAH, *n*
Review number	Screened, *n*	Normal TTE, *n*	RHC, *n*	PAH, *n*	Moderate TTE, *n*	RHC, *n*	PAH, *n*	High suspicion TTE, *n*	RHC, *n*	No. with PAH	High probability TTE, *n*	RHC, *n*	PAH, *n*	Positive screen[c], *n*	RHC, *n*	PAH, *n*	
1st screen	1363	470	19	4	358	38	11	121	36	25	101	83	72	313	24	10	122 (8.9%)
2nd screen	896	355	6	2	229	5	3	78	10	4	32	11	5	202	8	3	17 (1.9%)
3rd screen	679	272	0	0	167	4	1	65	5	3	20	7	6	155	3	1	11 (1.6%)
4th screen	482	199	0	0	125	3	0	42	7	2	13	5	3	103	1	0	5 (1.0%)
5th screen	361	149	0	0	104	0	0	25	1	1	9	4	1	74	1	0	2 (0.6%)
6th screen	235	91	0	0	72	1	1	25	1	1	6	0	0	41	0	0	2 (0.9%)
7th screen	162	66	0	0	48	0	0	14	0	0	3	0	0	31	1	0	0 (0.0%)
8th screen	104	48	0	0	27	1	1	10	0	0	1	0	0	18	0	0	0 (0.0%)
9th screen	43	20	0	0	11	1	1	6	0	0	1	0	0	5	0	0	1 (2.3%)
10th screen	1	0	0	0	1	0	0	0	0	0	0	0	0	0	0	0	0 (0.0%)
Total	4326	1670	25[b] (1.5%)	6[a] (24%)	1142	53[b] (4.6%)	17[a] (32.7%)	386	60[b] (15.5%)	36[a] (60%)	186	110[b] (59%)	87[a] (79.1%)	942	38[b] (4%)	14[a] (36.8%)	160 (11.7%)

[a]Probability of pulmonary arterial hypertension (PAH): no increased probability of PAH was indicated by systolic pulmonary arterial pressure (sPAP) <30 and diffusing capacity of the lung for carbon monoxide corrected for haemoglobin (DLCO) >50%, low probability of PAH was indicated by 30 ≤ sPAP <40 mmHg with normal forced vital capacity (FVC) and high-resolution computed tomography (HRCT), moderate probability of PAH was 40 ≤ sPAP <50 mmHg OR DLCO ≤50% and FVC <85% or annual fall in DLCO ≥20% or unexplained dyspnea and high probability of PAH was indicated by sPAP ≥50 mmHg.

[b]Percentage of patients who were detected by transthoracic echocardiogram (TTE) to be in a risk category and underwent right-heart catheterisation (RHC)

[c]Percentage of patients who underwent RHC and were diagnosed with World Health Organisation (WHO) Group I PAH

Table 4 Characteristics of patients with SSc by PAH status

	PAH mean ± SD or %	No PAH mean ± SD or %	*P* value
Number of patients	209	1283	
Age at recruitment, years	63.1 ± 10.4	56.3 ± 12.7	<0.001
Disease duration at recruitment, years[a]	13.6 ± 11.5	10.4 ± 9.9	<0.001
Female	87.1%	86.2%	0.88
Limited disease subtype	73.9%	70.3%	0.43
Anti-centromere pattern ANA	52.6%	44.1%	0.02
Scl 70 positive	6.9%	15.2%	0.003
RNA polymerase III positive	14.4%	12.9%	0.65
Digital ulcers ever	53.0%	41.9%	0.003
Telangiectasia ever	91.4%	82.4%	<0.001
Calcinosis ever	53.3%	34.7%	<0.001
Joint contractures ever	45.8%	35.7%	0.007
GORD	45.9%	45.3%	0.48
Bowel dysmotility	27.3%	22.7%	0.15
Anal incontinence	32.1%	25.7%	0.05
WHO Functional Class			
Class I	4 (2.1%)	467(39.1%)	<0.001
Class II	25 (12.9%)	469 (39.2%)	
Class III	106 (54.9%)	238 (19.9%)	
Class IV	58(30.1%)	22(1.8%)	
NT-pro-BNP	218.9 ± 285.7	75.1 ± 159.8	0.005

PAH pulmonary arterial hypertension, ANA antinuclear antibodies, *6MWD* six minute walk distance, *mPAP* mean pulmonary arterial pressure, *mRAP* mean right atrial pressure, *PVR* pulmonary vascular resistance, *GORD* gastro-oesphageal reflux disease, *WHO* World Health Organisation, *NT-pro-BNP* N-terminal pro b-type natriuretic peptide
[a]Disease duration defined as from first non-Raynaud's disease manifestation
Disease manifestations defined as present if ever present from systemic sclerosis (SSc) diagnosis

Table 5 Comparison of demographic, clinical and haemodynamic characteristics of patients with PAH diagnosed at first screen and PAH diagnosed at subsequent screens

Characteristic	PAH detected on first screening mean ± SD or %	PAH detected on subsequent screening mean ± SD or %	*P* value
Number of patients	122	38	
Age at PAH diagnosis	63.9 ± 11.0	62.7 ± 9.5	0.56
Disease duration at PAH diagnosis	13.4 ± 12.8	14.6 ± 8.7	0.62
Female	96 (85.7%)	32 (84.2%)	0.82
Disease subtype			
Limited	81 (75.7%)	23 (62.2%)	0.03
Diffuse	17 (15.9%)	13 (35.1%)	
MCTD	9 (8.4%)	1 (2.7%)	
Status			
Alive	54 (48.2%)	26 (68.4%)	0.03
Dead	55 (49.1%)	10 (26.3%)	
Withdrawn	3 (2.7%)	1 (2.6%)	
Unable to contact	0 (0%)	1 (2.6%)	
Follow up, years	3.3 ± 2.4	5.9 ± 1.9	<0.001
WHO class at PAH diagnosis			
Class I	4 (4.0%)	0 (0%)	0.01
Class II	16 (16.2%)	15 (40.5%)	
Class III	63 (75.9%)	20 (54.1%)	
Class IV	16 (16.2%)	2 (5.4%)	
6MWD at PAH diagnosis	295.9 ± 118.3	340.6 ± 115.6	0.05
mPAP on RHC	38.2 ± 11.4	32.5 ± 8.3	0.005
mRAP on RHC	9.7 ± 8.5	8.4 ± 3.9	0.40
PVR on RHC	5.5 ± 3.1	3.8 ± 1.7	0.005
CI on RHC	2.9 ± 1.6	2.9 ± 0.7	0.87
Pericardial effusion	16 (16.0%)	1 (2.7%)	0.03

Probability of PAH
PAH pulmonary arterial hypertension, *MCTD* mixed connective tissue disease, *WHO* World Health Organisation, *6MWD* six-minute walk distance, *mPAP* mean pulmonary arterial pressure, *RHC* right-heart catheterization, *mRAP* mean right atrial pressure, *PVR* pulmonary vascular resistance, *CI* cardiac index, *NT-pro-BNP* N-terminal pro b-type natriuretic peptide

from arranging RHC due to the presence of mild ILD that they felt accounted for the TTE or PFT result. The remaining justifications included a plan to repeat the TTE and/or PFT at a later date (4.2%), patient refusal to have RHC (2.1%), terminal malignancy (2.1%) and no access to RHC (1.1%).

Adherence to PAH screening guidelines by Australian rheumatologists after the establishment of the ASCS screening programme in 2007

Of 334 non-ASIG Australian rheumatologists, 52 responded to the survey on screening practices and barriers to screening (Additional file 1: Table S1). The majority (88.9%) reported screening asymptomatic patients for PAH regularly. Just over half of the respondents ordered annual screening for their asymptomatic patients with early SSc (lcSSc 58.9%, dcSSc 52.6%), with even fewer screening annually in late disease (lcSSc 38.5%, dcSSc 43.6%). All respondents (100%) would investigate their patients with symptoms consistent with PAH. In early symptomatic SSc (with breathlessness or reduced exercise tolerance), the majority of respondents would screen on a six-monthly (51.2%) or annual basis (33.6%). In late symptomatic SSc, 38.9% of respondents would screen their patients six-monthly and 41.2% of respondents would screen annually. Alarmingly, 17.5% of respondents would only screen symptomatic patients every two years.

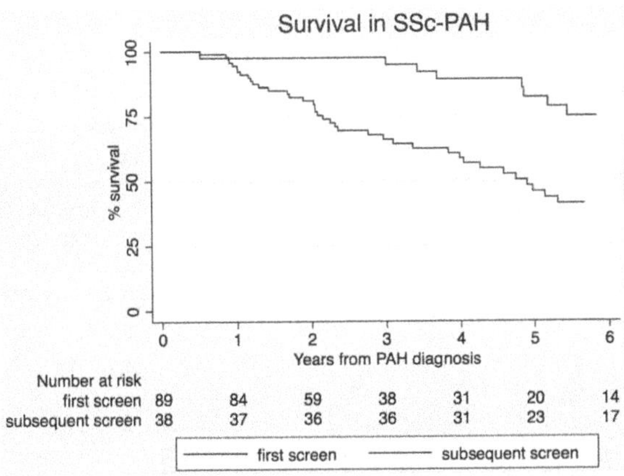

Fig. 2 Survival in systemic sclerosis (*SSc*) with pulmonary arterial hypertension (*PAH*) according to the screening visit when the diagnosis was made (first vs subsequent)

Explanations for not following guidelines for PAH screening included cost of screening (60%) and concerns about how to interpret the results (80%). In order to improve screening, 50% of respondents felt that they required better guidelines for the selection and frequency of screening tests, 44.7% wanted a reminder system, 42.1% wanted guideline simplification but only 31.6% felt that access to an experienced screening centre would be helpful. If reimbursed by Medicare Australia, 76.3% of respondents would consider the use of a blood test such as N-terminal pro B-type natriuretic peptide (NT-pro-BNP) a major advance.

Discussion

We present the ASCS as a model of multi-centre web--based data collection and decision support for applying a PAH screening algorithm in patients with SSc. Between 2007 and 2016, 1636 patients with SSc were recruited, an estimated 30.9% of all Australian patients with SSc based on a prevalence of 20 per 100,000 people. As Australia has such sparse population density and SSc is a low-frequency disease, such multicentre collaborations are required in order to recruit and retain sufficient patients for a longitudinal observational study.

The patient characteristics of our cohort are comparable to those of other large multi-centre cohorts indicating that a representative sample is being recruited [35]. As a result of screening, 160 patients were diagnosed with PAH over a ten-year period, providing an annual PAH of 1.4%, consistent with that of the French *ItinerAIR-Sclerodermie* Study of 0.6% [36] and a prevalence of 11.8% consistent with worldwide data [13, 36–39].

As in other cohorts [40, 41], patients with PAH were older, had longer disease duration from the first non-Raynaud's clinical manifestation, were more likely to be anti-centromere (ACA)-positive and to have digital ulcers, telangiectasia, calcinosis and joint contractures compared to those without PAH. Patients with PAH detected on the second or subsequent screen were more likely to have dcSSc, be in a better WHO Functional Class at PAH diagnosis and have less advanced PAH, which is consistent with the French data [36] but different from the classical teaching that PAH more commonly develops in patients with lcSSc [42].

Additionally, patients with PAH diagnosed on subsequent screen compared with first screen had significantly improved survival ($p < 0.001$) and a longer mean time to death (4.7 ± 2.3 vs 2.3 ± 2.3, $p < 0.001$), which may in part be due to lead-time bias. Our one-year and three- year survival in patients diagnosed with PAH on subsequent visits are similar to the survival rates in the PHAROS registry [14], one of the few other studies evaluating survival in incident SSc-PAH diagnosed on RHC. These survival rates are higher than those reported in other registries containing a mixture of patients with both incident and prevalent SSc-PAH or PAH diagnosed on TTE rather than RHC [38, 43, 44]. Diagnosis of early PAH is particularly important as patients with early PAH can progress rapidly, supporting the need for early treatment in this patient population [12].

Despite the majority of patients in the ASCS being screened annually, only 29.7% (170/572) of patients deemed at moderate or high risk of PAH were referred for RHC, predominantly due to preservation of functional class limiting patient eligibility for PBS-funded PAH therapy. Concern about the small but documented risk involved in RHC may also have deterred physicians from referring for RHC but this information was not specifically sought. These results highlight external factors that limit adherence to international screening recommendations.

The number of patients with no TR on TTE, and hence inestimable sPAP, was high at 21.8%, but consistent with the 20–30% reported in the literature [45]. Only 4% of these patients were referred for RHC, with 36.8% diagnosed with WHO Group 1 PAH. This highlights the need for a non-TTE dependent method of PAH screening and supports the emerging role of NT-pro-BNP, which is increased in PAH and in those at increased risk [46]. This test is not currently reimbursed for this indication in Australia and thus is not often performed.

Since the establishment of ASCS in 2007, Australian rheumatologists' adherence to screening guidelines has improved, with 88.9% of physicians regularly screening asymptomatic patients with SSc for PAH compared with 55.8% previously [29]. Of those who did not perform TTE for PAH screening, 50% reported this was due to difficulty assessing the right heart pressures with TTE. Referral of these patients to a tertiary screening centre may overcome this obstacle. To our knowledge, there have been no other studies addressing physicians' perceived barriers to SSc-PAH screening.

Limitations to our study include the potential for lead-time and length-time bias to impact on the survival benefit seen in PAH detected with screening. However, patients detected by screening were functionally impaired at the time of diagnosis and were all commenced on PAH therapy, indicating that their physician felt that their PAH required treatment. Our data analyses were conducted in patients who underwent all procedures listed in our screening algorithm; therefore, the incidence of PAH in our study may be an underestimate, although consistent with the literature. Additionally, only 15.6% of non-ASIG Australian rheumatologists responded to our survey on PAH screening adherence. Therefore these particular results may not be a true reflection of rheumatologists nationwide.

Conclusion

SSc-PAH is a tragic consequence of SSc, which despite advances in therapy, is the leading cause of SSc-related death. Screening with a web-based algorithm can identify patients with earlier PAH and improve outcomes. Identifying modifiable barriers to screening may improve adherence and ultimately patient outcomes.

Abbreviations

ASCS: Australian Scleroderma Cohort Study; ASIG: Australian Scleroderma Interest Group; DLCO: Diffusing capacity of the lung for carbon monoxide corrected for haemoglobin; dcSSc: Diffuse cutaneous systemic sclerosis; HRCT: High-resolution computed tomography; ILD: Interstitial lung disease; lcSSc: Limited cutaneous systemic sclerosis; MCTD: Mixed connective tissue disease; NT-pro-BNP: N-terminal pro B-type natriuretic peptide; PAH: Pulmonary arterial hypertension; PH: Pulmonary hypertension; RFTs: Respiratory function tests; RHC: Right-heart catheterisation; SSc: Systemic sclerosis (also known as systemic scleroderma); sPAP: Systolic pulmonary arterial pressure; TR: Tricuspid regurgitation; TTE: Transthoracic echocardiogram; WHO: World Health Organisation

Acknowledgements

We would like to acknowledge all investigators of the Australian Scleroderma Interest Group (ASIG) including Catherine Hill, Adelaide, South Australia; Sue Lester, Adelaide, South Australia; Peter Nash, Sunshine Coast, Queensland; Gian Ngian, Melbourne Victoria; Mandana Nikpour, Melbourne, Victoria; Susanna Proudman, Adelaide, South Australia; Maureen Rischmueller, Adelaide, South Australia; Janet Roddy, Perth, Western Australia; Joanne Sahhar, Melbourne, Victoria; Wendy Stevens, Melbourne, Victoria; Gemma Strickland, Geelong, Victoria; Vivek Thakkar, New South Wales; Jenny Walker, Adelaide, South Australia; Jane Zochling, Hobart, Tasmania.

Funding

This work was supported by Scleroderma Australia, Arthritis Australia, Actelion Australia, Bayer, CSL Biotherapies, GlaxoSmithKline Australia and Pfizer. Dr Morrisroe holds an NHMRC Scholarship (APP1113954). Dr Nikpour holds an NHMRC Fellowship (APP1071735).

Authors' contributions

KM: study design, data analysis, interpretation of results and preparation of the manuscript. WS: study design, data collection, interpretation of results and preparation of the manuscript. JS: data collection and preparation of the manuscript. CR: data analysis and preparation of the manuscript. SP: study design, data collection, interpretation of results and preparation of manuscript. MN: study design, data collection, data analysis, interpretation of results and preparation of the manuscript. All authors have read and approved the final manuscript.

Competing interests

All of the authors declare that they have no competing interests.

Author details

[1]Department of Medicine, The University of Melbourne at St Vincent's Hospital (Melbourne), 41 Victoria Parade, Fitzroy 3065, Victoria, Australia. [2]Departments of Rheumatology and Medicine, The University of Melbourne at St Vincent's Hospital (Melbourne), 41 Victoria Parade, Fitzroy 3065, Victoria, Australia. [3]Monash University and Monash Health, 246 Clayton Road, Clayton 3168, Victoria, Australia. [4]Rheumatology Unit, Royal Adelaide Hospital, North Terrace, SA 5000, Australia. [5]Discipline of Medicine, University of Adelaide, Adelaide, SA 5000, Australia.

References

1. Marie I, Jouen F, Hellot MF, Levesque H. Anticardiolipin and anti-beta2 glycoprotein I antibodies and lupus-like anticoagulant: prevalence and significance in systemic sclerosis. Br J Dermatol. 2008;158(1):141–4.
2. Thombs BD, Taillefer SS, Hudson M, Baron M. Depression in patients with systemic sclerosis: a systematic review of the evidence. Arthritis Rheum. 2007;57(6):1089–97.
3. Poole JL, Steen VD. The use of the Health Assessment Questionnaire (HAQ) to determine physical disability in systemic sclerosis. Arthritis Care Res. 1991;4(1):27–31.
4. Tyndall AJ, Bannert B, Vonk M, Airo P, Cozzi F, Carreira PE, et al. Causes and risk factors for death in systemic sclerosis: a study from the EULAR Scleroderma Trials and Research (EUSTAR) database. Ann Rheum Dis. 2010;69(10):1809–15.
5. Steen VD, Medsger TA. Changes in causes of death in systemic sclerosis, 1972-2002. Ann Rheum Dis. 2007;66(7):940–4.
6. Hao Y, Thakkar V, Stevens W, Morrisroe K, Prior D, Rabusa C, et al. A comparison of the predictive accuracy of three screening models for pulmonary arterial hypertension in systemic sclerosis. Arthritis Res Ther. 2015;17:7–18.
7. Humbert M, Sitbon O, Chaouat A, Bertocchi M, Habib G, Gressin V, et al. Pulmonary arterial hypertension in France: results from a national registry. Am J Respir Crit Care Med. 2006;173(9):1023–30.
8. D'Alonzo GE, Barst RJ, Ayres SM, Bergofsky EH, Brundage BH, Detre KM, et al. Survival in patients with primary pulmonary hypertension. Results from a national prospective registry. Ann Intern Med. 1991;115(5):343–9.
9. Lau EM, Humbert M, Celermajer DS. Early detection of pulmonary arterial hypertension. Nat Rev Cardiol. 2015;12(3):143–55.
10. Phung S, Strange G, Chung LP, Leong J, Dalton B, Roddy J, et al. Prevalence of pulmonary arterial hypertension in an Australian scleroderma population: screening allows for earlier diagnosis. Intern Med J. 2009;39:682–91.
11. Komocsi A, Vorobcsuk A, Faludi R, Pinter T, Lenkey Z, Kolto G, et al. The impact of cardiopulmonary manifestations on the mortality of SSc: a systematic review and meta-analysis of observational studies. Rheumatology (Oxford). 2012;51(6):1027–36.
12. Galie N, Rubin L, Hoeper M, Jansa P, Al-Hiti H, Meyer G, et al. Treatment of patients with mildly symptomatic pulmonary arterial hypertension with bosentan (EARLY study): a double-blind, randomised controlled trial. Lancet. 2008;371(9630):2093–100.
13. Humbert M, Yaici A, de Groote P, Montani D, Sitbon O, Launay D, et al. Screening for pulmonary arterial hypertension in patients with systemic sclerosis: clinical characteristics at diagnosis and long-term survival. Arthritis Rheum. 2011;63(11):3522–30.
14. Chung L, Domsic RT, Lingala B, Alkassab F, Bolster M, Csuka ME, et al. Survival and predictors of mortality in systemic sclerosis-associated pulmonary arterial hypertension: outcomes from the pulmonary hypertension assessment and recognition of outcomes in scleroderma registry. Arthritis Care Res (Hoboken). 2014;66(3):489–95.
15. Barst RJ, Gibbs JS, Ghofrani HA, Hoeper MM, McLaughlin W, Rubin LJ, et al. Updated evidence-based treatment algorithm in pulmonary arterial hypertension. J Am Coll Cardiol. 2009;54(1 Suppl):S78–84.
16. Galie N, Barbera JA, Frost AE, Ghofrani HA, Hoeper MM, McLaughlin W, et al. Initial use of ambrisentan plus tadalafil in pulmonary arterial hypertension. N Engl J Med. 2015;373(9):834–44.
17. Condliffe R, Kiely DG, Peacock AJ, Corris PA, Gibbs JS, Vrapi F, et al. Connective tissue disease-associated pulmonary arterial hypertension in the modern treatment era. Am J Respir Crit Care Med. 2009;179(2):151–7.

18. Launay D, Sitbon O, Hachulla E, Mouthon L, Gressin V, Rottat L, et al. Survival in systemic sclerosis-associated pulmonary arterial hypertension in the modern management era. Ann Rheum Dis. 2013;72(12):1940–6.
19. Morrisroe K HM, Stevens W, Rabusa C, Proudman S, Nikpour M, the Australian Scleroderma Interest Group (ASIG). Risk factors for development of pulmonary arterial hypertension in Australian systemic sclerosis patients: results from a large multicenter cohort study. BMC. 2016.
20. Shah AA, Wigley FM, Hummers LK. Telangiectases in scleroderma: a potential clinical marker of pulmonary arterial hypertension. J Rheumatol. 2010;37(1):98–104.
21. Proudman S, Stevens W, Sahhar J, Celermajer D. Pulmonary arterial hypertension in systemic sclerosis: the need for early detection and treatment. Intern Med J. 2007;37(7):485–94.
22. McLaughlin VV, Archer SL, Badesch DB, Barst RJ, Farber HW, Lindner JR, et al. ACCF/AHA 2009 expert consensus document on pulmonary hypertension a report of the American College of Cardiology Foundation Task Force on Expert Consensus Documents and the American Heart Association developed in collaboration with the American College of Chest Physicians; American Thoracic Society, Inc.; and the Pulmonary Hypertension Association. J Am Coll Cardiol. 2009;53(17):1573–619.
23. Pauling JD, McHugh NJ. Evaluating factors influencing screening for pulmonary hypertension in systemic sclerosis: does disparity between available guidelines influence clinical practice? Clin Rheumatol. 2012;31(2):357–61.
24. Mangat P, Conron M, Gabbay E, Proudman SM. Scleroderma lung disease, variation in screening, diagnosis and treatment practices between rheumatologists and respiratory physicians. Intern Med J. 2010;40(7): 494–502.
25. van den Hoogen F, Khanna D, Fransen J, Johnson SR, Baron M, Tyndall A, et al. 2013 classification criteria for systemic sclerosis: an American College of Rheumatology/European League against Rheumatism collaborative initiative. Arthritis Rheum. 2013;65(11):2737–47.
26. LeRoy EC, Medsger Jr TA. Criteria for the classification of early systemic sclerosis. J Rheumatol. 2001;28(7):1573–6.
27. Sharp GC, Irwin WS, Tan EM, et al. Mixed connective tissue disease: an apparently distinct rheumatic disease syndrome, associated with a specific antibody to extractable nuclear antigen (ENA). Am J Med. 1972;52(2):148–59.
28. Galiè N, Hoeper MM, Humbert M, Torbicki A, Vachiery J-L, Barbera JA, et al. Guidelines for the diagnosis and treatment of pulmonary hypertension. Eur Respir J. 2009;34(6):1219–63.
29. Chaisson NF, Hassoun PM, Chaisson NF, Hassoun PM. Systemic sclerosis-associated pulmonary arterial hypertension. Chest. 2013;144(4):1346–1356.
30. Simonneau G, Gatzoulis MA, Adatia I, Celermajer D, Denton C, Ghofrani A, et al. Updated clinical classification of pulmonary hypertension. J Am Coll Cardiol. 2013;62(25 Suppl):D34–41.
31. Englert H, Small-McMahon J, Davis K, O'Connor H, Chambers P, Brooks P. Systemic sclerosis prevalence and mortality in Sydney 1974-88. Aust NZ J Med. 1999;29(1):42–50.
32. Chandran G, Smith M, Ahern MJ, Roberts-Thomson PJ. A study of scleroderma in South Australia: prevalence, subset characteristics and nailfold capillaroscopy. Aust NZ J Med. 1995;25(6):688–94.
33. Statistics ABo. 2012.
34. Simonneau G, Gatzoulis MA, Adatia I, Celermajer D, Denton C, Ghofrani A, et al. Updated clinical classification of pulmonary hypertension. Turk Kardiyol Dern Ars. 2014;42 Suppl 1:45–54.
35. Fan X, Pope J, Baron M. What is the relationship between disease activity, severity and damage in a large Canadian systemic sclerosis cohort? Results from the Canadian Scleroderma Research Group (CSRG). Rheumatol Int. 2010;30(9):1205–10.
36. Hachulla E, de Groote P, Gressin V, Sibilia J, Diot E, Carpentier P, et al. The three-year incidence of pulmonary arterial hypertension associated with systemic sclerosis in a multicenter nationwide longitudinal study in France. Arthritis Rheum. 2009;60(6):1831–9.
37. Yang X, Mardekian J, Sanders KN, Mychaskiw MA, Thomas III J. Prevalence of pulmonary arterial hypertension in patients with connective tissue diseases: a systematic review of the literature. Clin Rheumatol. 2013;32(10):1519–31.
38. Mukerjee D, St George D, Coleiro B, Knight C, Denton CP, Davar J, et al. Prevalence and outcome in systemic sclerosis associated pulmonary arterial hypertension: application of a registry approach. Ann Rheum Dis. 2003; 62(11):1088–93.
39. Hachulla E, Gressin V, Guillevin L, Carpentier P, Diot E, Sibilia J, et al. Early detection of pulmonary arterial hypertension in systemic sclerosis: a French nationwide prospective multicenter study. Arthritis Rheum. 2005;52(12): 3792–800.
40. Yaqub A, Chung L. Epidemiology and risk factors for pulmonary hypertension in systemic sclerosis. Curr Rheumatol Rep. 2013;15(1):302.
41. Highland KB. Recent advances in scleroderma-associated pulmonary hypertension. Curr Opin Rheumatol. 2014;26(6):637–45.
42. Denton CP, Avouac J, Behrens F, Furst DE, Foeldvari I, Humbert M, et al. Systemic sclerosis-associated pulmonary hypertension: Why disease-specific composite endpoints are needed. Arthritis Res Ther. 2011;13(3):114.
43. Chung L, Liu J, Parsons L, Hassoun PM, McGoon M, Badesch DB, et al. Characterization of connective tissue disease-associated pulmonary arterial hypertension from REVEAL: identifying systemic sclerosis as a unique phenotype. Chest. 2010;138(6):1383–94.
44. Hachulla E, Clerson P, Airò P, Cuomo G, Allanore Y, Caramaschi P, et al. Value of systolic pulmonary arterial pressure as a prognostic factor of death in the systemic sclerosis EUSTAR population. Rheumatology (Oxford). 2015;54(7):1262–9.
45. Schwaiger JP, Khanna D, Gerry CJ. Screening patients with scleroderma for pulmonary arterial hypertension and implications for other at-risk populations. Eur Respir Rev. 2013;22(130):515–25.
46. Thakkar V, Stevens W, Prior D, Byron J, Patterson K, Hissaria P, et al. N-terminal pro-brain natriuretic peptide levels predict incident pulmonary arterial hypertension in SSc. Rheumatology. 2012;51:ii8.

Antibodies against chemokine receptors CXCR3 and CXCR4 predict progressive deterioration of lung function in patients with systemic sclerosis

Florian Weigold[1], Jeannine Günther[1,2], Moritz Pfeiffenberger[2], Otavio Cabral-Marques[3], Elise Siegert[1], Duska Dragun[4,5], Aurélie Philippe[4], Ann-Katrin Regensburger[6], Andreas Recke[6], Xinhua Yu[7], Frank Petersen[7], Rusan Catar[4,5], Robert Biesen[1], Falk Hiepe[1], Gerd R. Burmester[1], Harald Heidecke[8] and Gabriela Riemekasten[1,2,3,7*]

Abstract

Background: The chemokine receptors CXCR3 and CXCR4 are involved in the pathogenesis of fibrosis, a key feature of systemic sclerosis (SSc). It is hypothesized that immunoglobulin (Ig)G antibodies (abs) against these two receptors are present in patients with SSc and are associated with clinical findings.

Methods: Anti-CXCR3 and anti-CXCR4 ab levels were measured in 449 sera from 327 SSc patients and in 234 sera from healthy donors (HD) by enzyme-linked immunosorbent assay (ELISA). In SSc, ab levels were compared with clinical data in a cross-sectional and longitudinal setting. Protein expression of CXCR3 and CXCR4 on peripheral blood mononuclear cells (PBMCs) was analyzed in 17 SSc patients and 8 HD by flow cytometry.

Results: Anti-CXCR3 and anti-CXCR4 ab levels were different among SSc subgroups compared with HD and were highest in diffuse SSc patients. The ab levels strongly correlated with each other ($r = 0.85$). Patients with SSc-related interstitial lung disease (SSc-ILD) exhibited higher ab levels which negatively correlated with lung function parameters (e.g., $r = -0.5$ and $r = -0.43$ for predicted vital capacity, respectively). However, patients with deterioration of lung function showed lower anti-CXCR3/4 ab levels compared with those with stable disease. Frequencies and median fluorescence intensities (MFI) of $CXCR3^+$ and $CXCR4^+$ PBMCs were lower in SSc patients compared with HD and correlated with the severity of skin and lung fibrosis. They correlated with the severity of skin and lung fibrosis.

Conclusions: Anti-CXCR3/4 abs and their corresponding receptors are linked with the severity of SSc-ILD. Antibody levels discriminate patients with stable or decreasing lung function and could be used for risk stratification.

Keywords: Anti-CXCR3, Anti-CXCR4, Systemic sclerosis, Interstitial lung disease, GPCR

Background

Systemic sclerosis (SSc) is a severe autoimmune disease characterized by vasculopathy and fibrosis. In this disease, SSc-related interstitial lung disease (SSc-ILD) is one of the most frequent causes of mortality [1] due to activation and accumulation of T cells, neutrophils, and monocytes in the inflammation sites. C-X-C motif chemokine receptor (CXCR)3 and CXCR4 are G protein-coupled receptors (GPCRs) mediating the migration of different cells including lymphocytes, endothelial progenitor cells, and stem cells [2, 3]. CXCR3, which can bind to several proinflammatory chemokines, is induced on naive T cells upon activation by interferon gamma-inducible ligands present in inflamed tissues. As a result, $CXCR3^+$ T cells, predominantly Th1 cells, are recruited to sites of inflammation [4]. CXCR3 is also expressed on plasmacytoid dendritic and

* Correspondence: gabriela.riemekasten@uksh.de
[1]Department of Rheumatology and Clinical Immunology, Charité University Hospital, Berlin, Germany
[2]Cell Autoimmunity Group, German Rheumatism Research Center (DRFZ), Berlin, Germany
Full list of author information is available at the end of the article

natural killer (NK) cells [4, 5]. An increased number of CXCR3$^+$ cells were also found in lupus nephritis and in atherosclerotic lesions secondary to systemic lupus erythematosus (SLE) [6, 7]. CXCR4 is a specific receptor for stromal-derived factor 1 (SDF-1, also called C-X-C motif chemokine ligand 12 or CXCL12), a molecule with potent chemotactic activity for lymphocytes and neutrophils [5]. Involvement of the CXCR4/SDF-1 axis is discussed in several diseases including inflammatory bowel diseases, ischemia/reperfusion injury, and in idiopathic pulmonary fibrosis. CXCR4$^+$ cells as well as their ligands CXCL11 and CXCL12 have been shown to be associated with the pathogenesis of pulmonary complications in patients with autoimmune diseases [8–11]. Furthermore, CXCL11 levels in bronchoalveolar lavage fluid (BALF) from SSc patients predicted progressive SSc-ILD [12].

As recently reported by our group, immunoglobulin (Ig)G from SSc patients is able to induce ILD and vasculopathy in C57BL/6 mice indicating a pathogenic role of antibodies. IgG from SSc patients directly enhances *in vitro* migration of T cells and neutrophils correlating with anti-angiotensin II type I receptor (AT1R)/endothelin receptor type A (ETAR) antibody (ab) levels [13, 14]. In addition, anti-AT1R and anti-ETAR abs induced the production of different cytokines, Ca^{2+}, and chemokines by various cells, which were inhibited by AT1R or ETAR blockers [13–18]. However, the inhibition was partially incomplete or even absent indicating antibody-mediated activation of other receptors. In SSc patients, anti-AT1R and anti-ETAR ab levels were predictive for vascular complications such as pulmonary arterial hypertension (PAH) or digital ulcers [15–17, 19], but they were not able to predict deterioration of pulmonary fibrosis. Assuming the existence of antibodies against CXCR3 and CXCR4, our group has developed enzyme-linked immunosorbent assays (ELISAs) to measure their concentrations in sera. Here, we asked whether anti-CXCR3 and anti-CXCR4 antibodies or the receptors could be used as biomarkers for SSc or for SSc-related organ damage.

Methods

We analyzed 449 sera from 327 consecutive SSc patients from the Charité University Hospital for anti-CXCR3 abs; 425 sera from 312 SSc patients were analyzed for the presence of anti-CXCR4 abs. Epidemiologic data of the 327 SSc patients are shown in Additional file 1: Table S1 and baseline lung function parameters at the time point of anti-CXCR3/4 ab detection are given in Additional file 1: Table S2. The mean time between disease onset and determination of ab values is 8.5 ± 6.9 years for anti-CXCR3 and 8.4 ± 6.9 years for anti-CXCR4.

In comparison, sera from 234 healthy donors (HD) (68.4% male and 31.6% female, with a mean age of 36.6 ±12.8 years) were analyzed.

SSc patients were divided into different disease subsets according to the criteria of the EUSTAR and DNSS network [20–25]. Comorbidities were assessed in routine clinical practice as documented in the medical charts. Only those comorbidities that were present in at least 10 patients were analyzed. If multiple ab samples/clinical assessments were registered per patient, only the latest sample was considered in cross-sectional analyses. SSc patients with a follow-up period of at least 3 years were analyzed to identify the predictive capacity of the ab.

SSc-ILD was defined according to the guidelines from the German Network of Systemic Sclerosis and the definition has been applied and used for several studies. Accordingly, diagnosis of SSc-ILD was established when bilateral basal fibrosis occurred, confirmed by chest x-ray and/or high-resolution computed tomography (HR-CT) scan together with restrictive pulmonary abnormalities on pulmonary function tests (forced vital capacity (FVC) < 80%). Regularly, in patients with limited cutaneous disease and particularly in those with anti-Centromer ab and normal lung function, an HR-CT scan is not required and the x-ray is sufficient for primary diagnosis. Lung fibrosis was only quantified indirectly by lung function tests; quantitative analyses of HR-CT scans were not performed in our clinical routine setting.

Here, in our cross-sectional analyses for anti-CXCR3 ab, 35% of the patients have a diagnosed SSc-ILD, 23% of them with FVC < 70%. In analyses for anti-CXCR4 ab, 33% of the patients have a diagnosed SSc-ILD, 31% of them with FVC < 70%.

Detection of anti-CXCR3 and anti-CXCR4 IgG by solid-phase assay

Anti-CXCR3 and anti-CXCR4 IgG ab were measured by a commercially available sandwich ELISA (CellTrend GmbH Luckenwalde, Germany). Briefly, duplicate samples of a 1:100 serum dilution were incubated at 4 °C for 2 h. All sera were analyzed by personnel blinded to the clinical characteristics of the patients.

Isolation of peripheral blood mononuclear cells and flow cytometry

CXCR3 and CXCR4 protein expression was measured on peripheral blood mononuclear cell (PBMC) subpopulations from 17 SSc patients (eight diffuse cutaneous (d)SSc patients, 8 SSc patients with limited cutaneous (l)SSc, and one patient with overlap syndrome) and eight HD by flow cytometry. Epidemiologic data of the patients are given in Additional file 1: Table S1. PBMCs were isolated using Ficoll-Paque gradient centrifugation as described previously [18], identified by their corresponding CD surface antigens (CD4, T helper cells; CD8, cytotoxic T cells; CD19, B cells; CD14, monocytes), stained ex vivo or immediately after isolation, and fixed with 4% paraformaldehyde. Cytometric assays were performed using an LSR II flow cytometer (BD Biosciences) and analyzed with FlowJo software (TreeStar, Ashland, OR, USA). Frequencies were normalized to the corresponding isotype control, calculating the difference between isotype control (between 0 and 5%) and receptor-stained cells within the identical gate. For median of fluorescence intensity (MFI), the ratio of the MFI of receptor-stained cells and the MFI of isotype control was calculated. The other ab, as well as methods describing T-cell isolation and chemotaxis assays, are given in Additional file 1: Supplemental Material and Methods.

Statistical analysis

Associations between categorical data were measured using Chi squared or Fisher's exact test. Nonparametric Kruskal-Wallis test with Dunn-Bonferroni post-hoc tests, Mann-Whitney *U* test and Spearman's rho were used to examine noncategorical, non-normal distributed values. Receiver operating characteristic (ROC) analyses were performed to identify the best cut-off points for ab levels for patients with and without deterioration of lung function. Log-rank test and Cox proportional hazards model were performed to identify the predictive value of anti-CXCR3 and anti-CXCR4 ab regarding deterioration of lung function parameters (estimation of hazard ratios and baseline adjustment of lung function parameters, age, and sex).

For receptor expression, statistics were performed using Prism5 software (GraphPad Inc., La Jolla, USA). A value of $p \leq 0.05$ was interpreted as statistically significant.

Results

Anti-CXCR3 and anti-CXCR4 antibody levels show strong correlations with each other and are different among the different disease subsets

Anti-CXCR3 and anti-CXCR4 ab levels in sera from SSc patients were compared with those from HD (Additional file 1: Figure S1a, b). Median values of anti-CXCR3 abs were 3.5 Units (U) (95% confidence interval (CI) 2.9–3.8) in HD and 3.8 U in SSc patients (95% CI 3.2–4.2), showing no significant differences (p = 0.12). On the other hand, median values of anti-CXCR4 abs were higher in SSc patients (3.3 U, 95% CI 3–3.8) compared with HD (2.7 U, 95% CI 2.5–3; $p \leq 0.001$). However, 12.2% and 17.2% of the SSc patients displayed anti-CXCR3 and anti-CXCR4 ab levels above the 95th percentile in comparison to HD, respectively. The levels of anti-CXCR3 and anti-CXCR4 abs strongly correlate with each other in HD and in SSc patients (r = 0.89 and r = 0.85, respectively; $p \leq 0.001$, n = 198 and n = 312; Fig. 1). In SSc patients, anti-CXCR3 and anti-CXCR4 ab levels were weakly and negatively correlated with the corresponding ages at assessment (r = −0.2, $p \leq 0.001$; and r = −0.2, $p \leq 0.001$, respectively) and with the age at SSc diagnosis (r = −0.24, $p \leq 0.001$; and r = −0.27, $p \leq 0.001$, respectively), but not with disease duration (data not shown). In contrast, HD show positive correlations for both anti-CXCR3 and anti-CXCR4 ab levels with age (r = 0.13, $p \leq 0.05$; and r = 0.16, $p \leq 0.05$, respectively).

Anti-CXCR3 ab levels were higher in patients with diffuse cutaneous systemic sclerosis (dSSc) compared with patients with limited cutaneous systemic sclerosis (lSSc) ($p \leq 0.001$) and HD ($p \leq 0.001$; Fig. 2); 17.6% of the dSSc patients revealed anti-CXCR3 ab levels above the 95th percentile. Similarly, anti-CXCR4 ab levels were higher in dSSc patients compared with those in lSSc patients ($p \leq 0.05$) and HD ($p \leq 0.001$). In line with this, anti-topoisomerase I ab-positive patients have slightly higher anti-CXCR3 levels than anti-topoisomerase I ab-negative patients (median 4.1 vs. 4.7 U; $p \leq 0.05$, n = 252). No significant differences were observed for anti-CXCR4 abs. Patients with overlap syndromes revealed markedly increased ab levels compared with HD (p = 0.056); 25.5% of the dSSc patients have anti-CXCR4 ab levels above the 95th percentile of the HD.

Anti-CXCR3 and anti-CXCR4 antibodies are markers for lung involvement

The cross-sectional analyses showed that the subgroup of patients with confirmed SSc-ILD and FVC < 70% had

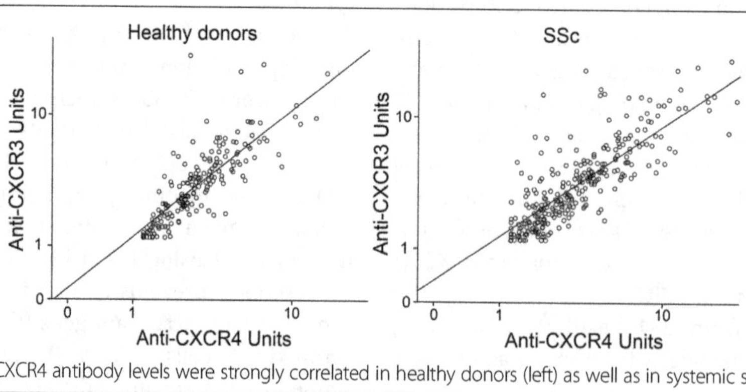

Fig. 1 Anti-CXCR3 and anti-CXCR4 antibody levels were strongly correlated in healthy donors (left) as well as in systemic sclerosis (SSc) patients (right)

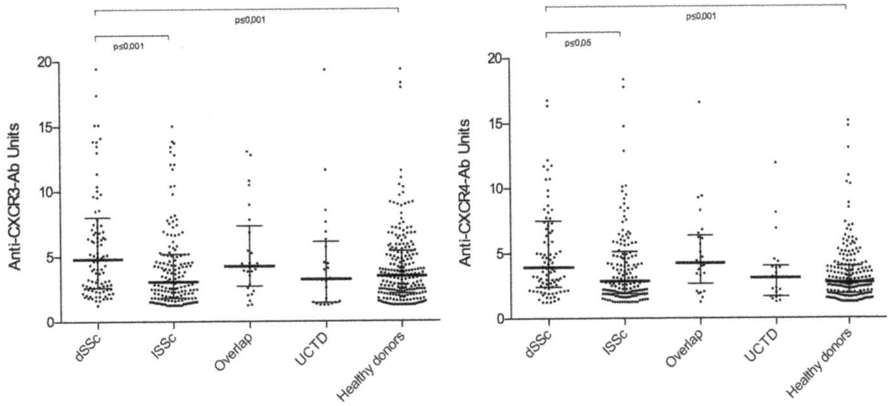

Fig. 2 Anti-CXCR3 (left) and anti-CXCR4 (right) antibody levels in diffuse cutaneous systemic sclerosis (dSSc), in patients with limited cutaneous systemic sclerosis (lSSc), with overlap syndromes (Overlap), with undifferentiated connective tissue disease (UCTD), and in healthy controls. *P* values with significant differences are shown

significantly lower median anti-CXCR3 and anti-CXCR4 ab levels than those with FVC ≥ 70% (2.9 U vs. 4.8 U, $p \leq 0.01$, $n = 82$; and 2.8 U vs. 5.0 U, $p \leq 0.05$, $n = 78$, respectively). In the next step, we studied correlations between ab levels and different metric clinical parameters of SSc patients. Significant negative correlations exist between anti-CXCR3 ab levels and the predicted percentages of vital capacity (VC), FVC, total lung capacity (TLC) and the diffusing capacity for carbon monoxide measured by a single breath (DLCO-SB). Anti-CXCR4 abs revealed similar correlations with lung function parameters (Table 1), indicating that high anti-CXCR3 and anti-CXCR4 ab levels are associated with more severely impaired lung function. In line with this, higher median anti-CXCR3 and anti-CXCR4 ab levels were present in patients with SSc-ILD compared with those without ILD (3.4 U vs. 4.1 U, $p \leq 0.05$; and 3.1 U vs. 3.9 U, $p \leq 0.05$, respectively).

Table 1 Correlations between anti-CXCR3 and anti-CXCR4 antibody levels and lung function parameters in systemic sclerosis patients

Lung function parameter	Anti-CXCR3			Anti-CXCR4		
	SRT-r	*p* values	*n*	SRT-r	*p* values	*n*
VC (%)	−0.50	≤ 0.001	71	−0.43	≤ 0.001	58
FVC (%)	−0.27	≤ 0.001	284	−0.2	≤ 0.001	271
TLC (%)	−0.25	≤ 0.001	253	−0.21	≤ 0.001	240
DLCO-SB (%)	−0.32	≤ 0.01	274	−0.26	≤ 0.05	64
DLCO/VA (%)	−0.20	= 0.08	245	−0.16	= 0.20	64
FEV1 (%)	−0.18	≤ 0.01	278	−0.17	≤ 0.01	265
FEV1/VC (%)	+0.25	≤ 0.05	71	+0.2	= 0.13	58

R values of Spearman's rho (SRT-r) as well as *p* values are shown
Vital capacity (VC), forced vital capacity (FVC), total lung capacity (TLC), the diffusing capacity for carbon monoxide (DLCO) measured by a single breath (DLCO-SB), DLCO/VA, forced expiratory volume in 1 s (FEV1), and Tiffeneau index (FEV1/VC) are given

No correlations were present between anti-CXCR3 and anti-CXCR4 ab levels and modified Rodnan Skin Score (mRSS), mean pulmonary arterial pressure (mPAP), systolic pulmonary arterial pressure (sPAP), or left ventricular ejection fraction (LVEF) (data not shown). For anti-CXCR3 ab levels, weak correlations existed with erythrocyte sedimentation rate (ESR) levels ($r = 0.16$, $p \leq 0.05$, $n = 251$), but not with C-reactive protein (CRP) values (data not shown).

Anti-CXCR3 and anti-CXCR4 antibodies were also associated with other clinical symptoms as shown in Additional file 1: Tables S3 and S4.

High anti-CXCR3/4 antibody levels correspond to and predict stable lung function

SSc patients with 3-year follow-up investigations were analyzed to identify the role of anti-CXCR3/4 abs to predict progression in SSc-ILD. SSc patients were grouped into those having > 10% deterioration in DCLO-SB, DLCO/VA, FVC, forced expiratory volume in 1 s (FEV1), and TLC values, and those with stable lung function parameters. Ab samples were obtained at the beginning of the 3-year follow-up. ROC analyses (Youden's-Index) were performed for all lung function parameters to identify the best cut-off values which can discriminate between stable and progressive diseases within 3 years. For clinical practicality, the median value (6.2 U for anti-CXCR3 and 5.18 U for anti-CXCR4) is used for all parameters.

In general, patients with lower levels of anti-CXCR3/CXCR4 abs have progressively impaired lung function during this follow-up period (Table 2).

Cumulative percentages of patients with deterioration > 10% of predicted FVC and FEV1 levels are shown in Fig. 3.

Within 12 months, 44% of the patients with anti-CXCR3 ab levels < 6.2 U showed a reduction in FVC values ≥ 10%, but this was only true for 13% of the patients with high ab levels. Similar results were

Table 2 Higher anti-CXCR3 and anti-CXCR4 antibody levels are associated with stable lung function parameters

Parameter	Patients above cut-off (%)		Patients below cut-off (%)		*p* values	Number of analyzed patients	Hazard ratios
	Deterioration ≥ 10%	No deterioration	Deterioration ≥ 10%	No deterioration			
Anti-CXCR3 antibodies							
FVC (%)	25.0	75.0	59.3	40.7	≤ 0.01	59	0.32
FEV1 (%)	23.5	76.5	71.1	28.9	≤ 0.001	72	0.22
DLCO-SB (%)	36.4	63.6	63.6	36.4	≤ 0.05	55	0.47
DLCO/VA (%)	42.4	57.6	70.4	29.6	≤ 0.05	60	0.38
Anti-CXCR4 antibodies							
FVC (%)	22.2	77.8	70.0	30.0	≤ 0.001	47	0.2
FEV1 (%)	33.3	66.7	78.6	21.4	≤ 0.001	61	0.27
TLC (%)	33.3	66.7	64.7	35.3	≤ 0.05	44	0.33
DLCO-SB (%)	43.3	56.7	75.0	25.0	≤ 0.05	46	0.46
DLCO/VA (%)	39.4	60.6	82.4	17.6	≤ 0.001	50	0.24

Patients with antibody levels above and below cut-off, with and without deterioration in forced vital capacity (FVC), forced expiratory volume in 1 s (FEV1), total lung capacity (TLC), the diffusing capacity for carbon monoxide (DLCO) measured by a single breath (DLCO-SB), and DLCO/VA within 3 years, *p* values (log-rank test) as well as number of analyzed patients are shown

Hazard ratios derived from the Cox proportional hazards model highlight the relationship between deterioration in lung function parameters and anti-CXCR3/anti-CXCR4 antibody levels

obtained at month 24 (56% versus 19%) and at month 36 (59% versus 25%). Baseline adjustment for lung function parameters, age, and sex did not reveal significant differences in the FVC deterioration. Anti-CXCR4 ab levels appear to discriminate better between patients with and without FVC deterioration. At month 12, 55% of the SSc patients with anti-CXCR4 ab levels < 5.18 U revealed deterioration in FVC values, but this was the case in only 11% of the patients with higher ab levels. Similar results were obtained at months 24 (70% versus 15%) and at months 36 (70% versus 22%). Low anti-CXCR3 and anti-CXCR4 ab levels were also predictive for deterioration in TLC, DLCO-SB, and DLCO/VA values.

CXCR3 and CXCR4 protein expressions are related to signs of fibrosis

The protein expressions of CXCR3 and CXCR4 were analyzed in PBMCs of SSc patients as well as HD. The percentages of peripheral blood monocytes, $CD8^+$ T cells, and B cells expressing CXCR3 as well as CXCR4 were lower in SSc patients compared with HD (Additional file 1: Figure S2 shows the percentages of cells expressing CXCR3). In addition, MFIs were reduced for CXCR3 and CXCR4 in monocytes, $CD8^+$ T cells, and B cells of SSc patients compared with those found in HD (Additional file 1: Figure S2).

In $CD14^+$ monocytes, both the percentage of CXCR3-expressing cells as well as their MFI inversely correlated with the FVC values (Fig. 4a, b). The MFI of CXCR4-positive $CD4^+$ T cells correlated well with the mRSS (Fig. 4c). The MFI of CXCR4 expression on monocytes correlated with the years since onset of Raynaud's phenomenon (r = 0.53, $p \le 0.05$), with years since the start of fibrosis (r = 0.52, $p \le 0.05$), and with years since the first organ involvement (r = 0.54, $p \le 0.05$) (Fig. 4f).

Discussion

In the present study, autoantibodies against the chemokine receptors CXCR3 and CXCR4 were mainly linked to the presence of SSc-ILD. Patients with dSSc and those with lung fibrosis revealed higher anti-CXCR3 and anti-CXCR4 ab levels compared with those with lSSc and without SSc-ILD. The ab levels weakly and negatively correlated with lung function parameters. In addition, CXCR3 and CXCR4 receptor expression in PBMCs correlated with the extent of lung and skin fibrosis. However, the deterioration of lung function parameters was associated with low anti-CXCR3 and anti-CXCR4 ab levels. In addition, low anti-CXCR3 and anti-CXCR4 ab levels predicted progressive impairment of lung function parameters.

The involvement of CXCR3 and CXCR4 has already been discussed in the pathogenesis of systemic sclerosis. Cipriani et al. have shown an upregulation of CXCR4 and SDF-1 in the skin of early systemic sclerosis patients [26, 27]. However, increased, normal, and decreased percentages of $CXCR3^+$ cells have been described in SSc [28–30]. Here, percentages of CXCR3 and $CXCR4^+$ cytotoxic T cells, B cells, and monocytes were lower in SSc patients compared with HD. This could reflect reduced activation of cells, downregulation of receptor expression by chronic stimulation, or migration of these cells from the blood stream into the tissue; this remains to be studied.

Here, anti-CXCR3 and anti-CXCR4 ab levels are shown to be very good markers of predicting lung fibrosis and are, therefore, candidates to stratify patients for

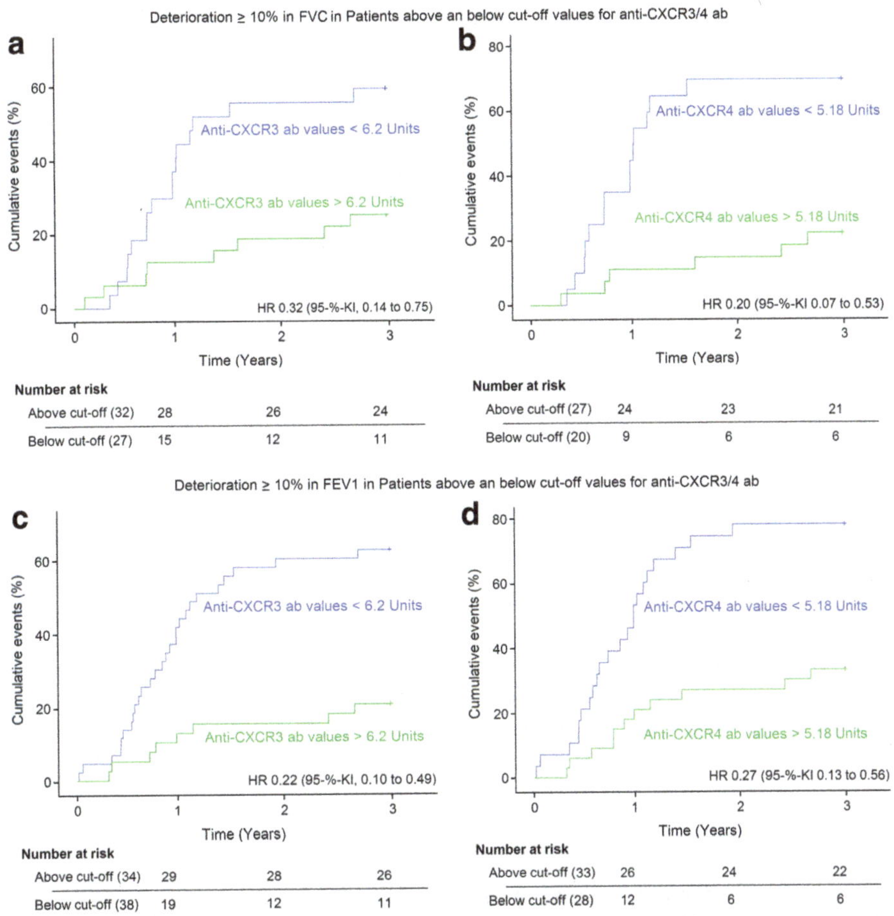

Fig. 3 Cumulative events indicate the capacity of anti-CXCR3 (**a,c**) and anti-CXCR4 (**b,d**) antibody (ab) levels to predict deterioration in forced vital capacity (FVC) (**a,b**) and forced expiratory volume in 1 s (FEV1) (**c,d**) by ≥ 10% within 3 years of follow-up. *P* values (log-rank test) are given in Table 2. HR hazard ratio, 95-%-KI 95% confidence interval

disease progression, e.g., in clinical studies. This is the main finding of our study. The association of high ab levels with signs of lung fibrosis and reduced progression of lung fibrosis seems to be a contradiction at first glance. A similar observation was found for regulatory T cells (Treg), which strongly correlate with disease activity in lupus [31]. This could be suggestive for their pathogenic role. Nevertheless, enrichment of Treg improved lupus activity illustrating that high Treg numbers do not necessarily indicate a pathogenic role of the Treg [31]. Similar to the beneficial role of Treg, the prediction of progressive deterioration of FVC values by low anti-CXCR3/4 levels suggests a protective effect of the antibodies, which needs to be further evaluated.

In our previous studies, anti-CXCR3/4 levels and anti-AT1R/ETAR ab levels were not able to predict progressive SSc-ILD (data not shown). Anti-CXCR3 and anti-CXCR4 ab levels correlate moderately with those of the anti-AT1R and anti-ETAR ab ($r = 0.39$ to $r = 0.43$, data not shown). Functionally, anti-AT1R/ETAR abs are stimulatory and agonistic to their natural ligands [32]. The previously described correlation between cell migration and the levels of anti-AT1R and anti-ETAR abs indicate a dominant role of anti-AT1R/ETAR abs in cell migration in SSc [14, 15]. As shown in the supplementary results (Additional file 1: Figure S3), IgG fractions from patients with high anti-CXCR3/4 abs also mediate migration via CXCR3 and probably via CXCR4 as suggested by blocking experiments with specific receptor blockers. Migration of lymphocytes was not dependent on the anti-CXCR3/4 ab levels (data not shown). Sequence identity between CXCR3 and CXCR4 abs and between anti-CXCR4 and anti-AT1R abs has been described [33, 34]. According to this, anti-CXCR3/4 ab levels as well as relative high receptor expressions could interfere with the effects of anti-AT1R/ETAR abs on cell migration. However, alterations in the anti-CXCR3/4 ab levels as well as in CXCR3 and CXCR4 expression were linked with fibrosis, suggesting a disturbed CXCR3/4 system in this condition.

Our study has some limitations. The assessment was performed in a routine clinical setting leading to some

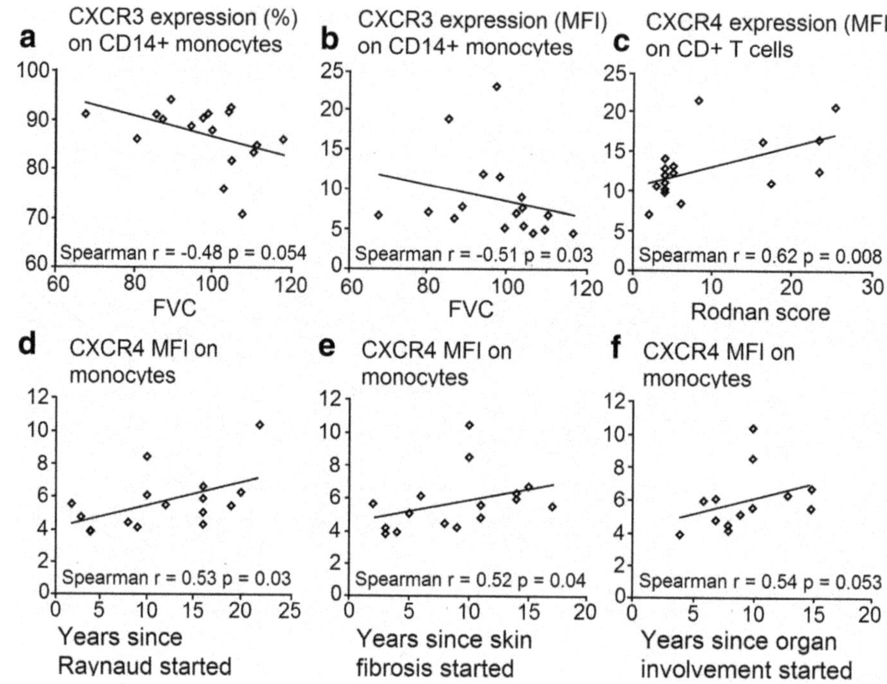

Fig. 4 Frequency of CXCR3-positive $CD14^+$ monocytes among $CD14^+$ monocytes (**a**) as well as CXCR3 density (**b**) on $CD14^+$ monocytes show a negative correlation with the predicted percentages of forced vital capacity (FVC). (**c**) CXCR4 density on $CD4^+$ T cells related to isotype controls correlated with modified Rodnan Skin Score (mRSS). Correlation between CXCR4 expressions on monocytes (MFIs) with years since diagnosis (**d**), start of fibrosis (**e**), and since first organ involvement (**f**, first non-Raynaud symptom). Statistical analyses were performed by Spearman's correlation; $*p \leq 0.05$. MFI median fluorescence intensity

missing clinical parameters. Based on the earlier availability of the CXCR3 ELISA, anti-CXCR4 abs were not measured in all patients. However, in the vast majority, anti-CXCR3 and anti-CXCR4 abs were measured in parallel in one individual. Also, we did not study patients with other diseases. This is a limitation that should be addressed in the future as well as analyzing cross-reactions of the antibodies. In addition, we used lung function parameters as surrogate markers for lung fibrosis and did not measure lung fibrosis by quantitative CT scans. In this study, we did not investigate the predictive value of these antibodies on mortality, nor did we investigate the effects of disease-modifying agents on the results. Finally, specific functions of the abs remain to be studied.

Conclusions

In conclusion, we have identified novel anti-GPCR abs against the chemokine receptors CXCR3 and CXCR4 in patients with systemic sclerosis linking autoimmunity with interstitial lung disease. Antibody levels discriminate patients with stable or decreasing lung function and could be used for risk stratification. We suggest a functional role of anti-CXCR3/4 abs and highlight their potential contribution to the orchestra of other antibodies.

Abbreviations

ab: Antibody; AT1R: Anti-angiotensin II type I receptor; BALF: Bronchoalveolar lavage fluid; CI: Confidence interval; CRP: C-reactive protein; CXCR: C-X-C motif chemokine receptor; DLCO-SB: Diffusing capacity for carbon monoxide by a single breath; dSSc: Diffuse cutaneous systemic sclerosis; ELISA: Enzyme-linked immunosorbent assay; ESR: Erythrocyte sedimentation rate; ETAR: Endothelin receptor type A; FEV1: Forced expiratory volume in one second; FVC: Forced vital capacity; GPCR: G protein-coupled receptor; HD: Healthy donors; HR-CT: High-resolution computed tomography; Ig: Immunoglobulin; ILD: Interstitial lung disease; lSSc: Limited cutaneous systemic sclerosis; LVEF: Left ventricular ejection fraction; MFI: Median fluorescence intensity; mPAP: Mean pulmonary arterial pressure; mRSS: Modified Rodnan Skin Score; PAH: Pulmonary arterial hypertension; PBMC: Peripheral blood mononuclear cell; ROC: Receiver operating characteristic; SDF-1: Stromal-derived factor 1; SLE: Systemic lupus erythematosus; sPAP: Systolic pulmonary arterial pressure; SSc: Systemic sclerosis; TLC: Total lung capacity; Treg: Regulatory T cells; VC: Vital capacity

Acknowledgments

The authors thank all the patients and healthy controls for their participation in this study.

Funding

We thank the Mirjam Lichy foundation for support as well as the DFG grant RI 1056-11-1/2 for financial support. We also thank Actelion Pharmaceutical GmbH, the Eppenauer/Gutzeit foundation, the German network of Systemic Sclerosis, as well as the EUSTAR network for their support. The study was promoted by the Charité University Hospital in Berlin and University Hospital of Schleswig-Holstein Campus Lübeck.

Authors' contributions

FW, JG, and GR designed the study, analyzed and interpreted the data, and wrote the manuscript. JG, MP, and AP performed the experiments. MP, OCM, ES, DD, AP, AKR, AR, XY, FP, RC, RB, FH, GRB, and HH made substantial contributions to data analysis, design, data interpretation, data acquisition, data assessment, statistics, and drafting of the manuscript. All authors read and approved the final manuscript.

Competing interests

GR is an advisor for CellTrend. HH is manager of CellTrend. The remaining authors declare that they have no competing interests.

Author details

[1]Department of Rheumatology and Clinical Immunology, Charité University Hospital, Berlin, Germany. [2]Cell Autoimmunity Group, German Rheumatism Research Center (DRFZ), Berlin, Germany. [3]Department of Rheumatology, University of Lübeck, Lübeck, Germany. [4]Department of Nephrology and Critical Care Medicine, Charité University Hospital, Campus Virchow, Berlin, Germany. [5]Berlin Institute of Health, Berlin, Germany. [6]Department of Dermatology, University of Lübeck, Lübeck, Germany. [7]Research Center Borstel, Airway Research Center North (ARCN), Members of the German Center for Lung Research (DZL), Borstel, Germany. [8]CellTrend GmbH, Luckenwalde, Brandenburg, Germany.

References

1. Tyndall AJ, Bannert B, Vonk M, Airo P, Cozzi F, Carreira PE, et al. Causes and risk factors for death in systemic sclerosis: a study from the EULAR Scleroderma Trials and Research (EUSTAR) database. Ann Rheum Dis. 2010;69:1809–15.
2. Groom JR, Luster AD. CXCR3 ligands: redundant, collaborative and antagonistic functions. Immunol Cell Biol. 2011;89:207–15.
3. Murdoch C. CXCR4: chemokine receptor extraordinaire. Immunol Rev. 2000; 177:175–84.
4. Lacotte S, Brun S, Muller S, Dumortier H. CXCR3, inflammation, and autoimmune diseases. Ann N Y Acad Sci. 2009;1173:310–7.
5. Hummel S, Van Aken H, Zarbock A. Inhibitors of CXC chemokine receptor type 4: putative therapeutic approaches in inflammatory diseases. Curr Opin Hematol. 2014;21:29–36.
6. Enghard P, Humrich JY, Rudolph B, Rosenberger S, Biesen R, Kuhn A, et al. CXCR3+CD4+ T cells are enriched in inflamed kidneys and urine and provide a new biomarker for acute nephritis flares in systemic lupus erythematosus patients. Arthritis Rheum. 2009;60:199–206.
7. Clement M, Charles N, Escoubet B, Guedj K, Chauveheid MP, Caligiuri G, et al. CD4+CXCR3+ T cells and plasmacytoid dendritic cells drive accelerated atherosclerosis associated with systemic lupus erythematosus. J Autoimmun. 2015;63:59–67.
8. Tourkina E, Bonner M, Oates J, Hofbauer A, Richard M, Znoyko S, et al. Altered monocyte and fibrocyte phenotype and function in scleroderma interstitial lung disease: reversal by caveolin-1 scaffolding domain peptide. Fibrogenesis Tissue Repair. 2011;4:15.
9. Andersson-Sjoland A, de Alba CG, Nihlberg K, Becerril C, Ramirez R, Pardo A, et al. Fibrocytes are a potential source of lung fibroblasts in idiopathic pulmonary fibrosis. Int J Biochem Cell Biol. 2008;40:2129–40.
10. Costello CM, McCullagh B, Howell K, Sands M, Belperio JA, Keane MP, et al. A role for the CXCL12 receptor, CXCR7, in the pathogenesis of human pulmonary vascular disease. Eur Respir J. 2012;39:1415–24.
11. Antoniou KM, Soufla G, Lymbouridou R, Economidou F, Lasithiotaki I, Manousakis M, et al. Expression analysis of angiogenic growth factors and biological axis CXCL12/CXCR4 axis in idiopathic pulmonary fibrosis. Connect Tissue Res. 2010;51:71–80.
12. Sfriso P, Cozzi F, Oliviero F, Caso F, Cardarelli S, Facco M, et al. CXCL11 in bronchoalveolar lavage fluid and pulmonary function decline in systemic sclerosis. Clin Exp Rheumatol. 2012;30:S71–5.
13. Günther J, Kill A, Becker MO, Heidecke H, Rademacher J, Siegert E, et al. Angiotensin receptor type 1 and endothelin receptor type A on immune cells mediate migration and the expression of IL-8 and CCL18 when stimulated by autoantibodies from systemic sclerosis patients. Arthritis Res Ther. 2014;16:R65.
14. Kill A, Tabeling C, Undeutsch R, Kühl AA, Günther J, Radic M, et al. Autoantibodies to angiotensin and endothelin receptors in systemic sclerosis induce cellular and systemic events associated with disease pathogenesis. Arthritis Res Ther. 2014;16:R29.
15. Becker MO, Kill A, Kutsche M, Guenther J, Rose A, Tabeling C, et al. Vascular receptor autoantibodies in pulmonary arterial hypertension associated with systemic sclerosis. Am J Respir Crit Care Med. 2014;190:808–17.
16. Günther J, Rademacher J, van Laar JM, Siegert E, Riemekasten G. Functional autoantibodies in systemic sclerosis. Semin Immunopathol. 2015;37:529–42.
17. Riemekasten G, Philippe A, Näther M, Slowinski T, Müller DN, Heidecke H, et al. Involvement of functional autoantibodies against vascular receptors in systemic sclerosis. Ann Rheum Dis. 2011;70:530–6.
18. Rademacher J, Kill A, Mattat K, Dragun D, Siegert E, Günther J, et al. Monocytic angiotensin and endothelin receptor imbalance modulate secretion of the profibrotic chemokine ligand 18. J Rheumatol. 2016;43: 587–91.
19. Avouac J, Riemekasten G, Meune C, Ruiz B, Kahan A, Allanore Y. Autoantibodies against endothelin 1 type A receptor are strong predictors of digital ulcers in systemic sclerosis. J Rheumatol. 2015;42:1801–7.
20. Walker UA, Tyndall A, Czirjak L, Denton C, Farge-Bancel D, Kowal-Bielecka O, et al. Clinical risk assessment of organ manifestations in systemic sclerosis: a report from the EULAR Scleroderma Trials and Research group. Ann Rheum Dis. 2007;66(6):754–63.
21. Hunzelmann N, Genth E, Krieg T, Lehmacher W, Melchers I, Meurer M, et al. The registry of the German network for systemic scleroderma: frequency of disease subsets and patterns of organ involvement. Rheumatology. 2008;47: 1185–92.
22. Carwile LeRoy E, Black C, Fleischmajer R, Jablonska S, Krieg T, Medsger TA, et al. Scleroderma (systemic sclerosis): classification, subsets and pathogenesis. J Rheumatol. 1988;15:202–5.
23. Bennett RM. Scleroderma overlap syndromes. Rheum Dis Clin N Am. 1990; 16:185–98.
24. Rodnan GP, Fennell RH. Progressive systemic sclerosis sine scleroderma. JAMA. 1962;180:665–70.
25. Mosca M, Neri R, Bombardieri S. Undifferentiated connective tissue diseases (UCTD): a review of the literature and a proposal for preliminary classification criteria. Clin Exp Rheumatol. 1999;17:615–20.
26. Cipriani P, Franca Milia A, Liakouli V, Pacini A, Manetti M, Marrelli A, et al. Differential expression of stromal cell-derived factor 1 and its receptor CXCR4 in the skin and endothelial cells of systemic sclerosis patients: pathogenetic implications. Arthritis Rheum. 2006;54:3022–33.
27. Makino H, Aono Y, Azuma M, Kishi M, Yokota Y, Kinoshita K, et al. Antifibrotic effects of CXCR4 antagonist in bleomycin-induced pulmonary fibrosis in mice. J Med Investig. 2013;60:127–37.
28. Jiang D, Liang J, Hodge J, Lu B, Zhu Z, Yu S, et al. Regulation of pulmonary fibrosis by chemokine receptor CXCR3. J Clin Invest. 2004;114:291–9.
29. Fujii H, Hasegawa M, Takehara K, Mukaida N, Sato S. Abnormal expression of intracellular cytokines and chemokine receptors in peripheral blood T lymphocytes from patients with systemic sclerosis. Clin Exp Immunol. 2002; 130:548–56.
30. Shimizu S, Yoshinouchi T, Niimi T, Ohtsuki Y, Fujita J, Maeda H, et al. Differing distributions of CXCR3- and CCR4-positive cells among types of interstitial pneumonia associated with collagen vascular diseases. Virchows Arch. 2007;450:51–8.
31. Humrich JY, Riemekasten G. Low-dose IL-2 therapy—a complex scenario that remains to be further explored. Nat Rev Rheumatol. 2017;13:386.
32. Cabral-Marques O, Riemekasten G. Vascular hypothesis revisited: role of stimulating antibodies against angiotensin and endothelin receptors in the pathogenesis of systemic sclerosis. Autoimmun Rev. 2016;15:690–4.
33. Schmidt D, Bernat V, Brox R, Tschammer N, Kolb P. Identifying modulators of CXC receptors 3 and 4 with tailored selectivity using multi-target docking. ACS Chem Biol. 2015;10:715–24.
34. Andrews SP, Cox RJ. Small Molecule CXCR3 Antagonists. J Med Chem. 2016; 59:2894–917.

19

Analysis of complement biomarkers in systemic sclerosis indicates a distinct pattern in scleroderma renal crisis

Marcin Okrój[1,2], Martin Johansson[3], Tore Saxne[4], Anna M. Blom[1*†] and Roger Hesselstrand[4†]

Abstract

Background: The complement system has been implicated in pathogenesis of systemic sclerosis (SSc). The goal of the present study was to evaluate improved complement biomarkers in SSc.

Methods: The presence of C4d, reflecting activation of the classical/lectin pathways, C3bBbP corresponding to activation of the alternative pathway, and soluble terminal complement complexes (all complement pathways), was measured in plasma samples by enzyme-linked immunosorbent assay and correlated to clinical parameters. The study included 81 patients with limited cutaneous SSc and 41 with diffuse cutaneous SSc, as well as 47 matched healthy controls and 81 patients with rheumatoid arthritis, 22 with psoriatic arthritis and 20 with ankylosing spondylitis. Skin and kidney biopsies of selected patients were stained to detect deposited C3b as a marker of local complement activation.

Results: Biomarkers of activation of all complement pathways were increased in SSc compared with healthy controls and were similar to those in other rheumatic diseases. When patients with SSc were divided into subgroups, a distinct pattern of complement markers was observed in individuals with scleroderma renal crisis (SRC). By functional assay, we confirmed a significant decrease in complement haemolytic activity in SRC vs. non-SRC patients, indicating complement consumption. Further, we detected glomerular deposits of C3b in some patients with SRC.

Conclusions: The data indicate that complement activation is an important feature of SRC.

Keywords: Scleroderma, Complement, Biomarkers, Renal crisis, Systemic sclerosis

Background

Scleroderma, also termed *systemic sclerosis* (SSc), is an autoimmune disease of connective tissue. Its pathology involves excessive collagen production, resulting in fibrosis of skin and internal organs [1, 2]. This condition is accompanied by microangiopathy of varying severity and locations, most obviously seen as Raynaud's phenomenon. The most widely accepted classification distinguishes two main subtypes: limited cutaneous SSc (lcSSc) and diffuse cutaneous SSc (dcSSc) [3]. In the latter case, internal organs, most typically the kidneys, gastrointestinal tract, heart and lungs, are more severely affected. There is an ongoing discussion about the primary cause of SSc because many molecular patterns and various pathways have been found to be involved in the pathogenesis. Importantly, 90% of patients with SSc present with autoantibodies to intracellular components such as topoisomerase, centromeres, histones, RNA polymerases or ribonucleases, and these patients also show an increase in surface density of CD19 on their B cells [2]. It has been shown that the presence of these autoantibodies represents specific phenotypes of the disease, but less is known about their pathogenic role.

Data from in vivo models show that low expression of CD19 affects B-cell proliferation, whereas overexpression potentiates antibody production and increases the degree of autoantibodies [4]. Indeed, whole-genome microarray analysis has demonstrated that gene expression patterns characteristic of plasma cells decreases more than 90%

* Correspondence: anna.blom@med.lu.se
†Equal contributors
[1]Department of Translational Medicine, Section of Medical Protein Chemistry, Lund University, Inga Marie Nilssons Street 53, Malmö S-20502, Sweden
Full list of author information is available at the end of the article

upon anti-CD19 treatment and correlates with inhibition of collagen expression [5]. Apart from intracellular components, protein complexes present on the surface of fibroblasts, lymphocytes and endothelial cells are also targets of autoantibodies in SSc [6]. These autoantibodies may activate fibroblasts to produce collagen, either directly or indirectly, by fuelling local inflammation and release of pro-inflammatory cytokines. However, it is unclear to what extent the complement system, for which antibodies are a main trigger, contributes to SSc pathogenesis. CD21 (CR2), a receptor on the surface of B cells, binds activation products of the main complement factor C3b. Following complement activation, C3b covalently binds target surfaces and forms transient enzymatic complexes: complement convertases such as C3bBbP, which fuel downstream events of the cascade such as release of the potent pro-inflammatory anaphylatoxin C5a, and formation of terminal complement complexes (TCCs), which can cause cell lysis. CD21 and CD19 associate and form a signal transduction complex capable of enhancing B-cell responses to antigen once CD21 binds complement degradation fragments [7].

In fact, over the last 30 years, researchers have tried to correlate the levels of complement proteins, markers of complement activation and circulating immune complexes in patients' bloodstream with severity of SSc and different subtypes of the disease. Elevated immune complexes were found only in some patients and were not associated with clinical or serological features [8, 9]. In another study, low-molecular-weight markers of complement activation—Ba, C3d and C4d—were measured by nephelometry in plasma of patients with SSc [10]. The results showed that C3d, C4d and Ba fragments, as well as C3d:C3 and C4d:C4 ratios, were clearly higher in patients with SSc than in healthy control subjects, indicating increased complement activation. Also, patients with dcSSc showed significantly higher values than those with lcSSc [10]. On the basis of observations of higher C4d values in patients with SSc and subendothelial deposition of immune complexes [11], the classical complement pathway may indeed play a role in the pathogenesis of SSc. However, this should be confirmed in a larger number of patients and with validated methods capable of specifically measuring products of complement activation.

We recently established a novel enzyme-linked immunosorbent assay (ELISA) that can reliably detect soluble C4d in plasma [12]. In the present study, we re-examined the usefulness of C4d as biomarker in a cohort of 122 patients with SSc. Also, we measured a soluble marker of alternative pathway activation, C3bBbP, and soluble TCC (sTCC), a marker of the final step of complement activation via any pathway in the same cohort. In order to compare the results obtained for patients with SSc with those for patients with other autoimmune diseases in whom activation of the complement system was previously reported, we performed the same analyses in patients with rheumatoid arthritis (RA) [13], psoriatic arthritis (PsoA) [14] and ankylosing spondylitis (AS) [15], as well as in healthy control subjects.

Methods

Patients

Plasma samples were collected from 122 patients who fulfilled the American College of Rheumatology (ACR) criteria for SSc [16]. The disease was classified as dcSSc ($n = 41$) or lcSSc ($n = 81$), based on the extent of skin involvement [3]. Samples were collected within a mean (±SD) of 7.5 (8.5) years of disease onset, which was defined as the first non-Raynaud's manifestation. A summary of baseline characteristics of patients with SSc is presented in Table 1. Healthy control plasma samples were collected from 47 age-matched (mean 52.3 ± 8.7 years) and sex-matched (14 males, 33 females) healthy volunteers with no history of rheumatologic disease. All plasma samples were retrieved in a standardised fashion (non-fasting) and were stored at −80 °C after centrifugation until the experiments. Additionally, we included plasma samples from age- and sex-matched patients with RA ($n = 81$), PsoA ($n = 22$) and AS ($n = 20$). All patients with RA fulfilled the 1987 ACR criteria [17]. Diagnoses of PsoA and AS were based on clinical judgment by the treating physician and included radiographic examinations when applicable. All patients with AS had axial involvement but no clinical signs of peripheral arthritis, whereas the patients with PsoA had peripheral arthritis but no clinical signs of axial involvement.

Clinical data

Anti-nuclear antibodies (ANA) and anti-centromeric antibodies (ACA) were analysed by an indirect immunofluorescence technique using the human Hep-2 cell line as a substrate; anti-topoisomerase I antibodies (ATA)

Table 1 Clinical features at the time of blood sampling of 122 patients with systemic sclerosis

Feature	Data
Age, years	56.4 (14.8)
Disease duration, years	7.5 (8.5)
mRSS, points	11.1 (11.0)
Sex, male/female, *n* (%)	22 (18)/100 (82)
Subset, lcSSc/dcSSc, *n* (%)	81 (66)/41 (34)
Ab, ACA/ATA/ARA/ANA$^+$/ANA$^-$, *n* (%)	34 (28)/22 (18)/17 (14)/40 (33)/9 (7)

Abbreviations: *Ab* Autoantibodies, *mRSS* Modified Rodnan skin score, *lcSSc* Limited cutaneous systemic sclerosis, *dcSSc* Diffuse cutaneous systemic sclerosis, *Ab* Autoantibodies, *ACA* Anti-centromere, *ATA* Anti-topoisomerase I, *ARA* Anti-RNA polymerase III, *ANA$^+$* Anti-nuclear but not anti-centromere, anti-topoisomerase I or anti-RNA polymerase III autoantibodies, *ANA$^-$* No anti-nuclear autoantibodies were analysed by ELISA; and anti-RNA polymerase III antibodies (ARA) were analysed by immunoprecipitation. Serum cartilage oligomeric matrix protein (COMP) was measured with a commercial sandwich ELISA using two monoclonal antibodies directed against separate antigenic determinants (AnaMar, Lund, Sweden) [18]. Subjects were classified as having dcSSc or lcSSc according to LeRoy et al.'s criteria [3]. The severity of skin involvement was determined by the modified Rodnan skin score (mRSS) [19]. Disease duration was determined as the time from the first non-Raynaud's manifestation.

Measurement of complement activation markers

Plasma concentrations of C4d [12], C3bBbP [20] and sTCC [20] were measured by specific sandwich ELISAs in plasma ethylenediaminetetraacetic acid (EDTA) samples as described previously. Readout of each of these assays was given in complement activation units (CAU), a defined arbitrary unit set for the International Complement Standard #2 (ICS#2) sample, which is serum-pooled from about 1000 healthy individuals and incubated with activators of all three complement pathways [20].

Haemolytic assays

Plasma EDTA samples collected from patients with SSc were tested for activity of classical or alternative complement pathways by haemolytic assays performed as described elsewhere [21], with small modifications. Briefly, the classical complement pathway was activated on antibody-sensitised sheep erythrocytes. To overcome the inhibitory effect of EDTA, plasma samples were diluted 1:100 in $DGVB^{2+}$ buffer (2.5 mM veronal buffer, pH 7.35, 72 mM NaCl, 140 mM glucose, 0.1% gelatin, 1 mM $MgCl_2$ and 0.15 mM $CaCl_2$). For the alternative pathway, plasma samples were diluted 1:20 in Mg-ethylene glycol-bis(2-aminoethylether)-*N,N,N′,N′*-tetraacetic acid (Mg-EGTA) buffer (2.5 mM veronal buffer, pH 7.3, 70 mM NaCl, 140 mM glucose, 0.1% gelatin, 7 mM $MgCl_2$ and 10 mM EGTA) and added directly to rabbit erythrocytes.

Immunohistochemical staining of C3

Kidney and skin biopsies collected from patients with SSc were fixed in formalin and embedded in paraffin. Sections of 4-μm thickness were cut and automatically pre-treated using the PT Link system (Dako/Agilent Technologies, Santa Clara, CA, USA) and then stained in an Autostainer Plus (Dako) with rabbit anti-human C3c polyclonal antibody (P0062; Dako) at a final dilution of 1:5000 for 30 minutes. Subsequently, the EnVision Flex HRP kit (Dako) was applied to the sections for 20 minutes to detect primary antibodies, followed by 3,3′-diaminobenzidine (DAB) reagent for visualisation.

Statistical analysis

Obtained data on the appearance of complement activation markers and haemolytic activity were not distributed normally; in each complement measurement there were outliers, and some patient subgroups were rather small. Therefore, we used non-parametric statistical methods throughout the whole analysis. The Kruskal-Wallis and Mann-Whitney *U* tests were used to compare multiple groups or two groups, respectively. Spearman's correlation was used to analyse relationships. p values <0.05 were considered significant. Calculations were performed with Prism 5.0 (GraphPad Software, La Jolla, CA, USA) and IBM SPSS Statistics version 20 (IBM, Armonk, NY, USA) software.

Results

The complement system is activated in patients with autoimmune diseases

We tested three different complement activation markers: (1) C4d, corresponding to activation of the classical pathway; (2) the fluid-phase alternative C3 convertase (C3bBbP), reflecting activation of the alternative pathway as well as the amplification loop enhancing the cascade at the level of convertases; and (3) sTCC, which evaluates the lytic (terminal) pathway (Fig. 1). All autoimmune patients, regardless of diagnosis, had 5- to 15-fold increased levels of all three markers, thus confirming ongoing complement activation. Regarding SSc, C4d was increased to a similar degree as for AS and PsoA, but to a lesser extent than in RA ($p = 0.05$ by Kruskal-Wallis test). Interestingly, the alternative pathway was activated significantly more strongly in patients with SSc than in patients with RA ($p < 0.001$). All groups of patients showed similar levels of sTCC. As expected, healthy control subjects showed low levels of all three markers.

Correlations of complement activation markers in patients with autoimmune diseases

Because sTCC is a marker of the terminal complement pathway, which is fuelled by all complement pathways, we analysed which of the early complement markers correlate to appearance of sTCC in patients with SSc and other autoimmune diseases. Only C3bBbP, and not C4d, was significantly correlated to sTCC in all groups of patients. However, in patients with RA, C4d was significantly correlated to C3bBbP, which may indicate the role of the amplification of the classical pathway via alternative convertases in overall complement activation in this patient group. Correlation coefficients and p values are given in Table 2.

Correlations of complement activation markers to mRSS and COMP

To find out whether complement activation correlates to the severity of fibrosis expressed by mRSS, we performed

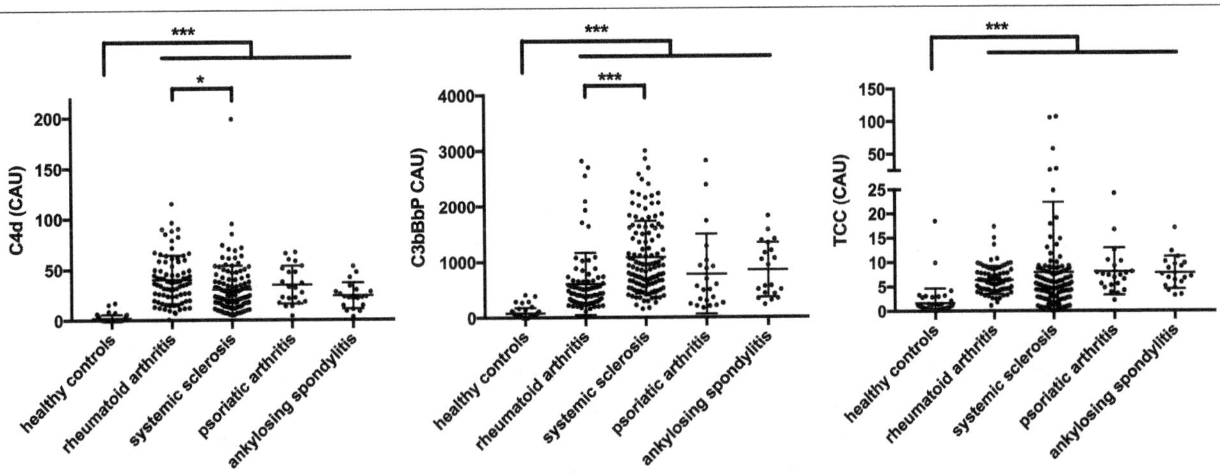

Fig. 1 Complement activation markers in systemic sclerosis and other autoimmune diseases. Graphs show mean and standard deviation of C4d (*left panel*), C3bBbP (*middle panel*) and soluble terminal complement complex (TCC) (*right panel*) concentrations. Value obtained for each patient (depicted with single points) is an average of two independent experiments. Statistical analysis was performed by Kruskal-Wallis test with Dunn's multiple comparisons post-test, and statistical significance was set at $^*p < 0.05$ and $^{***}p < 0.001$.Abbreviation: *CAU* Complement activation units

Spearman's correlation analysis and found weak, borderline significant correlation between mRSS and C4d (Table 3). Furthermore, COMP, which is expressed by fibroblasts in SSc, is associated with mRSS [22] (in the present cohort, Spearman's $r = 0.47$, $p = 0.0005$) and is known to activate the alternative pathway [23]. However, we did not observe a statistically significant correlation between complement activation markers and COMP levels in plasma, implying that it is likely not a major complement trigger in these patients, at least not when released into blood.

Analyses of complement activation markers in the subgroups of patients with SSc

We classified the patients into subgroups depending on the form of disease (lcSSc vs. dcSSc); typical complications, such as pulmonary arterial hypertension (PAH), scleroderma renal crisis (SRC), pitting scars, ulcers, telangiectasias; or the presence of certain types of anti-nuclear autoantibodies, including ACA, ATA, ARA, ANA without ACA, ATA or ARA, and finally ANA-negative. We did not observe significant differences in C4d, C3bBbP and sTCC levels between men and women or between patients with lcSSc and those with dcSSc (Table 4). Also, concentrations of these markers were equally distributed within patients with and without PAH, pitting scars, ulcers, and telangiectasias. Importantly, a different distribution of complement activation markers was detected in patients with SRC, who had significantly higher amounts of C4d ($p = 0.036$) and significantly lower levels of C3bBbP ($p < 0.001$) and sTCC ($p = 0.003$) than patients without kidney involvement. When overall distribution of autoantibodies was analysed by the Kruskal-Wallis test, we found a significant difference for sTCC ($p = 0.016$) and a difference on the border of significance for C3bBbP ($p = 0.055$). Although not statistically significant ($p = 0.095$), there was a trend for C4d, according to which patients without any antinuclear autoantibodies presented with low levels of this marker. Furthermore, patients with ARA positivity showed a pattern of complement activation markers similar to that of the patients with SRC (high C4d, low C3bBbP and TCC). Additional Kruskal-Wallis analysis performed for a single type of autoantibody revealed that the ARA-positive group differed

Table 2 Correlations between complement biomarkers C4d, C3bBbP and terminal complement complex in plasma samples from patients with autoimmune diseases

Disease	C4d-TCC correlation		C3bBbP-TCC correlation		C4d-C3bBbP correlation	
	Spearman's *r*	*p* value	Spearman's *r*	*p* value	Spearman's *r*	*p* value
SSc ($n = 122$)	−0.06	0.47	0.47	<0.0001[a]	0.099	0.27
RA ($n = 81$)	0.12	0.29	0.41	0.0001[a]	0.26	0.018[b]
PsoA ($n = 22$)	0.035	0.88	0.52	0.013[b]	0.086	0.70
AS ($n = 20$)	−0.33	0.15	0.52	0.019[b]	−0.20	0.40

Abbreviations: AS Ankylosing spondylitis, *PsoA* Psoriatic arthritis, *RA* Rheumatoid arthritis, *SSc* Systemic sclerosis, *TCC* Terminal complement complex

[a] $p < 0.001$

[b] $p < 0.05$

Table 3 Correlations of complement activation markers with age, modified Rodnan skin score and cartilage oligomeric matrix protein

	n	C4d	*p* value	C3bBbP	*p* value	TCC	*p* value
Age	122	−0.14	0.13	−0.083	0.36	0.017	0.86
mRSS	118	0.17	0.06	−0.16	0.087	−0.082	0.38
COMP	53	0.16	0.26	−0.052	0.71	0.092	0.51

Abbreviations: COMP Cartilage oligomeric matrix protein, *mRSS* Modified Rodnan skin score, *TCC* Terminal complement complex

significantly from patients without any antinuclear antibodies (ANA-negative) at a p level <0.05 for all complement markers. Also, the ARA-positive group had significantly lower amounts of C3bBbP and TCC than ARA-negative patients ($p < 0.01$). Interestingly, 8 (47%) of 17 patients with ARA presented also with SRC, a group that accounted only for 15% of all patients with SSc (18 of 122). Taken together, patients with ARA were, as expected, overrepresented among those with SRC and, importantly, manifested the same pattern of complement activation markers.

Haemolytic activity of plasma samples collected from patients with SSc

The levels of C3bBbP and sTCC in the SRC group (means 656 CAU and 4.22 CAU, respectively) were lower than in other patients with SSc; however, these levels were still considerably higher than analogous means for healthy control subjects (79.7 CAU and 1.64 CAU, respectively), indicating that complement activation takes place during the renal crisis. At the same time, C4d, which is a marker of classical pathway activation

Table 4 Analyses of complement activation markers in the subgroups of patients with systemic sclerosis

	n	C4d, mean (SD)	*p* value	C3bBbP, mean (SD)	*p* value	TCC, mean (SD)	*p* value
Sex			0.96		0.20		0.87
Male	22	35.6 (40.3)		913 (574)		5.80 (3.69)	
Female	100	29.2 (18.3)		1119 (661)		8.39 (15.8)	
Subset			0.88		0.11		0.36
lcSSc	81	30.1 (25.2)		1143 (655)		8.56 (16.4)	
dcSSc	41	30.8 (20.7)		962 (629)		6.66 (9.34)	
PAH			0.19		0.75		0.76
No	96	31.8 (25.3)		1069 (645)		7.50 (12.4)	
Yes	26	25.0 (16.0)		1131 (676)		9.49 (20.5)	
SRC			0.036		<0.001		0.003
No	104	28.9 (23.7)		1156 (655)		8.57 (15.4)	
Yes	18	38.6 (22.9)		656 (423)		4.22 (5.54)	
Ab			0.095		0.055		0.016
ACA	34	30.7 (16.9)		1029 (594)		5.83 (5.70)	
ATA	22	32.7 (18.8)		1140 (744)		10.8 (22.0)	
ARA	17	35.0 (22.5)		761 (560)		3.19 (2.59)	
ANA^{+}	40	29.5 (32.2)		1195 (642)		10.6 (18.0)	
ANA^{-}	9	18.1 (10.0)		1244 (705)		5.62 (3.36)	
Pitting scar			0.50		0.35		0.76
No	68	31.0 (26.1)		1071 (658)		9.30 (18.6)	
Yes	50	28.6 (19.0)		1155 (633)		6.53 (5.62)	
Ulcer			0.35		0.36		0.54
No	105	30.5 (23.9)		1090 (656)		8.31 (15.3)	
Yes	14	25.5 (17.8)		1183 (574)		6.19 (6.53)	
Telangiectasias			0.83		0.19		0.39
No	56	28.5 (17.8)		1003 (586)		6.07 (3.80)	
Yes	63	31.2 (27.2)		1189 (687)		9.84 (19.6)	

Abbreviations: *PAH* Pulmonary arterial hypertension, *SRC* Scleroderma renal crisis, *Ab* Autoantibodies, *ACA* Anti-centromere, *ATA* Anti-topoisomerase I, *ARA* Anti-RNA polymerase III, *ANA*$^{+}$ Anti-nuclear but not anti-centromere, anti-topoisomerase I or anti-RNA polymerase III, *ANA*$^{-}$ No anti-nuclear autoantibodies, *dcSSc* Diffuse cutaneous systemic sclerosis, *lcSSc* Limited cutaneous systemic sclerosis, *TCC* Terminal complement complex
Autoantibody analyses were by Kruskal-Wallis test; all others were by Mann-Whitney *U* test

and the end-degradation product of C4b component, increased to significantly higher levels than in the non-SRC group. One possible explanation for these observations is that during SRC the classical pathway is strongly initiated by autoantibodies, and then an amplification loop driven by the alternative pathway takes over the cascade, leading to systemic depletion of its components, including C3 and factor B proteins. Such depletion is also reflected in a reduction of soluble sTCC compared with patients with no SRC episodes. To confirm the scenario of ongoing complement consumption in SRC, we analysed haemolytic activity of plasma samples from patients with SSc. Residual complement activity was examined in assays testing the classical and alternative pathways (Fig. 2). Of all classifications made for the whole SSc cohort, only the SRC-positive group showed significantly lower haemolytic activity in the alternative pathway ($p = 0.0107$) and a borderline significant drop of haemolytic activity in the classical pathway ($p = 0.063$), which confirmed systemic complement depletion, most probably at the level of alternative convertases.

C3 staining in kidney biopsies from patients with SRC

Because the SRC subgroup showed a distinct pattern of complement activation markers, we searched for the primary source of a putative strong complement activation deduced from lower levels of C3bBbP and lower haemolytic activity of plasma samples. Kidney biopsies from 5 of 18 patients with SRC included in the study were available, and we examined these for C3b deposition by immunohistochemistry. C3b deposits were detected in glomeruli of two patients and in tubules of one more patient (Fig. 3), whereas C3b staining was negative for kidneys of two remaining patients. These findings indicate that ongoing complement activation in kidneys may be one of the hallmarks of SRC. However, it does not explain all cases, and other sources of activation are also plausible.

C3b staining in skin biopsies from ARA$^+$, ARA$^-$ and ARA$^-$/ACA$^+$ patients

Searching for further explanations for complement activation in patients with SRC, we followed the overrepresentation of ARA-positive patients in the SRC group

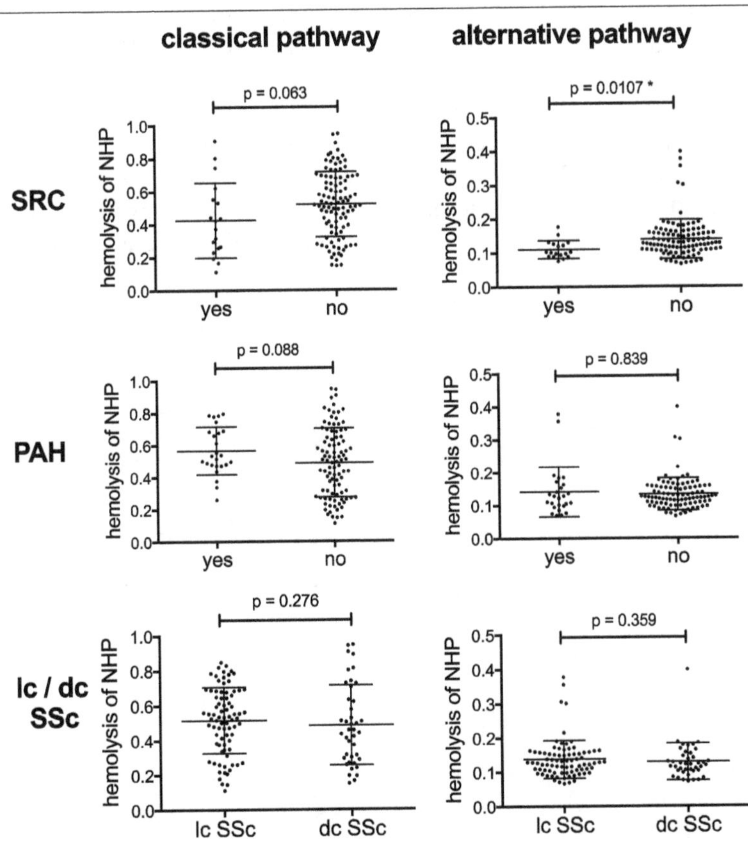

Fig. 2 Haemolytic activity of plasma samples collected from patients with systemic sclerosis. *Left column* shows classical pathway haemolytic activity of 1% plasma, and *right column* shows alternative pathway activity of 5% plasma. Value of 1 on *y*-axis corresponds to the readout of normal human plasma (NHP). Results are means ± standard deviation derived from two independent experiments, and statistical significance is set at $*p < 0.05$ according to Mann-Whitney *U* test.Abbreviations: *SRC* Scleroderma renal crisis, *PAH* Pulmonary arterial hypertension, *lcSSc* Limited cutaneous systemic sclerosis, *dcSSc* Diffuse cutaneous systemic sclerosis. Graphs comparing the patients with vs. without ulcers, pitting scars and telangiectasias are not shown, because the differences between groups did not reach statistical significance

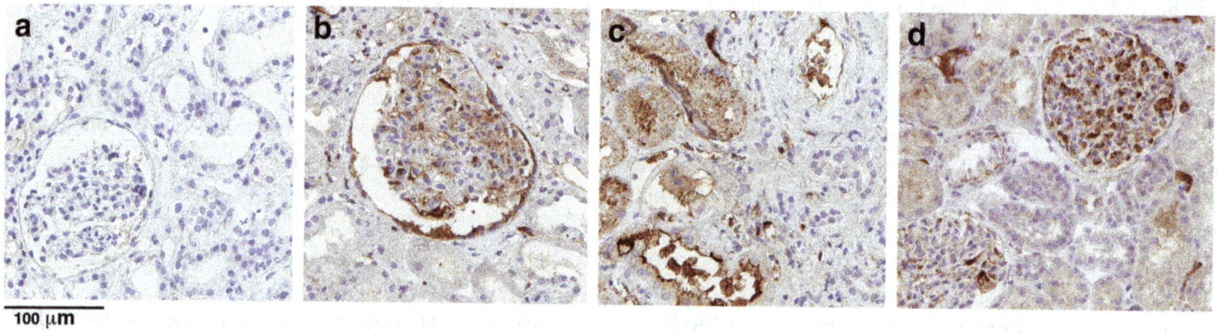

Fig. 3 C3b deposition in kidney biopsies from patients with scleroderma renal crisis (SRC). Shown are representative micrographs of kidney biopsy cores immunostained for C3b. **a** An example of a biopsy obtained from a patient with SRC, which was negative for C3b. **b** Example of a biopsy positive for C3b in glomeruli. **c** Example of a biopsy positive for C3b in tubules. **d** Positive control biopsy from patient diagnosed for immunoglobulin A nephropathy with distinct glomerular C3 positivity

and analysed C3b deposition in skin biopsies obtained from ARA^+, ARA^- and ARA^-/ACA^+ patients. Material from four patients in each group was available. We observed C3b deposition in skin tissue from all ARA^+ patients, but other groups also had at least two of four slides that were positive (Fig. 4), so there was no dramatic difference between the groups. The staining was localised to the dermal layer and most prominent in the endothelium of small dermal arteries. Less staining was associated with the collagenous fibres of the dermis. In the basal layer of the epidermis, cells were discovered containing what seemed to be stain. However, these cells were melanocytes, and the pigment was melanin, not DAB chromogen (Fig. 4).

Discussion

Reliable measurement of complement activation is not a trivial task. Of two possible strategies, measurement of native complement protein consumption and measurement of markers appearing only after complement activation, the latter seems to be more reliable. This is due partly to large interpersonal differences in some complement proteins, such as that normal concentration of the main complement protein C3 ranges from 0.8 to 1.8 mg/ml. On one hand, these levels are affected by both consumption and a changing rate of synthesis because many complement factors are acute-phase response proteins. On the other hand, challenges in the strategy of measuring products of activation relate to the specificity of

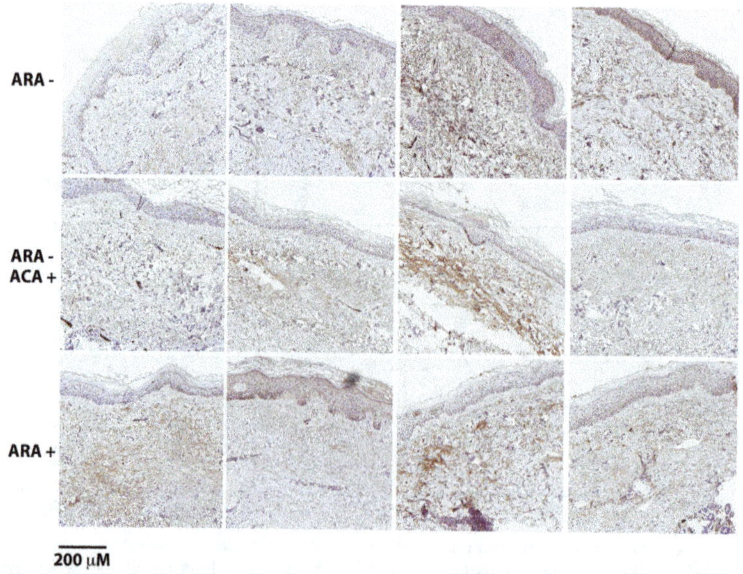

Fig. 4 C3b staining of skin biopsied from anti-RNA polymerase III (ARA^+), ARA^- and anti-centromere-positive (ACA^+)/ARA^- patients. Shown are representative micrographs of skin biopsies immunostained for C3b. Four patients per group (rows) were available for the study. In most images, the endothelium of the dermal arterioles is distinctly positive. There is also a fainter staining associated with the dermal collagen strands. In the basal layer of the epidermis, melanocytes are seen, filled with melanin pigment but negative for C3b

antibodies, which must target only neoepitopes localised on processed complement proteins and not epitopes on ubiquitous, native molecules. Previous studies performed with 34 patients with SSc revealed higher levels of C4d in blood of patients with dcSSc than in patients with lcSSc, suggesting that C4d content may be associated with clinical severity of SSc [10]. However, the authors of that study did not use specific anti-C4d antibodies; instead, they performed precipitation of high-molecular-weight plasma proteins and detected C4d in supernatant with whole antiserum by nephelometry. We re-examined this hypothesis using plasma samples of 122 patients with our recently designed C4d ELISA. The advantage of this method over nephelometry and other, previously used C4d immunoassays is that it uses a novel antibody specific to a 5-aa linear cleavage site neoepitope. Previously, we showed that the readout of this assay is unaffected by repeated freezing-thawing or heating of samples, which is not the case for some other techniques based on conformational neoepitopes [12]. We noticed a clear increase of C4d as well as the complement activation markers C3bBbP and sTCC in patients with SSc as well as in patients with other rheumatic diseases compared with healthy control subjects (Fig. 1). However, we could confirm neither a link between clinical severity of SSc and C4d content nor associations of complement activation markers with particular syndromes characteristic for SSc, except for SRC.

Renal crisis is reported typically in 5–10% patents with SSc [24, 25]. Historically, this group of patients had a high risk of death (up to 85% mortality after 1 year [26]), and even after introducing treatment with angiotensin-converting enzyme inhibitors, mortality remains relatively high at 18% after the first year and 41–58% after 5 years [27, 28]. To prevent loss of kidney function and other associated complications, such as systemic hypertension, retinopathy or pulmonary oedema, patients require early identification and aggressive treatment [25]. Therefore, increasing knowledge about underlying pathomechanisms of SRC is necessary. Our data suggest that activation of complement, which is a feature common to rheumatic and/or autoimmune diseases [13, 29], presents differently in patients with SSc with SRC. Another important observation was that the same pattern of complement activation markers seen in SRC was observed in the group of ARA-positive patients, which accounted for 44% of patients with SRC in our study and 33% [30] to 59% [27] in other studies. Trends and a significant increase of C4d marker in these two groups of patients linked to each other speak for enhanced activation of the classical pathway. C3bBbP is a marker that may indicate activation of the alternative pathway alone or as an amplification loop of the classical or lectin pathway. At first glance, elevated C4d and decreased C3bBbP levels in the same patients may appear contradictory, but the nature of these markers may provide a logical explanation. Whereas C4d is the end degradation product of an early component of the classical pathway C4b and may accumulate over time, C3bBbP is a fluid-phase convertase, an enzymatic complex that converts available C3 into C3b. Activation of the alternative pathway leads to depletion of C3 and factor B and, by doing so, limits de novo formation of C3bBbP. However, C3bBbP decays both spontaneously and with the aid of several complement inhibitors [20]. As a result of limited replacement of alternative pathway components and pathway exhaustion, patients with acute episodes of complement activation may present with lower C3bBbP content than those with chronic disease. The same is true for sTCC.

On the basis of our results, we hypothesised that acute complement activation takes place during the onset of SRC and that depletion of available complement is another consequence of such scenario. Our hypothesis was confirmed by haemolytic assays in which residual complement activity of plasma from patients with SRC was significantly lower than that in non-SRC subjects. In conjunction with a previous report showing increased C4d deposition in peritubular capillaries of patients with SSc with SRC compared with normotensive controls and hypertensive non-SRC control subjects [24], we should consider local complement activation as an important element of the SRC pathomechanism. This hypothesis is strengthened by presence of C3b deposits, which reflect complement activation via all pathways, in three of five analysed kidney biopsies from patients with SRC. We also tested whether ARA-positive patients overrepresented in the SRC group had increased C3b deposits in skin. Although all ARA-positive individuals showed C3b staining in skin biopsies, we also found it in some ARA-negative patients. Therefore, we hypothesise that local complement activation in kidneys and skin takes place during SRC, but that this phenomenon is probably not limited only to this subgroup and that other, distinct features may be characteristic for renal involvement. Nonetheless, complement activation may be a strongly contributing factor in some patients with SRC, and these patients could be considered for treatment with emerging complement inhibitors such as eculizumab, which is now used in therapy for another kidney disease with complement involvement: haemolytic uremic syndrome.

Conclusions

The present study shows that biomarkers of activation of all complement pathways measured with improved assays were increased in patients with SSc compared with healthy control subjects. Patients with SSc with SRC showed a distinct pattern of complement markers indicating ongoing complement consumption. This, finding, together with glomerular deposits of C3b found in some of these patients, indicates that complement activation is an important feature of SRC.

Abbreviations

ACA: Anti-centromere; ACR: American College of Rheumatology; ANA: Antinuclear; ARA: Anti-RNA polymerase III; AS: Ankylosing spondylitis; ATA: Antitopoisomerase I; CAU: Complement activation units; COMP: Cartilage oligomeric matrix protein; DAB: 3,3'-Diaminobenzidine; dcSSc: Diffuse cutaneous systemic sclerosis; EDTA: Ethylenediaminetetraacetic acid; EGTA: Ethylene glycol-bis(2-aminoethylether)-*N,N,N',N'*-tetraacetic acid; ELISA: Enzyme-linked immunosorbent assay; lcSSc: Limited cutaneous systemic sclerosis; mRSS: Modified Rodnan skin score; NHP: Normal human plasma; PAH: Pulmonary arterial hypertension; PsoA: Psoriatic arthritis; RA: Rheumatoid arthritis; SRC: Scleroderma renal crisis; SSc: Systemic sclerosis; sTCC: Soluble terminal complement complex; TCC: Terminal complement complex

Acknowledgements

We thank Marie Wildt for excellent technical assistance and Dr. Ben King for proofreading the manuscript.

Funding

This study was supported by the Swedish Research Council (K2012-66X-14928-09-5), the Polish National Science Centre (2014/14/E/NZ6/00182), the Alfred Österlund Foundation, the Kock Foundation, King Gustav V's 80th Birthday Fund, the Knut and Alice Wallenberg Foundation, and the IngaBritt and Arne Lundberg Foundation, as well as by grants for clinical research (Medical Training and Research Agreement [ALF] and Skåne University Hospital).

Authors' contributions

AMB, RH and MO were responsible for study conception and design. MO was responsible for the acquisition of experimental data. RH and TS recruited patients and provided samples and clinical data. MO, RH and MJ performed the data analysis and interpretation. All authors were involved in drafting the manuscript or revising it critically for important intellectual content, and all authors read and approved the final manuscript.

Competing interests

AMB and MO are named as inventors in a patent application (Antibodies specific for complement component C4d and uses thereof; application number PCT/EP2015/070526). The other authors state that they have no competing interests.

Author details

[1]Department of Translational Medicine, Section of Medical Protein Chemistry, Lund University, Inga Marie Nilssons Street 53, Malmö S-20502, Sweden. [2]Department of Medical Biotechnology, Intercollegiate Faculty of Biotechnology UG-MUG, Medical University of Gdańsk, Gdańsk 80210, Poland. [3]Department of Translational Medicine, Section of Clinical Pathology, Lund University, Jan Waldenströms street 59, Malmö S-20502, Sweden. [4]Department of Clinical Sciences, Lund, Section of Rheumatology, Lund University, Skåne University Hospital, Lund S-22185, Sweden.

References

1. Balbir-Gurman A, Braun-Moscovici Y. Scleroderma – new aspects in pathogenesis and treatment. Best Pract Res Clin Rheumatol. 2012;26:13–24.
2. Yoshizaki A, Sato S. Abnormal B lymphocyte activation and function in systemic sclerosis. Ann Dermatol. 2015;27:1–9.
3. LeRoy EC, Black C, Fleischmajer R, Jablonska S, Krieg T, Medsger Jr TA, et al. Scleroderma (systemic sclerosis): classification, subsets and pathogenesis. J Rheumatol. 1988;15:202–5.
4. Engel P, Zhou LJ, Ord DC, Sato S, Koller B, Tedder TF. Abnormal B lymphocyte development, activation, and differentiation in mice that lack or overexpress the CD19 signal transduction molecule. Immunity. 1995;3:39–50.
5. Streicher K, Morehouse CA, Groves CJ, Rajan B, Pilataxi F, Lehmann KP, et al. The plasma cell signature in autoimmune disease. Arthritis Rheumatol. 2014;66:173–84.
6. Chizzolini C, Raschi E, Rezzonico R, Testoni C, Mallone R, Gabrielli A, et al. Autoantibodies to fibroblasts induce a proadhesive and proinflammatory fibroblast phenotype in patients with systemic sclerosis. Arthritis Rheum. 2002;46:1602–13.
7. Tedder TF, Poe JC, Fujimoto M, Haas KM, Sato S. The CD19-CD21 signal transduction complex of B lymphocytes regulates the balance between health and autoimmune disease: systemic sclerosis as a model system. Curr Dir Autoimmun. 2005;8:55–90.
8. Swierczynska Z, Rdultowska H, Blaszczyk M, Jablonska S, Luft S. Circulating immune complexes in systemic scleroderma. Immunol Commun. 1984; 13:433–8.
9. Siminovitch K, Klein M, Pruzanski W, Wilkinson S, Lee P, Yoon SJ, et al. Circulating immune complexes in patients with progressive systemic sclerosis. Arthritis Rheum. 1982;25:1174–9.
10. Senaldi G, Lupoli S, Vergani D, Black CM. Activation of the complement system in systemic sclerosis: relationship to clinical severity. Arthritis Rheum. 1989;32:1262–7.
11. Chen M, Daha MR, Kallenberg CG. The complement system in systemic autoimmune disease. J Autoimmun. 2010;34:J276–86.
12. Blom AM, Osterborg A, Mollnes TE, Okroj M. Antibodies reactive to cleaved sites in complement proteins enable highly specific measurement of soluble markers of complement activation. Mol Immunol. 2015;66:164–70.
13. Okroj M, Heinegard D, Holmdahl R, Blom AM. Rheumatoid arthritis and the complement system. Ann Med. 2007;39:517–30.
14. Chimenti MS, Perricone C, Graceffa D, Di Muzio G, Ballanti E, Guarino MD, et al. Complement system in psoriatic arthritis: a useful marker in response prediction and monitoring of anti-TNF treatment. Clin Exp Rheumatol. 2012;30:23–30.
15. McGuigan LE, Geczy AF, Edmonds JP. The immunopathology of ankylosing spondylitis—a review. Semin Arthritis Rheum. 1985;15:81–105.
16. Subcommittee for scleroderma criteria of the American Rheumatism Association Diagnostic and Therapeutic Criteria Committee. Preliminary criteria for the classification of systemic sclerosis (scleroderma). Arthritis Rheum. 1980;23:581–90.
17. Arnett FC, Edworthy SM, Bloch DA, McShane DJ, Fries JF, Cooper NS, et al. The American Rheumatism Association 1987 revised criteria for the classification of rheumatoid arthritis. Arthritis Rheum. 1988;31:315–24.
18. Otteby KE, Holmquist E, Saxne T, Heinegard D, Hesselstrand R, Blom AM. Cartilage oligomeric matrix protein-induced complement activation in systemic sclerosis. Arthritis Res Ther. 2013;15:R215.
19. Clements P, Lachenbruch P, Siebold J, White B, Weiner S, Martin R, et al. Inter and intraobserver variability of total skin thickness score (modified Rodnan TSS) in systemic sclerosis. J Rheumatol. 1995;22:1281–5.
20. Bergseth G, Ludviksen JK, Kirschfink M, Giclas PC, Nilsson B, Mollnes TE. An international serum standard for application in assays to detect human complement activation products. Mol Immunol. 2013;56:232–9.
21. Okroj M, Holmquist E, Sjolander J, Corrales L, Saxne T, Wisniewski HG, et al. Heavy chains of inter alpha inhibitor (IαI) inhibit the human complement system at early stages of the cascade. J Biol Chem. 2012;287:20100–10.
22. Hesselstrand R, Kassner A, Heinegard D, Saxne T. COMP: a candidate molecule in the pathogenesis of systemic sclerosis with a potential as a disease marker. Ann Rheum Dis. 2008;67:1242–8.
23. Happonen KE, Saxne T, Aspberg A, Mörgelin M, Heinegård D, Blom AM. Regulation of complement by cartilage oligomeric matrix protein allows for a novel molecular diagnostic principle in rheumatoid arthritis. Arthritis Rheum. 2010;62:3574–83.
24. Batal I, Domsic RT, Shafer A, Medsger Jr TA, Kiss LP, Randhawa P, et al. Renal biopsy findings predicting outcome in scleroderma renal crisis. Hum Pathol. 2009;40:332–40.
25. Denton CP, Lapadula G, Mouthon L, Müller-Ladner U. Renal complications and scleroderma renal crisis. Rheumatology (Oxford). 2009;48 Suppl 3:iii32–5.
26. Steen VD, Costantino JP, Shapiro AP, Medsger Jr TA. Outcome of renal crisis in systemic sclerosis: relation to availability of angiotensin converting enzyme (ACE) inhibitors. Ann Intern Med. 1990;113:352–7.

Familial risk of systemic sclerosis and co-aggregation of autoimmune diseases in affected families

Chang-Fu Kuo[1,2], Shue-Fen Luo[2], Kuang-Hui Yu[2], Lai-Chu See[3], Weiya Zhang[1*] and Michael Doherty[1]

Abstract

Background: Systemic sclerosis (SSc) is a rare and devastating disease affecting skin and internal organs. Familial aggregation of SSc and co-aggregation with other autoimmune diseases is rarely reported.

Methods: We identified 23,658,577 beneficiaries registered with the National Health Insurance database in 2010, 1891 of whom had SSc. We identified 21,009,551 parent–child relationships and 17,168,340 full sibling pairs. The familial risks of SSc and other autoimmune diseases and familial transmission were estimated.

Results: The prevalence of SSc in the general population was 0.008 %. There are 3801 individuals had at least one first-degree relative with SSc, among them 3 people had SSc which was equivalent to a prevalence of 0.08 %. The adjusted relative risk (RR) (95 % CI) for SSc was 81.21 (11.40–579.72) for siblings of SSc patients. The familial transmission (genetic plus shared environmental contribution to total phenotypic variance of SSc) was 0.72. However, 84.1 % of patients were expected to be sporadic cases. The RR (95 % CI) in first-degree relatives of SSc patients was 2.64 (1.46–4.75) for rheumatoid arthritis, 6.51 (4.05–10.46) for systemic lupus erythematosus, 2.77 (1.04–7.35) for Sjögren's syndrome, 8.05 (2.03–31.92) for idiopathic inflammatory myositis, and 1.52 (1.15–2.01) for psoriasis.

Conclusions: The risks of SSc and other autoimmune diseases are increased in relatives of people with SSc, and family factors explain over two-thirds of the phenotypic variance of the disease. These findings may be useful in counselling families of patients with SSc and for further genetic studies.

Keyword: Systemic sclerosis, Familial aggregation, Familial transmission, Rheumatic diseases, Relative risk

Background

Systemic sclerosis (SSc) is an uncommon autoimmune disease characterized by the thickening of the skin and involvement of internal organs including blood vessels, heart, lung, kidney, and gastrointestinal tract. The prevalence and incidence of SSc are difficult to estimate because of its rarity and the difficulty to ascertain diagnosis. In the United States, the prevalence has been estimated at 24.2 cases per 100,000 adults [1]. In Taiwan, our group recently estimated the prevalence of SSc to be 5.6 per 100,000 people using the National Health Insurance (NHI) database, which contains health information of almost all the inhabitants in Taiwan [2, 3]. The outcome of SSc is generally thought to be poor, with a higher mortality and an increased risk for other severe comorbidity such as cancer [2–4].

SSc is thought to be a polygenic disorder which is contributed to by both genetic and environmental factors [5]. Evidence for familial aggregation has rarely been reported but indicates a possible familial or genetic contribution for SSc [6, 7]. The discovery of candidate genes located in both major histocompatibility complex (MHC) and non-MHC loci [8] has strengthened this concept; however, the relative contribution of genetic and shared environmental factors to SSc susceptibility (familial transmission) has not been adequately estimated. In addition, the precise estimates for familial relative risks (RRs) for the disease and other associated autoimmune diseases which are important parameters for genetic counselling have not been reported despite

* Correspondence: weiya.zhang@nottingham.ac.uk
[1]Division of Rheumatology, Orthopaedics and Dermatology, School of Medicine, University of Nottingham, NG51PDAcademic Rheumatology, Clinical Sciences Building, City Hospital, Nottingham NG51PB, Nottingham, UK
Full list of author information is available at the end of the article

evidence for familial aggregation of Raynaud's syndrome and an increased risk of SSc in individuals with a family history of systemic lupus erythematosus (SLE) [9, 10] and Sjögren's syndrome [11].

Therefore, we conducted this nationwide study using genealogy and linked health information derived from the NHI database comprising essentially the entire population of Taiwan in 2010 to determine familial aggregation of SSc and to assess the relative contribution of familial factors to susceptibility for the disease. In addition, we also investigated the co-aggregation of other autoimmune diseases with SSc.

Methods

Study population

This study was based on a cohort comprising all beneficiaries of the Taiwan National Health Insurance (NHI) system actively enrolled in 2010, which was constructed using data from the registry for beneficiaries, registry for catastrophic illness patients, and datasets of ambulatory care expenditures and details of ambulatory case orders, all of which are part of the NHI database. The enrolment in the NHI system is mandatory by law for all citizens and foreigners living longer than 6 months in Taiwan and this is a single payer system managed by the government. In 2010, over 99.5 % of the general population in Taiwan was insured by the system [12]. The NHI database is updated annually and records information on personal details, socioeconomic status, family relationships, dates of clinical visits, medical diagnoses, medical expenditures, prescription details, examinations, and procedures. All beneficiaries are given a unique identification which allows precise internal linkage of all data for a given individual. This identification was encrypted before being released for research to ensure confidentiality but the uniqueness of the encrypted identification is retained to ensure valid internal linkage.

Methods of identification of first-degree relatives and family ascertainment have been reported previously [10, 11]. The relationships recorded in the NHI database include spouse, parent, offspring, and grandparents, grandchildren, great grandparent, and great grandchildren on both paternal and maternal sides. The identification of siblings was based on sharing one or more common parents. In this study, half-siblings were excluded from the analysis. Twins were full siblings with the same date of birth (±1 day) but twin zygosity cannot be derived from the database. To consider the correlation among subjects from the same family, we grouped individuals into families according to their relationships. In total, 21,009,551 parent–child relationships, 17,168,340 full sibling pairs and 342,066 twin pairs were identified and these relationships were used to assemble 4,229,301 families with a mean family size of five persons spanning up to five generations.

Case definition of SSc and other autoimmune diseases

The case definition for SSc was a person with a catastrophic illness certificate for SSc (International Classification of Diseases, Ninth Revision (ICD-9) code 7101). The holders of a catastrophic illness certificate are entitled to a waiver of medical co-payments, which must be supported by comprehensive clinical and laboratory assessment. Relevant information is sent to the insurance administration for a formal review to confirm the diagnosis before approval of waivers. The panel reviews the diagnosis in compliance with the updated classification criteria. We also identified patients with other autoimmune diseases including rheumatoid arthritis, SLE, Sjögren's syndrome, idiopathic inflammatory myositis, type I diabetes mellitus, and multiple sclerosis using the catastrophic illness registry. The case definition of psoriasis was based on two recordings of rheumatologist or dermatologist diagnosis.

Statistical analysis

The prevalence of SSc was calculated for individuals with affected first-degree relatives and for the general population. Any individual with a valid insurance registration in 2010 who met the case definition of SSc between 1 January 1996 and 31 December 2010 was defined as a prevalent case. The number of individuals in the 2010 general population in Taiwan was used as the denominator for the prevalence of SSc. The recurrence risk for SSc was defined as the likelihood of having a diagnosis of SSc in an individual with affected first-degree relatives with a diagnosis of SSc. We calculated recurrence risk for a specific type of relative (sibling and offspring) of patients with SSc as the prevalence of SSc in individuals with a specific type of affected relative [13]. The adjusted prevalence ratio was used as a measure for relative risk (RR) for SSc [14], and was calculated as the prevalence of SSc among individuals with affected relatives divided by the prevalence of SSc in the general population. The RR estimated in this study is equivalent to the relative recurrence ratio (RRR) but for simplicity we refer it as RR throughout. The marginal Cox proportional hazard model with an equal follow-up time for all subjects was used to estimate the RR and the 95 % confidence interval (CI) [15]. We used the robust sandwich estimator to calculate corrected CIs to account for possible case clustering within the family [16]. This approach has been applied and validated previously in other diseases [17]. Covariates included age, gender, socioeconomic factors (place of residence, occupation, and income levels), and family size. A place of residence for each individual was categorised according to the level of urbanisation [18]. Occupations were classified into five categories and income levels were categorised into sex-specific income quintiles.

Heritability was defined as the proportion of phenotypic variance that is attributable to genetic factors, and familial transmission as the sum of heritability and the proportion attributable to shared environmental factors; both can be calculated using the polygenic liability model [19–21]. The familial transmission in this study was estimated as the function of the difference of normal deviation of the threshold from the mean liability between individuals with affected siblings and the normal population. The original model assumes zero common environmental variance and, therefore, familial transmission equals heritability. However, we consider this assumption not applicable in the case of SSc considering known environmental factors that may predispose to the disease and be shared among family members. In our previous paper, we further used spouses as a control to separate the shared environmental component and heritability [11]. As SSc is predominantly a female disease and its prevalence is low, it was not possible to identify enough affected spouse pairs to produce reliable estimates. Therefore, we only reported familial transmission. Next, we calculated the probability of a patient with SSc without a family history according to the formula based on a polygenic liability model developed by Yang et al. [22].

We further estimated the extent of familial co-aggregation of other autoimmune diseases in affected families. RRs and 95 % CIs for rheumatoid arthritis, SLE, Sjögren's syndrome, idiopathic inflammatory myositis, type I diabetes mellitus, multiple sclerosis, and psoriasis were estimated as the adjusted prevalence ratio of specified autoimmune diseases between individuals with a first-degree relative with SSc and the general population. We estimated the RR for other autoimmune diseases by a marginal Cox proportional hazards regression model with an equal follow-up time for all subjects. The RRs were adjusted for age, sex, and family size, and considered case clustering within families by using the robust sandwich estimate.

A two-sided p value ≤0.05 was considered statistically significant. All analyses were performed using SAS v.9.3 (SAS institute, Cary, NC, USA).

Results

Among 23,658,577 individuals enrolled in the NHI database in Taiwan in 2010, there were 1891 individuals (1495 women; 396 men) with SSc, equivalent to a prevalence of 0.008 % (women, 0.013 %; men, 0.003 %). In the general population of Taiwan in 2010, 3801 individuals had at least one first-degree relative with SSc. The baseline characteristics were shown in Table 1. Among people with a family history of SSc, three people had SSc which was equivalent to a prevalence of 0.08 %. Overall, having an affected first-degree relative with SSc was associated with an adjusted RR (95 % CI) of 13.23 (3.11–56.33) for the disease. For risks for specific kinship, RRs were 81.22 (11.40–578.72) for siblings and 9.17 (1.30–65.86) for offspring of patients with SSc. Using a polygenic liability model, we estimated that the familial transmission for SSc was 0.72. We estimated that 84.1 % of patients with SSc were expected to be sporadic cases.

Table 1 Baseline characteristics of individuals with affected relatives with systemic sclerosis and the general population

Variables	≥1 Affected relatives	General population	*P* value
No.	3801	23,658,577	
Male gender (*n* (%))	2037 (53.59)	11,732,064 (49.59)	<0.001
Age (years) (mean ± SD)	46.6 ± 16.2	37.5 ± 20.4	<0.001
Systemic sclerosis (*n* (%))	3 (0.08)	1891 (0.008)	<0.001
Place of residence (*n* (%))			
Urban	2421 (63.69)	13,935,055 (58.90)	<0.001
Suburban	991 (26.07)	6,581,657 (27.82)	
Rural	267 (7.02)	2,186,647 (9.24)	
Unknown	122 (3.21)	955,218 (4.04)	
Income levels (*n* (%))			
Quintile 1	594 (15.63)	4,077,139 (17.23)	<0.001
Quintile 2	529 (13.92)	3,334,917 (14.10)	
Quintile 3	881 (23.18)	6,296,926 (26.62)	
Quintile 4	830 (21.84)	4,547,059 (19.22)	
Quintile 5	847 (22.28)	4,437,878 (18.76)	
Unknown	120 (3.16)	964,658 (4.08)	
Occupation (*n* (%))			
Dependents of the insured individuals	1185 (31.18)	9,209,334 (38.93)	<0.001
Civil servants, teachers, military personnel and veterans	195 (5.13)	984,451 (4.16)	
Non-manual workers and professionals	1426 (3752)	6,357,208 (26.87)	
Manual workers	631 (16.60)	4,885,084 (20.65)	
Other	364 (9.58)	2,222,500 (9.39)	

Table 2 presents adjusted RR (95 % CIs) for other autoimmune diseases in individuals with affected first-degree relatives compared to the general population. The RR (95 % CI) in first-degree relatives of SSc patients was 2.64 (1.46–4.75) for rheumatoid arthritis, 6.51 (4.05–10.46) for SLE, 2.77 (1.04–7.35) for Sjögren's syndrome, 8.05 (2.03–31.92) for idiopathic inflammatory myositis, and 1.52 (1.15–2.01) for psoriasis.

Discussion

This study investigated the risk of SSc in individuals with affected first-degree relatives and estimated the familial transmission of SSc in a general population. We

Table 2 Relative risks of systemic sclerosis and other autoimmune diseases for individuals with affected first-degree relatives

Autoimmune diseases	With affected relatives		General population		Relative risk (95 % CI)[a]
	No. of cases	Prevalence (%)	No. of cases	Prevalence (%)	
Systemic sclerosis	3	0.08	1891	0.008	13.23 (3.11–56.33)
Rheumatoid arthritis	11	0.29	37,482	0.16	2.64 (1.46–4.75)
Systemic lupus erythematosus	20	0.53	18,915	0.08	6.51 (4.05–10.46)
Sjögren's syndrome	4	0.11	12,754	0.05	2.77 (1.04–7.35)
Idiopathic inflammatory myositis	2	0.05	1808	0.01	8.05 (2.03–31.92)
Type I diabetes mellitus	5	0.13	10,281	0.04	2.51 (0.90–7.07)
Multiple sclerosis	1	0.03	1252	0.01	5.16 (0.73–3665)
Psoriasis	47	1.24	196,333	0.83	1.52 (1.15–2.01)

[a] Adjusted for age, gender, place of residence, quintiles of income levels, occupations, and family size

found that the prevalence of SSc in relatives of patients with the disease is significantly higher than the general population and that the familial transmission of SSc was 0.72. Despite this, most cases of SSc are expected to be sporadic under the polygenic liability model. Furthermore, individuals with an affected first-degree relative with the disease also have a higher prevalence of other autoimmune diseases. These estimates are valuable for clinical counselling, and also for the preparation of future genetic studies to determine candidate susceptibility genes.

Formal evidence for familial aggregation and the magnitude of any familial or genetic contribution for SSc is rarely reported [6, 7, 23]. Englert et al. identified 710 Australian families with SSc and reported a prevalence of 1.4 % and a RR of 11 in people with affected family members [6]. Another study from the US reported a risk of 1.6 % in those with an affected first-degree relative and the RR was 13 [7]. The risk of SSc in an individual with an affected first-degree relative was estimated to be 1.1 %, which was 3.5-fold higher than the controls [23]. Another Canadian study reported that 2.8 % of individuals with a positive family history of SSc had the disease [24]. These studies in general indicate a high familial absolute and relative risk for SSc. However, the estimates vary over a wide range, probably due to variable study design, case ascertainment, and family member recruitment.

Estimates from both studies are similar to our study and indicate a high familiarity of SSc. Concordance of SSc in twins has been reported previously [25, 26]. In addition, monozygotic twins discordant for SSc were found to have a similar fibroblast gene expression pattern, suggesting a strong genetic predisposition to SSc at the molecular level in skin fibroblasts [27]. Interestingly, a small twin study comprising 24 monozygotic and 18 dizygotic twin pairs found a similar concordance rate for SSc between monozygotic (4.2 %) and dizygotic twin pairs (5.6 %). However, the concordance for a positive test for antinuclear antibody was very high (90 % in monozygotic and 40 % in dizygotic twins) [28]. In addition to twins, two reports have indicated familial forms of both diffuse cutaneous SSc [29, 30] and limited cutaneous SSc [31]. A positive family history of SSc is thought to represent the largest risk factor for this disease with a familial RR of 15 [7]. Using the Utah Population Database, the familial RR for SSc was approximately 2 to 3 in first- to third-degree relatives, but there is no apparent association between the magnitude of RR and genetic relatedness [32]. Heritability of SSc has not been assessed before; however, a twin study comprising 702 monozygotic and 727 dizygotic twin pairs reported a significant heritability (0.53) for Raynaud's phenomenon [33].

Our study provides several lines of evidence supporting the importance of familial factors, including both genes and environment, in the susceptibility of SSc. Firstly, the prevalence of SSc was significantly higher in first-degree relatives of SSc patients than in the general population, in addition to a high familial RR. Secondly, using the polygenic liability model, we estimated that 72 % of phenotypic variance can be explained by familial factors (familial transmission). Despite this apparent familial factor in the susceptibility of SSc, most patients are expected to be sporadic rather than familial under the polygenic liability model as with many common complex diseases [11, 22]. For example, 78–84 % of patients with rheumatoid arthritis, SLE [22], and Sjögren's syndrome [11] are expected to be sporadic cases depending on the parameters used [22].

In addition to SSc, other autoimmune diseases are more common in family members of patients with the disease, which suggest that some autoimmune diseases share part of the pathogenesis of SSc. Previous studies have documented that autoimmune diseases often co-aggregate within families. Several studies also found an increased risk of other autoimmune disease in family members of SSc patients [9–11, 23, 24, 34, 35]. A relatively large study investigating 4612 first-degree relatives of 1071 SSc probands found that the most prevalent autoimmune diseases among first-degree relatives of SSc patients were hypothyroidism, rheumatoid arthritis, hyperthyroidism, and SLE [34]. Collectively, our results provide useful information when counselling patients and their family members in which circumstances and details of genetic parameters related to SSc should be given and explained in full. An unselective screening for SSc and other autoimmune diseases in all asymptomatic family members of patients with SSc is not recommended given a low absolute risk of these conditions. On the contrary, a positive family history is an important hint for those suspected of having an autoimmune disease. However, further study should be undertaken to test the utility of family history as a tool to identify at-risk individuals.

Limitations and strengths

There are limitations to the present study. Firstly, the classification of cases was based on the diagnosis recorded in the registry of patients with catastrophic illnesses or based on records in primary care. Nevertheless, issuance of a catastrophic illness certificate requires strong medical evidence for a diagnosis of SSc that is agreed by an expert panel, and applications for these certificates are submitted almost exclusively by rheumatologists. Therefore, any misclassification is unlikely to affect our conclusions. However, some patients with milder disease may not have applied for the certificate and this might affect our results. Secondly, we are not able to differentiate different forms of SSc. Thirdly, our model cannot effectively separate contributions from genetic and shared environmental factors. Finally, whether these results apply to different populations and settings outside of Taiwan requires further study.

Conclusions

This nationwide study confirms that, in Taiwan, SSc clusters within families and familial factors contribute to a large proportion of the susceptibility to the disease. Relatives of patients with SSc tend to have an increased risk of other autoimmune diseases. These findings may also be useful in counselling families with patients with SSc.

Abbreviations

CI: Confidence interval; MHC: Major histocompatibility complex; NHI: National Health Insurance; RR: Relative risk; SLE: Systemic lupus erythematosus; SSc: Systemic sclerosis

Acknowledgements

This study is based in part on National Health Insurance Research database data provided by the National Health Insurance Administration, Ministry of Health and Welfare, and managed by the National Health Research Institute. The interpretation and conclusions contained herein do not represent positions of the National Health Insurance Administration or the National Health Research Institute.

Funding

The authors thank the Ministry of Science and Technology of Taiwan (project 103-2314-B-182A-070-MY2, 104-2314-B-182A-047) and Chang Gung Memorial Hospital (project CORP3E0141, CMRPG3F0841) for their financial support of this research.

Authors' contributions

CFK had full access to all of the data in the study and takes responsibility for the integrity of the data and the accuracy of the data analysis. CFK, WZ, and MD conceived and designed the study. CFK, SFL, and KHY obtained the funding and acquired the data. CFK, LCS, and WZ performed and supervised the statistical analysis. CFK, LCS, WZ, and MD analysed and interpreted the data. CFK and WZ drafted the manuscript. All authors contributed to the critical revision of the manuscript for important intellectual content. WZ and MD supervised the study. All authors read and approved the manuscript.

Competing interests

The authors declare that they have no competing interests.

Author details

[1]Division of Rheumatology, Orthopaedics and Dermatology, School of Medicine, University of Nottingham, NG51PDAcademic Rheumatology, Clinical Sciences Building, City Hospital, Nottingham NG51PB, Nottingham, UK. [2]Division of Rheumatology, Allergy and Immunology, Chang Gung Memorial Hospital, Taoyuan, Taiwan. [3]Department of Public Health, College of Medicine and Biostatistics Core Laboratory, Molecular Medicine Research Centre, Chang Gung University, Taoyuan, Taiwan.

References

1. Mayes MD, Lacey Jr JV, Beebe-Dimmer J, Gillespie BW, Cooper B, Laing TJ, Schottenfeld D. Prevalence, incidence, survival, and disease characteristics of systemic sclerosis in a large US population. Arthritis Rheum. 2003;48(8):2246–55.
2. Yu KH, See LC, Kuo CF, Chou IJ, Chou MJ. Prevalence and incidence in patients with autoimmune rheumatic diseases: a nationwide population-based study in Taiwan. Arthritis Care Res (Hoboken). 2013;65(2):244–50.
3. Kuo CF, See LC, Yu KH, Chou IJ, Tseng WY, Chang HC, Shen YM, Luo SF. Epidemiology and mortality of systemic sclerosis: a nationwide population study in Taiwan. Scand J Rheumatol. 2011;40(5):373–8.
4. Kuo CF, Luo SF, Yu KH, Chou IJ, Tseng WY, Chang HC, Fang YF, Chiou MJ, See LC. Cancer risk among patients with systemic sclerosis: a nationwide population study in Taiwan. Scand J Rheumatol. 2012;41(1):44–9.
5. Agarwal SK, Tan FK, Arnett FC. Genetics and genomic studies in scleroderma (systemic sclerosis). Rheum Dis Clin North Am. 2008;34(1):17–40. v.
6. Englert H, Small-McMahon J, Chambers P, O'Connor H, Davis K, Manolios N, White R, Dracos G, Brooks P. Familial risk estimation in systemic sclerosis. Aust N Z J Med. 1999;29(1):36–41.
7. Arnett FC, Cho M, Chatterjee S, Aguilar MB, Reveille JD, Mayes MD. Familial occurrence frequencies and relative risks for systemic sclerosis (scleroderma) in three United States cohorts. Arthritis Rheum. 2001;44(6):1359–62.
8. Mayes MD. The genetics of scleroderma: looking into the postgenomic era. Curr Opin Rheumatol. 2012;24(6):677–84.
9. Alarcon-Segovia D, Alarcon-Riquelme ME, Cardiel MH, Caeiro F, Massardo L, Villa AR, Pons-Estel BA, Grupo Latinoamericano de Estudio del Lupus E. Familial aggregation of systemic lupus erythematosus, rheumatoid arthritis, and other autoimmune diseases in 1,177 lupus patients from the GLADEL cohort. Arthritis Rheum. 2005;52(4):1138–47.
10. Kuo CF, Grainge MJ, Zhang W, Doherty M. Global epidemiology of gout: prevalence, incidence and risk factors. Nat Rev Rheumatol. 2015;11(11):649–62.
11. Kuo CF, Grainge MJ, Valdes AM, See LC, Luo SF, Yu KH, Zhang W, Doherty M. Familial risk of Sjogren's syndrome and co-aggregation of

autoimmune diseases in affected families: a nationwide population study. Arthritis Rheumatol. 2015;67(7):1904–12.

12. The National Health Insurance Statistics, 2010. http://www.nhi.gov.tw/English/webdata/webdata.aspx?menu=11&menu_id=296&webdata_id=1942&WD_ID=296. Accessed 5 Sept 2016.
13. Risch N. Linkage strategies for genetically complex traits. I. Multilocus models. Am J Hum Genet. 1990;46(2):222–8.
14. Chou CT, Pei L, Chang DM, Lee CF, Schumacher HR, Liang MH. Prevalence of rheumatic diseases in Taiwan: a population study of urban, suburban, rural differences. J Rheumatol. 1994;21(2):302–6.
15. Lee J, Chia KS. Estimation of prevalence rate ratios for cross sectional data: an example in occupational epidemiology. Br J Ind Med. 1993;50(9):861–2.
16. Lin DY. Cox regression analysis of multivariate failure time data: the marginal approach. Stat Med. 1994;13(21):2233–47.
17. Lichtenstein P, Yip BH, Bjork C, Pawitan Y, Cannon TD, Sullivan PF, Hultman CM. Common genetic determinants of schizophrenia and bipolar disorder in Swedish families: a population-based study. Lancet. 2009;373(9659):234–9.
18. Liu CYHY, Chuang YL, Chen YJ, Weng WS, Liu JS, Liang KY. Incorporating development stratification of Taiwan townships into sampling design of large scale health interview survey. J Health Manag. 2006;14:1–22.
19. Falconer DS. The inheritance of liability to diseases with variable age of onset, with particular reference to diabetes mellitus. Ann Hum Genet. 1967;31(1):1–20.
20. Reich T, James JW, Morris CA. The use of multiple thresholds in determining the mode of transmission of semi-continuous traits. Ann Hum Genet. 1972;36(2):163–84.
21. Reich T, Rice J, Cloninger CR, Wette R, James J. The use of multiple thresholds and segregation analysis in analyzing the phenotypic heterogeneity of multifactorial traits. Ann Hum Genet. 1979;42(3):371–90.
22. Yang J, Visscher PM, Wray NR. Sporadic cases are the norm for complex disease. Eur J Hum Genet. 2010;18(9):1039–43.
23. Koumakis E, Dieude P, Avouac J, Kahan A, Allanore Y, Association des Sclerodermiques de F. Familial autoimmunity in systemic sclerosis—results of a French-based case-control family study. J Rheumatol. 2012;39(3):532–8.
24. Hudson M, Rojas-Villarraga A, Coral-Alvarado P, Lopez-Guzman S, Mantilla RD, Chalem P, Canadian Scleroderma Research G, Colombian Scleroderma Research G, Baron M, Anaya JM. Polyautoimmunity and familial autoimmunity in systemic sclerosis. J Autoimmun. 2008;31(2):156–9.
25. Cook NJ, Silman AJ, Propert J, Cawley MI. Features of systemic sclerosis (scleroderma) in an identical twin pair. Br J Rheumatol. 1993;32(10):926–8.
26. De Keyser F, Peene I, Joos R, Naeyaert JM, Messiaen L, Veys EM. Occurrence of scleroderma in monozygotic twins. J Rheumatol. 2000;27(9):2267–9.
27. Zhou X, Tan FK, Xiong M, Arnett FC, Feghali-Bostwick CA. Monozygotic twins clinically discordant for scleroderma show concordance for fibroblast gene expression profiles. Arthritis Rheum. 2005;52(10):3305–14.
28. Feghali-Bostwick C, Medsger Jr TA, Wright TM. Analysis of systemic sclerosis in twins reveals low concordance for disease and high concordance for the presence of antinuclear antibodies. Arthritis Rheum. 2003;48(7):1956–63.
29. Soppi E, Lehtonen A, Toivanen A. Familial progressive systemic sclerosis (scleroderma): immunological analysis of two patients and six siblings from a single kindred. Clin Exp Immunol. 1982;50(2):275–82.
30. Greger RE, Greger RE. Familial progressive systemic scleroderma. Arch Dermatol. 1975;111(1):81–5.
31. Frayha RA, Tabbara KF, Geha RS. Familial CRST syndrome with sicca complex. J Rheumatol. 1977;4(1):53–8.
32. Frech T, Khanna D, Markewitz B, Mineau G, Pimentel R, Sawitzke A. Heritability of vasculopathy, autoimmune disease, and fibrosis in systemic sclerosis: a population-based study. Arthritis Rheum. 2010;62(7):2109–16.
33. Cherkas LF, Williams FM, Carter L, Howell K, Black CM, Spector TD, MacGregor AJ. Heritability of Raynaud's phenomenon and vascular responsiveness to cold: a study of adult female twins. Arthritis Rheum. 2007;57(3):524–8.
34. Arora-Singh RK, Assassi S, del Junco DJ, Arnett FC, Perry M, Irfan U, Sharif R, Mattar T, Mayes MD. Autoimmune diseases and autoantibodies in the first degree relatives of patients with systemic sclerosis. J Autoimmun. 2010;35(1):52–7.
35. Horimoto AM, Silveira AF, da Costa IP. Familial autoimmunity and polyautoimmunity in 60 Brazilian Midwest patients with systemic sclerosis. Rev Bras Reumatol Engl Ed. 2016;56(4):314–22.

Bosentan and macitentan prevent the endothelial-to-mesenchymal transition (EndoMT) in systemic sclerosis

Claudio Corallo[1*], Maurizio Cutolo[2], Bashar Kahaleh[3], Gianluca Pecetti[4], Antonio Montella[1], Chiara Chirico[1], Stefano Soldano[2], Ranuccio Nuti[1] and Nicola Giordano[1]

Abstract

Background: Systemic sclerosis (SSc) is characterized by early vascular abnormalities and subsequent fibroblast activation to myofibroblasts, leading to fibrosis. Recently, endothelial-to-mesenchymal transition (EndoMT), a complex biological process in which endothelial cells lose their specific markers and acquire a mesenchymal or myofibroblastic phenotype, has been reported in SSc. In the present study, we evaluated the ability of endothelin-1 (ET-1) dual receptor antagonists bosentan (BOS) and macitentan (MAC) to antagonize EndoMT in vitro.

Methods: Ten women with limited SSc were enrolled. They underwent double skin biopsy (affected and nonaffected skin). Fibroblasts and microvascular endothelial cells (MVECs) were isolated from biopsies. We performed mono- or coculture of MVECs (isolated from nonaffected skin) with fibroblasts (isolated from affected skin and stimulated with ET-1 and transforming growth factor beta [TGF-β]). In cocultures, the MVEC layer was left undisturbed or was preincubated with BOS or MAC. After 48 h of coculture, MVECs were analyzed for their tube formation ability and for messenger RNA and protein expression of different vascular (CD31, vascular endothelial growth factor-A [VEGF-A], VEGF-A165b) and profibrotic (alpha-smooth muscle actin [α-SMA], collagen type I [Col I], TGF-β) molecules.

Results: After 48 h, MVECs showed a reduced tube formation ability when cocultured with SSc fibroblasts. CD31 and VEGF-A resulted in downregulation, while VEGF-A165b, the antiangiogenic isoform, resulted in upregulation. At the same time, mesenchymal markers α-SMA, Col I, and TGF-β resulted in overexpression in MVECs. Tube formation ability was restored when MVECs were preincubated with BOS or MAC, also reducing the expression of mesenchymal markers and restoring CD31 expression and the imbalance between VEGF-A and VEGF-A165b.

Conclusions: With this innovative EndoMT in vitro model realized by coculturing nonaffected MVECs with affected SSc fibroblasts, we show that the presence of a myofibroblast phenotype in the fibroblast layer, coupled with an ET-1-TGF-β synergic effect, is responsible for EndoMT. BOS and MAC seem able to antagonize this phenomenon in vitro, confirming previous evidence of endothelium-derived fibrosis in SSc and possible pharmacological interference.

Keywords: Systemic sclerosis, EndoMT, Microvascular endothelial cells, Bosentan, Macitentan

* Correspondence: corallo.claudio@gmail.com
[1]Scleroderma Unit, Department of Medicine, Surgery and Neurosciences, University of Siena, 53100 Siena, Italy
Full list of author information is available at the end of the article

Background

Systemic sclerosis (SSc) is an autoimmune connective tissue disease characterized by cutaneous and visceral fibrosis coupled with widespread vascular pathology [1]. The first sign occurring in 90–98 % of patients with SSc is Raynaud's phenomenon, an abnormal reactivity of digital microvasculature under cold and other stimuli [2, 3], which highlights the central role of microvascular damage in the pathogenesis of SSc [4]. In SSc, imbalance of endothelial signals, such as increased release of vasoconstrictory endothelin 1 (ET-1), thromboxane, and thrombomodulin, and reduction of prostaglandin I_2 and nitric oxide are signs of the endothelial injury [5]. Although different molecules have been identified as key effectors of vascular remodeling in SSc, such as ET-1 and transforming growth factor beta (TGF-β), the mechanisms underlying SSc vasculopathy remain poorly understood [6]. There are two important issues: how the vascular damage can lead to the fibrotic process and the relationship between vessel disappearance and myofibroblast activation [7]. In fact, myofibroblasts in fibrotic tissues are derived from at least three sources: expansion and activation of resident tissue fibroblasts, transition of epithelial cells into mesenchymal cells (epithelial-to-mesenchymal transition [EMT]), and tissue migration of bone marrow-derived circulating fibrocytes [8]. Recently, endothelial-to-mesenchymal transition (EndoMT), a newly recognized type of cellular transdifferentiation, has emerged as another possible source of tissue myofibroblasts [9]. EndoMT is a complex biological process in which endothelial cells lose their specific markers and acquire a mesenchymal or myofibroblastic phenotype and express mesenchymal cell products such as alpha smooth muscle actin (α-SMA) and collagen type I (Col I) [8, 9]. Despite evidence suggesting that EndoMT is involved in not only pathological [10–12] but also physiological conditions [13], the underlying molecular mechanisms involved in this process are largely unknown. Similarly to EMT, EndoMT can be induced by TGF-β [14]. Of note, the same molecule is considered, together with ET-1, to be a pivotal player in the developmental of SSc fibrosis [15]. It is well documented that the activation of TGF-β intracellular transcription factors is responsible of the production of other fibrotic molecules, such as ET-1 [16]. Moreover, TGF-β-induced ET-1 release has been associated with the fibrotic response of skin and lung SSc fibroblasts [17]. In the present study, we established an in vitro model of EndoMT made up of fibroblast and microvascular endothelial cell (MVEC) cocultures. Considering the synergistic action of ET-1 and TGF-β to induce EndoMT, we investigated the potential of ET-1 dual receptor antagonists bosentan (BOS) and macitentan (MAC) to antagonize EndoMT in our in vitro coculture model.

Methods

Patient enrollment, skin biopsy, and cell isolation

Patients

We enrolled ten women (age 55.7 ± 12.3 years, disease duration 8.3 ± 1.8 years) affected by limited SSc (lSSc) in accordance with the description of LeRoy and colleagues [18] and who fulfilled the 2013 American College of Rheumatology/European League Against Rheumatism diagnostic criteria for SSc [19]. Table 1 shows the major demographic and clinical characteristics of these patients. We performed skin biopsies by using a 3-mm punch on affected skin graded as 2 according to modified Rodnan skin score (mRSS) [20]. Unaffected areas of midforearm skin from the same patients with lSSc were also taken. The unaffected skin of patients with lSSc was defined by clinical palpation (graded as 0 according to mRSS) and by histological examination that excluded SSc-related lesions.

Table 1 Clinical parameters of patients with limited systemic sclerosis

Patient	Age (years)	Sex	Disease duration (years)	Digital ulcers	PAH	mRSS/score at affected skin biopsy	ANA-ENA
1	64	F	8	no	no	10/2	Anticentromere-CenpB
2	35	F	9	no	no	09/2	Anticentromere-CenpB
3	72	F	11	yes	yes	13/2	Anticentromere-CenpB
4	49	F	7	no	no	10/2	Anticentromere-CenpB
5	37	F	5	no	no	10/2	Anticentromere-CenpB
6	52	F	10	no	no	11/2	Anticentromere-CenpB
7	59	F	8	yes	yes	13/2	Anticentromere-CenpB
8	66	F	9	no	no	09/2	Anticentromere-CenpB
9	58	F	6	no	no	10/2	Anticentromere-CenpB
10	65	F	10	no	no	10/2	Anticentromere-CenpB
Mean (SD)	55.7 (12.3)		8.3 (1.8)				

Abbreviations: *ANA* Antinuclear antibodies, *ENA* Extractable nuclear antigens, *CenpB* Centromere protein B, *mRSS* Modified Rodnan skin score, *PAH* Pulmonary arterial hypertension

Patients discontinued corticosteroids, oral vasodilators, intravenous prostanoids, and other disease-modifying drugs at least 1 month before skin biopsies

Fibroblast isolation and cultures

Fibroblasts were isolated from skin specimens by enzymatic digestion. Briefly, explants were de-epidermized using a dispase solution (dispase activity 14 U/ml; Sigma-Aldrich, St. Louis, MO, USA) for 2 h at 37 °C and then were dissolved into a collagenase III solution (2.4 U/ml; Sigma-Aldrich) for 30 minutes. Fibroblasts obtained were passaged twice and cultured at a density of 1×10^6 cells per flask in DMEM (Sigma-Aldrich) supplemented with penicillin (100 U/ml; Sigma-Aldrich), streptomycin (100 μg/ml; Sigma-Aldrich), amphotericin B (0.25 μg/ml; Sigma-Aldrich), glutamine (2 mM; Sigma-Aldrich), and 10 % FBS (Sigma-Aldrich), followed by incubation at 37 °C in an atmosphere of 5 % CO_2 and 95 % air until confluence (1 week) in 75-cm^2 flasks (BD Costar, Cambridge, MA, USA). Viability was estimated by trypan blue staining (Sigma-Aldrich). Fibroblasts were used at third passage (P3) for cocultures.

MVEC isolation and cultures

Biopsy samples were washed with PBS (Sigma-Aldrich) and placed into a 50-ml tube (BD Costar) containing 15 ml of trypsin (Sigma-Aldrich) for digestion at 37 °C for 45 minutes. Cells were cultured in EGM-MV microvascular endothelial cell growth medium (Lonza, Walkersville, MD, USA) at 37 °C in an atmosphere of 5 % CO_2 and 95 % air. Before reaching confluence, the heterogeneous pool of cells was exposed to a cluster of differentiation 31 (CD31)-positive selection by using the DynaBeads magnetic CD31 MicroBeads cell-sorting system (Invitrogen, Carlsbad, CA, USA) following the manufacturer's instructions. After removing CD31-negative cells, only cells positive for CD31 were collected. MVECs obtained were used at P3 for mono- and cocultures.

EndoMT coculture model

In order to set up an in vitro model of EndoMT, fibroblasts isolated from affected skin biopsies and MVECs isolated from unaffected skin areas were cocultured in Transwell® 12-well plate inserts (0.4-μm pore size; Corning, Corning, NY, USA). Fibroblasts and MVECs were seeded in cocultures in a 1:3 ratio: fibroblasts in transwell inserts and MVECs in the bottom of the wells. The following cocultures of affected fibroblasts with affected MVECs (positive control) and unaffected fibroblasts with unaffected MVECs (negative control) were also performed. The fibroblast layer of the EndoMT model was incubated with 100 nM ET-1 and 5 ng/ml TGF-β for 48 h to permanently maintain the myofibroblast phenotype in culture. The MVEC layer of the EndoMT model was left undisturbed for 48 h or preincubated with 10 μM BOS or 1 μM MAC [6] 1 h before treating the fibroblast layer with ET-1 and TGF-β.

Tube formation ability of MVECs

Tube formation ability was evaluated using a Matrigel assay. Matrigel (BD Biosciences, San Jose, CA, USA) was used at 8.6 mg/ml in a 1:1 dilution with EGM2-MV (Lonza), without any supplement. MVECs were labeled, before coculture in Matrigel, with the red fluorescent dye PKH26 (Sigma-Aldrich) following the manufacturer's instructions. After 48 h of mono- or coculture with fibroblasts, MVECs tube total length in each well, calculated as cells per millimeter, were calculated by using a Zeiss AxioPlan2 fluorescence microscope equipped with AxioVision 4.6 for Windows software (Carl Zeiss Vision GmbH, Hallbergmoos, Germany). The number of branching points was calculated using MetaMorph® software for Windows (Molecular Devices, Sunnyvale, CA, USA). The number of tubes formed was quantitated by an observer blinded to the experimental groups.

Western blot analysis

Collected MVECs were centrifuged at 1500 rpm for 10 minutes at room temperature. Pellets were then suspended in PBS buffer and centrifuged at 3000 rpm for 20 minutes at 4 °C. The obtained pellets were then suspended in radioimmunoprecipitation assay buffer (Sigma-Aldrich) containing protease inhibitor cocktail (Sigma-Aldrich) for 40 minutes in ice and then centrifuged at 15000 rpm for 30 minutes at 4 °C. After centrifugation, supernatants were collected, and protein concentration was calculated according to Bradford assay [21]. About 20 μg of cell lysate proteins for each lane were resolved in a 12 % SDS-PAGE buffer according to Laemmli [22]. The bands were transferred from the gels to polyvinyl difluoride membranes using the iBlot™ Dry Blotting System (Invitrogen). The endothelial markers chosen for MVECs were rabbit polyclonal anti-CD31 (Abcam, Cambridge, UK), rabbit polyclonal anti-vascular endothelial growth factor A (anti-VEGF-A) (Abcam), and rabbit polyclonal anti-VEGF-A165b (Abcam). The mesenchymal markers chosen for MVECs were rabbit polyclonal anti-α-SMA (Abcam), rabbit polyclonal anti-Col-I (Abcam), and rabbit polyclonal anti-TGF-β (Abcam). Incubation was carried out using iBlot® Western Detection Kit (Invitrogen). The load control protein used was beta actin (Abcam). The bound primary antibodies were detected using antirabbit immunoglobulin G alkaline phosphate conjugate (Invitrogen) and visualized using a ChemiDoc™ XRS 170-870 molecular imager (Bio-Rad Laboratories, Hercules, CA, USA) and quantified by using Quantity One software (Bio-Rad Laboratories).

RNA isolation and quantitative real-time polymerase chain reaction

MVECs were collected in TRIzol reagent (Sigma-Aldrich). Total RNA was extracted following the manufacturer's instructions. The total RNA content of the samples was quantified by measuring the absorbance at 260 nm using an Ultrospec 2000 spectrophotometer (Amersham Pharmacia Biotech, Piscataway, NJ, USA). The RNA was then reverse-transcribed using a random hexamer MultiScribe enzyme (Applied Biosystems, Foster City, CA, USA). Quantitative real-time polymerase chain reactions (qRT-PCR) were run in the StepOne Real-Time PCR System (Applied Biosystems) using TaqMan chemistry (Invitrogen). Two microliters of complementary DNA in a final volume of 20 μl were amplified using the 20× Assays-on-Demand gene expression assay mix (Applied Biosystems). Specific primers were designed on the basis of the reported sequences (National Center for Biotechnology Information PrimerBank): α-SMA: 5′-CGGT GCTGTCTCTCTATGCC-3′ (forward) and 5′-CGCTCA GTCAGGATCTTCA-3′ (reverse); Col I: 5′-AGGGCCAA GACGAAGACAGT-3′ (forward) and 5′-AGATCACGTC ATCGCACAACA-3′ (reverse); TGF-β: 5′-CTAATGGTG GAAACCCACAACG-3′ (forward) and 5′-TATCGCCAG GAATTGTTGCTG-3′ (reverse); CD31: 5′-AACAGTGT TGACATGAAGAGCC-3′ (forward) and 5′-TGTAAAA-CAGCACGTCATCCTT-3′ (reverse); VEGF-A: 5′-AGGG CAGAATCATCACGAAGT-3′ (forward) and 5′-GCTGC GCTGATAGACATCCA-3′ (reverse); VEGF-A165b: 5′-G AGCAAGACAAGAAAATCCC-3′ (forward) and 5′-GTGAGAGATCTGCAAGTACG-3′ (reverse). TaqMan probes, specific primers and ribosomal 18S, selected as a housekeeping gene, were purchased from Applied Biosystems. Messenger RNA (mRNA) levels were normalized to those of 18S.

Statistical analysis

Prism 6.0® for Windows software (GraphPad Software, La Jolla, CA, USA) was used for statistical analysis. Data regarding Western blot analyses are expressed as mean ± SD of three technical replicates evaluated by analysis of variance (ANOVA) and Tukey's multiple-comparisons test. Significance was set at $p < 0.05$. Data related to the number of branching points are expressed as mean ± SD, while those related to tube formation ability and to qRT-PCR are expressed as median (range) of six biological replicates. Because the data followed a nonparametric distribution, the Mann-Whitney *U* test was thought to be appropriate for the analyses. Significance was set at $p < 0.05$.

Results

Tube formation ability of MVECs

In our in vitro EndoMT model, MVECs cocultured with affected fibroblasts (stimulated with ET-1 and TGF-β) showed a significant impairment in tube formation, probably due to the persistent stimulation of the myofibroblast phenotype (Fig. 1a). After 48 h of coculture, MVECs statistically reduced their ability to form tubular structures in untreated samples. In fact, as shown in Fig. 1b, the analysis of tube formation ratio evidenced significant improvement in tube formation when MVECs were preincubated with BOS ($p < 0.01$) and MAC ($p < 0.01$).

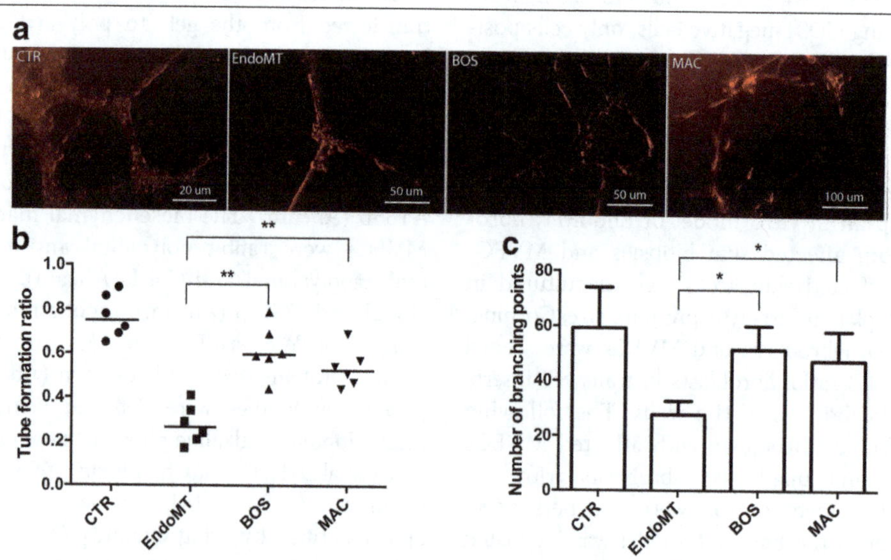

Fig. 1 **a** Tubular structure formation of microvascular endothelial cells (MVECs) in Matrigel after 48 h of culture alone (before endothelial-to-mesenchymal transition [EndoMT]) or cocultures with fibroblasts. The fluorescent *red* images show that MVECs (post-EndoMT) have a decreased tube formation ability with respect to those treated with bosentan (BOS) and macitentan (MAC), which show a well-organized tubelike network. **b** The tube formation ability was measured as cells per millimeter and is expressed as the ratio of total tube length in each culture condition to the length in the culture of untreated (CTR) MVECs. Data are expressed as median (range) of six biological replicates (*$p < 0.05$, **$p < 0.01$). **c** Number of branching points expressed as mean ± SD of six biological replicates (*$p < 0.05$)

These data were confirmed by analysis of the number of branching points (Fig. 1c) that were statistically increased when MVECs were incubated with BOS ($p < 0.05$) and MAC ($p < 0.05$).

Effect of BOS and MAC on endothelial marker expression in MVECs

As shown in Fig. 2, both BOS and MAC are able to antagonize the EndoMT process after 48 h. In particular, 1 h of preincubation with 10 μM BOS led to both protein ($p < 0.01$) and mRNA ($p < 0.01$) increases of CD31, and also of both protein ($p < 0.01$) and mRNA ($p < 0.05$) increases of VEGF-A. At the same time, the antiangiogenic VEGF-A165b protein ($p < 0.01$) but not mRNA levels statistically decreased. Conversely, 1 h of preincubation with 1 μM MAC led to both protein ($p < 0.01$) and mRNA ($p < 0.01$) increases of CD31, and also of both protein ($p < 0.01$) and mRNA ($p < 0.01$) increases of VEGF-A. VEGF-A165b protein ($p < 0.01$) and mRNA ($p < 0.05$) levels statistically decreased.

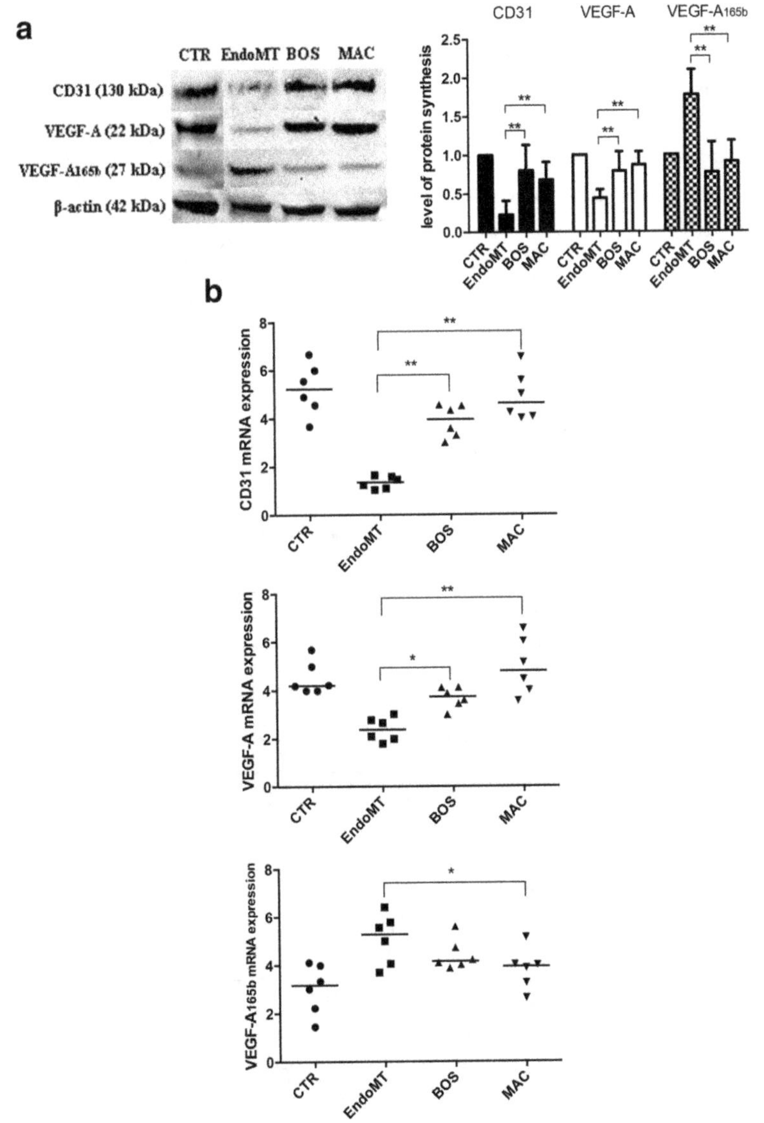

Fig. 2 a Western blot analyses (*left*) and the relative densitometric values (*right*) of cluster of differentiation 31 (CD31), vascular endothelial growth factor (VEGF)-A, and VEGF-A165b. Densitometric data are representative of three technical triplicates and are expressed as mean ± SD. The values of protein synthesis obtained for each treatment (bosentan [BOS] and macitentan [MAC]) were normalized to that of the untreated cells (CTR) taken as unit value by definition. Analysis of variance and Tukey's multiple-comparisons test were performed for each group (*$p < 0.05$, **$p < 0.01$). **b** Quantitative real-time polymerase chain reaction analyses for CD31 (*top*), VEGF-A (*middle*), and VEGF-A165b (*bottom*) confirm the results observed in Western blot analysis. The results are expressed as median (range) of six biological replicates (*$p < 0.05$, **$p < 0.01$). *mRNA* Messenger RNA; *EndoMT* Endothelial-to-mesenchymal transition

Effect of BOS and MAC on mesenchymal marker expression in MVECs

Figure 3 shows that BOS and MAC are able to antagonize the EndoMT through the expression of typical mesenchymal markers in MVECs. In particular, BOS is responsible for both protein ($p < 0.01$) and mRNA ($p < 0.05$) decreases of α-SMA, protein ($p < 0.01$) and mRNA ($p < 0.05$) decreases of Col I, and protein ($p < 0.01$) and mRNA ($p < 0.05$) decreases of TGF-β. MAC is responsible for both protein ($p < 0.05$) and mRNA ($p < 0.05$) decreases of α-SMA, protein ($p < 0.01$) and mRNA ($p < 0.01$) decreases of Col-1, and protein ($p < 0.05$) and mRNA ($p < 0.01$) decreases of TGF-β.

Discussion

The in vitro experimental model of EndoMT described in the present study provides evidence that the persistence of the myofibroblast phenotype in SSc and its mediators (ET-1 and TGF-β) are responsible for the transdifferentiation of MVECs toward the mesenchymal phenotype [23, 24]. As reported in the literature, the onset of SSc is represented mainly by vascular damage [4, 25], but

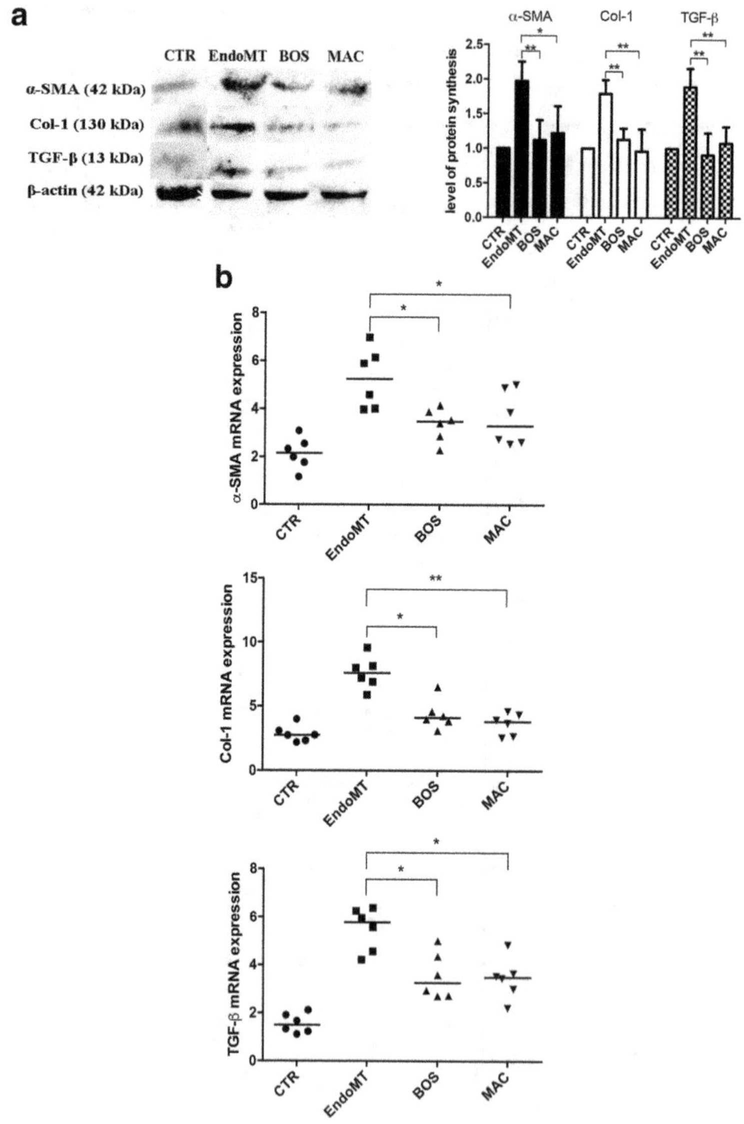

Fig. 3 a Western blot analyses (*left*) and the relative densitometric values (*right*) of alpha smooth muscle actin (α-SMA), collagen type I (Col I) and transforming growth factor beta (TGF-β). Densitometric data are representative of three technical replicates and are expressed as mean ± SD. The values of protein synthesis obtained for each treatment (bosentan [BOS] and macitentan [MAC]) were normalized to that of the untreated cells (CTR), taken as unit value by definition. Analysis of variance and Tukey's multiple-comparisons test were performed in each group (*$p < 0.05$, **$p < 0.01$). **b** Quantitative real-time polymerase chain reaction analyses for α-SMA (*top*), Col I (*middle*), and TGF-β (*bottom*) confirm results obtained by Western blot analysis. The results are expressed as median (range) of six biological replicates (*$p < 0.05$, **$p < 0.01$). *mRNA* Messenger RNA; *EndoMT* Endothelial-to-mesenchymal transition

this EndoMT in vitro model could explain the persistence of fibroblast-vascular crosstalk as a profibrotic loop-promoting condition in SSc. In fact, the recruitment of myofibroblasts in affected tissues, associated with their elevated biosynthetic functions, may be considered as pivotal determinants of the extent and progression rate of the fibrosis in SSc [26]. Using a tridimensional Matrigel model, we showed the reduction of MVECs' ability to form tubular structures when cocultured with affected fibroblasts incubated with ET-1 and TGF-β. In the same condition, it was possible to observe a switch from proangiogenic to antiangiogenic VEGF isoforms, as recently described in the literature [27, 28]. The overexpression of VEGF165b, an inhibitory splice variant of VEGF, leads to insufficient angiogenesis in patients with SSc [29]. Not only the VEGF family but also CD31, the specific endothelial marker, seems to be downregulated after 48 h of coculture during the EndoMT, a condition recently described in the literature [30, 31]. MVECs lose specific endothelial markers and increase mesenchymal profibrotic markers, such as α-SMA, Col I, and TGF-β [32]. This evidence allowed us to hypothesize that the above-mentioned profibrotic switch may be considered a normal response of MVECs in any physiological (wound healing) [33] and pathological (SSc) [34] conditions characterized by overexpression of ET-1 and TGF-β. In this setting, considering the synergistic action of ET-1 and TGF-β in triggering EndoMT [35], our study strengthens the fundamental therapeutic utility that blocking the ET-1 system, by using dual endothelin-1 receptor antagonists (ERA), could represent an important therapeutic strategy [36]. Our in vitro model demonstrates that both BOS and MAC are effective in inhibiting the ET-1/TGF-β-mediated EndoMT, supporting the hypothesis that ET-1 may represent the ultimate mediator of TGF-β actions [37, 38]. It is very important to highlight that not only MAC but also BOS is effective in EndoMT antagonism in vitro. Therefore, it could be hypothesized that the obtained results depend more on ET-1 receptor (ET_A and ET_B) blocking than on the physiochemical and pharmacokinetic properties of the ERA used, even though a functional in vitro assay demonstrated that the potency of MAC is tenfold higher than that of the parent compound BOS [39]. Translating these preclinical findings into clinical applications, we hypothesize that the therapeutic strategy of antagonizing EndoMT could contribute to counteract endothelial dysfunction in pulmonary arterial hypertension [40, 41], a frequent condition in patients with SSc [42], and to counteract the steps leading to SSc digital ulcerations [43]. In fact, the remodeling effects of ERA on microvascular damage progression in patients with SSc who have undergone long-term treatment have already been demonstrated by nailfold videocapillaroscopy and laser Doppler analysis of fingertip blood flow [44–46].

Conclusions

The present study provides further in vitro evidence of the use of ERA (BOS and MAC) in inhibiting the EndoMT process, supporting the clinical efficacy of these drugs in SSc therapy and their usefulness for interfering with progressive fibrosis.

Abbreviations

ANA: Antinuclear antibodies; ANOVA: Analysis of variance; BOS: Bosentan; CD31: Cluster of differentiation 31; CenpB: Centromere protein B; Col I: Collagen type I; EGM-MV: Microvascular endothelial cell growth medium; EMT: Epithelial-to-mesenchymal transition; ENA: Extractable nuclear antigen; EndoMT: Endothelial-to-mesenchymal transition; ERA: Dual endothelin 1 receptor antagonists; ET-1: Endothelin 1; lSSc: Limited systemic sclerosis; MAC: Macitentan; mRNA: Messenger RNA; mRSS: Modified Rodnan skin score; MVEC: Microvascular endothelial cell; P3: Third passage; PAH: Pulmonary arterial hypertension; qRT-PCR: Quantitative real-time polymerase chain reaction; SSc: Systemic sclerosis; TGF-β: Transforming growth factor beta; VEGF: Vascular endothelial growth factor; α-SMA: Alpha-smooth muscle actin

Acknowledgements

The authors thank Dr. Yongqing Wang of the University of Toledo Department of Medicine for his technical assistance.

Funding

Not applicable.

Authors' contributions

CCo conceived of and designed the study, performed the literature search, interpreted the data, created the figures, and wrote and revised the manuscript. MC conceived of and designed the study, interpreted the data, and wrote and revised the manuscript. BK conceived of and designed the study, interpreted the data, performed the literature search, and wrote and revised the manuscript. GP conceived of and designed the study, performed the literature search and statistical analysis, and revised the manuscript. AM collected and interpreted the data and revised the manuscript. CCh performed the literature search, collected and interpreted the data, and revised the manuscript. SS collected and interpreted the data, performed the statistical analysis, and revised the manuscript. RN designed the study, interpreted the data, and revised the manuscript. NG conceived of and designed the study, collected and interpreted the data, performed the literature search, and wrote and revised the manuscript. All authors read and approved the final manuscript, and all authors agree to be accountable for all aspects of the study.

Competing interests

The authors declare that they have no competing interests.

Author details

[1]Scleroderma Unit, Department of Medicine, Surgery and Neurosciences, University of Siena, 53100 Siena, Italy. [2]Research Laboratory and Academic Division of Clinical Rheumatology, Department of Internal Medicine, Institute for Research and Health Care (IRCCS), University of Genoa, San Martino, Genoa, Italy. [3]Division of Rheumatology and Immunology, College of Medicine, University of Toledo, Toledo, OH, USA. [4]Medical and Scientific Direction, Actelion Pharmaceuticals Italy, Imola, Italy.

References

1. Denton CP. Advances in pathogenesis and treatment of systemic sclerosis. Clin Med (Lond). 2016;16:55–60.
2. Cutolo M, Sulli A, Smith V. Evaluating microangiopathy in systemic sclerosis: what have we learnt and what is left to discover? Expert Rev Clin Immunol. 2011;7:395–7.
3. Allanore Y, Distler O. Systemic sclerosis in 2014: advances in cohort enrichment shape future of trial design. Nat Rev Rheumatol. 2015;11:72–4.
4. Matucci-Cerinic M, Kahaleh B, Wigley FM. Review: evidence that systemic sclerosis is a vascular disease. Arthritis Rheum. 2013;65:1953–62.
5. Herrick AL, Illingworth K, Blann A. von Willebrand factor, thrombomodulin, thromboxane, thromboglobulin and markers of fibrinolysis in primary Raynaud's phenomenon and systemic sclerosis. Ann Rheum Dis. 1996;55:122–27.
6. Cipriani P, Di Benedetto P, Ruscitti P, Capece D, Zazzeroni F, Liakouli V, et al. The endothelial-mesenchymal transition in systemic sclerosis is induced by endothelin-1 and transforming growth factor-β and may be blocked by macitentan, a dual endothelin-1 receptor antagonist. J Rheumatol. 2015;42:1808–16.
7. Cipriani P, Di Benedetto P, Ruscitti P, Campese AF, Liakouli V, Carubbi F, et al. Impaired endothelium-mesenchymal stem cells cross-talk in systemic sclerosis: a link between vascular and fibrotic features. Arthritis Res Ther. 2014;16:442.
8. Piera-Velazquez S, Li Z, Jimenez SA. Role of endothelial-mesenchymal transition (EndoMT) in the pathogenesis of fibrotic disorders. Am J Pathol. 2011;179:1074–80.
9. Piera-Velazquez S, Mendoza FA, Jimenez SA. Endothelial to mesenchymal transition (EndoMT) in the pathogenesis of human fibrotic diseases. J Clin Med. 2016;5:45.
10. Chen PY, Qin L, Baeyens N, Li G, Afolabi T, Budatha M, et al. Endothelial-to-mesenchymal transition drives atherosclerosis progression. J Clin Invest. 2015;125:4514–28.
11. Arciniegas E, Frid MG, Douglas IS, Stenmark KR. Perspectives on endothelial-to-mesenchymal transition: potential contribution to vascular remodeling in chronic pulmonary hypertension. Am J Physiol Lung Cell Mol Physiol. 2007;293:L1–8.
12. Li J, Bertram JF. Endothelial-myofibroblast transition, a new player in diabetic renal fibrosis. Nephrology (Carlton). 2010;15:507–12.
13. Fu Y, Chang A, Chang L, Niessen K, Eapen S, Setiadi A, et al. Differential regulation of transforming growth factor beta signaling pathways by Notch in human endothelial cells. J Biol Chem. 2009;284:19452–62.
14. Zeisberg EM, Potenta S, Xie L, Zeisberg M, Kalluri R. Discovery of endothelial to mesenchymal transition as a source for carcinoma-associated fibroblasts. Cancer Res. 2007;67:10123–8.
15. Lafyatis R. Transforming growth factor β—at the centre of systemic sclerosis. Nat Rev Rheumatol. 2014;10:706–19.
16. Rodríguez-Pascual F, Busnadiego O, González-Santamaría J. The profibrotic role of endothelin-1: is the door still open for the treatment of fibrotic diseases? Life Sci. 2014;118:156–64.
17. Ahmedat AS, Warnken M, Seemann WK, Mohr K, Kostenis E, Juergens UR, et al. Pro-fibrotic processes in human lung fibroblasts are driven by an autocrine/paracrine endothelinergic system. Br J Pharmacol. 2013;168:471–87.
18. Leroy EC, Black C, Fleischmajer R, Jablonska S, Krieg T, Medsger Jr TA, et al. Scleroderma (systemic sclerosis): classification, subsets and pathogenesis. J Rheumatol. 1988;15:202–5.
19. van den Hoogen F, Khanna D, Fransen J, Johnson SR, Baron M, Tyndall A, et al. 2013 classification criteria for systemic sclerosis: an American College of Rheumatology/European League against Rheumatism collaborative initiative. Arthritis Rheum. 2013;65:2737–47.
20. Clements PJ, Lachenruch PA, Nq SC, Simmons M, Sterz M, Furst DE. Skin score: a semiquantitative measure of cutaneous involvement that improves prediction of prognosis in systemic sclerosis. Arthritis Rheum. 1990;33:1256–63.
21. Bradford MM. A rapid and sensitive method for the quantitation of microgram quantities of protein utilizing the principle of protein-dye binding. Anal Biochem. 1976;72:48–254.
22. Laemmli UK. Cleavage of structural proteins during the assembly of the head of bacteriophage T4. Nature. 1970;227:680–5.
23. Frid MG, Kale VA, Stenmark KR. Mature vascular endothelium can give rise to smooth muscle cells via endothelial-mesenchymal transdifferentiation: in vitro analysis. Circ Res. 2002;90:1189–96.
24. Arciniegas E, Sutton AB, Allen TD, Schor AM. Transforming growth factor beta 1 promotes the differentiation of endothelial cells into smooth muscle-like cells in vitro. J Cell Sci. 1992;103:521–9.
25. Kahaleh B. The microvascular endothelium in scleroderma. Rheumatology (Oxford). 2008;47 Suppl 5:v14–5.
26. Jimenez SA. Role of endothelial to mesenchymal transition in the pathogenesis of the vascular alterations in systemic sclerosis. ISRN Rheumatol. 2013;2013:835948.
27. Manetti M, Guiducci S, Romano E, Bellando-Randone S, Lepri G, Bruni C, et al. Increased plasma levels of the VEGF165b splice variant are associated with the severity of nailfold capillary loss in systemic sclerosis. Ann Rheum Dis. 2013;72:1425–7.
28. Harris S, Craze M, Newton J, Fisher M, Shima DT, Tozer GM, et al. Do anti-angiogenic VEGF (VEGFxxxb) isoforms exist? A cautionary tale. PLoS One. 2012;7:e35231.
29. Manetti M, Guiducci S, Romano E, Ceccarelli C, Bellando-Randone S, Conforti ML, et al. Overexpression of VEGF165b, an inhibitory splice variant of vascular endothelial growth factor, leads to insufficient angiogenesis in patients with systemic sclerosis. Circ Res. 2011;109:e14–26.
30. Manetti M, Rosa I, Milia AF, Guiducci S, Carmeliet P, Ibba-Manneschi L, et al. Inactivation of urokinase-type plasminogen activator receptor (uPAR) gene induces dermal and pulmonary fibrosis and peripheral microvasculopathy in mice: a new model of experimental scleroderma? Ann Rheum Dis. 2014;73:1700–9.
31. Mendoza FA, Piera-Velazquez S, Farber JL, Feghali-Bostwick C, Jiménez SA. Endothelial cells expressing endothelial and mesenchymal cell gene products in lung tissue from patients with systemic sclerosis-associated interstitial lung disease. Arthritis Rheumatol. 2016;68:210–7.
32. Soldano S, Montagna P, Brizzolara R, Seriolo B, Sulli A, Cutolo M. Endothelial-to- mesenchymal transition in cultured human dermal microvascular endothelial cells: effects of endothelin-1 [abstract]. Ann Rheum Dis. 2013;72 Suppl 3:186.
33. Lagares D, García-Fernández RA, Jiménez CL, Magán-Marchal N, Busnadiego O, Lamas S, et al. Endothelin 1 contributes to the effect of transforming growth factor β1 on wound repair and skin fibrosis. Arthritis Rheum. 2010;62:878–89.
34. Cipriani P, Di Benedetto P, Ruscitti P, Verzella D, Fischietti M, Zazzeroni F, et al. Macitentan inhibits the transforming growth factor-β profibrotic action, blocking the signaling mediated by the ETR/TβRI complex in systemic sclerosis dermal fibroblasts. Arthritis Res Ther. 2015;17:247.
35. Horstmeyer A, Licht C, Scherr G, Eckes B, Krieg T. Signalling and regulation of collagen I synthesis by ET-1 and TGF-beta1. FEBS J. 2005;272:6297–309.
36. Cutolo M, Sulli A. Therapy: optimized treatment algorithms for digital vasculopathy in SSc. Nat Rev Rheumatol. 2015;11:569–71.
37. Shi-Wen X, Rodríguez-Pascual F, Lamas S, Holmes A, Howat S, Pearson JD, et al. Constitutive ALK5-independent c-Jun N-terminal kinase activation contributes to endothelin-1 overexpression in pulmonary fibrosis: evidence of an autocrine endothelin loop operating through the endothelin A and B receptors. Mol Cell Biol. 2006;26:5518–27.
38. Cutolo M, Sulli A, Pizzorni C, Paolino S, Smith V. Systemic sclerosis: markers and targeted treatments. Acta Reumatol Port. 2016;41:18–25.
39. Iglarz M, Binkert C, Morrison K, Fischli W, Gatfield J, Treiber A, et al. Pharmacology of macitentan, an orally active tissue-targeting dual endothelin receptor antagonist. J Pharmacol Exp Ther. 2008;327:736–45.
40. Good RB, Gilbane AJ, Trinder SL, Denton CP, Coghlan G, Abraham DJ, et al. Endothelial to mesenchymal transition contributes to endothelial dysfunction in pulmonary arterial hypertension. Am J Pathol. 2015;185:1850–8.
41. Ranchoux B, Antigny F, Rucker-Martin C, Hautefort A, Péchoux C, Bogaard HJ, et al. Endothelial-to-mesenchymal transition in pulmonary hypertension. Circulation. 2015;131:1006–18.
42. Jimenez SA, Piera-Velazquez S. Endothelial to mesenchymal transition (EndoMT) in the pathogenesis of systemic sclerosis-associated pulmonary fibrosis and pulmonary arterial hypertension: myth or reality? Matrix Biol. 2016;51:26–36.
43. Khanna D, Denton CP, Merkel PA, Krieg T, Le Brun FO, Marr A, et al. Effect of macitentan on the development of new ischemic digital ulcers in patients with systemic sclerosis: DUAL-1 and DUAL-2 randomized clinical trials. JAMA. 2016;15:1975–88.

Genetic susceptibility loci of idiopathic interstitial pneumonia do not represent risk for systemic sclerosis: a case control study in Caucasian patients

Minghua Wu[1*], Shervin Assassi[1], Gloria A. Salazar[1], Claudia Pedroza[2], Olga Y. Gorlova[3], Wei V. Chen[3], Julio Charles[1], Miranda L. Taing[1], Kelley Liao[1], Fredrick M. Wigley[4], Laura K. Hummers[4], Ami A. Shah[4], Monique Hinchcliff[5], Dinesh Khanna[6], Elena Schiopu[6], Kristine Phillips[6], Daniel E. Furst[7], Virginia Steen[8], Murray Baron[9], Marie Hudson[9], Xiaodong Zhou[1], Janet Pope[10], Niall Jones[11], Peter Docherty[12], Nader A. Khalidi[13], David Robinson[14], Robert W. Simms[15], Richard M. Silver[16], Tracy M. Frech[17], Barri J. Fessler[18], Marvin J. Fritzler[19], Jerry A. Molitor[20], Barbara M. Segal[20], Malahat Movahedian[1], Javier Martín[21], John Varga[5] and Maureen D. Mayes[1]

Abstract

Background: Systemic sclerosis (SSc)-related interstitial lung disease (ILD) has phenotypic similarities to lung involvement in idiopathic interstitial pneumonia (IIP). We aimed to assess whether genetic susceptibility loci recently identified in the large IIP genome-wide association studies (GWASs) were also risk loci for SSc overall or severity of ILD in SSc.

Methods: A total of 2571 SSc patients and 4500 healthy controls were investigated from the US discovery GWAS and additional US replication cohorts. Thirteen IIP-related selected single nucleotide polymorphisms (SNPs) were genotyped and analyzed for their association with SSc.

Results: We found an association of SSc with the SNP rs6793295 in the *LRRC34* gene (OR = 1.14, CI 95 % 1.03 to 1.25, p value = 0.009) and rs11191865 in the *OBFC1* gene (OR = 1.09, CI 95 % 1.00 to 1.19, p value = 0.043) in the discovery cohort. Additionally, rs7934606 in *MUC2* (OR = 1.24, CI 95 % 1.01 to 1.52, p value = 0.037) was associated with SSc-ILD defined by imaging. However, these associations failed to replicate in the validation cohort. Furthermore, SNPs rs2076295 in *DSP* (β = -2.29, CI 95 % -3.85 to -0.74, p value = 0.004) rs17690703 in *SPPL2C* (β = 2.04, CI 95 % 0.21 to 3.88, p value = 0.029) and rs1981997 in *MAPT* (β = 2.26, CI 95 % 0.35 to 4.17, p value = 0.02) were associated with percent predicted forced vital capacity (FVC%) even after adjusting for the anti-topoisomerase (ATA)-positive subset. However, these associations also did not replicate in the validation cohort.

Conclusions: Our results add new evidence that SSc and SSc-related ILD are genetically distinct from IIP, although they share phenotypic similarities.

Keywords: Idiopathic interstitial pneumonia (IIP), SSc-ILD, Genetic susceptibility

* Correspondence: Minghua.wu@uth.tmc.edu
[1]Division of Rheumatology and Clinical Immunogenetics, Department of Internal Medicine, University of Texas McGovern Medical School at Houston, 6431 Fannin Street, Houston, TX 77030, USA
Full list of author information is available at the end of the article

Background

Systemic sclerosis or scleroderma (SSc) is a complex autoimmune disease characterized by vasculopathy, autoantibody production and fibrosis in the skin and internal organs. The etiology of SSc remains unknown; effective treatments that target the underlying pathophysiology of SSc are unavailable and the disease-related mortality remains high [1]. Specifically, pulmonary fibrosis and pulmonary arterial hypertension (PAH) account for the majority of disease-related deaths in SSc [2]. SSc-associated interstitial lung disease (SSc-ILD) is usually characterized by a histologic pattern of nonspecific interstitial pneumonia (NSIP) or, less frequently, usual interstitial pneumonia (UIP). SSc-ILD has clinical and radiologic similarities to idiopathic interstitial pneumonia (IIP). A polymorphism in the MUC5B promoter region was strongly associated with familial and idiopathic pulmonary fibrosis (IPF; the most common IIP type) [3], but it has not been found to be a susceptibility locus for SSc or SSc-associated interstitial lung disease (SSc-ILD) [4–6].

Recently, large genome-wide association studies (GWASs) in fibrotic IIP (n = 1616 patients) and IPF (n = 542 patients and two validation cohorts n = 544 and n = 324) identified/confirmed susceptibility single nucleotide polymorphisms (SNPs) in *TERT, AZGP1, MUC2, IVD, DSP, MAPT, DPP9, LRRC34, FAM13A, OBFC1, CSMD1, ATP11A* [7] and *TOLLIP, MDGA2, SPPL2C* [8]. Given the clinical and radiologic similarities between SSc-ILD and IIP, we examined the association of the 13 SNPs among the listed genes, identified in the above IIP and IPF GWASs [7, 8] (*TOLLIP* and *MDGA2* genes were excluded because the related SNPs were not present on the Illumina BeadChip utilized in SSc GWAS) with SSc as a single disease entity, with SSc-ILD by imaging, or SSc-ILD severity (as determined by percent predicted forced vital capacity (FVC%)) in two large SSc patient samples.

Methods

Study population

Two non-Hispanic white populations (discovery and replication cohorts) were investigated. For the discovery cohort, we utilized data from our previously published SSc GWAS study consisting of 1486 SSc cases (patients from the US) and 3477 unaffected race- and ethnicity-matched controls [9]. Selected polymorphisms were genotyped in an independent replication cohort consisting of 1085 additional SSc cases (patients from the US and Canada) and 1023 additional unaffected controls. Patients were recruited at the University of Texas – Houston and from the following sites: the participating Canadian Scleroderma Research Group (CSRG) sites, University of California Los Angeles, University of Michigan, Georgetown University, Boston University, Medical University of South Carolina, Johns Hopkins University, University of Utah, Northwestern University, University of Alabama at Birmingham and University of Minnesota. All patients were enrolled in the National Scleroderma Family Registry and DNA Repository. All patients with SSc fulfilled the 1980 American College of Rheumatology classification criteria for SSc or had at least three of the five CREST (Calcinosis, Raynaud's phenomenon, Esophageal dysmotility, Sclerodactyly, Telangiectasias) features (Table 1).

The genotypes of unaffected controls for the discovery cohort were obtained from the Cancer Genetic Markers of Susceptibility (CGEMS; non-cancer healthy controls) studies and Illumina iControlDB database (www.illumina.com/iControlDB, Illumina, San Diego, CA, USA). The unaffected controls for the replication cohort were recruited through a nationwide effort by the Scleroderma Family Registry and DNA Repository.

Collection of blood samples and clinical information from case and control subjects was undertaken with fully informed consent and relevant ethical review board approval from each contributing center in accordance with the tenets of the Declaration of Helsinki.

SNP selection and genotyping assay

In the discovery cohort, genotyping was performed using the Illumina Bead-Array GWAS platform. Specifically, patients were genotyped using Illumina Human 610-Quad BeadChip and controls were genotyped on Illumina Hap550K-BeadChip [9]. The 13 single nucleotide polymorphisms (SNPs) identified/confirmed to be associated with IIP [7], rs2736100 (*TERT*), rs2076295 (*DSP*), rs4727443 (*AZGP1*), rs7934606 (*MUC2*), rs2034650 (*IVD*), rs1981997 (*MAPT*), rs12610495 (*DPP9*), rs6793295 (*LRRC34*), rs2609255 (*FAM13A*), rs11191865 (*OBFC1*), rs1278769 (*ATP11A*), rs1379326 (*CSMD1*) and an additional SNP rs17690703 (*SPPL2C*) [8], were investigated in the discovery cohort. We also investigated association of 13 SNPs with anti-topoisomerase 1 antibody (ATA) and anti-centromere

Table 1 Demographic and clinical features of SSc patients in the discovery and replication cohorts

	Discovery (n = 1486)	Replication (n = 1085)
Female	1307 (88.0 %)	934 (86.1 %)
Mean age ± years	54.5 ± 12.9 y	56.1 ± 12.8 y
Diffuse SSc	505 (34.0 %)	403 (37.1 %)
Disease duration	10.1 ± 8.7 y	10.9 ± 9.6 y
ACA	425 (28.6 %)	340 (31.3 %)
ATA	238 (16.0 %)	180 (16.6 %)
SSc-ILD		
Yes	185 (65.6 %)	313 (61.9 %)
No	97 (34.4 %)	193 (38.1 %)

ACA anti-centromere antibody, *ATA* anti-topoisomerase 1 antibody, *SSc* systemic sclerosis, *ILD* interstitial lung disease

antibody (ACA) positive subgroup patients. The SNPs reaching a nominal level of significance ($p < 0.05$) in the discovery cohort (rs6793295 and rs11191865) were genotyped in the replication cohort using TaqMan allele discrimination assays in a 7900HT fast real-time PCR system (Applied Biosystems, Foster City, CA, USA).

SSc-ILD and severity of SSc-ILD

We also investigated the association of the above SNPs with SSc-ILD by imaging. We compared the frequency of the above SNPs in patients with SSc-ILD to unaffected controls. SSc-ILD was defined by chest high-resolution computed tomography (HRCT)/chest X-ray images. SSc patients (total = 498; n = 185 in the discovery cohort and n = 313 in the replication cohort) were considered to have interstitial lung disease (ILD) by imaging if they had: (1) ground glass opacity or increased interstitial markings on chest HRCT; or (2) increased basilar reticular marking on chest X-ray (in total, 498 patients, 185 in the discovery cohort and 313 in the replication cohort had ILD). The number of patients with imaging-proven ILD is low because HRCT imaging results were available only n = 212 in the discovery cohort and n = 347 in the replication cohort patients. The case-case comparison in regard to presence of ILD was compared by the low number of patients with available HRCT imaging in the discovery cohort.

Furthermore, an association with severity of ILD was investigated. Percent predicted forced vital capacity (FVC%) (measured in a total of 1954 patients; n = 1072 in the discovery cohort and n = 882 in the replication cohort) as a continuous variable was used as a surrogate for severity of SSc-ILD as this has been demonstrated to be a validated outcome measure for severity of ILD in randomized controlled studies of patients with SSc [10]. SNPs reaching the nominal significance level ($p < 0.05$) in these two analyses were also genotyped in the replication cohort (rs7934606, rs2076295, rs17690703 and rs1981997).

Statistical analysis

We followed the same genetic inheritance modes for each specific SNP that was utilized in the IIP GWAS [7]. Specifically, all SNPs except for rs1379326 (*CSMD1*) were investigated in an additive model. Similar to the IIP GWAS [7], rs1379326 (*CSMD1*) was investigated in a recessive model. The additive model corresponds to the risk or protective effect conferred by the rarer (minor) allele (0, 1 or 2 copies) as a predictor of phenotypic status; and the recessive model corresponds to the effect conferred by only homozygous status for the rarer allele. Genotype data quality was verified for each SNP by testing for Hardy-Weinberg equilibrium (HWE). Hardy-Weinberg equilibrium was assessed by an x^2 test or Fisher's exact test. None of the included cohorts showed significant deviation from HWE for all the genotyped SNPs. Logistic regression that included both patients and controls was utilized to examine the association of the above SNPs with SSc overall and SSc-ILD. A linear regression model was used to investigate the association of these genetic variants with FVC% predicted (data was normally distributed) as a continuous variable, among patients only. FVC% predicted was investigated as a continuous rather than a dichotomous variable to increase our power to detect a difference in FVC levels conditional on the genotype. Anti-topoisomerase 1 antibody (ATA) status was included as a potential confounder in the multivariable regression model. The combined analysis of the discovery and the replication cohorts was performed via a random-effects meta-analysis model.

Results

Discovery cohort

We first investigated whether the 13 IIP-associated polymorphisms were associated with risk of SSc overall or with SSc-ILD. Several SNPs showed nominally significant associations with SSc in the discovery cohort (Table 2). Specifically, *LRRC34* rs6793295 (OR = 1.14, CI 95 % 1.03 to 1.25, p value = 0.009) and *OBFC1* rs11191865 (OR = 1.09, CI 95 % 1.00 to 1.19, p value = 0.043) were associated with SSc compared to controls (Table 2). There were no significant associations observed when the SNP frequencies in SSc antibody subgroups (ATA- or ACA-positive patients) were compared to controls (Table 3).

Next, we investigated the association in the discovery cohort between the above polymorphisms and SSc-ILD by imaging or FVC% predicted in order to investigate the relationship with SSc-ILD presence or severity. We also performed case-case comparison by presence of ILD with no ILD in SSc. Interestingly, rs7934606 in *MUC2* (OR = 1.24, CI 95 % 1.01 to 1.52, p value = 0.037) was associated with SSc-ILD by imaging when compared to controls (Table 4). Furthermore, three polymorphisms *DSP* rs2076295 (β = -2.29, CI 95 % -3.85 to -0.74, p value = 0.004) *SPPL2C* rs17690703 (β = 2.04, CI 95 % 0.21 to 3.88, p value = 0.029) and *MAPT* rs1981997 (β = 2.26, CI 95 % 0.35 to 4.17, p value = 0.02) were associated with FVC% predicted (Table 5). Of note, the minor allele (A) of *MAPT* rs1981997 and (T) of *SPPL2C* rs17690703 were associated with higher FVC% predicted, which is consistent with the IIP GWAS results with the minor allele being protective in that study (OR < 1) [7]. Even after adjustment for ATA status, the above three polymorphisms showed nominally significant associations with ILD severity in SSc patients (Table 5). *SPPL2C* rs17690703 was associated ILD-SSc compared to SSc with no ILD as determined by imaging in the discovery cohort (Table S1 in Additional file 1).

Table 2 Association between the investigated genotypes in SSc-versus-control comparisons in the discovery cohort

SNP	Gene	Minor allele*	MAF (case)**	OR (95 % CI)	*p* value
rs2736100	*TERT*	T	0.50	1.04 (0.95; 1.13)†	0.393
rs2076295	*DSP*	G	0.44	0.96 (0.88; 1.05)†	0.387
rs4727443	*AZGP1*	A	0.41	1.03 (0.95; 1.13)†	0.487
rs7934606	*MUC2*	A	0.41	1.08 (0.99; 1.18)†	0.084
rs2034650	*IVD*	G	0.49	1.03 (0.95; 1.13)†	0.458
rs1981997	*MAPT*	A	0.22	0.97 (0.88; 1.08)†	0.636
rs12610495	*DPP9*	G	0.28	1.00 (0.91; 1.10)†	0.967
rs6793295	***LRRC34***	**C**	**0.29**	**1.14 (1.03; 1.25)**†	**0.009**
rs2609255	*FAM13A*	G	0.22	1.01 (0.91; 1.12)†	0.851
rs11191865	***OBFC1***	**G**	**0.52**	**1.09 (1.00; 1.19)**†	**0.043**
rs1278769	*ATP11A*	A	0.24	0.95 (0.86; 1.06)†	0.365
rs1379326	*CSMD1*	G	0.26	0.86 (0.69; 1.08)‡	0.199
rs17690703	*SPPL2C*	T	0.26	1.03 (0.95; 1.11)	0.546

Gene names: *TERT*: telomerase reverse transcriptase; *DSP*: desmoplakin; *AZGP1*: alpha-2-glycoprotein 1, zinc-binding; *MUC2*: mucin 2; *IVD*: isovaleryl-CoA dehydrogenase; *MAPT*: microtubule-associated protein tau; *DPP9*: dipeptidyl-peptidase 9; *LRRC34*: leucine-rich repeat-containing 34; *FAM13A*: family with sequence similarity 13, member A; *OBFC1*: oligonucleotide/oligosaccharide-binding fold containing 1; *ATP11A*: ATPase, class VI, type 11A; *CSMD1*: CUB and Sushi multiple domains 1; *SPPL2C*: signal peptide peptidase-like 2C

SSc systemic sclerosis, *SNP* single nucleotide polymorphism, *MAF* minor allele frequency

*The minor allele is defined as the minor allele in the combined case and control group; **MAF is defined as the minor allele frequency in cases and controls; †Odds ratio for the minor allele in the additive model; ‡Odds ratio based on the recessive model

Replication cohort and combined analysis

We genotyped the samples from the validation set for the above six SNPs, which either showed nominally significant associations ($p < 0.05$) with risk of SSc overall (*LRRC34* rs6793295 and *OBFC1* rs11191865) or with SSc-ILD (rs7934606 in *MUC2*) and FVC% predicted (*DSP* rs2076295, *SPPL2C* rs17690703 and *MAPT* rs1981997). However, these associations were not found in the replication cohort (Table 4 and upper part of Table 6). Contrary to the discovery cohort, *MAPT*

Table 3 Association studies of investigated genotypes in comparison of ATA- or ACA-positive SSc patients to controls in the discovery cohort

		ATA (+)		ACA (+)	
SNP	Gene	OR (95 % CI)	*p* value	OR (95 % CI)	*p* value
rs2736100*	*TERT*	1.01 (0.84; 1.22)	0.881	1.14 (0.99; 1.31)	0.069
rs2076295*	*DSP*	1.01 (0.83; 1.21)	0.945	0.94 (0.82; 1.09)	0.423
rs4727443*	*AZGP1*	1.12 (0.93; 1.36)	0.226	0.96 (0.83; 1.11)	0.609
rs7934606*	*MUC2*	1.00 (0.83; 1.20)	0.992	1.07 (0.93; 1.23)	0.925
rs2034650*	*IVD*	0.99 (0.82; 1.19)	0.915	1.04 (0.90; 1.20)	0.584
rs1981997*	*MAPT*	0.92 (0.73; 1.16)	0.495	1.15 (0.97; 1.36)	0.100
rs12610495*	*DPP9*	0.98 (0.80; 1.20)	0.847	1.05 (0.90; 1.22)	0.572
rs6793295*	*LRRC34*	1.15 (0.94; 1.42)	0.172	1.15 (0.98; 1.35)	0.080
rs2609255*	*FAMI3A*	1.04 (0.83; 1.30)	0.736	1.00 (0.84; 1.19)	1.000
rs11191865*	***OBFC1***	**1.21 (1.00; 1.45)**	**0.048**	0.99 (0.86; 1.14)	0.898
rs1278769*	*ATP11A*	1.09 (0.89; 1.35)	0.394	0.96 (0.81; 1.14)	0.650
rs1379326†	*CSMD1*	0.78 (0.46; 1.31)	0.340	0.94 (0.65; 1.36)	0.736
rs17690703	*SPPL2C*	0.97 (0.76; 1.26)	0.870	1.14 (0.94; 1.38)	0.184

Gene names: *TERT*: telomerase reverse transcriptase; *DSP*: desmoplakin; *AZGP1*: alpha-2-glycoprotein 1, zinc-binding; *MUC2*: mucin 2; *IVD*: isovaleryl-CoA dehydrogenase; *MAPT*: microtubule-associated protein tau; *DPP9*: dipeptidyl-peptidase 9; *LRRC34*: leucine-rich repeat-containing 34; *FAMI3A*: family with sequence similarity 13, member A; *OBFC1*: oligonucleotide/oligosaccharide-binding fold containing 1; *ATP11A*: ATPase, class VI, type 11A; *CSMD1*: CUB and Sushi multiple domains 1; *SPPL2C*: signal peptide peptidase-like 2C

ATA anti-topoisomerase 1 antibody, *ACA* anti-centromere antibody, *SSc* systemic sclerosis, *SNP* single nucleotide polymorphism

*Additive model;,†Recessive model

Table 4 Association between the investigated genotypes in SSc-ILD (by imaging) patients compared to controls in the discovery and replication cohort

		SSc-ILD vs control (discovery cohort)		SSc-ILD vs control (replication cohort)	
SNP (coded allele)	Gene	OR (95 % CI)	*p* value	OR (95 % CI)	*p* value
rs2736100 (T)*	*TERT*	1.14 (0.93; 1.40)	0.199		
rs2076295 (G)*	*DSP*	1.13 (0.92; 1.39)	0.243		
rs4727443 (A)*	*AZGP1*	0.89 (0.71; 1.10)	0.270		
rs7934606 (A)*	***MUC2***	**1.24 (1.01; 1.52)**	**0.037**	1.14 (0.81; 1.63)	0.444
rs2034650 (C)*	*IVD*	0.86 (0.70; 1.06)	0.152		
rs1981997 (A)*	*MAPT*	0.81 (0.62; 1.06)	0.123		
rs12610495 (G)*	*DPP9*	1.17 (0.93; 1.46)	0.179		
rs6793295 (C)*	*LRRC34*	1.02 (0.80; 1.30)	0.863		
rs2609255 (G)*	*FAM13A*	0.99 (0.77; 1.27)	0.919		
rs11191865 (G)*	*OBFC1*	1.08 (0.87; 1.32)	0.496		
rs1278769 (A)*	*ATP11A*	1.00 (0.79; 1.28)	0.987		
rs1379326 (G)†	*CSMD1*	0.68 (0.37; 1.27)	0.224		
rs17690703 (T)*	*SPPL2C*	1.23 (0.87; 1.72)	0.238		

Gene names: *TERT*: telomerase reverse transcriptase; *DSP*: desmoplakin; *AZGP1*: alpha-2-glycoprotein 1, zinc-binding; *MUC2*: mucin 2; *IVD*: isovaleryl-CoA dehydrogenase; *MAPT*: microtubule-associated protein tau; *DPP9*: dipeptidyl-peptidase 9; *LRRC34*: leucine-rich repeat-containing 34; *FAM13A*: family with sequence similarity 13, member A; *OBFC1*: oligonucleotide/oligosaccharide-binding fold containing 1; *ATP11A*: ATPase, class VI, type 11A; *CSMD1*: CUB and Sushi multiple domains 1; *SPPL2C*: signal peptide peptidase-like 2C

SSc systemic sclerosis, *ILD* interstitial lung disease, *SNP* single nucleotide polymorphism

*Additive model; †Recessive model

rs1981997 (OR = 0.79; CI 95 % 0.68 to 0.91; *p* value = 0.002) and *SPPL2C* rs17690703 (OR = 0.64; CI 95 % 0.49 to 0.83; *p* value = 0.001) were associated with SSc susceptibility but not with ILD severity in the replication cohort (Table 6). Furthermore, *SPPL2C* rs17690703 was not associated with SSc-ILD when compared to SSc without ILD by imaging in the validation cohort (Table S1 in Additional file 1).

In the combined discovery and replication cohorts (lower part of Table 6), only the *LRRC34* rs6793295 was

Table 5 Association between the investigated genotypes and FVC% predicted in SSc patients in the discovery cohort

		FVC%		FVC% (adjusted for ATA status)	
SNP (Coded allele)	Gene	β (95 % CI)	*p* value	β (95 % CI)	*p* value
rs2736100 (T)*	*TERT*	0.51 (-1.04; 2.05)	0.521	0.76 (-0.81; 2.34)	0.343
rs2076295 (G)*	***DSP***	**−2.29 (-3.85; -0.74)**	**0.004**	**−2.52 (-4.09; -0.95)**	**0.002**
rs4727443 (A)*	*AZGP1*	−0.27 (-1.85; 1.32)	0.742	0.08 (-1.53; 1.70)	0.919
rs7934606 (A)*	*MUC2*	−0.55 (-2.16; 1.05)	0.499	−0.75 (-2.37; 0.86)	0.360
rs2034650 (C)*	*IVD*	0.67 (-0.90; 2.25)	0.402	0.37 (-1.22; 1.97)	0.646
rs1981997 (A)*	***MAPT***	**2.26 (0.35; 4.17)**	**0.020**	**3.19 (1.23; 5.14)**	**0.001**
rs12610495 (G)*	*DPP9*	0.57 (-1.18; 2.32)	0.523	1.05 (-0.72; 2.82)	0.246
rs6793295 (C)*	*LRRC34*	−0.46 (-2.19;1.27)	0.599	−1.05 (-2.82; 0.71)	0.242
rs2609255 (G)*	*FAM13A*	1.72 (-0.10; 3.55)	0.064	1.61 (-0.18; 3.41)	0.079
rs11191865 (G)*	*OBFC1*	−0.73 (-2.27; 0.82)	0.356	0.02 (-1.55; 1.60)	0.977
rs1278769 (A)*	*ATP11A*	−0.62 (-2.45; 1.20)	0.503	−0.74 (-2.60; 1.11)	0.433
rs1379326 (G)†	*CSMD1*	3.35 (-0.84; 7.54)	0.117	3.12 (-1.08; 7.31)	0.145
rs17690703 (T)*	***SPPL2C***	**2.04 (0.21; 3.88)**	**0.029**	**2.11 (0.30; 3.91)**	**0.022**

Gene names: *TERT*: telomerase reverse transcriptase; *DSP*: desmoplakin; *AZGP1*: alpha-2-glycoprotein 1, zinc-binding; *MUC2*: mucin 2; *IVD*: isovaleryl-CoA dehydrogenase; *MAPT*: microtubule-associated protein tau; *DPP9*: dipeptidyl-peptidase 9; *LRRC34*: leucine-rich repeat-containing 34; *FAM13A*: family with sequence similarity 13, member A; *OBFC1*: oligonucleotide/oligosaccharide-binding fold containing 1; *ATP11A*: ATPase, class VI, type 11A; *CSMD1*: CUB and Sushi multiple domains 1; *SPPL2C*: signal peptide peptidase-like 2C

FVC% percent predicted forced vital capacity, *SSc* systemic sclerosis, *ATA* anti-topoisomerase 1 antibody, *SNP* single nucleotide polymorphism

*Additive model; †Recessive model

Table 6 Association analysis of investigated genotypes in SSc versus control comparison as well as FVC% in the replication and combined cohorts

			Allele frequency		FVC%		FVC%–adjusted for ATA	
	SNPs	Gene	OR (95 % CI)	*p* value	β (95 % CI)	*p* value	β (95 % CI)	*p* value
Replication	rs2076295 (G)[†]	*DSP*	0.93 (0.82; 1.05)	0.252	0.32 (-1.49; 2.13)	0.729	0.39 (-1.40; 2.17)	0.671
	rs1981997 (A)[†]	***MAPT***	**0.79 (0.68; 0.91)**	**0.002**	0.15 (-2.05; 2.35)	0.894	−0.01 (-2.17; 2.15)	0.994
	rs6793295 (C)[†]	*LRRC34*	1.06 (0.92; 1.21)	0.435	−0.54 (-2.53;1.45)	0.593	−0.55 (-2.51; 1.41)	0.581
	rs11191865 (G)[†]	*OBFC1*	0.90 (0.80; 1.01)	0.093	−0.34 (-2.11; 1.44)	0.710	−0.30 (-2.05; 1.45)	0.736
	rs17690703 (T)[†]	***SPPL2C***	**0.64 (0.49; 0.83)**	**0.001**	2.20 (-1.38; 5.78)	0.227	3.11 (-0.45; 6.66)	0.086
Combined	rs2076295 (G)[†]	*DSP*	0.95 (0.89; 1.02)	0.171	−1.02 (-3.58; 1.54)	0.579	−1.07 (-3.94; 1.80)	0.079
	rs1981997 (A)[†]	*MAPT*	0.89 (0.78; 1.02)	0.091	1.26 (-0.81; 3.32)	0.445	1.59 (-1.56; 4.74)	0.503
	rs6793295 (C)[†]	***LRRC34***	**1.11 (1.03; 1.20)**	**0.010**	−0.50 (-1.80; 0.81)	0.590	−0.81 (-2.12; 0.50)	0.440
	rs11191865 (G)[†]	*OBFC1*	1.01 (0.90; 1.13)	0.912	−0.55 (-1.72; 0.61)	0.524	−0.13 (-1.30; 1.04)	0.868
	rs17690703 (T)[†]	***SPPL2C***	1.04 (0.97; 1.13)	0.221	**2.32 (0.68; 3.96)**	**0.006**	−1.03 (-4.67; 2.60)	0.575

Gene names: *TERT*: telomerase reverse transcriptase; *DSP*: desmoplakin; *AZGP1*: alpha-2-glycoprotein 1, zinc-binding; *MUC2*: mucin 2; *IVD*: isovaleryl-CoA dehydrogenase; *MAPT*: microtubule-associated protein tau; *DPP9*: dipeptidyl-peptidase 9; *LRRC34*: leucine-rich repeat-containing 34; *FAMI3A*: family with sequence similarity 13, member A; *OBFC1*: oligonucleotide/oligosaccharide-binding fold containing 1; *ATP11A*: ATPase, class VI, type 11A; *CSMD1*: CUB and Sushi multiple domains 1; *SPPL2C*: signal peptide peptidase-like 2C

SSc systemic sclerosis, *FVC %* percent predicted forced vital capacity, *ATA* anti-topoisomerase 1 antibody, *SNP* single nucleotide polymorphism

[†]Additive model

associated with risk of SSc overall (OR = 1.11; CI 95 % 1.03 to 1.2; *p* value = 0.01). However, the observed significance level was not stronger in the combined cohort than in the discovery cohort and this association did not withstand correction for multiple comparisons. Specifically, the *p* value = 0.13 in the combined cohort after Bonferroni correction for multiple comparisons. Furthermore, *LRRC34* rs6793295 was not associated with FVC% predicted in the combined cohort. *SPPL2C* rs17690703 was associated with FVC% predicted in the combined cohort but not after ATA adjustment or with overall SSc risk (Table 6). The observed association of *SPPL2C* rs17690703 with FVC% did not withstand correction for multiple comparison (p_{corr} = 0.078).

Discussion

The aim of this study was to assess genetic components of SSc and SSc-related ILD, specifically to determine if SSc-ILD and IIP share common genetic risk factors. We analyzed 13 SNPs which showed robust association with IIP in a previous GWAS report [7, 8]. However, we failed to replicate these associations with SSc or SSc-related ILD in a large North American cohort.

Interstitial lung disease (ILD) is the most common pulmonary manifestation in patients with SSc [11] and is the most frequent cause of SSc disease-related death [12]. ILD occurs with greater frequency and increased severity in patients with diffuse cutaneous SSc (dc-SSc) and in ATA-positive patients. In SSc-ILD, loss of lung function and extent of fibrosis are the most important prognostic factors. It is known that genetic factors contribute not only to SSc susceptibility, but also to predisposition to SSc clinical phenotypes including disease type (limited versus diffuse cutaneous disease) and autoantibody status [13]. Recently, several lines of evidence have suggested that, even though SSc-ILD has phenotypic similarities to IIP, the genetic risk factors for these two conditions are quite different. For example the MUC5B promoter region polymorphism (rs868903), which was strongly associated with familial and idiopathic pulmonary fibrosis [3, 7], was not identified as a susceptibility locus for SSc or SSc–associated interstitial lung disease [4–6]. In addition, the two large SSc GWAS reports (each with independent discovery and validation cohorts) identified the major histocompatibility complex (MHC) class II region as being the most strongly associated region with SSc [9, 14], whereas MHC loci were not found to be risk factors in the IIP GWAS [7].

The present study has some limitations. In our study, only a subgroup of SSc patients had undergone HRCT. We performed a case-case comparison in regard to presence of SSc-ILD versus no SSc-ILD in the low number of patients because HRCT results were not available in the remainder of patients. The genotype results for *TOLLIP* and *MDGA2* genes were not available on our GWAS platform and could not be investigated. Furthermore, this is a cross-sectional study, thus, we cannot examine whether the investigated genetic loci have predictive significance for ILD progression. However, mean disease duration of this study was more than 10 years and most of the SSc-ILD cases had been already established. Therefore, we believe the cross-sectional FVC% is a reasonable surrogate for severity of ILD.

Conclusions

In this study, we confirm that genetic susceptibility loci for IIP are not risk loci for SSc or severity of SSc-ILD in two validation SSc cohorts of non-Hispanic white ethnic background. Our findings and those of previous genetic susceptibility studies in SSc [15] implicate pathways in innate and adaptive immunity, whereas susceptibility loci for IIP relate to epithelial cell injury/dysfunction and abnormal wound healing [16]. Future challenges will be to identify the functional relevance of these variants for the final common pathway that results in the phenotype of fibrotic lung disease. This study represents an important step forward toward a better understanding of the complex genetic association of SSc particularly with lung involvement. We add new evidence that SSc and SSc-ILD are genetically distinct from IIP.

Abbreviations

ACA: Anti-centromere antibody; ATA: Anti-topoisomerase 1 antibody; CGEMS: Cancer Genetic Markers of Susceptibility; CREST: Calcinosis, Raynaud's phenomenon, Esophageal dysmotility, Sclerodactyly, Telangiectasias; dcSSc: Diffuse cutaneous SSc; FVC%: Percent predicted forced vital capacity; GWAS: Genome-wide association study; HRCT: High-resolution computed tomography; HWE: Hardy-Weinberg equilibrium; IIP: Idiopathic interstitial pneumonia; ILD: Interstitial lung disease; IPF: Idiopathic pulmonary fibrosis; MHC: Major histocompatibility complex; NSIP: Nonspecific interstitial pneumonia; PAH: Pulmonary arterial hypertension; SNP: Single nucleotide polymorphisms; SSc: Systemic sclerosis; SSc-ILD: SSc-associated interstitial lung disease; UIP: Usual interstitial pneumonia.

Competing interests

The authors declare that they have no competing interests.

Authors' contributions

MW, SA, JV, and MDM contributed to study conception and design, MW, SA, GAS, JC, MLT, KL, FMW, LKH, AAS, MH, DK, ES, KP, DEF, VS, MB, MH, XZ, JP, NJ, PD, NAK, DR, RWS, RMS, TMF, BJF, MJF, JAM, BMS, MM, JM, JV, and MDM contributed to acquisition of data. MW, SA, GAS, CP, OYG, WVC, JC, MLT, KL, FMW, LKH, AAS, MH, DK, ES, KP, DEF, VS, MB, MH, XZ, JP, NJ, PD, NAK, DR, RWS, RMS, TMF, BJF, MJF, JAM, BMS, MM, JM, JV, and MDM contributed to analysis and interpretation of data. MW had full access to all of the data in the study and takes responsibility for the integrity of the data and accuracy of the data analysis. All authors were involved in drafting the manuscript or revising it critically for important intellectual content, and all authors approved the final version to be submitted for publication.

Acknowledgements

The authors thank Marilyn Perry and Yuxiao Du for their work as Registry coordinators and we are grateful for the generous participation of our subjects. This work was supported by the Scleroderma Foundation New Investigator Award to Dr. Wu, and by the National Institutes of Health (NIH) National Institute of Arthritis and Musculoskeletal and Skin Diseases (NIAMS) Centers of Research Translation (CORT) grant P50AR054144 to Dr. Mayes, NIH grant K23AR061436 to Dr. Assassi, NIH/NIAMS Scleroderma Family Registry and DNA Repository grant N01-AR02251 to Dr. Mayes, NIH/NIAMS grant AR055258 to Dr. Mayes, NIH National Center for Clinical and Translational Sciences grant 3UL1RR024148, Department of Defense Congressionally Directed Medical Research Program W81XWH-13-1-0452, Proposal number PR120687 to Dr. Mayes.

Author details

[1]Division of Rheumatology and Clinical Immunogenetics, Department of Internal Medicine, University of Texas McGovern Medical School at Houston, 6431 Fannin Street, Houston, TX 77030, USA. [2]Department of Pediatrics, The University of Texas Mcgovern Medical School at Houston, 6431 Fannin Street, Houston, TX 77030, USA. [3]Department of Community and Family Medicine, Geisel School of Medicine at Dartmouth, 1 Rope Ferry Road, Hanover, NH 03755, USA. [4]Division of Rheumatology, Johns Hopkins University School of Medicine, 5501 Hopkins Bayview circle, Baltimore, MD 21224, USA. [5]Division of Rheumatology, Northwestern University Feinberg School of Medicine, 240 East Huron Street, Chicago, IL 60611, USA. [6]Department of Internal Medicine, Division of Rheumatology, University of Michigan Health Center, 300 North Ingalls Street, Ann Arbor, MI 48109, USA. [7]Division of Rheumatology, University of California Los Angeles, 1000 Veterans Avenue, Los Angeles, CA 90024, USA. [8]Division of Rheumatology, Georgetown University Medical Center, 3800 Reservoir Road, Washington, MD 20007, USA. [9]Division of Rheumatology, McGill University, 1650 Cedar Avenue, Montreal, QC H3G 1A4, Canada. [10]Division of Rheumatology, St. Joseph's Health Care, University of Western Ontario, 268 Grosvenor Street, London, ON, Canada. [11]Division of Rheumatology, University of Alberta, 11405-87 Avenue, Edmonton, AB T6G 1C9, Canada. [12]Division of Rheumatology, Moncton Hospital, 135 MacBeath Avenue, Moncton, NB E1C 6Z8, Canada. [13]Division of Rheumatology, McMaster University at Hamilton, 1280 Main Street West, Hamilton, ON L8S 4L8, Canada. [14]Division of Rheumatology, University of Manitoba, 820 Sherbrook Street, Winnipeg, MB R3A 1R9, Canada. [15]Division of Rheumatology, Boston University School of Medicine, 72 East Concord Street, Boston, MA 02118, USA. [16]Division of Rheumatology, Medical University of South Carolina, 171 Ashley Avenue, Charleston, SC 29425, USA. [17]Division of Rheumatology, University of Utah, 30 North 1900 East, Salt Lake City, UT 84132, USA. [18]Division of Clinical Immunology and Rheumatology, University of Alabama at Birmingham, 1825 University Boulevard, Birmingham, AB 35294, USA. [19]Division of Rheumatology, University of Calgary Cumming School of Medicine, 3330 Hospital Drive NW, Calgary, AB T2N 4N1, Canada. [20]Division of Rheumatology, University of Minnesota, 420 Delaware Street SE, Minneapolis, MN 55455, USA. [21]Instituto de Parasitología y Biomedicina López-Neyra, Consejo Superior de Investigaciones Cientıficas, C/Ventanilla 11, 18001 Granada, Spain.

References

1. Elhai M, Meune C, Avouac J, Kahan A, Allanore Y. Trends in mortality in patients with systemic sclerosis over 40 years: a systematic review and meta-analysis of cohort studies. Rheumatology (Oxford). 2012;51:1017–26.
2. Tyndall AJ, Bannert B, Vonk M, Airo P, Cozzi F, Carreira PE, et al. Causes and risk factors for death in systemic sclerosis: a study from the EULAR Scleroderma Trials and Research (EUSTAR) database. Ann Rheum Dis. 2010;69:1809–15.
3. Seibold MA, Wise AL, Speer MC, Steele MP, Brown KK, Loyd JE, et al. A common MUC5B promoter polymorphism and pulmonary fibrosis. N Engl J Med. 2011;364:1503–12.
4. Stock CJ, Sato H, Fonseca C, Banya WA, Molyneaux PL, Adamali H, et al. Mucin 5B promoter polymorphism is associated with idiopathic pulmonary fibrosis but not with development of lung fibrosis in systemic sclerosis or sarcoidosis. Thorax. 2013;68:436–41.
5. Borie R, Crestani B, Dieude P, Nunes H, Allanore Y, Kannengiesser C, et al. The MUC5B variant is associated with idiopathic pulmonary fibrosis but not with systemic sclerosis interstitial lung disease in the European Caucasian population. PLoS One. 2013;8:e70621.
6. Peljto AL, Steele MP, Fingerlin TE, Hinchcliff ME, Murphy E, Podlusky S, et al. The pulmonary fibrosis-associated MUC5B promoter polymorphism does not influence the development of interstitial pneumonia in systemic sclerosis. Chest. 2012;142:1584–8.
7. Fingerlin TE, Murphy E, Zhang W, Peljto AL, Brown KK, Steele MP, et al. Genome-wide association study identifies multiple susceptibility loci for pulmonary fibrosis. Nat Genet. 2013;45:613–20.

8. Noth I, Zhang Y, Ma SF, Flores C, Barber M, Huang Y, et al. Genetic variants associated with idiopathic pulmonary fibrosis susceptibility and mortality: a genome-wide association study. Lancet Respir Med. 2013;1:309–17.
9. Radstake TR, Gorlova O, Rueda B, Martin JE, Alizadeh BZ, Palomino-Morales R, et al. Genome-wide association study of systemic sclerosis identifies CD247 as a new susceptibility locus. Nat Genet. 2010;42:426–9.
10. Furst D, Khanna D, Matucci-Cerinic M, Clements P, Steen V, Pope J, et al. Systemic sclerosis - continuing progress in developing clinical measures of response. J Rheumatol. 2007;34:1194–200.
11. Ramirez A, Varga J. Pulmonary arterial hypertension in systemic sclerosis: clinical manifestations, pathophysiology, evaluation, and management. Treat Respir Med. 2004;3:339–52.
12. Steen VD, Medsger TA. Changes in causes of death in systemic sclerosis, 1972-2002. Ann Rheum Dis. 2007;66:940–4.
13. Gorlova O, Martin JE, Rueda B, Koeleman BP, Ying J, Teruel M, et al. Identification of novel genetic markers associated with clinical phenotypes of systemic sclerosis through a genome-wide association strategy. PLoS Genet. 2011;7:e1002178.
14. Allanore Y, Saad M, Dieude P, Avouac J, Distler JH, Amouyel P, et al. Genome-wide scan identifies TNIP1, PSORS1C1, and RHOB as novel risk loci for systemic sclerosis. PLoS Genet. 2011;7:e1002091.
15. Wu M, Mayes MD. Insights into the genetic basis of systemic sclerosis: immunity in human disease and in mouse models. Adv Genomics Genet. 2014;4:143–51.
16. Spagnolo P, Grunewald J, du Bois RM. Genetic determinants of pulmonary fibrosis: evolving concepts. Lancet Respir Med. 2014;2:416–28.

Permissions

All chapters in this book were first published in AR&T, by BioMed Central; hereby published with permission under the Creative Commons Attribution License or equivalent. Every chapter published in this book has been scrutinized by our experts. Their significance has been extensively debated. The topics covered herein carry significant findings which will fuel the growth of the discipline. They may even be implemented as practical applications or may be referred to as a beginning point for another development.

The contributors of this book come from diverse backgrounds, making this book a truly international effort. This book will bring forth new frontiers with its revolutionizing research information and detailed analysis of the nascent developments around the world.

We would like to thank all the contributing authors for lending their expertise to make the book truly unique. They have played a crucial role in the development of this book. Without their invaluable contributions this book wouldn't have been possible. They have made vital efforts to compile up to date information on the varied aspects of this subject to make this book a valuable addition to the collection of many professionals and students.

This book was conceptualized with the vision of imparting up-to-date information and advanced data in this field. To ensure the same, a matchless editorial board was set up. Every individual on the board went through rigorous rounds of assessment to prove their worth. After which they invested a large part of their time researching and compiling the most relevant data for our readers.

The editorial board has been involved in producing this book since its inception. They have spent rigorous hours researching and exploring the diverse topics which have resulted in the successful publishing of this book. They have passed on their knowledge of decades through this book. To expedite this challenging task, the publisher supported the team at every step. A small team of assistant editors was also appointed to further simplify the editing procedure and attain best results for the readers.

Apart from the editorial board, the designing team has also invested a significant amount of their time in understanding the subject and creating the most relevant covers. They scrutinized every image to scout for the most suitable representation of the subject and create an appropriate cover for the book.

The publishing team has been an ardent support to the editorial, designing and production team. Their endless efforts to recruit the best for this project, has resulted in the accomplishment of this book. They are a veteran in the field of academics and their pool of knowledge is as vast as their experience in printing. Their expertise and guidance has proved useful at every step. Their uncompromising quality standards have made this book an exceptional effort. Their encouragement from time to time has been an inspiration for everyone.

The publisher and the editorial board hope that this book will prove to be a valuable piece of knowledge for researchers, students, practitioners and scholars across the globe.

List of Contributors

Michael E. Johnson, Andrew V. Grassetti, Jaclyn N. Taroni, Devin Schweppe and Scott A. Gerber
Department of Genetics, Geisel School of Medicine at Dartmouth, Hanover, NH, USA

Michael L. Whitfield
Department of Genetics, Geisel School of Medicine at Dartmouth, Hanover, NH, USA
Dartmouth Medical School, Hinman Hanover, NH 03755, USA

Shawn M. Lyons and Paul J. Anderson
Division of Rheumatology, Immunology, and Allergy, Brigham and Women's Hospital, Boston, MA, USA

Jessica K. Gordon and Robert F. Spiera
Department of Rheumatology, Hospital for Special Surgery, New York, NY, USA

Robert Lafyatis
Boston University School of Medicine, Boston, MA, USA

Yves Francès and Fanny Bernard-Guervilly
Internal Medicine Department, Assistance Publique-Hôpitaux de Marseille (APHM), CHU Nord, 13015 Marseilles, France

Audrey Benyamine
Internal Medicine Department, Assistance Publique-Hôpitaux de Marseille (APHM), CHU Nord, 13015 Marseilles, France
Haematology and Vascular Biology Laboratory, APHM, CHU Conception, 13005 Marseilles, France
Vascular Research Centre of Marseille (VRCM) UMR-S1076, INSERM, Aix-Marseille Université, 13385 Marseilles, Cedex, France

Brigitte Granel and Pascal Rossi
Internal Medicine Department, Assistance Publique-Hôpitaux de Marseille (APHM), CHU Nord, 13015 Marseilles, France
Vascular Research Centre of Marseille (VRCM) UMR-S1076, INSERM, Aix-Marseille Université, 13385 Marseilles, Cedex, France

Laurent Arnaud
Haematology and Vascular Biology Laboratory, APHM, CHU Conception, 13005 Marseilles, France

Sylvie Cointe, Romaric Lacroix, Françoise Dignat-George and Pascale Paul
Haematology and Vascular Biology Laboratory, APHM, CHU Conception, 13005 Marseilles, France
Vascular Research Centre of Marseille (VRCM) UMR-S1076, INSERM, Aix-Marseille Université, 13385 Marseilles, Cedex, France

Jérémy Magalon and Florence Sabatier
Vascular Research Centre of Marseille (VRCM) UMR-S1076, INSERM, Aix-Marseille Université, 13385 Marseilles, Cedex, France
Culture and Cell Therapy Laboratory, CICBT 1409, APHM, CHU Conception, 13005 Marseilles, France

Nathalie Bardin
Vascular Research Centre of Marseille (VRCM) UMR-S1076, INSERM, Aix-Marseille Université, 13385 Marseilles, Cedex, France
Immunology Laboratory, APHM, CHU Conception, 13005 Marseilles, France

Gilles Kaplanski
Vascular Research Centre of Marseille (VRCM) UMR-S1076, INSERM, Aix-Marseille Université, 13385 Marseilles, Cedex, France
Internal Medicine Department, APHM, CHU Conception, 13005 Marseilles, France

Jean-Robert Harlé and Pierre-Jean Weiller
Internal Medicine Department, APHM, CHU Timone, 13005 Marseilles, France

Philippe Berbis
Dermatology Department, APHM, CHU Nord, 13015 Marseilles, France

David Braunstein, Elisabeth Jouve, Nathalie Lesavre and Françoise Couranjou
Centre d'Investigation Clinique Centre de Pharmacologie Clinique et d'Evaluations Thérapeutiques, APHM, CHU Timone, CHU Nord, Marseille, France

Alfredo Guillén-Del Castillo, Eduardo L. Callejas-Moraga, Vicente Fonollosa-Plá and Carmen Pilar Simeón-Aznar
Department of Systemic Autoimmune Diseases, Hospital Universitari Vall d'Hebron, Universitat Autònoma de Barcelona, Passeig Vall d'Hebron 119-129, PC: 08035 Barcelona, Spain

Gabriela García, José F. Rodríguez-Palomares and Enric Domingo
Department of Cardiology, Hospital Universitari Vall d'Hebron, Universitat Autònoma de Barcelona, Barcelona, Spain

Antonio Román, Cristina Berastegui and Manuel López-Meseguer
Department of Pneumology, Hospital Universitari Vall d'Hebron, Universitat Autònoma de Barcelona, Barcelona, Spain

Barbara Vigone, Monica Caronni, Adriana Severino, Chiara Bellocchi, Gaia Montanelli, Alessandro Santaniello and Lorenzo Beretta
Scleroderma Unit, Referral Center for Systemic Autoimmune Diseases, Fondazione IRCCS Ca' Granda Ospedale Maggiore Policlinico di Milano, Via Pace 9, 20122 Milano, Italy

Anna Rita Baldassarri and Mirella Fraquelli
Gastroenterology and Endoscopy Unit, Fondazione IRCCS Ca' Granda Ospedale Maggiore Policlinico di Milano, Via Francesco Sforza 35, Milano, Italy

Romina Andracco, Eleonora Zaccara, Wanda Maglione, Francesca Pignataro, Domenico Sambataro, Gianluca Sambataro and Nicoletta Del Papa
UOC Day Hospital of Rheumatology, Department of Rheumatology, ASST G. Pini-CTO, Milan, Italy

Rosaria Irace, Serena Vettori, Antonella Riccardi, Roberta Ferrara and Gabriele Valentini
Rheumatology Unit, Department of Internal Medicine, 2nd University of Naples, Naples, Italy

Claudio Vitali
Section of Rheumatology, Villa San Giuseppe, Istituto Santo Stefano, Como, Italy

Katsunari Makino, Tomoko Makino, Lukasz Stawski and Maria Trojanowska
Arthritis Center, Boston University School of Medicine, 72 East Concord Street, E-5, Boston, MA 02118, USA

Kenneth E. Lipson
FibroGen, Inc, San Francisco, CA, USA

Andrew Leask
Departments of Dentistry and Physiology and Pharmacology, Schulich School of Medicine and Dentistry, University of Western Ontario, Dental Sciences Building, London, ON, Canada

Pierre-Yves Hatron, Éric Hachulla, David Launay, Sébastien Sanges, Jonathan Giovannelli, Vincent Sobanski and Marc Lambert
University of Lille, INSERM U995, LIRIC—Lille Inflammation Research International Center, F-59000 Lille, France
INSERM U995, F-59000 Lille, France
CHU Lille, Département de Médecine Interne et Immunologie Clinique, F-59000 Lille, France
Centre National de Référence Maladies Systémiques et Auto-immunes Rares (Sclérodermie Systémique), F-59000 Lille, France
Health Care Provider of the European Reference Network on Rare Connective Tissue and Musculoskeletal Diseases Network (ReCONNET), F-59000 Lille, France

Céline Podevin
CHU Lille, Département de Médecine Interne et Immunologie Clinique, F-59000 Lille, France
Centre National de Référence Maladies Systémiques et Auto-immunes Rares (Sclérodermie Systémique), F-59000 Lille, France

Sandrine Morell-Dubois and Hélène Maillard
CHU Lille, Département de Médecine Interne et Immunologie Clinique, F-59000 Lille, France
Centre National de Référence Maladies Systémiques et Auto-immunes Rares (Sclérodermie Systémique), F-59000 Lille, France
Health Care Provider of the European Reference Network on Rare Connective Tissue and Musculoskeletal Diseases Network (ReCONNET), F-59000 Lille, France

Nicolas Lamblin and Pascal De Groote
CHU Lille, Service de Cardiologie, F-59000 Lille, France

Jean-François Bervar
CHU Lille, Service de Pneumologie, F-59000 Lille, France

Thierry Perez and Régis Matran
CHU Lille, Service d'Explorations Fonctionnelles Respiratoires, F-59000 Lille, France

Martine Rémy-Jardin
CHU Lille, Département d'Imagerie Thoracique, F-59000 Lille, France

Ryosuke Saigusa, Yoshihide Asano, Takashi Taniguchi, Megumi Hirabayashi, Kouki Nakamura, Shunsuke Miura, Takashi Yamashita, Takehiro Takahashi, Yohei Ichimura, Tetsuo Toyama, Ayumi Yoshizaki and Shinichi Sato
Department of Dermatology, University of Tokyo Graduate School of Medicine, 7-3-1 Hongo, Bunkyo-ku, Tokyo 113-8655, Japan

Maria Trojanowska
Arthritis Center, Boston University School of Medicine, Boston, MA, USA

Vu Huy Luong, Takenao Chino, Noritaka Oyama and Minoru Hasegawa
Department of Dermatology, Division of Medicine, Faculty of Medical Sciences, University of Fukui, Fukui, Japan

Takashi Matsushita
Department of Dermatology, Faculty of Medicine, Institute of Medical, Pharmaceutical and Health Sciences, Kanazawa University, Kanazawa, Japan

Yoko Sasaki, Dai Ogura and Shin-ichiro Niwa
Link Genomics, Inc., Tokyo, Japan

Tanima Biswas, Akiyuki Hamasaki, Okamoto and Masami Otsuka
Department of Bioorganic Medicinal Chemistry, Kumamoto University, Kumamoto, Japan

Mikako Fujita
Research Institute for Drug Discovery, Kumamoto University, Kumamoto, Japan

Yoshinari Hironobu Ihn
Department of Dermatology and Plastic Surgery, Faculty of Life Sciences, Kumamoto University, Kumamoto, Japan

Elizabeth R. Volkmann, Donald P. Tashkin, Michael D. Roth, Philip J. Clements, Daniel E. Furst and Chi-Hong Tseng
Department of Medicine, University of California, David Geffen School of Medicine, Los Angeles, CA, USA

Dinesh Khanna
Department of Medicine, University of Michigan Medical School, Ann Arbor, MI, USA

Maureen Mayes, Julio Charles and Shervin Assassi
Department of Medicine, University of Texas Health Science Center at Houston, Houston, TX, USA

Robert M. Elashoff
Department of Biomathematics, University of California, Los Angeles, CA, USA

Maurizio Cutolo, Barbara Ruaro, Paola Montagna, Renata Brizzolara, Amelia Chiara Trombetta, Sabrina Paolino, Carmen Pizzorni, Alberto Sulli and Stefano Soldano
Research Laboratory and Academic Division of Clinical Rheumatology, Department of Internal Medicine, University of Genova, Polyclinic San Martino Hospital, Genoa, Italy

Emanuela Stratta and Stefano Scabini
Oncologic Surgery, Department of Surgery, Polyclinic San Martino Hospital, Genoa, Italy

Pier Paolo Tavilla and Aurora Parodi
Department of Health Science, Unit of Dermatology, University of Genova, Polyclinic San Martino Hospital, Genoa, Italy

Claudio Corallo and Nicola Giordano
Department of Medicine, Surgery and Neurosciences, Scleroderma Unit, University of Siena, Siena, Italy

Vanessa Smith
Department of Rheumatology, Ghent University Hospital, Ghent, Belgium

Hongtao Jin, Chao Sun, Xiaoping Wang, Lin Yang, Jingjing He, Yanru Wang and Aijing Liu
Department of Immunology and Rheumatology, the Second Hospital of Hebei Medical University, Shijiazhuang, Hebei, China

Hongyan Li
Department of Immunology and Rheumatology, the Second Hospital of Hebei Medical University, Shijiazhuang, Hebei, China
The Affiliated Jiangning Hospital of Nanjing Medical University, Nanjing, Jiangsu, China

Daniel E. Furst
Department of Rheumatology, Geffen School of Medicine, University of California, Los Angeles, CA, USA

Elena Schiopu
Department of Internal Medicine, University of Michigan, 1500 E Medical Center Dr, SPC 5370, Ann Arbor, MI 48109, USA

Soumya Chatterjee
Department of Rheumatologic and Immunologic Diseases, Cleveland Clinic, 9500 Euclid Ave, Cleveland, OH 44195, USA

Vivien Hsu
Clinical Research Center, Rutgers-Robert Wood Johnson Medical School, 125 Paterson St, New Brunswick, NJ 0890, USA

Armando Flor, Daniel Cimbora, Kaushik Patra, Wenliang Yao, Katie Streicher Eliezer Katz, Jorn Drappa, Sarah Sweeny and Ronald Herbst
Departments of Research and Clinical Biologics, MedImmune, 1 MedImmune Way, Gaithersburg, MD 20878, USA

Kathleen McKeever
Departments of Research and Clinical Biologics, MedImmune, 1 MedImmune Way, Gaithersburg, MD 20878, USA
Ultragenyx Pharmaceutical, 60 Leveroni Ct, Novato, CA 94949, USA

Barbara White
Departments of Research and Clinical Biologics, MedImmune, 1 MedImmune Way, Gaithersburg, MD 20878, USA
Corbus Pharmaceuticals, 100 River Ridge Dr, Norwood, MA 02062, USA

Jing Li
Department of Clinical Pharmacology and Drug Metabolism and Pharmacokinetics, MedImmune, 319 North Bernardo Ave, Mountain View, CA 94043, USA

Octavio Aravena, Ashley Ferrier, Juan Carlos Aguillón and Diego Catalán
Programa Disciplinario de Inmunología, Instituto de Ciencias Biomédicas (ICBM), Facultad de Medicina, Universidad de Chile, and Millennium Institute in Immunology and Immunotherapy, Santiago, Chile

Lilian Soto
Programa Disciplinario de Inmunología, Instituto de Ciencias Biomédicas (ICBM), Facultad de Medicina, Universidad de Chile, and Millennium Institute in Immunology and Immunotherapy, Santiago, Chile
Departamento de Medicina, Hospital Clínico, Universidad de Chile, Santiago, Chile

Madhvi Menon and Claudia Mauri
Centre for Rheumatology Research, Department of Medicine, University College London, London, UK

Yosuke Kanno and Ayaka Matsuda
Department of Clinical Pathological Biochemistry, Faculty of Pharmaceutical Science, Doshisha Women's Collage of Liberal Arts, 97-1 Kodo, Kyotanabe, Kyoto 610-0395, Japan

En Shu, Hiroyuki Kanoh and Mariko Seishima
Department of Dermatology, Gifu University Graduate School of Medicine, 1-1 Yanagido, Gifu 501-119, Japan

Celestina Mazzotta, Eloisa Romano,Jelena Blagojevic, Silvia Bellando-Randone, Cosimo Bruni, Gemma Lepri, Serena Guiducci and Marco Matucci-Cerinic
Department of Experimental and Clinical Medicine, Division of Rheumatology, University of Florence, AOUC, Largo Brambilla 3, 50134 Florence, Italy

Irene Rosa
Department of Experimental and Clinical Medicine, Division of Rheumatology, University of Florence, AOUC, Largo Brambilla 3, 50134 Florence, Italy
Department of Experimental and Clinical Medicine, Section of Anatomy and Histology, University of Florence, Largo Brambilla 3, 50134 Florence, Italy

Mirko Manetti and Lidia Ibba-Manneschi
Department of Experimental and Clinical Medicine, Section of Anatomy and Histology, University of Florence, Largo Brambilla 3, 50134 Florence, Italy

Kathleen Morrisroe and Mandana Nikpour
Department of Medicine, The University of Melbourne at St Vincent's Hospital (Melbourne), 41 Victoria Parade, Fitzroy 3065, Victoria, Australia
Departments of Rheumatology and Medicine, The University of Melbourne at St Vincent's Hospital (Melbourne), 41 Victoria Parade, Fitzroy 3065, Victoria, Australia

Wendy Stevens and Candice Rabusa
Departments of Rheumatology and Medicine, The University of Melbourne at St Vincent's Hospital (Melbourne), 41 Victoria Parade, Fitzroy 3065, Victoria, Australia

Joanne Sahhar
Monash University and Monash Health, 246 Clayton Road, Clayton 3168, Victoria, Australia

Susanna Proudman
Rheumatology Unit, Royal Adelaide Hospital, North Terrace, SA 5000, Australia
Discipline of Medicine, University of Adelaide Adelaide, SA 5000, Australia

Florian Weigold, Elise Siegert, Robert Biesen, Falk Hiepe and Gerd R. Burmester
Department of Rheumatology and Clinical Immunology, Charité University Hospital, Berlin, Germany

Gabriela Riemekasten
Department of Rheumatology and Clinical Immunology, Charité University Hospital, Berlin, Germany
Cell Autoimmunity Group, German Rheumatism Research Center (DRFZ), Berlin, Germany
Department of Rheumatology, University of Lübeck, Lübeck, Germany
Research Center Borstel, Airway Research Center North (ARCN), Members of the German Center for Lung Research (DZL), Borstel, Germany

Jeannine Günther
Department of Rheumatology and Clinical Immunology, Charité University Hospital, Berlin, Germany
Cell Autoimmunity Group, German Rheumatism Research Center (DRFZ), Berlin, Germany

Moritz Pfeiffenberger
Cell Autoimmunity Group, German Rheumatism Research Center (DRFZ), Berlin, Germany

Otavio Cabral-Marques
Department of Rheumatology, University of Lübeck, Lübeck, Germany

Aurélie Philippe
Department of Nephrology and Critical Care Medicine, Charité University Hospital, Campus Virchow, Berlin, Germany

Duska Dragun and Rusan Catar
Department of Nephrology and Critical Care Medicine, Charité University Hospital, Campus Virchow, Berlin, Germany
Berlin Institute of Health, Berlin, Germany

Ann-Katrin Regensburger and Andreas Recke
Department of Dermatology, University of Lübeck, Lübeck, Germany

Xinhua Yu and Frank Petersen
Research Center Borstel, Airway Research Center North (ARCN), Members of the German Center for Lung Research (DZL), Borstel, Germany

Harald Heidecke
CellTrend GmbH, Luckenwalde, Brandenburg, Germany

Anna M. Blom
Department of Translational Medicine, Section of Medical Protein Chemistry, Lund University, Inga Marie Nilssons Street 53, Malmö S-20502, Sweden

Marcin Okrój
Department of Translational Medicine, Section of Medical Protein Chemistry, Lund University, Inga Marie Nilssons Street 53, Malmö S-20502, Sweden
Department of Medical Biotechnology, Intercollegiate Faculty of Biotechnology UG-MUG, Medical University of Gdańsk, Gdańsk 80210, Poland

Martin Johansson
Department of Translational Medicine, Section of Clinical Pathology, Lund University, Jan Waldenströms street 59, Malmö S-20502, Sweden

Tore Saxne and Roger Hesselstrand
Department of Clinical Sciences, Lund, Section of Rheumatology, Lund University, Skåne University Hospital, Lund S-22185, Sweden

Weiya Zhang and Michael Doherty
Division of Rheumatology, Orthopaedics and Dermatology, School of Medicine, University of Nottingham, NG51PDAcademic Rheumatology, Clinical Sciences Building, City Hospital, Nottingham NG51PB, Nottingham, UK

Chang-Fu Kuo
Division of Rheumatology, Orthopaedics and Dermatology, School of Medicine, University of Nottingham, NG51PDAcademic Rheumatology, Clinical Sciences Building, City Hospital, Nottingham NG51PB, Nottingham, UK
Division of Rheumatology, Allergy and Immunology, Chang Gung Memorial Hospital, Taoyuan, Taiwan

Shue-Fen Luo and Kuang-Hui Yu
Division of Rheumatology, Allergy and Immunology, Chang Gung Memorial Hospital, Taoyuan, Taiwan

Lai-Chu See
Department of Public Health, College of Medicine and Biostatistics Core Laboratory, Molecular Medicine Research Centre, Chang Gung University, Taoyuan, Taiwan

Claudio Corallo, Antonio Montella, Chiara Chirico, Ranuccio Nuti and Nicola Giordano
Scleroderma Unit, Department of Medicine, Surgery and Neurosciences, University of Siena, 53100 Siena, Italy

Maurizio Cutolo and Stefano Soldano
Research Laboratory and Academic Division of Clinical Rheumatology, Department of Internal Medicine, Institute for Research and Health Care (IRCCS), University of Genoa, San Martino, Genoa, Italy

Bashar Kahaleh
Division of Rheumatology and Immunology, College of Medicine, University of Toledo, Toledo, OH, USA

Gianluca Pecetti
Medical and Scientific Direction, Actelion Pharmaceuticals Italy, Imola, Italy

Minghua Wu, Shervin Assassi, Gloria A. Salazar, Julio Charles, Miranda L. Taing, Kelley Liao and Malahat Movahedian
Division of Rheumatology and Clinical Immunogenetics, Department of Internal Medicine, University of Texas McGovern Medical School at Houston, 6431 Fannin Street, Houston, TX 77030, USA

Claudia Pedroza
Department of Pediatrics, The University of Texas Mcgovern Medical School at Houston, 6431 Fannin Street, Houston, TX 77030, USA

Olga Y. Gorlova and Wei V. Chen
Department of Community and Family Medicine, Geisel School of Medicine at Dartmouth, 1 Rope Ferry Road, Hanover, NH 03755, USA

Fredrick M. Wigley, Laura K. Hummers and Ami A. Shah
Division of Rheumatology, Johns Hopkins University School of Medicine, 5501 Hopkins Bayview circle, Baltimore, MD 2122, USA

Barri J. Fessler
Division of Clinical Immunology and Rheumatology, University of Alabama at Birmingham, 1825 University Boulevard, Birmingham, AB 3529, USA

Marvin J. Fritzler
Division of Rheumatology, University of Calgary Cumming School of Medicine, 3330 Hospital Drive NW, Calgary, AB T2N 4N, Canada

Jerry A. Molitor and Barbara M. Segal
Division of Rheumatology, University of Minnesota, 420 Delaware Street SE, Minneapolis, MN 55455, USA

Javier Martín
Instituto de Parasitología y Biomedicina López-Neyra, Consejo Superior de Investigaciones Cientıficas, C/Ventanilla 1,18001 Granada, Spain

Index

www.ingramcontent.com/pod-product-compliance
Lightning Source LLC
LaVergne TN
LVHW080808220926
848485LV00011B/453